Neurodegenerative Diseases: Neurobiology, Pathogenesis and Therapeutics

Neurodegenerative Diseases: Neurobiology, Pathogenesis and Therapeutics

Editor: Jennifer Wagner

AMERICAN
MEDICAL PUBLISHERS
www.americanmedicalpublishers.com

AMERICAN
MEDICAL PUBLISHERS
www.americanmedicalpublishers.com

Cataloging-in-Publication Data

Neurodegenerative diseases : neurobiology, pathogenesis and therapeutics / edited by Jennifer Wagner.
p. cm.
Includes bibliographical references and index.
ISBN 979-8-88740-303-8
1. Nervous system--Degeneration. 2. Neurobiology. 3. Nervous system--Degeneration--Pathogenesis.
4. Nervous system--Degeneration--Treatment. 5. Nervous system--Diseases. 6. Neurology. I. Wagner, Jennifer.
RC365 .N48 2023
616.804 7--dc23

American Medical Publishers,
41 Flatbush Avenue,
1st Floor, New York,
NY 11217, USA

ISBN 979-8-88740-303-8 (Hardback)

Contents

Preface

This book has been an outcome of determined endeavour from a group of educationists in the field. The primary objective was to involve a broad spectrum of professionals from diverse cultural background involved in the field for developing new researches. The book not only targets students but also scholars pursuing higher research for further enhancement of the theoretical and practical applications of the subject.

The diseases which affect neurons and lead to the loss of function or structure within them are known as neurodegenerative diseases. Some of the major examples of these diseases are Parkinson's disease, Alzheimer's disease, amyotrophic lateral sclerosis and multiple sclerosis. The mechanisms of these diseases range from epigenetic to genetic and intracellular. There is another class of neurodegenerative diseases known as proteopathies which are caused due to the aggregation of misfolded proteins. The research on the therapeutics for these diseases is still ongoing as no cure has been found yet. There are similarities between these diseases at the subcellular level, which suggests that the development of a cure for a particular disease will be beneficial to people suffering from other neurodegenerative diseases. This book is a valuable compilation of topics, comprising neurobiological and therapeutic studies on neurodegenerative diseases. It will serve as a valuable source of reference for graduate and post graduate students.

It was an honour to edit such a profound book and also a challenging task to compile and examine all the relevant data for accuracy and originality. I wish to acknowledge the efforts of the contributors for submitting such brilliant and diverse chapters in the field and for endlessly working for the completion of the book. Last, but not the least; I thank my family for being a constant source of support in all my research endeavours.

Editor

1

TREM2/DAP12 Complex Regulates Inflammatory Responses in Microglia via the JNK Signaling Pathway

Li Zhong [1†], Zhen-Lian Zhang [1†], Xinxiu Li [1†], Chunyan Liao [1†], Pengfei Mou [1], Tingting Wang [1], Zongqi Wang [1], Zhe Wang [1], Min Wei [1], Huaxi Xu [1,2], Guojun Bu [1,3] and Xiao-Fen Chen [1,4]**

[1] Fujian Provincial Key Laboratory of Neurodegenerative Disease and Aging Research, Institute of Neuroscience, Medical College, Xiamen University, Xiamen, China, [2] Neuroscience and Aging Research Center, Sanford-Burnham-Prebys Medical Discovery Institute, La Jolla, CA, United States, [3] Department of Neuroscience, Mayo Clinic, Jacksonville, FL, United States, [4] Shenzhen Research Institute of Xiamen University, Shenzhen, China

***Correspondence:**
Guojun Bu
bu.guojun@mayo.edu
Xiao-Fen Chen
chenxf@xmu.edu.cn

† Co-first authors. These authors have contributed equally to this work.

DNAX-activating protein of 12 kDa (DAP12) is a signaling adapter protein expressed in cells that participate in innate immune responses. By pairing with different triggering receptors expressed on myeloid cell (TREM) proteins, DAP12 can mediate both positive and negative cellular responses. In particular, TREM1 acts as an amplifier of the immune response, while TREM2 functions as a negative regulator. TREM2 has also been shown to stimulate the phagocytosis of apoptotic neurons and define the barrier function in microglia. Notably, loss-of-function mutations of either *DAP12* or *TREM2* result in a disorder known as Nasu-Hakola disease (NHD); and mutations of these genes have been associated with the risk for Alzheimer's disease (AD), suggesting that TREM2 and DAP12 may regulate common signaling pathways in the disease pathogenesis. In this study, we demonstrated an anti-inflammatory role of DAP12 in murine microglia that depends on the presence of TREM2. We also uncovered the JNK signaling pathway as the underlying molecular mechanism by which the TREM2/DAP12 complex suppresses the hyperactivation of microglia upon LPS stimulation. Interestingly, LPS down-regulates the expression of *Trem2* via the activation of JNK and NF-κB signaling pathways, resulting in a vicious cycle that synergistically promotes the inflammatory responses. Our study provides insights into mechanism-based therapy for neuroinflammatory disorders.

Keywords: DAP12, TREM2, JNK, LPS, microglia, inflammation

INTRODUCTION

DNAX-activating protein of 12 kDa (DAP12; also known as TYROBP and KARAP) is a signaling adapter protein expressed by a variety of innate immune cells including macrophages, microglia, monocytes, dendritic cells and natural killer (NK) cells (Lanier, 2009). The broad distribution of DAP12 suggests a general function in immune responses. DAP12 consists of a minimal extracellular domain, a transmembrane segment and a cytoplasmic region containing a single immunoreceptor tyrosine-based activation motif (ITAM). An aspartic acid in the transmembrane domain of DAP12 allows its association with cell surface receptors via an electrostatic interaction. The receptors usually have an oppositely charged amino acid (arginine or lysine) embedded within their transmembrane region that allows the formation of non-covalent complexes with DAP12 (Lanier and Bakker, 2000; Humphrey et al., 2005). Ligation of a DAP12-associated receptor to its ligand leads to the activation of SRC-family kinases and subsequent phosphorylation of tyrosine residues in the ITAM of DAP12 (Mason et al., 2006). DAP12 was originally shown to trigger the activation of NK cells (Lanier et al., 1998). Since then, more than 20 DAP12-associated receptors have been identified (Turnbull and Colonna, 2007). Triggering receptors expressed on myeloid cells (TREMs) are a family of cell surface receptors expressed broadly on myeloid cells that have been identified to associate with DAP12 (Bouchon et al., 2000; Daws et al., 2001; Chung et al., 2002). In particular, TREM1 is a potent amplifier of the inflammatory responses; while TREM2 has an anti-inflammatory function (Bouchon et al., 2000; Gibot et al., 2004; Takahashi et al., 2005; Turnbull et al., 2006).

TREM2 is a DAP12-coupled receptor that acts as a sensor for a wide array of lipids and apolipoprotein E (ApoE) in the central nervous system (CNS; Atagi et al., 2015; Bailey et al., 2015; Wang et al., 2015; Yeh et al., 2016). Notably, loss-of-function mutations of either *DAP12* or *TREM2* result in a disorder known as Nasu-Hakola disease (NHD; Paloneva et al., 2000, 2002). Furthermore, both *TREM2* (Guerreiro et al., 2013; Jonsson et al., 2013) and *DAP12* (Pottier et al., 2016) mutations have been found to be associated with the risk for Alzheimer's disease (AD). These observations suggest that TREM2 and DAP12 may regulate common signaling pathways in the disease pathogenesis. TREM2 and DAP12 are both preferentially expressed in microglia within the CNS (Sessa et al., 2004). Together, they regulate functions in microglia including inhibition of pro-inflammatory responses and stimulation of phagocytosis of apoptotic neurons (Takahashi et al., 2005; Hamerman et al., 2006; Turnbull et al., 2006; Zhong et al., 2015). Recently, TREM2/DAP12 complex has also been demonstrated to regulate the barrier function in microglia that prevents the outward extension of amyloid fibrils and axonal dystrophy (Sirkis et al., 2016; Yuan et al., 2016).

Despite intense interest in the function of TREM2/DAP12 complex in microglia, current understanding of the relevant molecular, cellular and biophysical mechanisms is limited. Studies elucidating such mechanisms may uncover targetable pathways for AD therapy. In this study, we demonstrated an anti-inflammatory role of DAP12 in murine microglia that requires the function of TREM2. Mechanistically, TREM2/DAP12 suppressed the hyperactivation of JNK signaling pathway upon LPS stimulation. Consequently, a JNK inhibitor, SP600125, eliminated the hypersensitivity of *Dap12*-deficient microglia to LPS. Together, our data suggest that TREM2/DAP12 complex negatively regulates LPS-induced inflammatory responses by modulating the JNK signaling pathway in microglia.

MATERIALS AND METHODS

Reagents and Antibodies

Amaxa® Cell Line Nucleofector® Kit T and Amaxa® Glia Cell Nucleofector® Kit T were purchased from LONZA. Primers for quantitative RT-PCR were synthesized by Life Technologies. SYBR Green for quantitative RT-PCR was

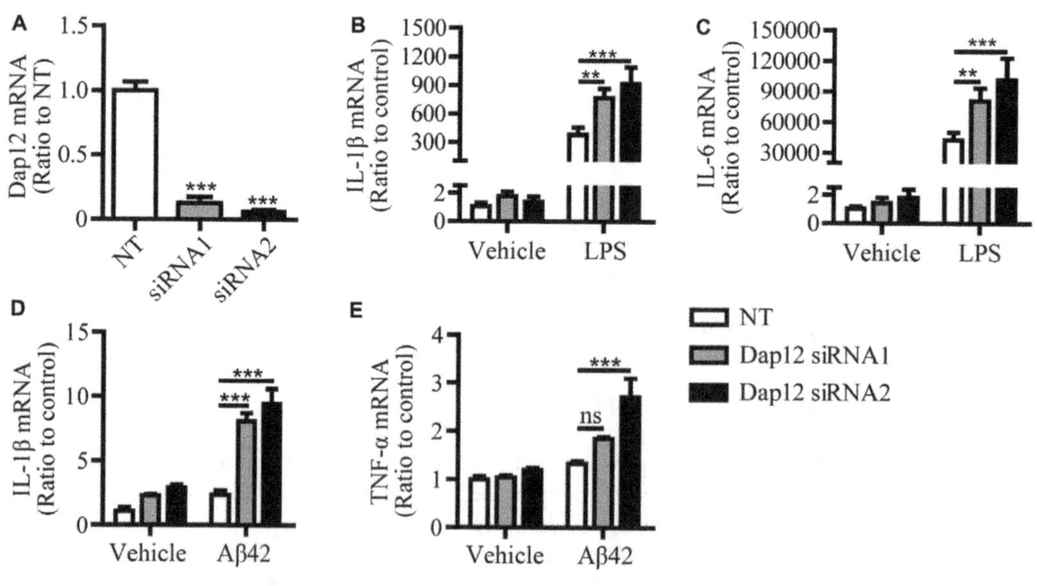

FIGURE 1 | Knockdown of *Dap12* exacerbates LPS- or Aβ42-oligomer-stimulated production of pro-inflammatory cytokines. **(A)** Primary microglia cells were transiently transfected with non-targeting siRNA (NT) or *Dap12*-specific siRNAs for 48 h. The relative mRNA levels of *Dap12* were determined by quantitative RT-PCR and shown as bar graph ($n = 3$, 1-way ANOVA). **(B,C)** Cells from **(A)** were treated with 500 ng/mL LPS or vehicle control for 4 h. RNA was extracted and the relative mRNA levels of IL-1β **(B)** and IL-6 **(C)** shown as bar graph were determined by quantitative RT-PCR ($n = 3$, two-way ANOVA). **(D–E)** Cells from **(A)** were treated with 10 μM oligomeric-Aβ42 or vehicle control for 4 h. RNA was extracted and the relative mRNA levels of IL-1β and TNF-α shown as bar graph were determined by quantitative RT-PCR ($n = 3$, two-way ANOVA). β-actin was used as an internal control. Data represent mean ± SEM. $^{**}p < 0.01$; $^{***}p < 0.001$; ns, not significant.

purchased from Roche. SP600125, Bay11-7082, SB203580, U0126 and LPS were purchased from Sigma. Amyloid-β 42 (Aβ42) peptide was purchased from AnaSpec. Oligomeric Aβ42 was prepared as previously described (Huang et al., 2015). Antibodies used in this study are as followed: anti-phospho-p38-MAPK, anti-total-p38-MAPK, anti-phospho-ERK1/2, anti-total-ERK1/2, anti-phospho-JNK, anti-total-JNK, anti-phospho-IκBα, anti-total-IκBα, anti-phosho-NF-κB, anti-total-NF-κB, anti-phospho-c-Jun, anti-total-c-Jun and anti-β-actin were purchased from Cell Signaling Technology; anti-tubulin (Millipore); anti-mouse IgG and anti-rabbit IgG antibody conjugated with horseradish peroxidase (ThermoFisher Scientific).

Isolation and Culture of Mouse Primary Microglia

Trem2 knockout mice (*Trem2*-KO on C57BL/6N background) and wild-type (WT) C57BL/6N mice were obtained from the UC Davis Knockout Mouse Project (KOMP) repository. The exons 2–4 of the *Trem2* gene were replaced with a LacZ reporter which is identical to the line recently reported (Jay et al., 2015). Primary microglial cultures were prepared as previously described (Zhu et al., 2010; Atagi et al., 2015). All animal experiments were conducted in compliance with the protocols approved by the Institutional Animal Care and Use Committee of Xiamen University. Briefly, WT or *Trem2*-KO mice (3–4 pups) at postnatal day 1–2 were used to prepare mixed glial cultures. Cells were plated onto flasks and grown in DMEM supplemented with 10% heat-inactivated fetal bovine serum (FBS; Gibco). Three days later, medium was changed to that containing 25 ng/mL GM-CSF and 10% FBS. Primary microglia were harvested by shaking (200 rpm, 20 min) after 10–12 days in culture and once every 3 days thereafter (up to three harvests).

Western Blotting

BV2 microglial cells or primary microglia were lysed at the indicated times with lysis buffer (1% NP-40, 50 mM Tris-HCl, pH 8.0, 150 mM sodium chloride) supplemented with protease and phosphotase inhibitor cocktails. BCA protein assay kit was used to determine the protein concentration according to the manufacturer's instruction (ThermoFisher

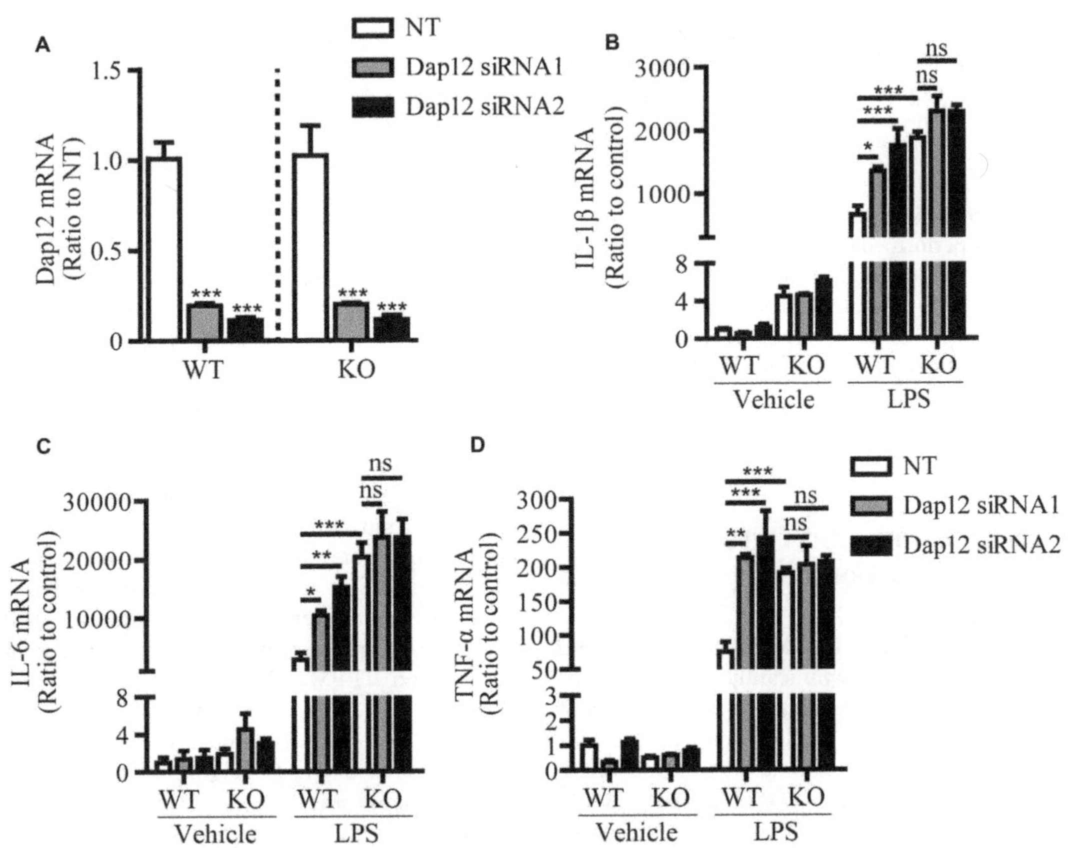

FIGURE 2 | DAP12 regulates inflammatory responses in a manner that depends on the presence of TREM2. **(A)** Primary microglia cells from wild-type (WT) or *Trem2*- knockout (KO) mice were transiently transfected with NT or *Dap12*-specific siRNAs for 48 h. The relative mRNA levels of *Dap12* were determined by quantitative RT-PCR and shown as bar graph ($n = 3$, one-way ANOVA). **(B–D)** Cells from **(A)** were treated with 100 ng/mL LPS or vehicle control for 4 h. RNA was extracted and the relative mRNA levels of IL-1β **(B)** IL-6 **(C)** TNF-α **(D)** shown as bar graph were determined by quantitative RT-PCR ($n = 3$, two-way ANOVA). β-actin was used as an internal control. Data represent mean ± SEM. *$p < 0.05$; **$p < 0.01$; ***$p < 0.001$; ns, not significant.

Scientific). Equal amounts of total proteins were analyzed by sodium dodecyl sulfate-polyacrylamide gel electrophoresis (SDS-PAGE) and Western blotting using appropriate antibodies and HRP-conjugated secondary antibodies. Proteins were visualized using ECL Western blotting detection reagents (Millipore). Immunoreactive bands were quantified using ImageJ.

Quantitative RT-PCR

Total RNAs were extracted using TRIzol reagent (Invitrogen). One microgram RNA was reverse-transcribed into first-strand cDNA using TransScript All-in-One First-Strand cDNA Synthesis SuperMix (TRANSGEN BIOTECH, Beijing, China) according to the manufacturer's protocol. Quantitative PCR was performed using the FastStart Universal SYBR Green Master (Roche). The primer sequences used for Dap12, Trem2, IL-1β, TNF-α, IL-6 and β-Actin were the same as previously described (Zhong et al., 2015, 2017).

RNA Interference

siRNA at a concentration of 300 nM was transfected into BV2 cells using Amaxa® Cell Line Nucleofector® Kit T or primary microglia cells using Amaxa® Glia Cell Nucleofector® Kit T. Cells were harvested 48 h later, followed by RNA extraction for quantitative RT-PCR analysis or protein extraction for Western blotting analysis. The siRNA sequences for Dap12 were the same as previously described (Zhong et al., 2015).

Statistical Analyses

Statistical analyses were performed using GraphPad Prism and all data were presented as mean ± SEM. At least three independent experiments were analyzed by unpaired *t*-test, one-way ANOVA or two-way ANOVA test. To classify and indicate significant values, the following *p*-values were used: $^{*}p < 0.05$; $^{**}p < 0.01$; $^{***}p < 0.001$; ns, not significant.

RESULTS

DAP2 Inhibits LPS-Induced Cytokines Production Dependent on TREM2 Receptor

In our previous study, we found that knockdown of *Dap12* gene in microglial BV2 cells significantly increased the mRNA levels of pro-inflammatory cytokines in the presence of LPS (Zhong et al., 2015). To further confirm the role of DAP12 in mediating the inflammatory responses to pathogenic stimuli, we employed two *Dap12*-specific siRNAs to knockdown the expression of *Dap12* in primary microglia and examined its impacts on cytokine expression (**Figure 1A**). Consistently, the knockdown of *Dap12* significantly increased the mRNA levels of IL-1β and IL-6 in LPS-stimulated primary microglia (**Figures 1B,C**). The production of IL-1β and TNF-α were also elevated in response to treatment with Aβ42 oligomers in *Dap12*-knockdown primary microglia

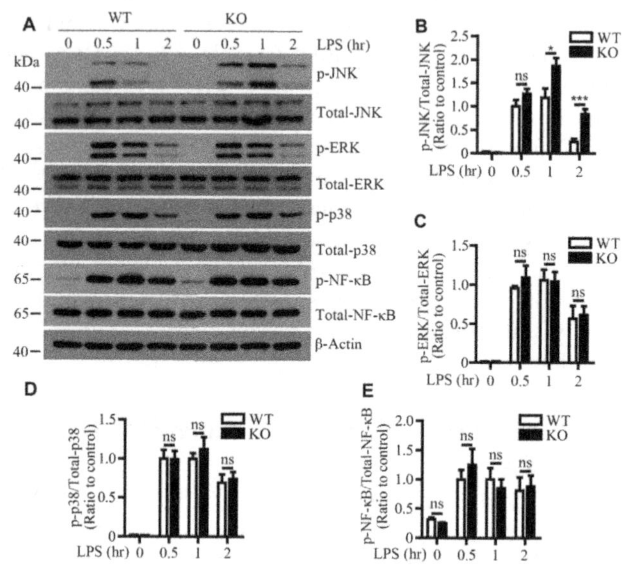

FIGURE 3 | LPS-induced JNK phosphorylation is increased in *Trem2*-deficient microglia. **(A)** Primary microglia cells from WT or *Trem2*- knockout (KO) mice were stimulated with 100 ng/ml LPS for the indicated time. Cell lysates at each time point were analyzed by Western blotting using antibodies specific for either total proteins or phosphorylated form of JNK, P38-MAPK, ERK1/2 and NF-κB. **(B–E)** Bar graphs show the quantification of Western blots as ratios of phospho-JNK/total JNK **(B)** phospho-ERK1/2/total ERK1/2 **(C)** phospho-p38-MAPK/total p38-MAPK **(D)** and phospho-NF-κB/total NF-κB **(E)**, respectively. β-actin was used as an internal control. The ratio at "0.5 h" time point of WT cells served as a control ($n \geq 3$, unpaired Student's *t*-test). Data represent mean ± SEM. $^{*}p < 0.05$; $^{***}p < 0.001$; ns, not significant.

(**Figures 1D,E**). These data suggest that DAP12 is essential for suppressing the production of pro-inflammatory cytokines when microglial cells are exposed to pathogenic stimuli.

In cells of myeloid origin, TREM1 and TREM2 are two receptors that signal through DAP12 to oppositely regulate the inflammatory response. TREM1 has been shown to function as an amplifier of the inflammatory response (Bouchon et al., 2000), whereas TREM2 has an anti-inflammatory function (Turnbull et al., 2006). Since we observed an anti-inflammation function of DAP12 in microglia, we further investigated whether DAP12 suppresses the production of inflammatory cytokines in a manner that depends on TREM2. Primary microglia were isolated from both WT and *Trem2*-knockout (KO) mice and further subjected to siRNA treatment that specifically knock down the expression of *Dap12* (**Figure 2A**). Although the deficiency of *Dap12* significantly enhanced the production of inflammatory cytokines IL-1β, IL-6 and TNF-α in LPS-stimulated WT primary microglia, the effects were abolished in *Trem2*-KO microglia (**Figures 2B–D**). It is noteworthy that the amounts of these inflammatory cytokines were significantly higher in *Trem2*-KO microglia than WT microglia, which is consistent with our previous reports (Zheng et al., 2016). Taken together, we conclude that DAP12 suppresses the production

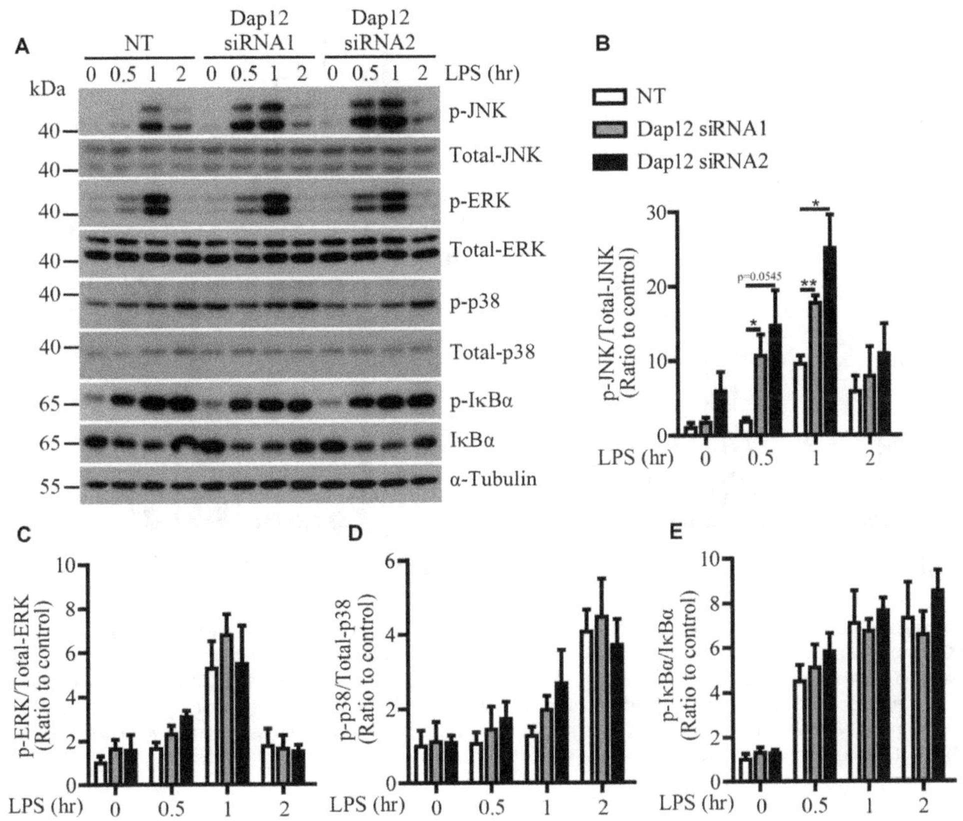

FIGURE 4 | LPS-induced JNK phosphorylation is increased in *Dap12*-knockdown BV2 cells. **(A)** BV2 cells were transiently transfected with NT or *Dap12*-specific siRNAs for 48 h, then stimulated with 500 ng/mL LPS for the indicated times. **(B–E)** Bar graphs show the quantification of Western blots as ratios of phospho-JNK/total JNK **(B)** phospho-ERK1/2/total ERK1/2 **(C)** phospho-p38-MAPK/total p38-MAPK **(D)** and phospho-IκBα/total IκBα **(E)**, respectively. α-Tubulin was used as an internal control. The ratio at "0" time point of NT cells served as a control (n = 3, unpaired Student's t-test). Data represent mean ± SEM. $^*p < 0.05$; $^{**}p < 0.01$.

of pro-inflammatory cytokines in microglia in a manner that depends on TREM2 receptor.

Enhanced JNK Phosphorylation in *Trem2*- and *Dap12*-Deficient Microglia

To identify the signaling pathway(s) that mediates the inflammatory responses induced by LPS in the absence of *Trem2*/*Dap12*, we first examined the activation kinetics of the transcription factor NF-κB and the major MAPKs subtypes (ERK1/2, p38-MAPK and JNK) in both WT and *Trem2*-KO primary microglia. The activation kinetics and magnitude of phosphorylated ERK1/2, p38-MAPK and NF-κB were similar in LPS-stimulated WT and *Trem2*-KO primary microglia (**Figures 3A,C–E**). In contrast, the phosphorylation of JNK was more pronounced in primary microglia from *Trem2*-KO mice compared with WT mice (**Figures 3A,B**). Similarly, knockdown of *Dap12* in microglial BV2 cells significantly increased the phosphorylation of JNK (**Figures 4A,B**), whereas no effects were observed for phosphorylated ERK1/2, p38-MAPK and IκBα, a key regulator in the NF-κB signaling pathway (**Figures 4C–E**). We therefore conclude that the TREM2/DAP12 complex regulates the inflammatory responses in microglia by specifically blocking the activation of JNK signaling pathway.

JNK Inhibitor Eliminates the Hypersensitivity of *Dap12*-Deficient Microglia to LPS

To further explore the molecular mechanism by which *Dap12* down-regulation affects the pro-inflammatory responses induced by LPS, a specific inhibitor (SP600125) was used to block the activation of JNK signaling pathway. Microglial BV2 cells were pre-treated with SP600125 before LPS stimulation. At a dose of 10 or 20 μM, SP600125 inhibits the phosphorylation of c-Jun which is a downstream target of JNK pathway (**Figures 5A,B**). The mRNA levels of pro-inflammatory cytokines IL-1β and IL-6 were increased upon knockdown of *Dap12*; however, the effect was abolished by pre-treatment with the JNK inhibitor (**Figures 5C,D**). Taken together, these data indicated that DAP12 negatively regulates LPS-induced inflammatory responses in microglia by modulating the activity of JNK signaling pathway.

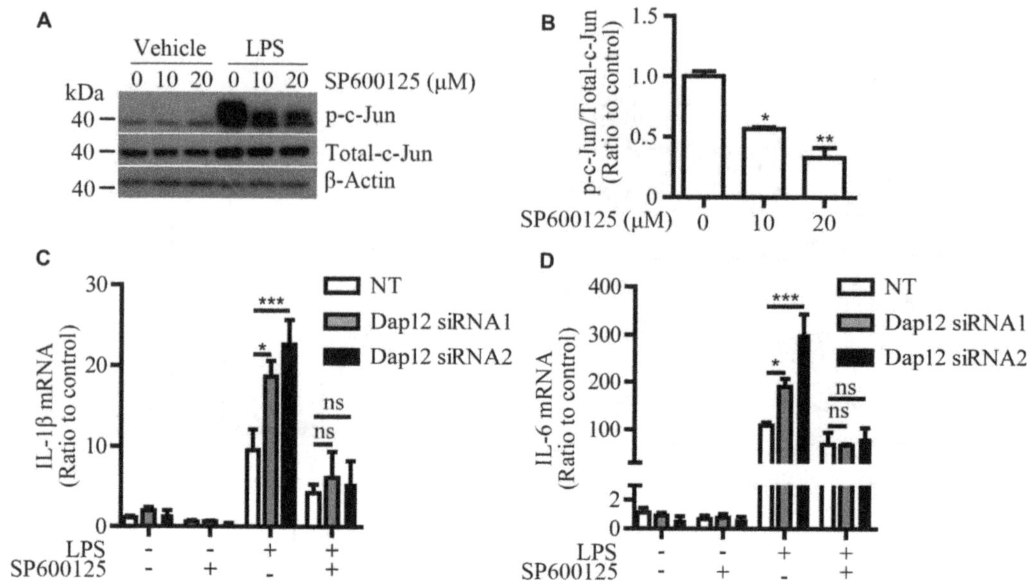

FIGURE 5 | JNK inhibitor reverses the increased pro-inflammatory cytokines in *Dap12*-knockdown BV2 cells. **(A)** BV2 cells were pretreated with indicated concentrations of SP600125 for 30 min, and then stimulated with 500 ng/mL LPS or vehicle control for 1 h. Cell lysates were analyzed by Western blotting. **(B)** Bar graphs show the quantification of Western blots as ratios of phospho-c-Jun/total c-Jun ($n = 3$, one-way ANOVA). **(C,D)** BV2 cells were transiently transfected with non-targeting siRNA (NT) or *Dap12*-specific siRNAs for 48 h, and then stimulated with 500 ng/mL LPS or vehicle control for 4 h in the presence or absence of 20 μM SP600125 (pretreated for 30 min). RNA was extracted and the relative mRNA levels of IL-1β and IL-6 shown as bar graph were determined by quantitative RT-PCR ($n = 3$, two-way ANOVA). β-actin was used as an internal control. *$p < 0.05$; **$p < 0.01$; ***$p < 0.001$; ns, not significant.

LPS-Induced Down-Regulation of *Trem2* is Rescued by JNK and NF-κB Inhibitors

We have previously shown that LPS stimulation significantly suppressed *Trem2* expression in primary microglia and mouse brain (Zheng et al., 2016). Consistently, the mRNA levels of *Trem2* were significantly down-regulated in LPS stimulated microglial BV2 cells (**Figure 6A**). However, the expression of *Dap12* was unaffected even upon the stimulation with 1 μg/mL LPS (**Figure 6B**). To further dissect the molecular pathway that modulates *Trem2* expression, we pretreated BV2 cells with various compounds that specifically block individual signaling pathways downstream of LPS, including NF-κB and each of the major MAP kinase subtypes. The mRNA level of *Trem2* was similarly down-regulated by LPS in the presence or absence of p38-MAPK and ERK1/2 inhibitors (**Figures 6D,E**). However, the LPS down-regulated *Trem2* expression was restored by the presence of inhibitors for either JNK or NF-κB (**Figures 6C,F**). Taken together, our data suggest that both JNK and NF-κB signaling pathways downstream of LPS modulate the expression of *Trem2* in microglia.

DISCUSSION

In this study, we showed that DAP12 suppresses the production of pro-inflammatory cytokines when microglial cells are exposed to LPS. Importantly, the negative modulation of inflammatory response by DAP12 depends on the presence of TREM2. In view of the underlying molecular mechanism, we revealed that the TREM2/DAP12 axis suppresses the activity of JNK signaling pathway to reduce the inflammatory response in microglia (**Figure 7**). Intriguingly, LPS down-regulates the expression of *Trem2* via the activation of JNK and NF-κB signaling pathways (**Figure 7**), resulting in a vicious cycle that synergistically promotes the inflammatory responses.

As a signaling adaptor protein, DAP12 couples with a variety of cell-surface receptors to modulate the threshold for cellular activation in response to pathogenic stimuli (Turnbull and Colonna, 2007). For instance, the association of DAP12 with TREM1 has been shown to amplify the inflammatory response (Bouchon et al., 2000; Gibot et al., 2004); while the association with TREM2 dampens the production of pro-inflammatory cytokines (Takahashi et al., 2005; Turnbull et al., 2006). Therefore, the roles of DAP12 in different cell types could be varied depending on the presence of specific cell surface receptors. DAP12 is preferentially expressed in microglia within the CNS (Hickman et al., 2013). In our previous work and in current study, we have demonstrated that DAP12 inhibits the production of pro-inflammatory cytokines in LPS-stimulated microglia by using both immortalized cell line and primary cultures (Zhong et al., 2015). We further demonstrated that DAP12 exerts its anti-inflammatory function by coupling with TREM2 which is the highest expressed DAP12-associated receptor in microglia among TREM family members (Zhang et al., 2014). Interestingly, the DAP12 signaling has been shown to amplify inflammation during sepsis (Turnbull et al., 2005). The receptors that are involved remain unknown; TREM1, for instance, might be needed for DAP12 to signal

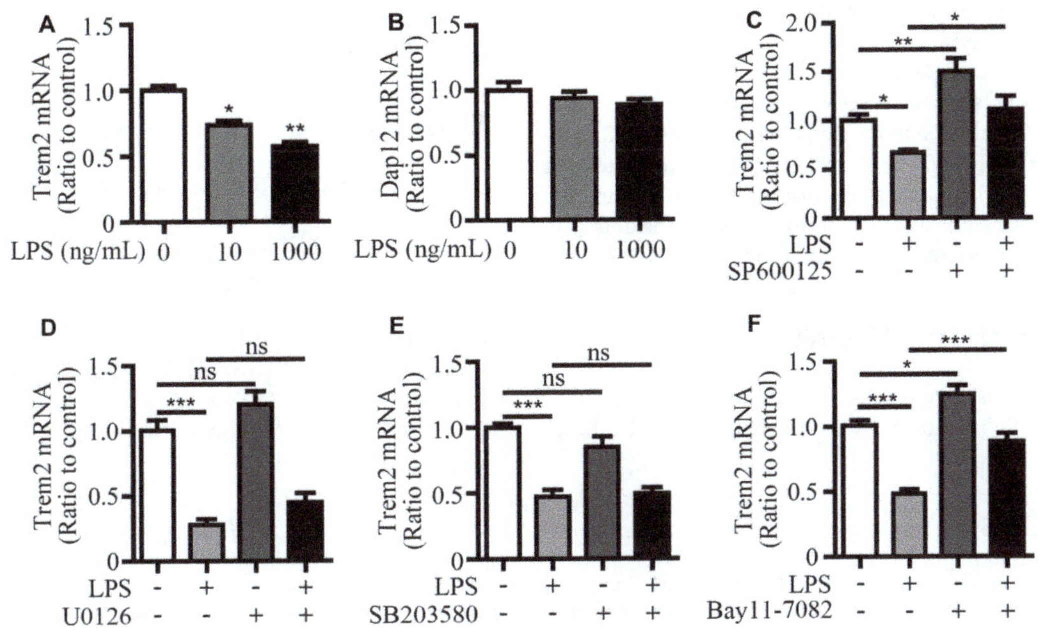

FIGURE 6 | Inhibitors for JNK and NF-κB restore *Trem2* expression suppressed by LPS. **(A,B)** BV2 cells were treated with indicated concentrations of LPS (0, 10 and 1000 ng/mL) for 4 h. RNA was extracted and the relative mRNA levels of *Trem2* **(A)** or *Dap12* **(B)** shown as bar graph was determined by quantitative RT-PCR ($n = 3$, one-way ANOVA). **(C–F)** BV2 cells were pretreated with 10 μM SP600125 **(C)**, 5 μM U0126 **(D)**, 5 μM SB203580 **(E)** or 5 μM Bay11–7082 **(F)** for 30 min, followed by treatment with 500 ng/mL LPS or vehicle control for 12 h. RNA was extracted and the relative mRNA levels of *Trem2* shown as bar graph were determined by quantitative RT-PCR ($n \geq 3$, one-way ANOVA). β-actin was used as an internal control. $^{*}p < 0.05$; $^{**}p < 0.01$; $^{***}p < 0.001$; ns, not significant.

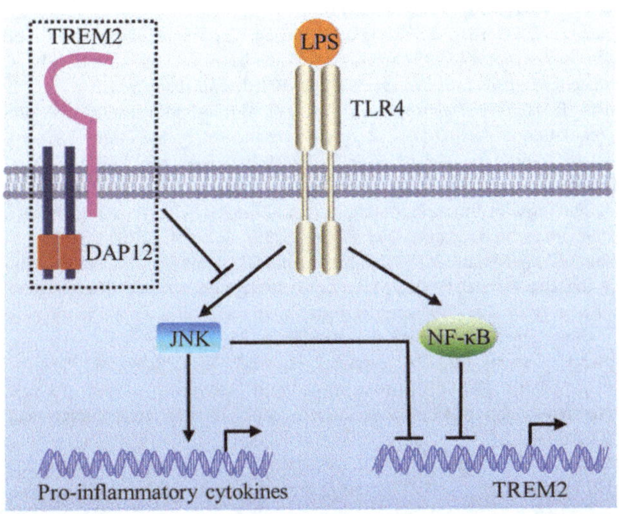

FIGURE 7 | Schematic model of the interplay between TREM2/DAP12 complex and LPS-induced inflammation. The TREM2/DAP12 complex suppresses the activity of JNK signaling pathway to reduce LPS-triggered inflammatory response in microglia. LPS down-regulates the expression of *Trem2* via the activation of JNK and NF-κB signaling pathways.

in a pro-inflammatory manner. The activating and inhibitory functions of DAP12 in inflammation are proposed to be modulated by the avidity of the interaction between the DAP12-associated receptor and its ligand (Turnbull and Colonna, 2007).

In accordance with our findings in microglia, *Dap12*-deficient macrophages have been reported to express higher amounts of inflammatory cytokines in response to a variety of pathogenic stimuli (Hamerman et al., 2005). However, the signaling mechanism by which Dap12 regulates cytokine production was distinct between microglia and macrophages. Upon LPS stimulation, ERK1/2 signaling was more pronounced in *Dap12*-deficient macrophages than in WT cells (Hamerman et al., 2005). In contrast, we observed the activation of JNK signaling pathway in *Trem2*- and *Dap12*-deficient microglia. It remains uncharacterized how DAP12 regulates the phosphorylation of either ERK1/2 in macrophages or JNK in microglia. Further study is needed to define the precise molecular pathway downstream of DAP12 actions.

We and others have consistently shown that LPS stimulation significantly suppressed microglial *Trem2* expression both *in vitro* and *in vivo* (Schmid et al., 2002; Zheng et al., 2016). The decrease in *Trem2* expression further augments the production of inflammatory cytokines, leading to detrimental exaggeration of neuroinflammation (Zhong et al., 2015; Zheng et al., 2016). Therefore, understanding the molecular mechanism by which LPS or other pathogenic stimuli regulate *Trem2* expression would provide insights into eliminating the source of inflammation cascade. Our current study showed that applying either JNK or NF-κB inhibitor restored *Trem2* expression down-regulated by LPS, implicating a potentially beneficial effect of those inhibitors for treating neurological diseases with an inflammatory component. The precise molecular pathways downstream of JNK and NF-κB require further investigation. It would be intriguing to examine whether the transcription factors activated by JNK and NF-κB regulate *Trem2* expression via direct binding to its proximal promoter.

Collectively, our studies revealed that DAP12 possesses an anti-inflammatory function in murine microglia that is TREM2-dependent. The TREM2/DAP12 axis negatively regulates the activity of JNK signaling pathway downstream of LPS to suppress the inflammatory responses. Our study provides insights into mechanism-based therapy for neuroinflammatory disorders.

AUTHOR CONTRIBUTIONS

LZ, X-FC and GB: designed research; LZ, Z-LZ, XL, CL, PM, TW, ZQW, ZW and MW: performed experiments; LZ, Z-LZ, XL, CL and X-FC: analyzed data; X-FC and LZ: wrote the manuscript; HX and GB: reviewed the manuscript. All authors read and approved the final manuscript.

FUNDING

Research by the authors was supported by grants from the National Natural Science Foundation of China 81370459, 31400914 (to X-FC) and U1505227 (to GB), a grant from the Fundamental Research Funds for the Central Universities (20720150051 to X-FC), a grant from the Guangdong Natural Science Foundation (2016A030306005 to X-FC), NIH grants R01AG035355 and P01NS074969 (to GB), a grant from the Cure Alzheimer's Fund (to GB), a grant from the China Postdoctoral Science Foundation (2016M600503 to LZ).

REFERENCES

Atagi, Y., Liu, C. C., Painter, M. M., Chen, X. F., Verbeeck, C., Zheng, H., et al. (2015). Apolipoprotein E is a ligand for triggering receptor expressed on myeloid cells 2 (TREM2). *J. Biol. Chem.* 290, 26043–26050. doi: 10.1074/jbc.M115.679043

Bailey, C. C., DeVaux, L. B., and Farzan, M. (2015). The triggering receptor expressed on myeloid cells 2 binds apolipoprotein E. *J. Biol. Chem.* 290, 26033–26042. doi: 10.1074/jbc.M115.677286

Bouchon, A., Dietrich, J., and Colonna, M. (2000). Cutting edge: inflammatory responses can be triggered by TREM-1, a novel receptor expressed on neutrophils and monocytes. *J. Immunol.* 164, 4991–4995. doi: 10.4049/jimmunol.164.10.4991

Chung, D. H., Seaman, W. E., and Daws, M. R. (2002). Characterization of TREM-3, an activating receptor on mouse macrophages: definition of a family of single Ig domain receptors on mouse chromosome 17. *Eur. J. Immunol.* 32, 59–66. doi: 10.1002/1521-4141(200201)32:1<59::AID-IMMU59>3.0.CO;2-U

Daws, M. R., Lanier, L. L., Seaman, W. E., and Ryan, J. C. (2001). Cloning and characterization of a novel mouse myeloid DAP12-associated receptor family. *Eur. J. Immunol.* 31, 783–791. doi: 10.1002/1521-4141(200103)31:3<783::AID-IMMU783>3.0.CO;2-U

Gibot, S., Kolopp-Sarda, M. N., Béné, M. C., Bollaert, P. E., Lozniewski, A., Mory, F., et al. (2004). A soluble form of the triggering receptor expressed on myeloid cells-1 modulates the inflammatory response in murine sepsis. *J. Exp. Med.* 200, 1419–1426. doi: 10.1084/jem.20040708

Guerreiro, R., Wojtas, A., Bras, J., Carrasquillo, M., Rogaeva, E., Majounie, E., et al. (2013). TREM2 variants in Alzheimer's disease. *N. Engl. J. Med.* 368, 117–127. doi: 10.1056/NEJMoa1211851

Hamerman, J. A., Jarjoura, J. R., Humphrey, M. B., Nakamura, M. C., Seaman, W. E., and Lanier, L. L. (2006). Cutting edge: inhibition of TLR and FcR responses in macrophages by triggering receptor expressed on myeloid cells (TREM)-2 and DAP12. *J. Immunol.* 177, 2051–2055. doi: 10.4049/jimmunol.177.4.2051

Hamerman, J. A., Tchao, N. K., Lowell, C. A., and Lanier, L. L. (2005). Enhanced Toll-like receptor responses in the absence of signaling adaptor DAP12. *Nat. Immunol.* 6, 579–586. doi: 10.1038/ni1204

Hickman, S. E., Kingery, N. D., Ohsumi, T. K., Borowsky, M. L., Wang, L. C., Means, T. K., et al. (2013). The microglial sensome revealed by direct RNA sequencing. *Nat. Neurosci.* 16, 1896–1905. doi: 10.1038/nn.3554

Huang, D., Zimmerman, M. I., Martin, P. K., Nix, A. J., Rosenberry, T. L., and Paravastu, A. K. (2015). Antiparallel β-sheet structure within the C-terminal region of 42-residue Alzheimer's amyloid-β peptides when they form 150-kDa oligomers. *J. Mol. Biol.* 427, 2319–2328. doi: 10.1016/j.jmb.2015.04.004

Humphrey, M. B., Lanier, L. L., and Nakamura, M. C. (2005). Role of ITAM-containing adapter proteins and their receptors in the immune system and bone. *Immunol. Rev.* 208, 50–65. doi: 10.1111/j.0105-2896.2005.00325.x

Jay, T. R., Miller, C. M., Cheng, P. J., Graham, L. C., Bemiller, S., Broihier, M. L., et al. (2015). TREM2 deficiency eliminates TREM2+ inflammatory macrophages and ameliorates pathology in Alzheimer's disease mouse models. *J. Exp. Med.* 212, 287–295. doi: 10.1084/jem.20142322

Jonsson, T., Stefansson, H., Steinberg, S., Jonsdottir, I., Jonsson, P. V., Snaedal, J., et al. (2013). Variant of TREM2 associated with the risk of Alzheimer's disease. *N. Engl. J. Med.* 368, 107–116. doi: 10.1056/NEJMoa1211103

Lanier, L. L. (2009). DAP10- and DAP12-associated receptors in innate immunity. *Immunol. Rev.* 227, 150–160. doi: 10.1111/j.1600-065x.2008.00720.x

Lanier, L. L., and Bakker, A. B. (2000). The ITAM-bearing transmembrane adaptor DAP12 in lymphoid and myeloid cell function. *Immunol. Today* 21, 611–614. doi: 10.1016/s0167-5699(00)01745-x

Lanier, L. L., Corliss, B. C., Wu, J., Leong, C., and Phillips, J. H. (1998). Immunoreceptor DAP12 bearing a tyrosine-based activation motif is involved in activating NK cells. *Nature* 391, 703–707. doi: 10.1038/35642

Mason, L. H., Willette-Brown, J., Taylor, L. S., and McVicar, D. W. (2006). Regulation of Ly49D/DAP12 signal transduction by Src-family kinases and CD45. *J. Immunol.* 176, 6615–6623. doi: 10.4049/jimmunol.176.11.6615

Paloneva, J., Kestilá, M., Wu, J., Salminen, A., Böhling, T., Ruotsalainen, V., et al. (2000). Loss-of-function mutations in TYROBP (DAP12) result in a presenile dementia with bone cysts. *Nat. Genet.* 25, 357–361. doi: 10.1038/77153

Paloneva, J., Manninen, T., Christman, G., Hovanes, K., Mandelin, J., Adolfsson, R., et al. (2002). Mutations in two genes encoding different subunits of a receptor signaling complex result in an identical disease phenotype. *Am. J. Hum. Genet.* 71, 656–662. doi: 10.1086/342259

Pottier, C., Ravenscroft, T. A., Brown, P. H., Finch, N. A., Baker, M., Parsons, M., et al. (2016). TYROBP genetic variants in early-onset Alzheimer's disease. *Neurobiol. Aging* 48, 222.e9–222.e15. doi: 10.1016/j.neurobiolaging.2016.07.028

Schmid, C. D., Sautkulis, L. N., Danielson, P. E., Cooper, J., Hasel, K. W., Hilbush, B. S., et al. (2002). Heterogeneous expression of the triggering receptor expressed on myeloid cells-2 on adult murine microglia. *J. Neurochem.* 83, 1309–1320. doi: 10.1046/j.1471-4159.2002.01243.x

Sessa, G., Podini, P., Mariani, M., Meroni, A., Spreafico, R., Sinigaglia, F., et al. (2004). Distribution and signaling of TREM2/DAP12, the receptor system mutated in human polycystic lipomembraneous osteodysplasia with sclerosing leukoencephalopathy dementia. *Eur. J. Neurosci.* 20, 2617–2628. doi: 10.1111/j.1460-9568.2004.03729.x

Sirkis, D. W., Bonham, L. W., Aparicio, R. E., Geier, E. G., Ramos, E. M., Wang, Q., et al. (2016). Rare TREM2 variants associated with Alzheimer's disease display reduced cell surface expression. *Acta Neuropathol. Commun.* 4:98. doi: 10.1186/s40478-016-0367-7

Takahashi, K., Rochford, C. D., and Neumann, H. (2005). Clearance of apoptotic neurons without inflammation by microglial triggering receptor expressed on myeloid cells-2. *J. Exp. Med.* 201, 647–657. doi: 10.1084/jem.20041611

Turnbull, I. R., and Colonna, M. (2007). Activating and inhibitory functions of DAP12. *Nat. Rev. Immunol.* 7, 155–161. doi: 10.1038/nri2014

Turnbull, I. R., Gilfillan, S., Cella, M., Aoshi, T., Miller, M., Piccio, L., et al. (2006). Cutting edge: TREM-2 attenuates macrophage activation. *J. Immunol.* 177, 3520–3524. doi: 10.4049/jimmunol.177.6.3520

Turnbull, I. R., McDunn, J. E., Takai, T., Townsend, R. R., Cobb, J. P., and Colonna, M. (2005). DAP12 (KARAP) amplifies inflammation and increases mortality from endotoxemia and septic peritonitis. *J. Exp. Med.* 202, 363–369. doi: 10.1084/jem.20050986

Wang, Y., Cella, M., Mallinson, K., Ulrich, J. D., Young, K. L., Robinette, M. L., et al. (2015). TREM2 lipid sensing sustains the microglial response in an Alzheimer's disease model. *Cell* 160, 1061–1071. doi: 10.1016/j.cell.2015.01.049

Yeh, F. L., Wang, Y., Tom, I., Gonzalez, L. C., and Sheng, M. (2016). TREM2 binds to apolipoproteins, including APOE, and CLU/APOJ and thereby facilitates uptake of amyloid-β by microglia. *Neuron* 91, 328–340. doi: 10.1016/j.neuron.2016.06.015

Yuan, P., Condello, C., Keene, C. D., Wang, Y., Bird, T. D., Paul, S. M., et al. (2016). TREM2 haplodeficiency in mice and humans impairs the microglia barrier function leading to decreased amyloid compaction and severe axonal dystrophy. *Neuron* 92, 252–264. doi: 10.1016/j.neuron.2016.09.016

Zhang, Y., Chen, K., Sloan, S. A., Bennett, M. L., Scholze, A. R., O'Keeffe, S., et al. (2014). An RNA-sequencing transcriptome and splicing database of glia, neurons and vascular cells of the cerebral cortex. *J. Neurosci.* 34, 11929–11947. doi: 10.1523/JNEUROSCI.1860-14.2014

Zheng, H., Liu, C. C., Atagi, Y., Chen, X. F., Jia, L., Yang, L., et al. (2016). Opposing roles of the triggering receptor expressed on myeloid cells 2 and triggering receptor expressed on myeloid cells-like transcript 2 in microglia activation. *Neurobiol. Aging* 42, 132–141. doi: 10.1016/j.neurobiolaging.2016.03.004

Zhong, L., Chen, X. F., Wang, T., Wang, Z., Liao, C., Wang, Z., et al. (2017). Soluble TREM2 induces inflammatory responses and enhances microglial survival. *J. Exp. Med.* 214, 597–607. doi: 10.1084/jem.20160844

Zhong, L., Chen, X. F., Zhang, Z. L., Wang, Z., Shi, X. Z., Xu, K., et al. (2015). DAP12 stabilizes the C-terminal fragment of the triggering receptor expressed on myeloid cells-2 (TREM2) and protects against LPS-induced Pro-inflammatory response. *J. Biol. Chem.* 290, 15866–15877. doi: 10.1074/jbc.M115.645986

Zhu, W., Zheng, H., Shao, X., Wang, W., Yao, Q., and Li, Z. (2010). Excitotoxicity of TNFα derived from KA activated microglia on hippocampal neurons *in vitro* and *in vivo*. *J. Neurochem.* 114, 386–396. doi: 10.1111/j.1471-4159.2010.06763.x

2

Curcumin Protects against Ischemic Stroke by Titrating Microglia/Macrophage Polarization

*Zongjian Liu[1,2†], Yuanyuan Ran[1,2†], Shuo Huang[1,2], Shaohong Wen[2], Wenxiu Zhang[2], Xiangrong Liu[3], Zhili Ji[2], Xiaokun Geng[1], Xunming Ji[1,3], Huishan Du[1], Rehana K. Leak[4] and Xiaoming Hu[1,5]**

[1]China-America Institute of Neuroscience, Beijing Luhe Hospital, Capital Medical University, Beijing, China, [2]Central Laboratory, Beijing Luhe Hospital, Capital Medical University, Beijing, China, [3]Institute of Hypoxia Medicine, Xuanwu Hospital, Xuan Wu Hospital of the Capital Medical University, Beijing, China, [4]Division of Pharmaceutical Sciences, Duquesne University, Pittsburgh, PA, United States, [5]Pittsburgh Institute of Brain Disorders and Recovery, and Department of Neurology, University of Pittsburgh School of Medicine, Pittsburgh, PA, United States

***Correspondence:**
Xiaoming Hu
hux2@upmc.edu

†These authors have contributed equally to this work.

Stroke is the most common type of cerebrovascular disease and is a leading cause of disability and death. Ischemic stroke accounts for approximately 80% of all strokes. The remaining 20% of strokes are hemorrhagic in nature. To date, therapeutic options for acute ischemic stroke are very limited. Recent research suggests that shifting microglial phenotype from the pro-inflammatory M1 state toward the anti-inflammatory and tissue-reparative M2 phenotype may be an effective therapeutic strategy for ischemic stroke. The dietary phytochemical curcumin has shown promise in experimental stroke models, but its effects on microglial polarization and long-term recovery after stroke are unknown. Here we address these gaps by subjecting mice to distal middle cerebral artery occlusion (dMCAO) and administering curcumin intraperitoneally (150 mg/kg) immediately after ischemia and 24 h later. Histological studies revealed that curcumin post-treatment significantly reduced cerebral ischemic damage 3 days after dMCAO. Sensorimotor functions—as measured by the adhesive removal test and modified Garcia scores—were superior in curcumin-treated mice at 3, 5, 7 and 10 days after stroke. RT-PCR measurements revealed an elevation of M2 microglia/macrophage phenotypic markers and a reduction in M1 markers in curcumin-treated brains 3 days after dMCAO. Immunofluorescent staining further showed that curcumin treatment significantly increased the number of $CD206^+Iba1^+$ M2 microglia/macrophages and reduced the number of $CD16^+Iba1^+$ M1 cells 10 days after stroke. *In vitro* studies using the BV2 microglial cell line confirmed that curcumin inhibited lipopolysaccharide (LPS) and interferon-γ (IFN-γ)-induced M1 polarization. Curcumin treatment concentration-dependently reduced the expression of pro-inflammatory cytokines, including TNF-α, IL-6 and IL-12p70, in the absence of any toxic effect on microglial cell survival. In conclusion, we demonstrate that curcumin has a profound regulatory effect on microglial responses, promoting M2 microglial polarization and inhibiting microglia-mediated pro-inflammatory responses. Curcumin post-treatment reduces ischemic stroke-induced brain damage and improves functional outcomes, providing new evidence that curcumin might be a promising therapeutic strategy for stroke.

Keywords: curcumin, microglial polarization, ischemic stroke, inflammation, neuroprotection

INTRODUCTION

Stroke remains one of the leading causes of death and disability worldwide (Huuskonen et al., 2017; Mijajlović et al., 2017). Ischemic stroke accounts for approximately 80% of all strokes. The remaining 20% of strokes are hemorrhagic in nature. Thrombolytic therapy with recombinant tissue plasminogen activator (rtPA) is the only FDA-approved clinical treatment for acute ischemic stroke. A large number of neuroprotective agents have been investigated in the past few decades and shown promising results in animal models of stroke; all of them, however, failed in subsequent clinical trials (Cook et al., 2012; Guekht et al., 2017). Thus, rescuing neurons without improving the microenvironment in the injured brain is not sufficient to achieve long-term protection and functional recovery after stroke. Therefore, new therapeutic strategies that re-establish brain homeostasis and foster a permissive environment for cell survival or regeneration are being actively explored.

Microglia and infiltrated macrophages play critical roles in regulating immune and inflammatory responses after brain injuries (Perry et al., 2010). Accumulating evidence shows that microglia/macrophages assume different phenotypes with distinct functions during the course of ischemic brain injury (Hu et al., 2012). For example, alternatively activated M2 microglia protect neighboring cells by removing cell debris and releasing trophic factors for brain repair. However, classically activated M1 microglia may exacerbate brain injury by producing neurotoxic substances when overactivated for prolonged times, even if they participate in clearing cell debris at early stages after stroke (Hu et al., 2012, 2015). These two microglia/macrophage phenotypes probably lie along a continuum of activation status. Such phenotypic plasticity and diversity support the view that microglia serve a unique and important role in maintaining brain homeostasis under physiological and pathological conditions. Several agents known to be protective against ischemic stroke, such as Ginkgolide B (Shu et al., 2016), Malibatol A (Pan et al., 2015), thiamet G (He et al., 2016), and Exendin-4 (Darsalia et al., 2014) have the capacity to promote M2 polarization in microglia. Thus, balancing microglia/macrophage phenotype is a promising therapeutic strategy for stroke treatment.

Curcumin (1,7-bis[4-hydroxy-3-methoxyphenyl]-1,6-heptadiene-3,5-dione) is a major component of the rhizomes of *Curcuma longa* and a well-established polyphenolic antioxidant (Gupta et al., 2012). A number of studies have demonstrated that curcumin can protect against ischemic stroke in experimental models (Thiyagarajan and Sharma, 2004; Lapchak, 2011; Shah et al., 2016). Pre-/post-stroke treatment with curcumin was found to effectively reduce infarct volumes and improve functional outcomes. Curcumin has also been proposed as a promising agent for stroke prevention in humans (Ovbiagele, 2008). Manifold mechanisms are involved in the protective effects of curcumin, including anti-oxidative, anti-inflammatory (Thiyagarajan and Sharma, 2004; Yang et al., 2009; Wu et al., 2013), and anti-apoptotic mechanisms (Zhao et al., 2008, 2010; Altinay et al., 2017), as well as neurogenesis (Liu S. et al., 2016). However, the effect of curcumin on microglial phenotypic polarization after ischemic stroke has not been explored.

In the present study, we assessed the effects of curcumin on microglial polarization and inflammatory responses both *in vitro* and in a mouse model of ischemic stroke. Our results demonstrate that curcumin promoted microglial M2 polarization and inhibited M1 polarization, both *in vivo* and *in vitro*. Furthermore, curcumin treatment ameliorated post-stroke brain injury and improved functional outcomes. These findings support the view that curcumin improves functional recovery after stroke by adjusting the balance between M1 and M2 microglial states.

MATERIALS AND METHODS

Animals

Adult male C57BL/6 mice (8–10 weeks, 23–25 g) were purchased from the Vital River Laboratory Animal Technology Co., Ltd (Beijing, China). All animal experiments were approved by the Institutional Animal Care and Use Committee of Capital Medical University. Food and water were available *ad libitum*. All efforts were made to minimize animal suffering and the number of animals used. Animals were randomly divided into: (1) sham; (2) stroke plus vehicle; and (3) stroke plus curcumin groups. In this study, a total of 80 mice were used for infarct volume measurements (23 mice), behavioral tests and immunohistochemical examinations (42 mice), and mRNA or protein expression measurements (15 mice).

Distal Middle Cerebral Artery Occlusion (dMCAO) Model

Anesthesia was induced with 2% isoflurane in 70% nitrogen/30% oxygen gas mixture. Rectal temperature was maintained at 37 ± 0.5°C with a heating pad. A ∼2 cm incision was made between the right eye and ear. Using a surgical microscope, the temporal muscle was dissected to expose right zygomatic arches and squamosal bone. A craniotomy was performed and the right MCA was occluded distal to the lenticulostriate branches with bipolar electrocautery (Goldbov Photoelectronics CO. Ltd, Wuhan, China). The middle cerebral artery occlusion (MCAO) was accompanied by 15-min bilateral occlusion of the common carotid artery (CCA). Regional cerebral blood flow (rCBF) was monitored with a two-dimensional laser speckle imager (Perimed AB, Järfälla, Sweden). Mice with rCBF reduction less than 30% of baseline levels were excluded from further experiments. Sham-operated mice were manipulated in the same way, but the MCA and CCA were not occluded.

Drug Preparation and Treatments

Curcumin (Sigma-Aldrich) was dissolved in 5 mol/L NaOH, titrated to pH 7.4 using 1 mol/L HCl, and then diluted with saline. Ischemic mice were subjected to intraperitoneal injections of 150 mg/kg curcumin or the same volume of vehicle. Injections were performed 0 h and 24 h after reperfusion of the CCA.

Measurements of Infarct Volume

At 72 h after cerebral ischemia, mice were decapitated and brains were rapidly removed on ice. Brains were sliced into 1 mm-thick coronal sections and stained with 2% 2, 3, 5-triphenyltetrazolium chloride (TTC, Sigma-Aldrich), as previously described (Liu X. et al., 2016). The infarct area was calculated as the area of the contralateral hemisphere minus the noninfarcted area of the ipsilateral hemisphere by a person blinded to the experiment group. Infarct volumes were determined using National institutes of Health ImageJ software. The total infarct areas were multiplied by the thickness of the brain sections to obtain the infarct volumes.

Adhesive Removal Test

Sensorimotor functional recovery after stroke was measured before or 3, 5, 7 and 10 days after stroke with the adhesive removal test, as described in prior studies (Wang et al., 2017). In brief, a mouse was placed in a cage for 1 min. An adhesive tape (50 mm^2) was applied to the distal radial region of the right forelimb as a tactile stimulus. The time to contact and the time to remove the tape were both recorded. Each animal was tested three times with a cutoff time of 120 s per trial. The data are presented as the mean time to contact and the mean time to remove the tape on each testing day. The investigators performing the assessments were blinded to experimental group assignments.

Modified Garcia Score Test

The Modified Garcia Score system was used to assess sensorimotor functions at 3, 5, 7 and 10 days after dMCAO by an observer blinded to the experimental groups. Five tests were performed: body proprioception, vibrissae touch, limb symmetry, lateral turning and forelimb walking with scores of 0–3 for each test, as previously reported studies (Wang et al., 2017). The data from pre-stroke tests were defined as the baseline.

Immunohistochemistry and Cell Counting

Brain slices were prepared and subjected to immunohistochemistry, as previously published (Pan et al., 2015). Mice were perfused with saline and 4% paraformaldehyde. Brains were then removed, followed by cryoprotection in 30% sucrose. The brains were sliced into 20 μm-thick coronal sections at −25°C using a freezing microtome (CM3050S, Leica, German). The slices were then subjected to immunofluorescent staining. Non-specific staining was blocked with 10% normal serum. Next, brain slices were incubated with mouse anti-CD16 (1:100, BD Pharmingen, San Jose, CA, USA), goat anti-CD206 (1:100, R&D Systems, Minneapolis, MN, USA), and rabbit anti-Iba-1 (1:100, Wako, Richmond, VA, USA) overnight at 4°C. The sections were then treated with fluorophore-conjugated secondary antibodies (Invitrogen Corporation, Carlsbad, CA, USA)—goat anti-rabbit antibody conjugated to Alexa 594 (1:400), goat anti-mouse antibody conjugated to Alexa 488 (1:400), and donkey anti-goat antibody conjugated to Alexa 488 (1:400), at room temperature for 2 h. All images were captured with a fluorescence microscope (DM4000 B LED, Leica Microsystem, Germany) and analyzed by a blinded observer with ImageJ. Cell numbers were calculated from three randomly-selected microscopic fields, and three consecutive sections were analyzed for each brain.

BV2 Microglia Cell Line Cultures

The BV2 microglia cell line (Cell Center, Institute of Basic Medical Sciences, CAMS and PUMC, Beijing, China) was cultured in RPMI 1640 (Cat No.: C11875500BT, Gibco), supplemented with 10% fetal bovine serum (Cat No.: 16000-044, Gibco) and 1% penicillin-streptomycin (Cat No.: 15070-063, Gibco). Cells were incubated at 37°C in a humidified atmosphere containing 5% CO_2 and the medium was changed every 2 days. For M1 stimulation, lipopolysaccharide (LPS, 100 ng/mL) and IFN-γ (20 ng/mL) were added to BV2 microglia cultures. Different concentrations of curcumin were added to the cultures immediately following the application of M1 inducers. After 48 h of treatment, cells were collected for RT-PCR and the supernatant was harvested for the detection of cytokines by ELISA.

The cytotoxicity of curcumin against BV2 microglia cell line was analyzed by a lactate dehydrogenase (LDH) cytotoxicity assay kit (Cat No.: C0017, Beyotime, Shanghai, China) according to the manufacturer's protocol. Absorbance was measured at 490 nm by a microplate reader (Cat No.: Synergy HT, Biotek, Winooski, VT, USA). All cell culture experiments were performed in duplicate and repeated six times.

Real-Time PCR

Total RNA was extracted from the cortex of C57BL/6 mice or from the BV2 microglia cell line (Cell Center, Institute of Basic Medical Sciences, CAMS and PUMC, Beijing, China) by RNeasy® Lipid Tissue Mini Kit (Cat No.: 74804, QIAGEN) according to manufacturer's instructions. Three microgram RNA were reverse-transcribed into cDNA using the SuperScript™ III First-Strand Synthesis SuperMix for qRT-PCR (Cat No.: 11752-250, Invitrogen). RT-PCR was performed using quantitative PCR systems (Applied Biosystems® 7500 Real-Time PCR Systems, Thermo Fisher Scientific, Waltham, MA, USA) with corresponding primers (**Table 1**,

TABLE 1 | Primers for RT-PCR.

Genes		Primers (5′-3′)
GAPDH	Forward	AGGTCGGTGTGAACGGATTTG
	Reverse	GGGGTCGTTGATGGCAACA
IL-12	Forward	AAATGAAGCTCTGCATCCTGC
	Reverse	TCACCCTGTTGATGGTCACG
TNF-α	Forward	GATCTCAAAGACAACCAACTAGTG
	Reverse	CTCCAGCTGGAAGACTCCTCCCAG
iNOS	Forward	CAAGCACCTTGGAAGAGGAG
	Reverse	AAGGCCAAACACAGCATACC
CD16	Forward	TTTGGACACCCAGATGTTTCAG
	Reverse	GTCTTCCTTGAGCACCTGGATC
CD32	Forward	AATCCTGCCGTTCCTACTGATC
	Reverse	GTGTCACCGTGTCTTCCTTGAG
CD206	Forward	CAAGGAAGGTTGGCATTTGT
	Reverse	CCTTTCAGTCCTTTGCAAGC
Arg1	Forward	TCACCTGAGCTTTGATGTCG
	Reverse	CTGAAAGGAGCCCTGTCTTG
Ym1/2	Forward	CAGGGTAATGAGTGGGTTGG
	Reverse	CACGGCACCTCCTAAATTGT

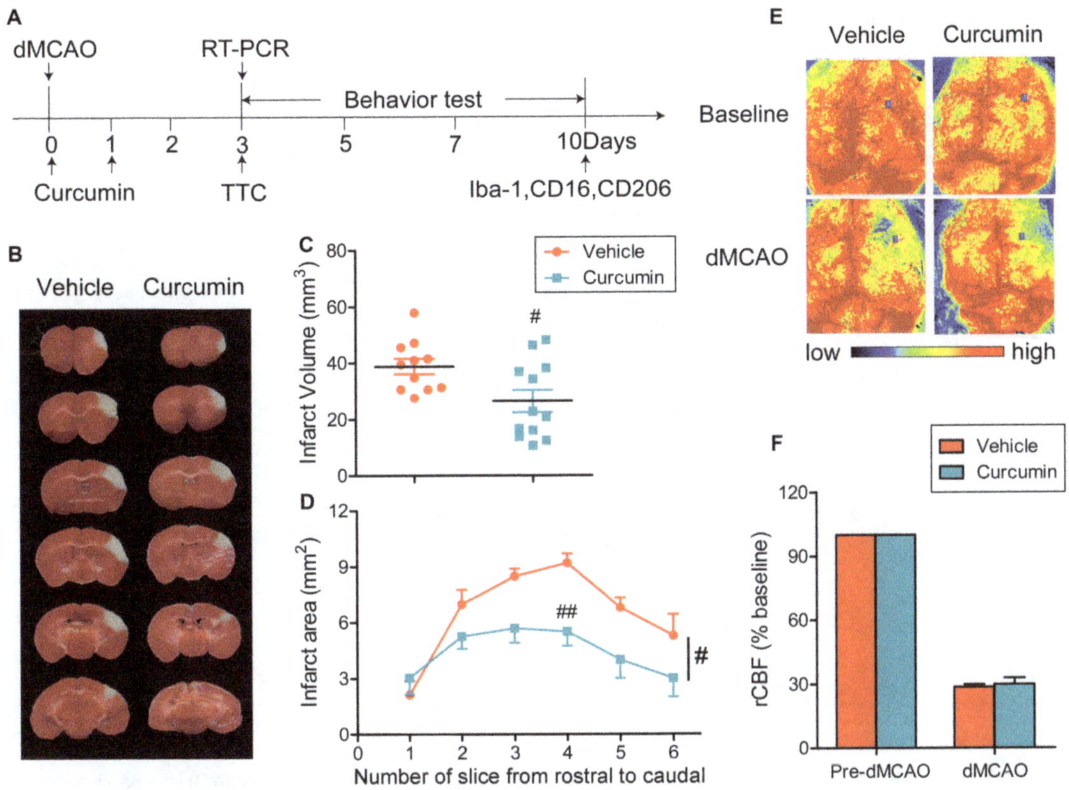

FIGURE 1 | Curcumin treatment reduces infarct volume 3 days after distal middle cerebral artery occlusion (dMCAO). **(A)** Timeline for *in vivo* experiments. Stroke was induced in mice with permanent occlusion of the dMCAO. Curcumin was intraperitoneally injected (150 mg/kg) at 0 and 24 h after ischemia. At 3 days after stroke, RT-PCR was performed to determine the mRNA expression of M1/M2 microglia markers and infarct volume was measured after 2,3,5-triphenyltetrazolium chloride (TTC) staining. Adhesive removal tests and modified Garcia scores were used to measure post-stroke sensorimotor functions at 0, 3, 5, 7 and 10 days after cerebral ischemia. To confirm whether curcumin regulates microglial polarization in the brain after dMCAO, brain sections were double-stained for Iba-1 (microglia) with CD206 (M2 marker) or CD16 (M1 marker) at 10 days after stroke. **(B)** Representative TTC staining at 3 days after dMCAO. **(C)** Infarct volume in vehicle (red) and curcumin-treated (blue) dMCAO mice. **(D)** Infarct areas in TTC-stained slices. **(E)** Representative two-dimensional laser speckle images for regional cerebral blood flow (rCBF) in curcumin and vehicle-treated mice. **(F)** Changes in rCBF in infarct regions. Data are expressed as a percentage of pre-dMCAO rCBF. $n = 11$ animals per group. Data are means ± SEM. $^{\#}p < 0.05$, $^{\#\#}p < 0.01$ vs. vehicle-treated group, Student's two-tailed t test **(C)** and two-way ANOVA followed by Bonferroni *post hoc* test **(D)**.

Invitrogen) and a fluorescent dye (RT2 SYBR® Green FAST Mastermixes, Cat No.: 330603, QIAGEN). The cycle time (CT) was normalized to GAPDH in the same sample. The expression levels of mRNAs were reported as fold changes vs. sham control.

ELISA Measurements

Cytokine production (IL-1β, IL-2, IL-12p70, IL-13 and TNF-α) in the BV2 culture media was determined by ELISA (Cusabio Co., Ltd., Wuhan, China), according to the manufacturer's instructions. Each sample was assayed in triplicate.

Statistical Analyses

Power analyses were used to determine the number of mice within each experimental group, according to our past experience with similar measurements ($\alpha = 0.05$ and $\beta = 0.20$). All data are presented as mean ± SEM. The Student's two tailed t-test was used for comparisons of two experimental groups. Differences in means across multiple groups were analyzed using one-way or two-way ANOVA, depending on the number of independent variables. Differences in means across multiple groups with multiple measurements over time were analyzed using two-way repeated measures ANOVA. When the ANOVA revealed significant differences, the Bonferroni *post hoc* test was used for pairwise comparisons between means.

RESULTS

Curcumin Treatment Significantly Reduces Infarct Volumes 3 days after dMCAO

Curcumin (150 mg/kg) was administered intraperitoneally immediately after dMCAO and 24 h after surgery (**Figure 1A**). As shown in **Figures 1B–D**, curcumin treatment significantly reduced infarct volumes compared to vehicle. rCBF was measured before and after dMCAO with a two-dimensional laser speckle imager (**Figure 1E**). For all animals assigned to curcumin or vehicle groups, the rCBF after dMCAO was reduced to about

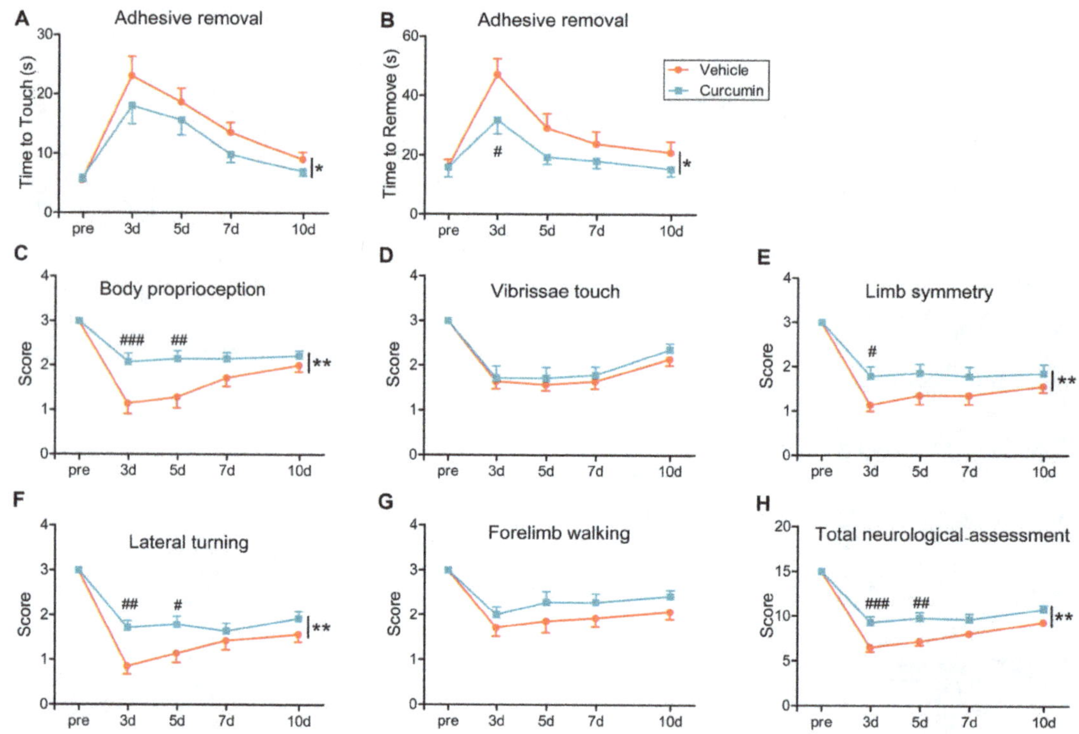

FIGURE 2 | Curcumin treatment significantly improves sensorimotor functions early after dMCAO. Adhesive removal test **(A,B)** and modified Garcia scores **(C–H)** were used to evaluate sensorimotor functions pre-surgery or 3, 5, 7 and 10 days after dMCAO in mice treated with vehicle or curcumin. **(A)** Time to touch adhesive tape. **(B)** Time to remove adhesive tape. **(C)** Body proprioception. **(D)** Vibrissae touch. **(E)** Limb symmetry. **(F)** Lateral turning. **(G)** Forelimb walking. **(H)** Total neurologic assessment score. $n = 14$ animals per group. Data are means ± SEM. $^{*}p < 0.05$, $^{**}p < 0.01$ between vehicle-treated group and curcumin-treated group. $^{\#}p < 0.05$, $^{\#\#}p < 0.01$, $^{\#\#\#}p < 0.001$ at a particular time point between vehicle-treated and curcumin-treated group. Two way repeated measures ANOVA followed by Bonferroni *post hoc* test.

30% of pre-ischemic baseline values (**Figure 1E**). There was no statistical difference in rCBF reduction between curcumin and vehicle-treated groups (**Figure 1F**), verifying that outcome differences between the experimental and control groups cannot be attributed to different degrees of the original ischemic injury.

Curcumin Treatment Significantly Improves Sensorimotor Functions after dMCAO

To evaluate the effects of curcumin treatment on functional outcomes after dMCAO, sensorimotor deficits were measured by the adhesive removal test and modified Garcia score system at 3, 5, 7 and 10 days post-stroke. Curcumin treatment significantly improved neurological performance in the adhesive removal test after dMCAO, as manifested by a consistent reduction in the times to contact and then remove the tape from the compromised limb (**Figures 2A,B**, respectively). In addition, sensorimotor functions such as body proprioception (**Figure 2C**), limb symmetry (**Figure 2E**), and lateral turning (**Figure 2F**) were all significantly improved in curcumin-treated mice compared to vehicle-treated mice, resulting in an increase in the total neurological score, especially at day 3–5 after stroke (**Figure 2H**). There was no significant difference in vibrissae touch (**Figure 2D**) or forelimb walking (**Figure 2G**) between vehicle and curcumin-treated groups. These data reveal improvements in some aspects of neurological function at early timepoints after stroke with curcumin.

Curcumin Treatment Inhibits M1 Polarization and Promotes M2 Polarization of Microglia

Polarization of microglia plays a critical role in the pathological progression of ischemic stroke (Hu et al., 2012). Thus, the effect of curcumin on microglial polarization was examined by RT-PCR. RNA samples were prepared from dMCAO mice treated with curcumin or vehicle. As shown in **Figure 3**, the expression of M1 markers (TNF-α, IL-12, CD16, CD32 and iNOS) and M2 markers (Arg-1 and YM1/2) were all significantly increased in vehicle-treated stroke mice 3 days after dMCAO. Curcumin treatment significantly inhibited this increase of M1 markers and enhanced the expression of M2 markers 3 days after dMCAO (**Figure 2**).

To further assess whether curcumin regulates microglial polarization in the brain after dMCAO, brain sections were double-stained for Iba-1 (microglial marker) and CD16 (M1 marker) or CD206 (M2 marker). As shown in **Figures 4A,C**, the percentage of $CD16^{+}Iba\text{-}1^{+}$ cells among total $Iba\text{-}1^{+}$ microglia/macrophages was significantly higher in

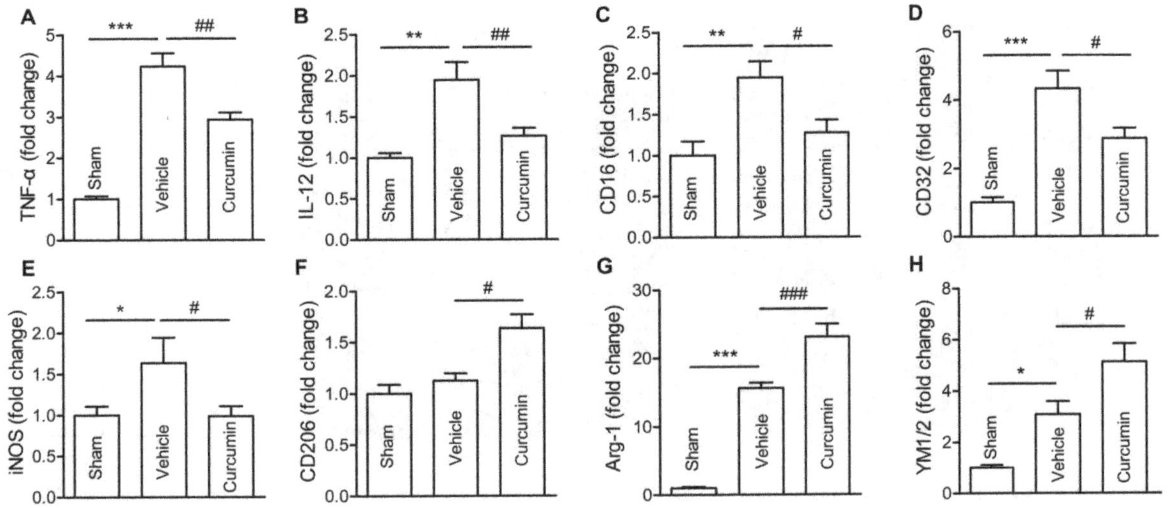

FIGURE 3 | Curcumin treatment inhibits M1 polarization and promotes M2 polarization of microglia/macrophages 3 days after dMCAO. Mice were subjected to dMCAO. Curcumin (150 mg/kg) or the same volume of vehicle was intraperitoneally injected into mice at 0h and 24 h after dMCAO. Brain samples were collected 3 days after dMCAO. mRNA expression of M1 microglia/macrophage signature genes (TNF-α **(A)**, IL-12 **(B)**, CD16 **(C)**, CD32 **(D)**, and iNOS **(E)**) and M2 signature genes (CD206 **(F)**, Arg-1**(G)**, and YM1/2 **(H)**) were measured by RT-PCR. Data are means ± SEM. $n = 5$ animals per group. *$p < 0.05$, **$p < 0.01$, ***$p < 0.001$ vs. sham; #$p < 0.05$, ##$p < 0.01$, ###$p < 0.001$ vs. vehicle-treated, one-way ANOVA followed by Bonferroni *post hoc* test.

vehicle-treated mice compared to curcumin-treated stroke mice. Moreover, curcumin administration significantly increased the percentage of $CD206^{+}Iba\text{-}1^{+}$ M2 microglia/macrophages after dMCAO (**Figures 4B,D**). Taken together, these results demonstrate that curcumin treatment promotes M2 polarization and inhibits M1 polarization after stroke, consistent with its neuroprotective properties.

Administration of Curcumin Promotes M2 Polarization and Inhibits M1 Polarization *In Vitro*

The BV2 microglial cell line was used to further determine the effects of curcumin on microglial polarization. First, we performed the LDH assay to determine curcumin cytotoxicity in BV2 microglia cells (**Figure 5A**). Treatment with 6.25, 12.5 and 25 μmmol/L curcumin showed no significant effects on microglial survival. Treatment with 35 μmmol/L curcumin exerted a significantly cytotoxic effect on BV2 microglia cells. Therefore, the 12.5 and 25 μmol/L concentrations were selected for further experiments.

BV2 microglial cells were treated with LPS (100 ng/mL) and IFN-γ (20 ng/mL) for 48 h to induce the M1 phenotype. As shown in **Figures 5B–E**, the mRNA expression of M1 markers (TNF-α, IL-12, CD16 and CD32) was increased significantly in BV2 microglia after stimulation with LPS and IFN-γ, but markedly reduced after treatment with 12.5 or 25 μmmol/L curcumin. However, the mRNA expression of iNOS (M1 marker, **Figure 5F**) was drastically upregulated by LPS and IFN-γ and not significantly reduced with curcumin. In contrast to the upregulation of M1 markers with LPS and IFN-γ, the mRNA expression of M2 markers (CD206 and Arg-1) was reduced by these two pro-inflammatory stimuli. The 12.5 or 25 μmmol/L concentrations of curcumin partially reversed this reduction of CD206 expression (**Figure 5G**), but showed only marginal effects on Arg-1 expression (**Figure 5H**). We conclude that most, but not all, M1 markers are almost completely inhibited by curcumin treatment in stimulated microglial cells, whereas M2 markers are partially upregulated.

Administration of Curcumin Significantly Reduces Pro-Inflammatory Cytokines in LPS + IFN-γ-Stimulated BV2 Cells

Next, we performed ELISAs to measure the release of pro-inflammatory cytokines in LPS + IFN-γ-stimulated BV2 cells. LPS and IFN-γ dramatically increased the production of pro-inflammatory cytokines from BV2 cells, including TNF-α, IL-12p70, IL-6, IL-2 and IL-1β (**Figure 6**). Curcumin treatment significantly reduced the production of pro-inflammatory cytokines including TNF-α, IL-12p70 and IL-6. However, the secretion of IL-1β and IL-2 was not dramatically attenuated with curcumin administration at 12.5 or 25 μmmol/L. Taken together, our *in vitro* data demonstrate that curcumin promotes M2 polarization and inhibits M1 polarization of microglia, and inhibits production of pro-inflammatory cytokines from M1-stimulated microglia. Collectively, these findings suggest a titration of polarization status by curcumin, both *in vivo* and *in vitro*.

DISCUSSION

Curcumin is a natural compound deemed as safe for ingestion by animals and humans by the Food and

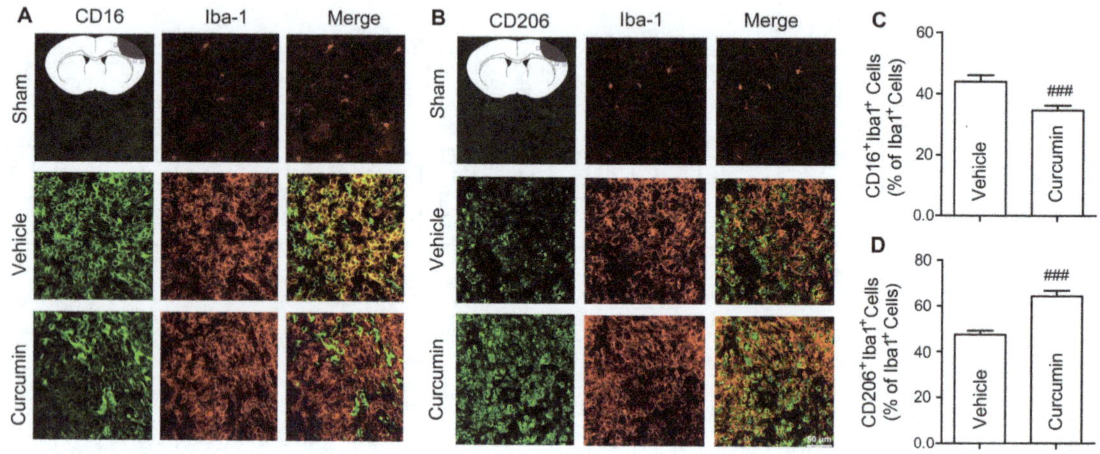

FIGURE 4 | Curcumin treatment enhances M2 polarization and suppresses M1 polarization of microglia in the ischemic cortex at 10 days after dMCAO. Representative double-immunofluorescence staining for CD16 or CD206 and Iba-1 markers in brain sections obtained from curcumin or vehicle-treated mice 10 days after dMCAO, or from sham-operated mice. Scale bar: 50 μm. Blue squares in the schematic diagram illustrate the anatomical location of images in the ipsilateral peri-infarct cortex. **(A)** Cortex sections co-stained for CD16 (M1 marker) (green) and Iba-1(red). **(B)** Cortex sections co-stained for CD206 (M2 marker) (green) and Iba-1 (red). **(C)** Quantification of the percentage of $CD16^+Iba\text{-}1^+$ cells among total $Iba\text{-}1^+$ cells. **(D)** Quantification of the percentage of $CD206^+/Iba\text{-}1^+$ cell among total $Iba\text{-}1^+$ cells. Data are means ± SEM. $n = 6$ animals per group. $^{###}p < 0.001$ vs. vehicle-treated group, Student's two-tailed t test.

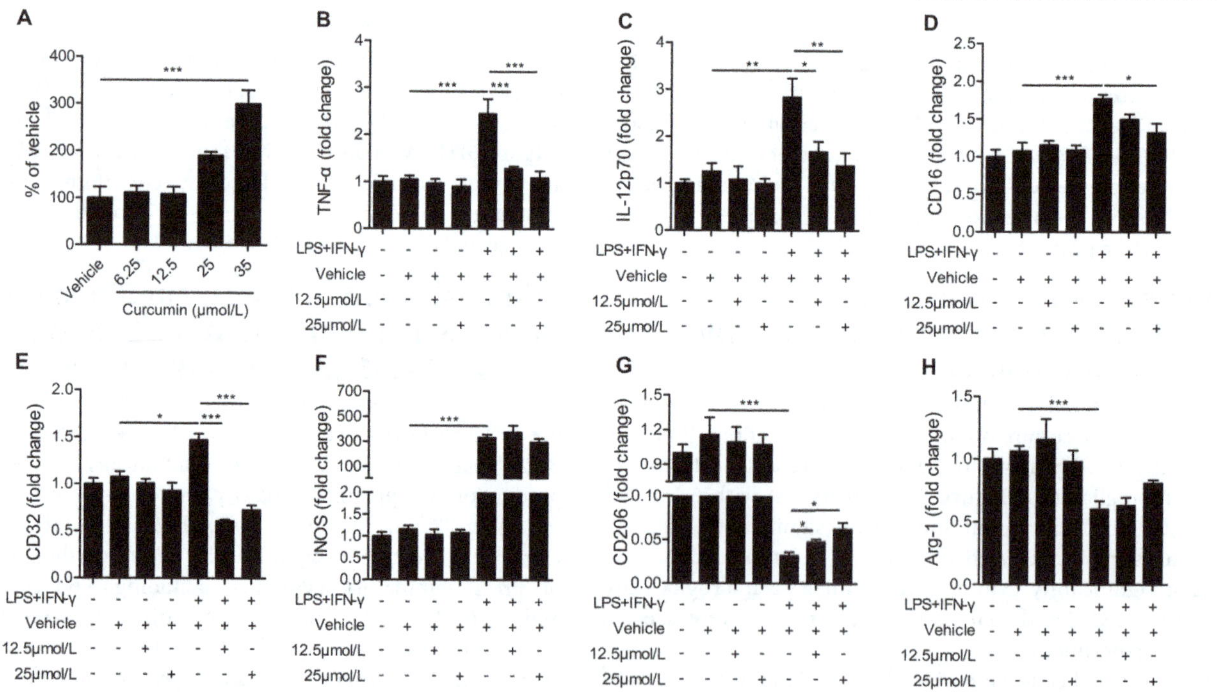

FIGURE 5 | Curcumin inhibits M1 polarization and promotes M2 polarization in lipopolysaccharide (LPS) and interferon-γ (IFN-γ)-activated BV2 microglial cells. **(A)** lactate dehydrogenase (LDH) cell cytotoxicity assay in BV2 cells cultured with vehicle or 6.25, 12.5, 25 and 35 μmmol/L curcumin. **(B–H)** BV2 microglia were stimulated with LPS (100 ng/mL) and IFN-γ (20 ng/mL), and then treated with vehicle or 12.5 and 25 μmmol/L curcumin. The mRNA expression of M1 markers (TNF-α **(A)**, IL-12p70 **(B)**, CD16 **(C)**, CD32 **(D)** and iNOS **(E)**) and M2 markers (CD206 **(G)** and Arg-1 **(H)**) were examined by RT-PCR. Data are means ± SEM. $n = 6$ per group. Samples were collected from six independent experiments, each performed in duplicate. $^{*}p < 0.05$, $^{**}p < 0.01$, $^{***}p < 0.001$, one-way ANOVA followed by Bonferroni *post hoc* test.

Drug Administration (FDA). The therapeutic potential of curcumin has been reported in many diseases, including cancer and neurodegenerative disorders (Pluta et al., 2015; Panda et al., 2017). A growing number of reports suggest that curcumin can protect against stroke-induced brain damage (Thiyagarajan and Sharma, 2004; Lin et al., 2016;

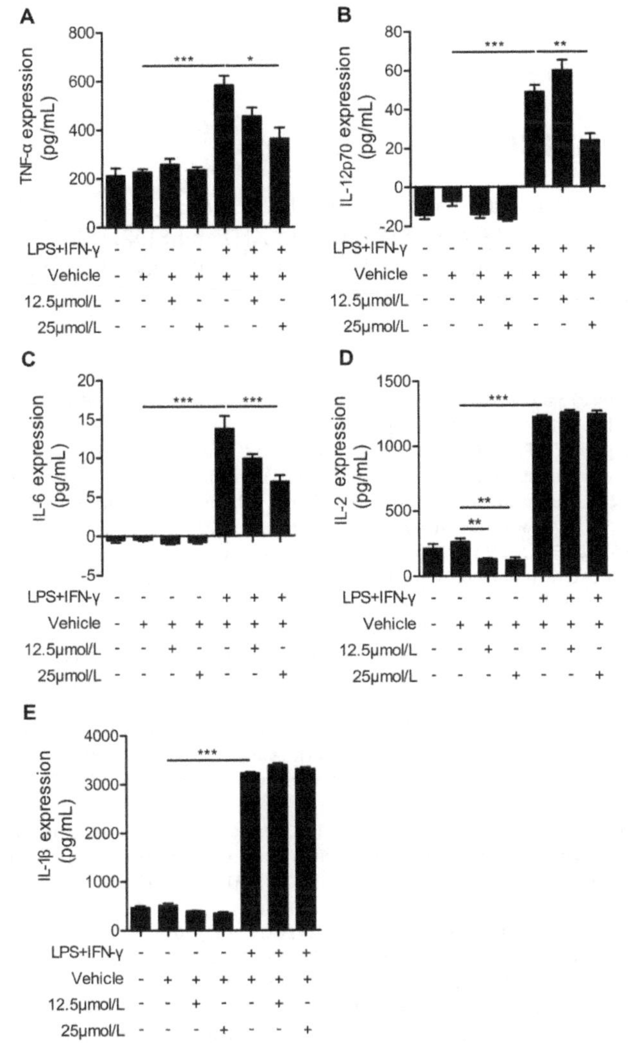

FIGURE 6 | Curcumin suppresses inflammatory cytokines in LPS and IFN-γ-treated BV2 microglia. BV2 microglia were stimulated with LPS (100 ng/mL) and IFN-γ (20 ng/mL), and then treated with vehicle or 12.5 and 25 μmmol/L curcumin. The concentrations of inflammatory cytokines (TNF-α **(A)**, IL-12p70 **(B)**, IL-6 **(C)**, IL-2 **(D)**, and IL-1β **(E)**) were measured by ELISA. Data are means ± SEM. Samples were collected from six independent experiments, each performed in duplicate. $^{*}p < 0.05$, $^{**}p < 0.01$, $^{***}p < 0.001$, one-way ANOVA followed by Bonferroni *post hoc* test.

Miao et al., 2016; Altinay et al., 2017). In the present study, we reported that curcumin treatment not only ameliorated infarct volumes, but also improved multiple aspects of neurological function at early timepoints after ischemic stroke.

Our previous study revealed an elevation of both M1 and M2 markers in microglia/macrophages after ischemic stroke, with an early M2-dominant phenotype and a later transition into M1-dominant responses (Hu et al., 2012). Different microglial phenotypes are well known to exert distinct effects on stroke pathology and brain repair (Hu et al., 2012, 2015). M1 microglia are known to release inflammatory cytokines (TNF-α, IL-1β, IL-6, iNOS and IL-12), which accelerate cell death and aggravate local inflammation (Girard et al., 2013). In contrast, M2 polarization upregulates anti-inflammatory or reparative factors and protects the ischemic brain. The lack of necessary endogenous signals for M2 induction is known to worsen outcomes after cerebral ischemia (Lee et al., 2016; Liu X. et al., 2016; Yang et al., 2017). For example, IL-4 deficient mice display less long-term functional recovery after ischemic stroke (Liu X. et al., 2016). Thus, shifting microglia from the M1 phenotype toward M2 may be an effective therapeutic strategy for ischemic stroke. Notably, we discovered that curcumin can shift microglia/macrophage polarization toward the neuroprotective and tissue-reparative M2 phenotype in the ischemic brain. *In vitro* studies in a microglial cell line confirm a direct effect on microglial polarization. Similarly, curcumin treatment inhibited cerebral inflammation in the ischemic brain *in vivo*. In agreement with our results, several recent studies demonstrated that curcumin induced macrophage polarization toward M2, and this was accompanied by an inhibition of local inflammatory responses (Gao et al., 2015; Karuppagounder et al., 2016).

Although the mechanisms whereby curcumin promotes microglial M2 polarization are not yet clear, several signaling pathways critical for microglial phenotype regulation may be activated by curcumin. For example, curcumin inhibited the phosphorylation and activation of STAT1 and STAT3 (Qin et al., 2012)—known to be important for microglial M1 polarization—in gangliosides, LPS, or IFN-γ activated microglia (Kim et al., 2003). In addition, miRNA 155 enhances M1 polarization and suppresses the expression of M2 signature genes (Cai et al., 2012; Moore et al., 2013) and is downregulated by curcumin treatment in LPS-treated macrophages and LPS-treated mice (Ma et al., 2017). Further studies are warranted to confirm the involvement of these mechanisms in curcumin-afforded neuroprotection and microglial phenotypic regulations in stroke models.

Similar to other polyphenols, curcumin is known to possess pleiotropic activities (Gupta et al., 2012). Previous studies performed in stroke models have shown that curcumin exerts diverse neuroprotective functions, including antioxidative effects (Thiyagarajan and Sharma, 2004; Yang et al., 2009; Wu et al., 2013), regulation of neuronal (and other cell) apoptosis (Zhao et al., 2008, 2010; Altinay et al., 2017), promotion of mitochondrial biogenesis (Liu et al., 2014), and enhancement of neurogenesis (Liu S. et al., 2016). The present study demonstrates that curcumin reduces ischemic stroke-induced brain damage and improves several functional outcomes. Our *in vivo* and *in vitro* studies suggest that curcumin has a profound regulatory effect on microglial responses, promoting M2 microglial polarization and inhibiting microglia-mediated pro-inflammatory responses. Thus, curcumin and perhaps other polyphenols may be "physiology tuners" that, among other beneficial functions, balance the equilibrium between M1 and M2 polarization states to elicit a wide range of protective effects. This multi-targeting characteristic of curcumin may underlie its efficacy in models of ischemic brain injury and justifies further investigation. Finally, the advent of new delivery systems might help increase the bioavailability and pharmacokinetic activity of curcumin (Panda et al., 2017), which would facilitate the translation of this compound to the clinic.

AUTHOR CONTRIBUTIONS

ZL and SH are responsible for the animal experiments. YR is responsible for the data acquisition and RT-PCR experiments. SW and XL performed the cell culture, ELISA and RT-PCR experiments. WZ performed the immunohistochemical staining experiments. XH, RKL, XG, ZJ, XJ and HD are responsible for the conception or design of the work. All authors drafted the work or revisited it critically and approved the final version of the manuscript.

FUNDING

This work was supported by the National Natural Science Foundation of China, 81571152 (to XH) and 81671161 (to ZL), and the Natural Science Foundation of Beijing Municipality, 7163219 (to ZL).

REFERENCES

Altinay, S., Cabalar, M., Isler, C., Yildirim, F., Celik, D. S., Zengi, O., et al. (2017). Is chronic curcumin supplementation neuroprotective against ischemia for antioxidant activity, neurologic deficit score, or neuronal apoptosis in an experimental stroke model? *Turk. Neurosurg.* 27, 537–545. doi: 10.5137/1019-5149.JTN.17405-16.0

Cai, X., Yin, Y., Li, N., Zhu, D., Zhang, J., Zhang, C. Y., et al. (2012). Re-polarization of tumor-associated macrophages to pro-inflammatory M1 macrophages by microRNA-155. *J. Mol. Cell Biol.* 4, 341–343. doi: 10.1093/jmcb/mjs044

Cook, D. J., Teves, L., and Tymianski, M. (2012). Treatment of stroke with a PSD-95 inhibitor in the gyrencephalic primate brain. *Nature* 483, 213–217. doi: 10.1038/nature10841

Darsalia, V., Hua, S., Larsson, M., Mallard, C., Nathanson, D., Nyström, T., et al. (2014). Exendin-4 reduces ischemic brain injury in normal and aged type 2 diabetic mice and promotes microglial M2 polarization. *PLoS One* 9:e103114. doi: 10.1371/journal.pone.0103114

Gao, S., Zhou, J., Liu, N., Wang, L., Gao, Q., Wu, Y., et al. (2015). Curcumin induces M2 macrophage polarization by secretion IL-4 and/or IL-13. *J. Mol. Cell. Cardiol.* 85, 131–139. doi: 10.1016/j.yjmcc.2015.04.025

Girard, S., Brough, D., Lopez-Castejon, G., Giles, J., Rothwell, N. J., and Allan, S. M. (2013). Microglia and macrophages differentially modulate cell death after brain injury caused by oxygen-glucose deprivation in organotypic brain slices. *Glia* 61, 813–824. doi: 10.1002/glia.22478

Guekht, A., Skoog, I., Edmundson, S., Zakharov, V., and Korczyn, A. D. (2017). ARTEMIDA trial (A randomized trial of efficacy, 12 months international double-blind actovegin): a randomized controlled trial to assess the efficacy of actovegin in poststroke cognitive impairment. *Stroke* 48, 1262–1270. doi: 10.1161/STROKEAHA.116.014321

Gupta, S. C., Patchva, S., Koh, W., and Aggarwal, B. B. (2012). Discovery of curcumin, a component of golden spice and its miraculous biological activities. *Clin. Exp. Pharmacol. Physiol.* 39, 283–299. doi: 10.1111/j.1440-1681.2011.05648.x

He, Y., Ma, X., Li, D., and Hao, J. (2016). Thiamet G mediates neuroprotection in experimental stroke by modulating microglia/macrophage polarization and inhibiting NF-κB p65 signaling. *J. Cereb. Blood Flow Metab.* doi: 10.1177/0271678x16679671 [Epub ahead of print].

Hu, X., Leak, R. K., Shi, Y., Suenaga, J., Gao, Y., Zheng, P., et al. (2015). Microglial and macrophage polarization—new prospects for brain repair. *Nat. Rev. Neurol.* 11, 56–64. doi: 10.1038/nrneurol.2014.207

Hu, X., Li, P., Guo, Y., Wang, H., Leak, R. K., Chen, S., et al. (2012). Microglia/macrophage polarization dynamics reveal novel mechanism of injury expansion after focal cerebral ischemia. *Stroke* 43, 3063–3070. doi: 10.1161/STROKEAHA.112.659656

Huuskonen, M. T., Tuo, Q. Z., Loppi, S., Dhungana, H., Korhonen, P., McInnes, L. E., et al. (2017). The copper bis(thiosemicarbazone) complex cuII(atsm) is protective against cerebral ischemia through modulation of the inflammatory milieu. *Neurotherapeutics* 14, 519–532. doi: 10.1007/s13311-016-0504-9

Karuppagounder, V., Arumugam, S., Thandavarayan, R. A., Sreedhar, R., Giridharan, V. V., Afrin, R., et al. (2016). Curcumin alleviates renal dysfunction and suppresses inflammation by shifting from M1 to M2 macrophage polarization in daunorubicin induced nephrotoxicity in rats. *Cytokine* 84, 1–9. doi: 10.1016/j.cyto.2016.05.001

Kim, H. Y., Park, E. J., Joe, E. H., and Jou, I. (2003). Curcumin suppresses Janus kinase-STAT inflammatory signaling through activation of Src homology 2 domain-containing tyrosine phosphatase 2 in brain microglia. *J. Immunol.* 171, 6072–6079. doi: 10.4049/jimmunol.171.11.6072

Lapchak, P. A. (2011). Neuroprotective and neurotrophic curcuminoids to treat stroke: a translational perspective. *Expert Opin. Investig. Drugs* 20, 13–22. doi: 10.1517/13543784.2011.542410

Lee, J. H., Wei, Z. Z., Cao, W., Won, S., Gu, X., Winter, M., et al. (2016). Regulation of therapeutic hypothermia on inflammatory cytokines, microglia polarization, migration and functional recovery after ischemic stroke in mice. *Neurobiol. Dis.* 96, 248–260. doi: 10.1016/j.nbd.2016.09.013

Lin, B., Yu, H., Lin, Y., Cai, C., Lu, H., and Zhu, X. (2016). Suppression of GRASP65 phosphorylation by tetrahydrocurcumin protects against cerebral ischemia/reperfusion injury via ERK signaling. *Mol. Med. Rep.* 14, 4775–4780. doi: 10.3892/mmr.2016.5816

Liu, L., Zhang, W., Wang, L., Li, Y., Tan, B., Lu, X., et al. (2014). Curcumin prevents cerebral ischemia reperfusion injury via increase of mitochondrial biogenesis. *Neurochem. Res.* 39, 1322–1331. doi: 10.1007/s11064-014-1315-1

Liu, S., Cao, Y., Qu, M., Zhang, Z., Feng, L., Ye, Z., et al. (2016). Curcumin protects against stroke and increases levels of Notch intracellular domain. *Neurol. Res.* 38, 553–559. doi: 10.1080/01616412.2016.1187804

Liu, X., Liu, J., Zhao, S., Zhang, H., Cai, W., Cai, M., et al. (2016). Interleukin-4 is essential for microglia/macrophage M2 polarization and long-term recovery after cerebral ischemia. *Stroke* 47, 498–504. doi: 10.1161/STROKEAHA.115.012079

Ma, F., Liu, F., Ding, L., You, M., Yue, H., Zhou, Y., et al. (2017). Anti-inflammatory effects of curcumin are associated with down regulating microRNA-155 in LPS-treated macrophages and mice. *Pharm. Biol.* 55, 1263–1273. doi: 10.1080/13880209.2017.1297838

Miao, Y., Zhao, S., Gao, Y., Wang, R., Wu, Q., Wu, H., et al. (2016). Curcumin pretreatment attenuates inflammation and mitochondrial dysfunction in experimental stroke: the possible role of Sirt1 signaling. *Brain Res. Bull.* 121, 9–15. doi: 10.1016/j.brainresbull.2015.11.019

Mijajlović, M. D., Aleksić, V. M., Šternić, N. M., Mirković, M. M., and Bornstein, N. M. (2017). Role of prediabetes in stroke. *Neuropsychiatr. Dis. Treat.* 13, 259–267. doi: 10.2147/NDT.S128807

Moore, C. S., Rao, V. T., Durafourt, B. A., Bedell, B. J., Ludwin, S. K., Bar-Or, A., et al. (2013). miR-155 as a multiple sclerosis-relevant regulator of myeloid cell polarization. *Ann. Neurol.* 74, 709–720. doi: 10.1002/ana.23967

Ovbiagele, B. (2008). Potential role of curcumin in stroke prevention. *Expert Rev. Neurother.* 8, 1175–1176. doi: 10.1586/14737175.8.8.1175

Pan, J., Jin, J. L., Ge, H. M., Yin, K. L., Chen, X., Han, L. J., et al. (2015). Malibatol A regulates microglia M1/M2 polarization in experimental stroke in a PPARgamma-dependent manner. *J. Neuroinflammation* 12:51. doi: 10.1186/s12974-015-0270-3

Panda, A. K., Chakraborty, D., Sarkar, I., Khan, T., and Sa, G. (2017). New insights into therapeutic activity and anticancer properties of curcumin. *J. Exp. Pharmacol.* 9, 31–45. doi: 10.2147/JEP.S70568

Perry, V. H., Nicoll, J. A., and Holmes, C. (2010). Microglia in neurodegenerative disease. *Nat. Rev. Neurol.* 6, 193–201. doi: 10.1038/nrneurol.2010.17

Pluta, R., Bogucka-Kocka, A., Ułamek-Koziol, M., Furmaga-Jabłońska, W., Januszewski, S., Brzozowska, J., et al. (2015). Neurogenesis and neuroprotection in postischemic brain neurodegeneration with Alzheimer phenotype: is there a role for curcumin? *Folia Neuropathol.* 53, 89–99. doi: 10.5114/fn.2015.52405

Qin, H., Holdbrooks, A. T., Liu, Y., Reynolds, S. L., Yanagisawa, L. L., and Benveniste, E. N. (2012). SOCS3 deficiency promotes M1 macrophage polarization and inflammation. *J. Immunol.* 189, 3439–3448. doi: 10.4049/jimmunol.1201168

Shah, F. A., Gim, S. A., Sung, J. H., Jeon, S. J., Kim, M. O., and Koh, P. O. (2016). Identification of proteins regulated by curcumin in cerebral ischemia. *J. Surg. Res.* 201, 141–148. doi: 10.1016/j.jss.2015.10.025

Shu, Z. M., Shu, X. D., Li, H. Q., Sun, Y., Shan, H., Sun, X. Y., et al. (2016). Ginkgolide B protects against ischemic stroke via modulating microglia polarization in mice. *CNS Neurosci. Ther.* 22, 729–739. doi: 10.1111/cns.12577

Thiyagarajan, M., and Sharma, S. S. (2004). Neuroprotective effect of curcumin in middle cerebral artery occlusion induced focal cerebral ischemia in rats. *Life Sci.* 74, 969–985. doi: 10.1016/j.lfs.2003.06.042

Wang, J., Ye, Q., Xu, J., Benedek, G., Zhang, H., Yang, Y., et al. (2017). DRα1-MOG-$_{35-55}$ reduces permanent ischemic brain injury. *Transl. Stroke Res.* 8, 284–293. doi: 10.1007/s12975-016-0514-2

Wu, J., Li, Q., Wang, X., Yu, S., Li, L., Wu, X., et al. (2013). Neuroprotection by curcumin in ischemic brain injury involves the Akt/Nrf2 pathway. *PLoS One* 8:e59843. doi: 10.1371/journal.pone.0059843

Yang, C., Zhang, X., Fan, H., and Liu, Y. (2009). Curcumin upregulates transcription factor Nrf2, HO-1 expression and protects rat brains against focal ischemia. *Brain Res.* 1282, 133–141. doi: 10.1016/j.brainres.2009.05.009

Yang, Y., Liu, H., Zhang, H., Ye, Q., Wang, J., Yang, B., et al. (2017). ST2/IL-33-dependent microglial response limits acute ischemic brain injury. *J. Neurosci.* 37, 4692–4704. doi: 10.1523/JNEUROSCI.3233-16.2017

Zhao, J., Yu, S., Zheng, W., Feng, G., Luo, G., Wang, L., et al. (2010). Curcumin improves outcomes and attenuates focal cerebral ischemic injury via antiapoptotic mechanisms in rats. *Neurochem. Res.* 35, 374–379. doi: 10.1007/s11064-009-0065-y

Zhao, J., Zhao, Y., Zheng, W., Lu, Y., Feng, G., and Yu, S. (2008). Neuroprotective effect of curcumin on transient focal cerebral ischemia in rats. *Brain Res.* 1229, 224–232. doi: 10.1016/j.brainres.2008.06.117

3

Pharmacological Modulation of Functional Phenotypes of Microglia in Neurodegenerative Diseases

Gyun Jee Song and Kyoungho Suk*

BK21 Plus KNU Biomedical Convergence Program, Department of Pharmacology, Brain Science & Engineering Institute, School of Medicine, Kyungpook National University, Daegu, South Korea

***Correspondence:**
Kyoungho Suk
ksuk@knu.ac.kr

Microglia are the resident innate immune cells of the central nervous system that mediate brain homeostasis maintenance. Microglia-mediated neuroinflammation is a hallmark shared by various neurodegenerative diseases, including Alzheimer's disease, Parkinson's disease, and multiple sclerosis. Numerous studies have shown microglial activation phenotypes to be heterogeneous; however, these microglial phenotypes can largely be categorized as being either M1 or M2 type. Although the specific classification of M1 and M2 functionally polarized microglia remains a topic for debate, the use of functional modulators of microglial phenotypes as potential therapeutic approaches for the treatment of neurodegenerative diseases has garnered considerable attention. This review discusses M1 and M2 microglial phenotypes and their relevance in neurodegenerative disease models, as described in recent literature. The modulation of microglial polarization toward the M2 phenotype may lead to development of future therapeutic and preventive strategies for neuroinflammatory and neurodegenerative diseases. Thus, we focus on recent studies of microglial polarization modulators, with a particular emphasis on the small-molecule compounds and their intracellular target proteins.

Keywords: pharmacological modulator, microglial polarization, neurodegenerative diseases, neuroinflammation, neuroprotective

INTRODUCTION: DIVERSITY OF MICROGLIAL PHENOTYPES AND DISEASE RELEVANCE

Microglia, the resident immune cells of the central nervous system (CNS), are highly specialized macrophages that play a fundamental role in neurodegenerative diseases such as Alzheimer's disease (AD), Parkinson's disease (PD), and multiple sclerosis (MS) (Mandrekar-Colucci and Landreth, 2010; Colonna and Butovsky, 2017). Microglia have been traditionally classified as either of the following: (1) resting with branched morphology and present in healthy brains or (2) activated with amoeboid morphology and present in diseased brains. Recent microglia classifications are more complex. Activated microglia are now recognized as being heterogeneous and plastic, and exist in various phenotypes in the CNS. Microglia can be divided into at least two types (neurotoxic or neuroprotective) based on their function (Kettenmann et al., 2013). Microglia can promote neurotoxicity via the release of several pro-inflammatory mediators, such as nitric oxide, interleukin (IL)-1β, and tumor necrosis factor-alpha (TNF-α) (Hanisch, 2002; Block et al., 2007). Conversely, they can be neuroprotective and neurosupportive, via several mechanisms under certain conditions. For example, neuroprotective roles of microglia include glutamate uptake (Byrnes et al., 2009), removal of dead cell debris and abnormally accumulated proteins (Diaz-Aparicio et al., 2016), and production of neurotrophic factors such as insulin-like growth factor-1 (IGF-1) (Thored et al., 2009), glial cell-derived neurotrophic factor (GDNF) (Lu et al., 2005), and brain-derived neurotrophic factor (BDNF) (Batchelor et al., 1999).

The dual nature of microglial functional polarization is consistent with the general classification of macrophages as being either the M1 (classic pro-inflammatory) or M2 (anti-inflammatory) phenotype (Michelucci et al., 2009). Specific environmental cues induce macrophages to adopt a given functionality. For example, stimulation with either lipopolysaccharide (LPS) or interferon (IFN)-γ induces activation of the classical M1 phenotype, whereas stimulation with either IL-4 or IL-13 induces the M2 activation (Cherry et al., 2014; Loane and Kumar, 2016). Microglia are critical to immune response in the CNS, and unsurprisingly, microglial functional polarization has been implicated in almost all CNS disorders, and in the progression of neurodegenerative diseases (Tang and Le, 2016). Microglia also play key functional roles in recovery from brain injury and in the maintenance of homeostasis in the brain.

Microglia in Neurodegenerative Disease

Neurodegenerative diseases such as AD, PD, amyotrophic lateral sclerosis (ALS), and MS, are characterized by neuronal degeneration in specific regions of the CNS, sharing common pathophysiological mechanisms including inflammation and abnormal protein deposition (Heppner et al., 2015; Chen et al., 2016). AD is the most prevalent neurodegenerative disorder that is characterized by progressive focal cortical atrophy, cognitive dysfunction, β-amyloid deposition, and neuronal degeneration that initiates with neurons of the hippocampus and cortex. PD is the second-most prevalent disorder, and is characterized by a progressive loss of the dopaminergic neurons in the substantia nigra and accumulation of α-synuclein and other abnormal proteins in Lewy bodies. ALS is a chronic degenerative disease characterized by the progressive degeneration of motor neurons. The accumulation of abnormal proteins such as superoxide dismutase (SOD)1 and transactive response (TAR) DNA binding protein 43 kDa (TDP-43) in motor neurons is the major pathological feature. MS is an inflammatory and degenerative disease of the CNS characterized by autoimmunity, monocyte infiltration, microglial activation, demyelination, and neuronal death. Inflammatory mediators, such as IL-1β, IL-6 TNF-α, chemokines, matrix metalloproteinase 2 (MMP2), nitric oxide, and nuclear factor kappa-B (NF-κB), contribute to neurodegeneration and myelin damage in these neurodegenerative diseases. Activated microglia and macrophages produce these inflammatory mediators, orchestrating neuroinflammation, and neurodegeneration. Neuroinflammation is initially a protective response in the brain, however, uncontrolled inflammatory responses are detrimental as they induce the release of high levels of neurotoxic factors such as ROS and TNF-α, and block neuronal regeneration (Chen et al., 2016).

Therefore, demonstrating a microglial functional polarization would potentially uncover new prospects for understanding the way in which neurodegeneration can be promoted by local CNS inflammation. In AD, inflammation is considered to be a pathology that occurs in response to β-amyloid accumulation. Classical (M1) activation of microglia is considered the initial defense mechanism in AD, and is characterized by the release of proinflammatory cytokines. Conversely, alternative (M2) activation is associated with angiogenesis, neurogenesis, anti-inflammatory effects, and the degradation of β-amyloid deposits. Thus, modulation of microglial activation toward the M2 phenotype has been proposed as a novel therapeutic strategy for patients with AD. Indeed, Latta et al. (2015) showed that an enhanced M2 phenotype, induced either by IL-4 overexpression, or treatment with exogenous IL-4, decreased β-amyloid deposition both *in vitro* and in an animal model. Similarly, M1 polarization of microglia induced by expression of IFN-γ has been shown to increase the amyloid burden in an amyloid precursor protein/presenilin1 (APP/PS1) AD mouse model (Weekman et al., 2014).

Microglia-mediated neuroinflammation is also a hallmark of PD. In the brains of PD patients, microglia exert both neurotoxic and neuroprotective effects depending on the surrounding microenvironment. Persistent microglial activation by damaged neurons and α-synuclein deposition is generally detrimental. Reactive microglia release a range of reactive oxygen species, such as nitric oxide and superoxide-anion and pro-inflammatory cytokines, which exacerbate motor deficits in PD. Therefore, many anti-inflammatory agents have been proposed as promising PD therapeutic agents. Indeed, non-steroidal anti-inflammatory drugs and minocycline have been used in clinical studies for PD patients (Gao and Hong, 2008).

Accumulation of the misfolded ALS-linked mutant SOD1 or TDP-43 is tightly associated with the neurotoxic M1 inflammatory microglial activation (Boillee et al., 2006; Swarup et al., 2011; Huang et al., 2012). Primary microglia isolated from SOD^{G93A} transgenic mice are more neurotoxic compared to wild-type microglia, due to an increased production of superoxide and nitric oxide as well as the decreased expression of IGF-I (Xiao et al., 2007). Furthermore, IL-4-induced M2 microglia reduced LPS-induced microglia-mediated motor neuron injury (Zhao et al., 2006) and disease stage-dependent microglial switch from neuroprotective to neurotoxic phenotype has been observed in an ALS mouse model.

Microglia isolated from ALS mice at disease onset expressed higher levels of M2 markers and lower levels of the M1 marker, NADPH oxidase (NOX)2, compared with those isolated at the end-stage of ALS, indicating a diminished function of neuroprotective microglia in the late stage of the disease (Liao et al., 2012). Thus, the administration of minocycline delays the pathogenesis of SOD^{G93A} mice by selectively attenuating the induction of M1 microglia markers during the progressive phase, without affecting the transient enhancement of M2 microglia markers at the early stage (Kobayashi et al., 2013).

Microglial activation has also been studied extensively in MS patients and in the experimental autoimmune encephalomyelitis (EAE) mouse model. In this pathological condition, microglia release neurotoxic and neurotrophic molecules, pro- and anti-inflammatory cytokines, playing both beneficial and detrimental roles during the demyelination and recovery stages (Correale, 2014). Miron et al. (2013) examined whether M2 phenotypes contribute to regenerative response in the CNS. In their study, the M1 to M2 switch was observed at the initiation of remyelination, 10 days post-injection of lyso-phosphatidylcholine (lecithin). Oligodendrocyte differentiation for regeneration was enhanced by M2 microglia-conditioned medium. M2 polarization of microglia has been proposed to preserve myelin homeostasis after white matter injury in traumatic brain injury (TBI) or cuprizone-induced demyelination models (Chen et al., 2014c; Wang et al., 2015). Furthermore, the protective mechanisms exerted by alternatively activated (M2) microglia have been discussed in recent review articles (Cherry et al., 2014; Du et al., 2016; Tang and Le, 2016). Thus, enhancing the neuroprotective effects of these M2 microglia may be a promising therapeutic approach.

Prion disease is another progressive neurodegenerative disorder, and like many other neurodegenerative diseases, it is characterized by misfolded protein aggregates and neuroinflammation (Burchell and Panegyres, 2016; Stopschinski and Diamond, 2017). In prion disease, misfolded prion protein aggregates propagate by the conversion of normal cellular prion protein (PrPC) to abnormal isoforms, designated pathogenic conformers of the prion protein (PrPSc), which causes rapid neurodegeneration accompanied by spongiform change and neuronal loss in the brain. Furthermore, the crosstalk between misfolded proteins in animal models of Alzheimer's and prion diseases has been proposed in recent studies (Morales et al., 2010; Fernandez et al., 2017), suggesting that one protein misfolding process may be an important risk factor for the development of other protein aggregation-induced diseases. Importantly, microglial proliferation, activation, and phenotype conversion have been associated with overall prion disease progression (Aguzzi et al., 2013; Grizenkova et al., 2014; Lins et al., 2016).

Specific Markers for the M1 and M2 Phenotypes

M1-type microglia release diverse proinflammatory mediators and free radicals that inhibit brain repair and regeneration. Conversely, microglia of the M2 phenotype improve brain repair and regeneration by enhancing phagocytosis, releasing trophic factors, and reducing brain inflammation. Following stimulation with LPS or IFN-γ, M1 microglia express high levels of inducible nitric oxide synthase (iNOS) and pro-inflammatory cytokines/chemokines such as TNF-α, IL-1β, and CC chemokine ligand (CCL)2. IL-4- or IL-13-stimulated microglia express Argl, Ym-1, CD200R, IL-10, transforming growth factor (TGF)-β and Fizzl-1, which serve as specific markers for M2 microglia. M1 and M2 microglia represent a spectrum of various activation phenotype rather than single phenotype of each status. Three subtypes of M2 microglia have been proposed, such as M2a (wound-healing and anti-inflammatory phenotype expressing CD206, Fizz-1, Argl, Yml), M2b (inflammation modulatory phenotype expressing IL-10, COX2) and M2c (immunosuppressive phenotype expressing CD163) (Franco and Fernandez-Suarez, 2015; Du et al., 2016). More recently, Kumar et al. (2016) proposed a mixed transitional phenotype of microglia called Mtran, co-expressing M1 makers (iNOS and IL-12) and M2 markers (TGF-β and Argl). In their study, up to 42% of Argl (M2 marker)-positive cells co-express the M1 marker iNOS at 7 days post-TBI indicating a significant mixed population of microglia during recovery after injury (Kumar et al., 2016), which was confirmed in the middle cerebral artery occlusion (MCAo) model (Moretti et al., 2016). Furthermore, it is difficult to discriminate between M1 or each M2 subtype *in vitro*, and even more so *in vivo*. Recent technical advancements, including the fluorescent analysis of activation markers, cell sorting, and single-cell RNA-seq analysis, have helped to define microglia-specific genes compared to those specific to macrophages and other glia (Butovsky et al., 2014; Crotti and Ransohoff, 2016). However, M1/M2 phenotypes of microglia do not precisely match the microglial classification based on a transcriptomic analysis such as RNA-seq (Yamasaki et al., 2014). Although the binary concept of microglial M1/M2 classification has been recently debated (Ransohoff, 2016), the functional classification of microglia as being either neurotoxic (M1) or neuroprotective (M2) is a useful for illustrating the pathobiology of inflammatory and degenerative CNS disorders. Therefore, we used the M1 and M2 phenotypic classification for activated microglia in this review.

PHARMACOLOGICAL APPROACHES FOR MODULATING MICROGLIAL PHENOTYPES

Currently available medication is incapable of repairing degenerated neurons, inducing regeneration, and/or preventing further neuronal death in AD, PD, ALS, and/or MS patients. Current drugs are used to reduce the severity of disease-related symptoms by limiting the extent of neuroinflammation in patients (Glass et al., 2010). Nevertheless, although these drugs reduce symptoms, and thus increase the quality of life for these patients, they are not able to repair or regenerate damaged neurons.

Given that the balance of microglial M1/M2 phenotypes has been implicated in the pathogenesis of neurodegenerative diseases, several small-molecule compounds have recently been studied to ascertain their ability to regulate microglial functional polarization, and thereby exert neuroprotection against neurodegenerative diseases in animal models. Elucidating the underlying mechanisms of action and identifying the target proteins of these small-molecule compounds may be essential to design better chemical modulators of microglial polarization and thus effective neuroprotective drugs.

The microglial microenvironment (for example, infection, ischemic injury, β-amyloid depositions, and/or pro-inflammatory mediators such as TNF-α, IL-1β, and nitric oxide), has been shown to play a critical role in determining the microglial polarization state. Several soluble factors released from neurons and astrocytes are suggested to contribute to the determination of microglial phenotypes, as demonstrated by the M2 to M1 microglial phenotypic switch induced by exposure to cell culture medium conditioned by damaged neurons or activated astrocytes. Furthermore, many intracellular molecules are involved in controlling microglial/macrophage polarization. For example, nuclear receptors [peroxisome proliferator-activated receptor (PPAR)γ, PPARδ, retinoid X receptor (RXR)], redox signaling molecules [NOX2, hypoxia-inducible factor (HIF)-1α], NF-κB signaling molecules, and metabolic shift-mediated proteins are all known to control the phenotypic switching of microglia and macrophages (Sica and Mantovani, 2012). Thus, potential exploitation of these molecules may be a promising method for developing novel therapeutic drugs for neurodegenerative diseases.

Gene therapies, including BDNF- or IL4-overexpressing viruses, recombinant proteins such as IL-4, IL-10, IL-13, and/or TGF-β, Etanercept (a TNF-α-antagonist fusion protein), and cell therapies (M2 microglia and macrophages) have been applied as therapeutic tools. However, due to the blood–brain barrier, these therapeutic strategies have limited efficacy, leading to the screening of small synthetic chemical and/or natural compounds as treatments for various brain diseases. In this review, we focus on the effect and the target proteins of these small-molecule compounds that modulate M1/M2 microglial polarization (**Table 1**).

Nuclear Receptors

The nuclear hormone receptor PPAR is a key regulator of the M2 phenotype in macrophages and microglia (Bouhlel et al., 2007; Chawla, 2010). PPAR activation increases phagocytic uptake of amyloid-β plaques, and is neuroprotective in an AD mouse model (Mandrekar-Colucci et al., 2012; Yamanaka et al., 2012). Accordingly, treatment with the PPARγ agonist, pioglitazone, results in the phenotypic switch of proinflammatory M1 to anti-inflammatory M2 microglia. Furthermore, pioglitazone treatment dramatically reduces the levels of soluble and insoluble β-amyloid, and reverses the cognitive deficits in 12-month-old APP/PS1 mice (Toba et al., 2016). A novel selective-PPAR modulator, DSP-8658, was shown to enhance the microglial phagocytosis and improve the spatial memory performance in an AD mouse model (Yamanaka et al., 2012). Similarly, a PPARγ agonist called rosiglitazone has also been shown to induce IL-4 expression in the rat brain as well as age-dependent M1 microglial activation in an IL-4 dependent manner (Loane et al., 2009). A novel compound, MDG548, was found to induce neuroprotection in MPTP-treated mice and decrease LPS-induced NF-κB activation in a dose-dependent manner (Lecca et al., 2015). Finally, an *N*-carbamolylated urethane compound (SNU-BP) has been identified as a novel PPARγ agonist, and inhibits LPS-induced pro-inflammatory cytokine and nitric oxide production as well as potentiates IL-4-induced M2 marker expression in microglia and astrocytes. SNU-BP was also shown to exhibit an anti-neuroinflammatory effect in an LPS-injected mouse model, probably via the M1/M2 switch (Song et al., 2016).

Alzheimer's disease (AD) is strongly associated with the impaired clearance of β-amyloid from the brain. The RXR agonist bexarotene (Targretin) has been shown to enhance β-amyloid clearance by activating PPARγ/RXR and liver X receptors (LXRs)/RXR, inducing apoE expression, and promoting microglial phagocytosis (Cramer et al., 2012). It is a highly selective, synthetic retinoid analog with specific affinity for the RXR, which is able to cross the blood–brain barrier and has a favorable FDA-approved safety profile (Skalak et al., 1987; Cramer et al., 2012).

Malibatol A (MA) is a natural resveratrol oligomer extracted from the leaves of the Chinese plant *Hopea hainanensis*. MA has an anti-inflammatory effect on MCAo mice and LPS-stimulated microglia. MA treatment was found to decrease the expression of M1 (CD16, CD32, and CD86), while increasing that of M2 markers (CD206 and YM-1), in a PPARγ-dependent manner (Pan et al., 2015).

Metabolism-Associated Proteins

Evidence suggests a role for metabolic reprogramming in the modulation of M1/M2 microglial phenotypes (Orihuela et al., 2016). Various studies support the belief that mitochondrial metabolic shifts are associated with microglial polarization. Under normoxic conditions, ATP (energy) production is achieved via oxidative phosphorylation; in contrast, anaerobic glycolysis converts pyruvate into lactate under hypoxic conditions. In the context of the peripheral immune cells, a shift in the cellular metabolism from oxidative phosphorylation to aerobic glycolysis favors the polarization of microglia toward the M1 phenotype. This metabolic switch is promoted by PI3K/AKT and inhibited by AMP-activated protein kinase (AMPK) and IL-10.

AMP-activated protein kinase activation is associated with neuroprotection after stroke (Jin et al., 2014; Venna et al., 2014) via enhanced neurogenesis and lowered blood glucose levels. The AMPK activator metformin promotes both functional recovery and tissue repair following stroke. Mice that administered metformin daily after MCAo exhibited more M2-polarized microglia and macrophages, as well as increased angiogenesis and neurogenesis (Jin et al., 2014). The same study also demonstrated metformin-induced M2 polarization of BV-2 microglial cells dependent upon AMPK activation. Patil et al. (2014) similarly demonstrated the neuroprotective effect of metformin in a PD mouse model, such that impaired locomotor activities and the loss of TH-positive cells were both significantly improved in metformin (500 mg/kg for 21 days)-treated PD mice, compared to controls.

Pyruvate dehydrogenase kinases (PDKs) are mitochondrial metabolic regulators that modulate pyruvate dehydrogenase (PDH) activity to convert pyruvate either aerobically to acetyl-CoA, or anaerobically to lactate (Jha et al., 2015). *In vitro* studies support the role of PDK2/4 as promoters of the classical proinflammatory (M1) activation of macrophages. Moreover, the pharmacological PDK inhibitor dichloroacetate (DCA) diminishes complete Freund's adjuvant (CFA)-induced inflammation and pain via an induced M1-M2 switch (Jha et al., 2015). This suggests that a pathological metabolic shift,

TABLE 1 | Pharmacological tools for modulating microglial polarization.

Targets	Small-molecules	Models	Effects	Reference
Nuclear receptors				
PPARγ (agonist)	Pioglitazone	AD mice	M1 to M2 switch, reverse cognitive deficits	Toba et al., 2016
	DSP-8658	AD mice	Enhanced microglial phagocytosis, improved memory	Yamanaka et al., 2012
	MDG548	PD mice *in vitro*	Neuroprotection, reduction of NF-κB activation	Lecca et al., 2015
	SNU-BP	LPS model	Increased M2 and decreased M1	Song et al., 2016
RXR (agonist)	Bexarotene	AD mice and *in vitro*	Clearance of β-amyloid, reverse cognitive deficits	Cramer et al., 2012
Metabolism-associated molecules				
AMPK (activator)	Metformin	MCAo PD mice	M2 polarization, angiogenesis, neurogenesis, improved locomotor activity	Jin et al., 2014; Patil et al., 2014
PDK (inhibitor)	DCA	CFA inflammation model, *in vitro*	M1/M2 switch, reduced pain and inflammation	Jha et al., 2015
Aldose reductase (inhibitor)	Fidarestat (SNK-860)	SCI model *In vitro*	M2 polarization Reduced LPS-induced inflammation	Zhang et al., 2016; Reddy et al., 2010
cAMP-dependent pathway for M2 polarization				
PKA (activator)	Db-cAMP	SCI model	Induce M2 phenotype	Ghosh et al., 2016
PDE4 (inhibitor)	Rolipram PDE4D-NAM	Aged mice and primates	Neuroprotective, anti-inflammatory Memory consolidation	Barad et al., 1998; Burgin et al., 2010
PDE5 (inhibitor)	Sildenafil	MCAo AD mice EAE model	M1/M2 modulation Clearance of β-amyloid prevent axonal loss promote re-myelination	Puzzo et al., 2009; Pifarre et al., 2011; Moretti et al., 2016
Redox signaling molecules for microglial M1/M2 balance				
NOX (inhibitor)	Apocynin	*In vitro* PD mice	Induce M2 polarization protect from dopaminergic neuron degeneration	Choi et al., 2012; Hernandes et al., 2013a
	GKT137831	Diabetic retinopathy, *in vitro*	Hypoxia-induced ROS production and the expression of inflammatory cytokines in retinal microglia	Deliyanti and Wilkinson-Berka, 2015
M1 polarization for inhibiting glioma cell growth				
mTOR (inhibitor)	Rad	Glioma	M1 polarization, prevented glioma growth	Lisi et al., 2014
–	Chlorogenic acid	Glioma	Increased M1 and decreased M2 reduction of tumor size	Xue et al., 2017
Other signaling molecules				
HDAC (inhibitor)	Scriptaid	TBI *In vitro* model	M2 polarization, protect white brain matter, suppress LPS-induced cytokine expression	Wang et al., 2015; Kannan et al., 2013
ROCK (inhibitor)	FSD-C10 Y-39983	EAE model EAE model	Inhibit neuroinflammation Attenuation of demyelination	Li et al., 2014; Gao et al., 2013
	Fasudil	*In vitro*	M2 polarization	Chen et al., 2014a

AD, Alzheimer's disease; PD, Parkinson's disease; MS, multiple sclerosis; MCAo, middle cerebral artery occlusion; SCI, spinal cord injury; TBI, traumatic brain injury; EAE, experimental allergic encephalomyelitis; CFA, complete Freund's adjuvant; LPS, lipopolysaccharide; PDE4D-NAM, PDE4D negative allosteric modulator.

and subsequent lactic acid production, each contribute to neuroinflammatory disease progression.

Fidarestat (SNK-860) is an aldose reductase (AR) inhibitor used for the treatment of diabetic neuropathy (Kuzumoto et al., 2006). A recent study showed the incubation of macrophages with LPS to cause a significant increase (6-fold) in the uptake of glucose in a time dependent manner. In contrast, the inhibition of AR via fidarestat treatment decreased LPS-induced glucose uptake by 30% (Reddy et al., 2010). AR expression is enhanced in microglia/macrophages after spinal cord injury (SCI). The study further demonstrated that AR inhibition and/or deficiency in microglia/macrophages favors a phenotype switch toward the M2, rather than the M1 phenotype, and that AR inhibition induces the phosphorylation of cAMP response element-binding protein (CREB) leading to the enhanced expression of the M2 marker, Arg-1 (Zhang et al., 2016).

cAMP-Dependent Pathways and their Regulators

Cyclic adenosine monophosphate (cAMP) is a well-known regulator of microglial function and activation (Ghosh et al., 2012, 2015, 2016). The elevation of cAMP in microglia or macrophages via the application of an adenylyl cyclase activator, synthetic cyclic AMP analoges or phosphodiesterase (PDE) inhibitors, inhibits the production of pro-inflammatory molecules (Gerlo et al., 2011). Interestingly, proinflammatory cytokines such as TNF-α and IL-1β both rapidly reduced cAMP, and increased PDE4 expression in microglia (Ghosh et al., 2012). The protective effect of cAMP on neuronal regeneration has been reported in rat SCI (Neumann et al., 2002) and cerebral ischemia-reperfusion injury models (Niu et al., 2010). Dibutyryl (db)-cAMP is a membrane-permeable derivative of cAMP that exhibits a prolonged response time. Ghosh et al. (2016) investigated the effect of cAMP on the modulation of microglial phenotypes and found that co-treatment of microglial cells with cAMP and IL-4 induced an M2 phenotype (Arg-1+/iNOS−) with concomitant expression of various M2-specific markers including TG2 and FIZZ1. Administration of db-cAMP and IL-4 also promoted M2 phenotypes in the lesions of SCI model mice (Ghosh et al., 2016). Together, these data strongly support that cAMP is a critical determinant of M1-M2 polarization.

PDE4 is an enzyme that negatively regulates cAMP signaling by hydrolyzing cAMP in immune and brain cells. PDE4 inhibitors (including rolipram) are reported to have precognitive, neuroprotective, and anti-inflammatory effects (Barad et al., 1998; Dinter, 2000; Block et al., 2001). PDE4-negative allosteric modulators (NAMs) have been recently developed for specific inhibition of each PDE4 subtype (i.e., PDE4A, B, C, and D). PDE4D-NAM has been shown to improve cognitive performance in healthy rodents (Burgin et al., 2010) and primates (Sutcliffe et al., 2014). PDE4D-NAMs (including D158681, D159153, D159404, and D159687) have also been demonstrated to produce potent cognitive benefits by augmenting signaling via the cAMP/protein kinase A/CREB pathway for memory consolidation (Burgin et al., 2010; Gurney et al., 2015).

PDE4 subtypes are known to modulate the inflammatory response in the brain, such that TNF-α increases PDE4B expression and nuclear translocation in microglia (Ghosh et al., 2012). Of the PDE4 subtypes, PDE4B in particular is highly expressed in activated microglia after TBI and SCI. Importantly, this observation promotes the potential application of therapeutic modulators for the treatment of neuroinflammatory diseases including AD.

PDE5 inhibitor sildenafil has been recently developed as a first-line drug for diabetic patients with erectile dysfunction. Recently PDE5 inhibitors have been proposed as potential therapeutic agents for neuroinflammatory, degenerative, and memory-loss diseases including AD, PD, and MS (Puzzo et al., 2009; Pifarre et al., 2011; Fiorito et al., 2013; Peixoto et al., 2015). Possible underlying mechanisms for the beneficial effects of PDE5 inhibitors include a neuroprotective effect exerted via the cGMP and/or cAMP signaling pathways and an anti-inflammatory-related effect. In an *in vitro* study of microglia, PDE5 inhibitors were shown to inhibit LPS-induced M1 polarization by decreasing the production of nitric oxide, TNF-α, and IL-1β (Zhao et al., 2016). M2 polarization induced by sildenafil has been shown to provide protection against lesion extension in the late phase of MCAo in neonatal mice (Moretti et al., 2016). Furthermore, the chronic inhibition of PDE-5 has been shown to facilitate the shift from classic (M1) to alternative (M2) macrophage polarization in streptozotocin-induced diabetic mice (Venneri et al., 2015).

Redox Signaling Molecules

Activated microglia-derived oxidative stress is implicated in numerous CNS diseases. The redox status modulates the acquisition of classical microglia activation phenotypes by various mechanisms, including the NOX and NOS-dependent pathways (Bermudez et al., 2016; Haslund-Vinding et al., 2016; Seredenina et al., 2016; Vilhardt et al., 2016). NOX induces M1 polarization of microglia, and thus unsurprisingly, either a NOX inhibitor (apocynin) or genetic depletion has been reported to induce M2 polarization. Choi et al. (2012) showed that pharmacological inhibition of NOX changed microglia from an M1 to an M2 phenotype. Moreover, NOX2 gene-deficient mice (gp91phox$^{-/-}$) have been found to be completely protected against glial M1 over-activation and dopaminergic neuron degeneration in the 6-hydroxydopamine (6-OHDA)-induced PD mouse model (Hernandes et al., 2013a,b). GKT137831 (NOX1 and NOX4 inhibitor), originally developed for diabetic nephropathy, has been shown to significantly reduce both hypoxia-induced ROS production, and the expression of inflammatory cytokines in retinal microglia (Deliyanti and Wilkinson-Berka, 2015), suggesting that NOX inhibitors may be promising therapeutic agents for diabetic retinopathy and/or neuropathy.

Resveratrol (3,5,4′-trihydroxy-*trans*-stilbene) is a natural phytoalexin found in grape-skin that exerts anti-inflammatory and antioxidant, as well as various other biological effects. Recently, resveratrol has been suggested to have neuroprotective effects against many neurological diseases (Porro et al., 2015; Abdel-Aleem et al., 2016; Ghaiad et al., 2016; Jeong et al., 2016; Shi et al., 2016; Xu et al., 2017), and several underlying mechanisms for this effect have been suggested. For example, resveratrol attenuates hypoxia-induced neurotoxicity by inhibiting microglial activation (Zhang et al., 2015), and similarly constrains amyloid-β-induced microglial activation via NOX (Yao et al., 2015).

mTOR Inhibitors and Chlorogenic Acid: M1 Polarization for Inhibiting Glioma Cell Growth

The mammalian target of rapamycin (mTOR) is a serine/threonine protein kinase involved in many cellular processes such as transcription and translation, ribosomal biogenesis, energy metabolism, and autophagy (Laplante and Sabatini, 2012). The inhibition of mTOR has been recently suggested to prevent glioblastoma, the most common and aggressive primary CNS tumor-type, originating from glial cells (Rolle et al., 2012). Rad, an inhibitor of mTOR, was recently found to significantly increase iNOS expression, and to reduce IL-10 expression, suggesting that Rad prevents the acquisition of an M2 phenotype in response to glioma factors promoting classic M1 activation. Thus, mTOR inhibition prevented glioma growth by inhibiting M2 polarization of microglial cells, thereby increasing their anti-tumor cytotoxic potential (Lisi et al., 2014).

Chlorogenic acid, a phenolic compound extracted from natural products, has been shown to exert anti-tumor effects on multiple malignant tumors (Bandyopadhyay et al., 2004; Belkaid et al., 2006). Previous studies on the anti-tumor effects of chlorogenic acid focused on its direct cytotoxic or antioxidant effect (Lewandowska et al., 2016); however, a recent report suggested a novel anti-tumorigenic mechanism for the chlorogenic acid-induced effects, in which it promotes M1 polarization to inhibit tumor growth (Xue et al., 2017). In glioma xenograft mice, chlorogenic acid was shown to increase CD11-positive M1 and decrease CD206-positive M2 cells in tumor tissues, leading to a reduction of the overall tumor size.

Epigenetic Regulators and Other Signaling Molecules

Previous studies have shown that histone deacetylase (HDACs) inhibitors preferentially promote the transcription of neuroprotective genes, and protect against TBI-induced neuronal damage (Lazo-Gomez et al., 2013; Wang et al., 2013) and strongly suppress LPS-induced cytokine expression and release by microglia (Kannan et al., 2013). Recently, Wang et al. (2015) showed that a novel HDAC inhibitor, scriptaid, protected white brain matter from damage by TBI via polarization of microglia/macrophages toward the beneficial M2 phenotype. Scriptaid induced the expression of microglial glycogen synthase kinase 3 beta (GSK3β) and the microglial phenotypic switch from M1 to M2. Media conditioned by Scriptaid treated-microglia conferred a greater protective effect against oxygen and glucose deprivation-induced cell death in oligodendrocytes, as compared to media conditioned by vehicle-treated microglia (Wang et al., 2015).

Rho-associated kinase (ROCK) has been proposed as another potential regulator of the microglial phenotype. ROCK is a serine/threonine kinase and a key regulator in controlling formation of the actin cytoskeleton, as well as cell motility, and cell adhesion. Selective ROCK inhibitors, such as FSD-C10 or Y-39983, have been shown to exhibit therapeutic potential in an EAE model via attenuation of demyelination and neuroinflammation (Gao et al., 2013; Li et al., 2014). More recently, microglial treatment with a ROCK inhibitor Fasudil induced alteration in microglial phenotype polarization and functional plasticity, shifting the M1 to a M2 phenotype (Chen et al., 2014a).

CONCLUSION

Here, we summarized the current research on pharmacological modulators of microglial phenotypes and their cellular targets. We focused on the effects of these modulators both *in vivo*, and in *in vitro* models of neurodegenerative diseases. We divided the cellular targets into groups according to their original functions, these being nuclear receptors, metabolism-associated proteins, proteins regulating the cAMP pathway, redox signaling molecules, and others. These target proteins are potential therapeutic candidates for the effective treatment of neurodegenerative diseases. Furthermore, an improved characterization of target protein functions will enable the design of novel pharmacological compounds to modulate cytotoxic and/or neurotrophic microglial phenotypes at specific stages of neurodegenerative disease. This is owing to the time-dependent microglial activation in the switch from neuroprotective to neurotoxic profiles in chronic diseases. Thus, further studies are essential in cultured cells and animal models, as well as in human patients, to enable the translation of these preliminary findings into clinically applicable interventions for AD, PD, MS, and other neurodegenerative diseases.

AUTHOR CONTRIBUTIONS

Both authors have made a substantial intellectual contribution to this work, and approved submission of the manuscript. GS and KS formulated the focus of this review focus. GS conducted the literature review and summarized the discussed studies. KS evaluated the manuscript and contributed to the final version.

ACKNOWLEDGMENTS

This work was supported by the National Research Foundation of Korea (NRF) grant funded by the Korean government (MSIP) (Grant Nos. 2015R1A2A1A10051958, 2016M3C7A1904148, 2016R1D1A1B01009186), and by the Korean Health Technology R&D Project, Korean Ministry of Health & Welfare (Grant No. HI14C3331).

REFERENCES

Abdel-Aleem, G. A., Khaleel, E. F., Mostafa, D. G., and Elberier, L. K. (2016). Neuroprotective effect of resveratrol against brain ischemia reperfusion injury in rats entails reduction of DJ-1 protein expression and activation of PI3K/Akt/GSK3b survival pathway. *Arch. Physiol. Biochem.* 122, 200–213.

Aguzzi, A., Nuvolone, M., and Zhu, C. (2013). The immunobiology of prion diseases. *Nat. Rev. Immunol.* 13, 888–902. doi: 10.1038/nri3553

Bandyopadhyay, G., Biswas, T., Roy, K. C., Mandal, S., Mandal, C., Pal, B. C., et al. (2004). Chlorogenic acid inhibits Bcr-Abl tyrosine kinase and triggers p38 mitogen-activated protein kinase-dependent apoptosis in chronic myelogenous leukemic cells. *Blood* 104, 2514–2522.

Barad, M., Bourtchouladze, R., Winder, D. G., Golan, H., and Kandel, E. (1998). Rolipram, a type IV-specific phosphodiesterase inhibitor, facilitates the establishment of long-lasting long-term potentiation and improves memory. *Proc. Natl. Acad. Sci. U.S.A.* 95, 15020–15025.

Batchelor, P. E., Liberatore, G. T., Wong, J. Y., Porritt, M. J., Frerichs, F., Donnan, G. A., et al. (1999). Activated macrophages and microglia induce dopaminergic sprouting in the injured striatum and express brain-derived neurotrophic factor and glial cell line-derived neurotrophic factor. *J. Neurosci.* 19, 1708–1716.

Belkaid, A., Currie, J. C., Desgagnes, J., and Annabi, B. (2006). The chemopreventive properties of chlorogenic acid reveal a potential new role for the microsomal glucose-6-phosphate translocase in brain tumor progression. *Cancer Cell Int.* 6:7.

Bermudez, S., Khayrullina, G., Zhao, Y., and Byrnes, K. R. (2016). NADPH oxidase isoform expression is temporally regulated and may contribute to microglial/macrophage polarization after spinal cord injury. *Mol. Cell. Neurosci.* 77, 53–64. doi: 10.1016/j.mcn.2016.10.001

Block, F., Schmidt, W., Nolden-Koch, M., and Schwarz, M. (2001). Rolipram reduces excitotoxic neuronal damage. *Neuroreport* 12, 1507–1511.

Block, M. L., Zecca, L., and Hong, J. S. (2007). Microglia-mediated neurotoxicity: uncovering the molecular mechanisms. *Nat. Rev. Neurosci.* 8, 57–69.

Boillee, S., Vande Velde, C., and Cleveland, D. W. (2006). ALS: a disease of motor neurons and their nonneuronal neighbors. *Neuron* 52, 39–59.

Bouhlel, M. A., Derudas, B., Rigamonti, E., Dievart, R., Brozek, J., Haulon, S., et al. (2007). PPARgamma activation primes human monocytes into alternative M2 macrophages with anti-inflammatory properties. *Cell Metab.* 6, 137–143.

Burchell, J. T., and Panegyres, P. K. (2016). Prion diseases: immunotargets and therapy. *Immunotargets Ther.* 5, 57–68. doi: 10.2147/ITT.S64795

Burgin, A. B., Magnusson, O. T., Singh, J., Witte, P., Staker, B. L., Bjornsson, J. M., et al. (2010). Design of phosphodiesterase 4D (PDE4D) allosteric modulators for enhancing cognition with improved safety. *Nat. Biotechnol.* 28, 63–70. doi: 10.1038/nbt.1598

Butovsky, O., Jedrychowski, M. P., Moore, C. S., Cialic, R., Lanser, A. J., Gabriely, G., et al. (2014). Identification of a unique TGF-beta-dependent molecular and functional signature in microglia. *Nat. Neurosci.* 17, 131–143. doi: 10.1038/nn.3599

Byrnes, K. R., Loane, D. J., and Faden, A. I. (2009). Metabotropic glutamate receptors as targets for multipotential treatment of neurological disorders. *Neurotherapeutics* 6, 94–107. doi: 10.1016/j.nurt.2008.10.038

Chawla, A. (2010). Control of macrophage activation and function by PPARs. *Circ. Res.* 106, 1559–1569. doi: 10.1161/CIRCRESAHA.110.216523

Chen, C., Li, Y. H., Zhang, Q., Yu, J. Z., Zhao, Y. F., Ma, C. G., et al. (2014a). Fasudil regulates T cell responses through polarization of BV-2 cells in mice experimental autoimmune encephalomyelitis. *Acta Pharmacol. Sin.* 35, 1428–1438. doi: 10.1038/aps.2014.68

Chen, S., Zhang, H., Pu, H., Wang, G., Li, W., Leak, R. K., et al. (2014c). n-3 PUFA supplementation benefits microglial responses to myelin pathology. *Sci. Rep.* 4:7458. doi: 10.1038/srep07458

Chen, W. W., Zhang, X., and Huang, W. J. (2016). Role of neuroinflammation in neurodegenerative diseases (Review). *Mol. Med. Rep.* 13, 3391–3396. doi: 10.3892/mmr.2016.4948

Cherry, J. D., Olschowka, J. A., and O'Banion, M. K. (2014). Neuroinflammation and M2 microglia: the good, the bad, and the inflamed. *J. Neuroinflammation* 11:98. doi: 10.1186/1742-2094-11-98

Choi, S. H., Aid, S., Kim, H. W., Jackson, S. H., and Bosetti, F. (2012). Inhibition of NADPH oxidase promotes alternative and anti-inflammatory microglial activation during neuroinflammation. *J. Neurochem.* 120, 292–301. doi: 10.1111/j.1471-4159.2011.07572.x

Colonna, M., and Butovsky, O. (2017). Microglia function in the central nervous system during health and neurodegeneration. *Annu. Rev. Immunol.* 35, 441–468. doi: 10.1146/annurev-immunol-051116-052358

Correale, J. (2014). The role of microglial activation in disease progression. *Mult. Scler.* 20, 1288–1295. doi: 10.1177/1352458514533230

Cramer, P. E., Cirrito, J. R., Wesson, D. W., Lee, C. Y., Karlo, J. C., Zinn, A. E., et al. (2012). ApoE-directed therapeutics rapidly clear beta-amyloid and reverse deficits in AD mouse models. *Science* 335, 1503–1506. doi: 10.1126/science.1217697

Crotti, A., and Ransohoff, R. M. (2016). Microglial physiology and pathophysiology: insights from genome-wide transcriptional profiling. *Immunity* 44, 505–515. doi: 10.1016/j.immuni.2016.02.013

Deliyanti, D., and Wilkinson-Berka, J. L. (2015). Inhibition of NOX1/4 with GKT137831: a potential novel treatment to attenuate neuroglial cell inflammation in the retina. *J. Neuroinflamm.* 12:136. doi: 10.1186/s12974-015-0363-z

Diaz-Aparicio, I., Beccari, S., Abiega, O., and Sierra, A. (2016). Clearing the corpses: regulatory mechanisms, novel tools, and therapeutic potential of harnessing microglial phagocytosis in the diseased brain. *Neural Regen. Res.* 11, 1533–1539.

Dinter, H. (2000). Phosphodiesterase type 4 inhibitors: potential in the treatment of multiple sclerosis? *BioDrugs* 13, 87–94.

Du, L., Zhang, Y., Chen, Y., Zhu, J., Yang, Y., and Zhang, H. L. (2016). Role of microglia in neurological disorders and their potentials as a therapeutic target. *Mol. Neurobiol.* doi: 10.1007/s12035-016-0245-0 [Epub ahead of print].

Fernandez, M. R., Batlle, C., Gil-Garcia, M., and Ventura, S. (2017). Amyloid cores in prion domains: key regulators for prion conformational conversion. *Prion* 11, 31–39. doi: 10.1080/19336896.2017.1282020

Fiorito, J., Saeed, F., Zhang, H., Staniszewski, A., Feng, Y., Francis, Y. I., et al. (2013). Synthesis of quinoline derivatives: discovery of a potent and selective phosphodiesterase 5 inhibitor for the treatment of Alzheimer's disease. *Eur. J. Med. Chem.* 60, 285–294. doi: 10.1016/j.ejmech.2012.12.009

Franco, R., and Fernandez-Suarez, D. (2015). Alternatively activated microglia and macrophages in the central nervous system. *Prog. Neurobiol.* 131, 65–86. doi: 10.1016/j.pneurobio.2015.05.003

Gao, C., Huang, L., Long, Y., Zheng, J., Yang, J., Pu, S., et al. (2013). Y-39983, a selective Rho-kinase inhibitor, attenuates experimental autoimmune encephalomyelitis via inhibition of demyelination. *Neuroimmunomodulation* 20, 334–340. doi: 10.1159/000353568

Gao, H. M., and Hong, J. S. (2008). Why neurodegenerative diseases are progressive: uncontrolled inflammation drives disease progression. *Trends Immunol.* 29, 357–365. doi: 10.1016/j.it.2008.05.002

Gerlo, S., Kooijman, R., Beck, I. M., Kolmus, K., Spooren, A., and Haegeman, G. (2011). Cyclic AMP: a selective modulator of NF-kappaB action. *Cell Mol. Life. Sci.* 68, 3823–3841. doi: 10.1007/s00018-011-0757-8

Ghaiad, H. R., Nooh, M. M., El-Sawalhi, M. M., and Shaheen, A. A. (2016). Resveratrol promotes remyelination in cuprizone model of multiple sclerosis: biochemical and histological study. *Mol. Neurobiol.* doi: 10.1007/s12035-016-9891-5 [Epub ahead of print].

Ghosh, M., Aguirre, V., Wai, K., Felfly, H., Dietrich, W. D., and Pearse, D. D. (2015). The interplay between cyclic AMP, MAPK, and NF-kappaB pathways in response to proinflammatory signals in microglia. *Biomed. Res. Int.* 2015:308461. doi: 10.1155/2015/308461

Ghosh, M., Garcia-Castillo, D., Aguirre, V., Golshani, R., Atkins, C. M., Bramlett, H. M., et al. (2012). Proinflammatory cytokine regulation of cyclic AMP-phosphodiesterase 4 signaling in microglia in vitro and following CNS injury. *Glia* 60, 1839–1859. doi: 10.1002/glia.22401

Ghosh, M., Xu, Y., and Pearse, D. D. (2016). Cyclic AMP is a key regulator of M1 to M2a phenotypic conversion of microglia in the presence of Th2 cytokines. *J. Neuroinflammation* 13:9. doi: 10.1186/s12974-015-0463-9

Glass, C. K., Saijo, K., Winner, B., Marchetto, M. C., and Gage, F. H. (2010). Mechanisms underlying inflammation in neurodegeneration. *Cell* 140, 918–934. doi: 10.1016/j.cell.2010.02.016

Grizenkova, J., Akhtar, S., Brandner, S., Collinge, J., and Lloyd, S. E. (2014). Microglial Cx3cr1 knockout reduces prion disease incubation time in mice. *BMC Neurosci.* 15:44. doi: 10.1186/1471-2202-15-44

Gurney, M. E., D'Amato, E. C., and Burgin, A. B. (2015). Phosphodiesterase-4 (PDE4) molecular pharmacology and Alzheimer's disease. *Neurotherapeutics* 12, 49–56. doi: 10.1007/s13311-014-0309-7

Hanisch, U. K. (2002). Microglia as a source and target of cytokines. *Glia* 40, 140–155.

Haslund-Vinding, J., McBean, G., Jaquet, V., and Vilhardt, F. (2016). NADPH oxidases in microglia oxidant production: activating receptors, pharmacology, and association with disease. *Br. J. Pharmacol.* doi: 10.1111/bph.13425 [Epub ahead of print].

Heppner, F. L., Ransohoff, R. M., and Becher, B. (2015). Immune attack: the role of inflammation in Alzheimer disease. *Nat. Rev. Neurosci.* 16, 358–372. doi: 10.1038/nrn3880

Hernandes, M. S., Cafe-Mendes, C. C., and Britto, L. R. (2013a). NADPH oxidase and the degeneration of dopaminergic neurons in parkinsonian mice. *Oxid. Med. Cell. Longev.* 2013:157857. doi: 10.1155/2013/157857

Hernandes, M. S., Santos, G. D., Cafe-Mendes, C. C., Lima, L. S., Scavone, C., Munhoz, C. D., et al. (2013b). Microglial cells are involved in the susceptibility of NADPH oxidase knockout mice to 6-hydroxy-dopamine-induced neurodegeneration. *PLoS ONE* 8:e75532. doi: 10.1371/journal.pone.0075532

Huang, C., Tong, J., Bi, F., Zhou, H., and Xia, X. G. (2012). Mutant TDP-43 in motor neurons promotes the onset and progression of ALS in rats. *J. Clin. Invest.* 122, 107–118. doi: 10.1172/JCI59130

Jeong, S. I., Shin, J. A., Cho, S., Kim, H. W., Lee, J. Y., Kang, J. L., et al. (2016). Resveratrol attenuates peripheral and brain inflammation and reduces ischemic brain injury in aged female mice. *Neurobiol. Aging* 44, 74–84. doi: 10.1016/j.neurobiolaging.2016.04.007

Jha, M. K., Song, G. J., Lee, M. G., Jeoung, N. H., Go, Y., Harris, R. A., et al. (2015). Metabolic connection of inflammatory pain: pivotal role of a pyruvate dehydrogenase kinase-pyruvate dehydrogenase-lactic acid axis. *J. Neurosci.* 35, 14353–14369. doi: 10.1523/JNEUROSCI.1910-15.2015

Jin, Q., Cheng, J., Liu, Y., Wu, J., Wang, X., Wei, S., et al. (2014). Improvement of functional recovery by chronic metformin treatment is associated with enhanced alternative activation of microglia/macrophages and increased angiogenesis and neurogenesis following experimental stroke. *Brain Behav. Immun.* 40, 131–142. doi: 10.1016/j.bbi.2014.03.003

Kannan, V., Brouwer, N., Hanisch, U. K., Regen, T., Eggen, B. J., and Boddeke, H. W. (2013). Histone deacetylase inhibitors suppress immune activation in primary mouse microglia. *J. Neurosci. Res.* 91, 1133–1142. doi: 10.1002/jnr.23221

Kettenmann, H., Kirchhoff, F., and Verkhratsky, A. (2013). Microglia: new roles for the synaptic stripper. *Neuron* 77, 10–18. doi: 10.1016/j.neuron.2012.12.023

Kobayashi, K., Imagama, S., Ohgomori, T., Hirano, K., Uchimura, K., Sakamoto, K., et al. (2013). Minocycline selectively inhibits M1 polarization of microglia. *Cell Death Dis.* 4:e525. doi: 10.1038/cddis.2013.54

Kumar, A., Alvarez-Croda, D. M., Stoica, B. A., Faden, A. I., and Loane, D. J. (2016). Microglial/macrophage polarization dynamics following traumatic brain injury. *J. Neurotrauma* 33, 1732–1750.

Kuzumoto, Y., Kusunoki, S., Kato, N., Kihara, M., and Low, P. A. (2006). Effect of the aldose reductase inhibitor fidarestat on experimental diabetic neuropathy in the rat. *Diabetologia* 49, 3085–3093.

Laplante, M., and Sabatini, D. M. (2012). mTOR signaling in growth control and disease. *Cell* 149, 274–293. doi: 10.1016/j.cell.2012.03.017

Latta, C. H., Sudduth, T. L., Weekman, E. M., Brothers, H. M., Abner, E. L., Popa, G. J., et al. (2015). Determining the role of IL-4 induced neuroinflammation in microglial activity and amyloid-beta using BV2 microglial cells and APP/PS1 transgenic mice. *J. Neuroinflammation* 12:41. doi: 10.1186/s12974-015-0243-6

Lazo-Gomez, R., Ramirez-Jarquin, U. N., Tovar, Y. R. L. B., and Tapia, R. (2013). Histone deacetylases and their role in motor neuron degeneration. *Front. Cell. Neurosci.* 7:243. doi: 10.3389/fncel.2013.00243

Lecca, D., Nevin, D. K., Mulas, G., Casu, M. A., Diana, A., Rossi, D., et al. (2015). Neuroprotective and anti-inflammatory properties of a novel non-thiazolidinedione PPARgamma agonist in vitro and in MPTP-treated mice. *Neuroscience* 302, 23–35. doi: 10.1016/j.neuroscience.2015.04.026

Lewandowska, H., Kalinowska, M., Lewandowski, W., Stepkowski, T. M., and Brzoska, K. (2016). The role of natural polyphenols in cell signaling and cytoprotection against cancer development. *J. Nutr. Biochem.* 32, 1–19. doi: 10.1016/j.jnutbio.2015.11.006

Li, Y. H., Yu, J. Z., Liu, C. Y., Zhang, H., Zhang, H. F., Yang, W. F., et al. (2014). Intranasal delivery of FSD-C10, a novel Rho kinase inhibitor, exhibits therapeutic potential in experimental autoimmune encephalomyelitis. *Immunology* 143, 219–229. doi: 10.1111/imm.12303

Liao, B., Zhao, W., Beers, D. R., Henkel, J. S., and Appel, S. H. (2012). Transformation from a neuroprotective to a neurotoxic microglial phenotype in a mouse model of ALS. *Exp. Neurol.* 237, 147–152. doi: 10.1016/j.expneurol.2012.06.011

Lins, N., Mourao, L., Trevia, N., Passos, A., Farias, J. A., Assuncao, J., et al. (2016). Virus infections on prion diseased mice exacerbate inflammatory microglial response. *Oxid. Med. Cell. Longev.* 2016:3974648. doi: 10.1155/2016/3974648

Lisi, L., Laudati, E., Navarra, P., and Dello Russo, C. (2014). The mTOR kinase inhibitors polarize glioma-activated microglia to express a M1 phenotype. *J. Neuroinflammation* 11:125. doi: 10.1186/1742-2094-11-125

Loane, D. J., Deighan, B. F., Clarke, R. M., Griffin, R. J., Lynch, A. M., and Lynch, M. A. (2009). Interleukin-4 mediates the neuroprotective effects of rosiglitazone in the aged brain. *Neurobiol. Aging* 30, 920–931.

Loane, D. J., and Kumar, A. (2016). Microglia in the TBI brain: The good, the bad, and the dysregulated. *Exp. Neurol.* 275(Pt 3), 316–327. doi: 10.1016/j.expneurol.2015.08.018

Lu, Y. Z., Lin, C. H., Cheng, F. C., and Hsueh, C. M. (2005). Molecular mechanisms responsible for microglia-derived protection of Sprague-Dawley rat brain cells during in vitro ischemia. *Neurosci. Lett.* 373, 159–164.

Mandrekar-Colucci, S., Karlo, J. C., and Landreth, G. E. (2012). Mechanisms underlying the rapid peroxisome proliferator-activated receptor-gamma-mediated amyloid clearance and reversal of cognitive deficits in a murine model of Alzheimer's disease. *J. Neurosci.* 32, 10117–10128. doi: 10.1523/JNEUROSCI.5268-11.2012

Mandrekar-Colucci, S., and Landreth, G. E. (2010). Microglia and inflammation in Alzheimer's disease. *CNS Neurol. Disord. Drug Targets* 9, 156–167.

Michelucci, A., Heurtaux, T., Grandbarbe, L., Morga, E., and Heuschling, P. (2009). Characterization of the microglial phenotype under specific pro-inflammatory and anti-inflammatory conditions: effects of oligomeric and fibrillar amyloid-beta. *J. Neuroimmunol.* 210, 3–12. doi: 10.1016/j.jneuroim.2009.02.003

Miron, V. E., Boyd, A., Zhao, J. W., Yuen, T. J., Ruckh, J. M., Shadrach, J. L., et al. (2013). M2 microglia and macrophages drive oligodendrocyte differentiation during CNS remyelination. *Nat. Neurosci.* 16, 1211–1218. doi: 10.1038/nn.3469

Morales, R., Estrada, L. D., Diaz-Espinoza, R., Morales-Scheihing, D., Jara, M. C., Castilla, J., et al. (2010). Molecular cross talk between misfolded proteins in animal models of Alzheimer's and prion diseases. *J. Neurosci.* 30, 4528–4535. doi: 10.1523/JNEUROSCI.5924-09.2010

Moretti, R., Leger, P. L., Besson, V. C., Csaba, Z., Pansiot, J., Di Criscio, L., et al. (2016). Sildenafil, a cyclic GMP phosphodiesterase inhibitor, induces microglial modulation after focal ischemia in the neonatal mouse brain. *J. Neuroinflammation* 13, 95. doi: 10.1186/s12974-016-0560-4

Neumann, S., Bradke, F., Tessier-Lavigne, M., and Basbaum, A. I. (2002). Regeneration of sensory axons within the injured spinal cord induced by intraganglionic cAMP elevation. *Neuron* 34, 885–893.

Niu, L., Zhou, J., Huang, Y., Chen, Y., and Li, C. (2010). db-Cyclic adenosine monophosphate promotes axon regeneration and motor function recovery in cerebral ischemia-reperfusion rats. *Neurol. India* 58, 195–200. doi: 10.4103/0028-3886.63786

Orihuela, R., McPherson, C. A., and Harry, G. J. (2016). Microglial M1/M2 polarization and metabolic states. *Br. J. Pharmacol.* 173, 649–665. doi: 10.1111/bph.13139

Pan, J., Jin, J. L., Ge, H. M., Yin, K. L., Chen, X., Han, L. J., et al. (2015). Malibatol A regulates microglia M1/M2 polarization in experimental stroke in a PPARgamma-dependent manner. *J. Neuroinflamm.* 12, 51. doi: 10.1186/s12974-015-0270-3

Patil, S. P., Jain, P. D., Ghumatkar, P. J., Tambe, R., and Sathaye, S. (2014). Neuroprotective effect of metformin in MPTP-induced Parkinson's disease in mice. *Neuroscience* 277, 747–754. doi: 10.1016/j.neuroscience.2014.07.046

Peixoto, C. A., Nunes, A. K., and Garcia-Osta, A. (2015). Phosphodiesterase-5 inhibitors: action on the signaling pathways of neuroinflammation, neurodegeneration, and cognition. *Mediat. Inflamm.* 2015:940207. doi: 10.1155/2015/940207

Pifarre, P., Prado, J., Baltrons, M. A., Giralt, M., Gabarro, P., Feinstein, D. L., et al. (2011). Sildenafil (Viagra) ameliorates clinical symptoms and neuropathology in a mouse model of multiple sclerosis. *Acta Neuropathol.* 121, 499–508. doi: 10.1007/s00401-010-0795-6

Porro, C., Cianciulli, A., Calvello, R., and Panaro, M. A. (2015). Reviewing the role of resveratrol as a natural modulator of microglial activities. *Curr. Pharm. Des.* 21, 5277–5291.

Puzzo, D., Staniszewski, A., Deng, S. X., Privitera, L., Leznik, E., Liu, S., et al. (2009). Phosphodiesterase 5 inhibition improves synaptic function, memory, and amyloid-beta load in an Alzheimer's disease mouse model. *J. Neurosci.* 29, 8075–8086. doi: 10.1523/JNEUROSCI.0864-09.2009

Ransohoff, R. M. (2016). A polarizing question: do M1 and M2 microglia exist? *Nat. Neurosci.* 19, 987–991. doi: 10.1038/nn.4338

Reddy, A. B., Srivastava, S. K., and Ramana, K. V. (2010). Aldose reductase inhibition prevents *lipopolysaccharide-induced glucose uptake and glucose transporter 3 expression in RAW264.7 macrophages. Int. J. Biochem. Cell Biol.* 42, 1039–1045. doi: 10.1016/j.biocel.2010.03.014

Rolle, C. E., Sengupta, S., and Lesniak, M. S. (2012). Mechanisms of immune evasion by gliomas. *Adv. Exp. Med. Biol.* 746, 53–76. doi: 10.1007/978-1-4614-3146-6_5

Seredenina, T., Nayernia, Z., Sorce, S., Maghzal, G. J., Filippova, A., Ling, S. C., et al. (2016). Evaluation of NADPH oxidases as drug targets in a mouse model of familial amyotrophic lateral sclerosis. *Free Radic. Biol. Med.* 97, 95–108. doi: 10.1016/j.freeradbiomed.2016.05.016

Shi, N., Zhu, C., and Li, L. (2016). Rehabilitation Training and Resveratrol Improve the Recovery of Neurological and Motor Function in Rats after Cerebral Ischemic Injury through the Sirt1 Signaling Pathway. *Biomed Res. Int.* 2016:1732163. doi: 10.1155/2016/1732163

Sica, A., and Mantovani, A. (2012). Macrophage plasticity and polarization: in vivo veritas. *J. Clin. Invest.* 122, 787–795. doi: 10.1172/JCI59643

Skalak, R., Soslowsky, L., Schmalzer, E., Impelluso, T., and Chien, S. (1987). Theory of filtration of mixed blood suspensions. *Biorheology* 24, 35–52.

Song, G. J., Nam, Y., Jo, M., Jung, M., Koo, J. Y., Cho, W., et al. (2016). A novel small-molecule agonist of PPAR-gamma potentiates an anti-inflammatory M2 glial phenotype. *Neuropharmacology* 109, 159–169. doi: 10.1016/j.neuropharm.2016.06.009

Stopschinski, B. E., and Diamond, M. I. (2017). The prion model for progression and diversity of neurodegenerative diseases. *Lancet Neurol.* 16, 323–332. doi: 10.1016/S1474-4422(17)30037-6

Sutcliffe, J. S., Beaumont, V., Watson, J. M., Chew, C. S., Beconi, M., Hutcheson, D. M., et al. (2014). Efficacy of selective PDE4D negative allosteric modulators in the object retrieval task in female cynomolgus monkeys (Macaca fascicularis). *PLoS ONE* 9:e102449. doi: 10.1371/journal.pone.0102449

Swarup, V., Phaneuf, D., Dupre, N., Petri, S., Strong, M., Kriz, J., et al. (2011). Deregulation of TDP-43 in amyotrophic lateral sclerosis triggers nuclear factor kappaB-mediated pathogenic pathways. *J. Exp. Med.* 208, 2429–2447. doi: 10.1084/jem.20111313

Tang, Y., and Le, W. (2016). Differential Roles of M1 and M2 Microglia in Neurodegenerative Diseases. *Mol. Neurobiol.* 53, 1181–1194. doi: 10.1007/s12035-014-9070-5

Thored, P., Heldmann, U., Gomes-Leal, W., Gisler, R., Darsalia, V., Taneera, J., et al. (2009). Long-term accumulation of microglia with proneurogenic phenotype concomitant with persistent neurogenesis in adult subventricular zone after stroke. *Glia* 57, 835–849. doi: 10.1002/glia.20810

Toba, J., Nikkuni, M., Ishizeki, M., Yoshii, A., Watamura, N., Inoue, T., et al. (2016). PPARgamma agonist pioglitazone improves cerebellar dysfunction at pre-Abeta deposition stage in APPswe/PS1dE9 Alzheimer's disease model mice. *Biochem. Biophys. Res. Commun.* 473, 1039–1044. doi: 10.1016/j.bbrc.2016.04.012

Venna, V. R., Li, J., Hammond, M. D., Mancini, N. S., and McCullough, L. D. (2014). Chronic metformin treatment improves post-stroke angiogenesis and recovery after experimental stroke. *Eur. J. Neurosci.* 39, 2129–2138. doi: 10.1111/ejn.12556

Venneri, M. A., Giannetta, E., Panio, G., De Gaetano, R., Gianfrilli, D., Pofi, R., et al. (2015). Chronic Inhibition of PDE5 Limits Pro-Inflammatory Monocyte-Macrophage Polarization in Streptozotocin-Induced Diabetic Mice. *PLoS ONE* 10:e0126580. doi: 10.1371/journal.pone.0126580

Vilhardt, F., Haslund-Vinding, J., Jaquet, V., and McBean, G. (2016). Microglia antioxidant systems and redox signaling. *Br. J. Pharmacol.* doi: 10.1111/bph.13426 [Epub ahead of print].

Wang, G., Jiang, X., Pu, H., Zhang, W., An, C., Hu, X., et al. (2013). Scriptaid, a novel histone deacetylase inhibitor, protects against traumatic brain injury via modulation of PTEN and AKT pathway : scriptaid protects against TBI via AKT. *Neurotherapeutics* 10, 124–142. doi: 10.1007/s13311-012-0157-2

Wang, G., Shi, Y., Jiang, X., Leak, R. K., Hu, X., Wu, Y., et al. (2015). HDAC inhibition prevents white matter injury by modulating microglia/macrophage polarization through the GSK3beta/PTEN/Akt axis. *Proc. Natl. Acad. Sci. U.S.A.* 112, 2853–2858. doi: 10.1073/pnas.1501441112

Weekman, E. M., Sudduth, T. L., Abner, E. L., Popa, G. J., Mendenhall, M. D., Brothers, H. M., et al. (2014). Transition from an M1 to a mixed neuroinflammatory phenotype increases amyloid deposition in APP/PS1 transgenic mice. *J. Neuroinflammation* 11, 127. doi: 10.1186/1742-2094-11-127

Xiao, Q., Zhao, W., Beers, D. R., Yen, A. A., Xie, W., Henkel, J. S., et al. (2007). Mutant SOD1(G93A) microglia are more neurotoxic relative to wild-type microglia. *J. Neurochem.* 102, 2008–2019.

Xu, P., Zhang, M., Sheng, R., and Ma, Y. (2017). Synthesis and biological evaluation of deferiprone-resveratrol hybrids as antioxidants, Abeta1-42 aggregation inhibitors and metal-chelating agents for Alzheimer's disease. *Eur. J. Med. Chem.* 127, 174–186. doi: 10.1016/j.ejmech.2016.12.045

Xue, N., Zhou, Q., Ji, M., Jin, J., Lai, F., Chen, J., et al. (2017). Chlorogenic acid inhibits glioblastoma growth through repolarizating macrophage from M2 to M1 phenotype. *Sci. Rep.* 7:39011. doi: 10.1038/srep39011

Yamanaka, M., Ishikawa, T., Griep, A., Axt, D., Kummer, M. P., and Heneka, M. T. (2012). PPARgamma/RXRalpha-induced and CD36-mediated microglial amyloid-beta phagocytosis results in cognitive improvement in amyloid precursor protein/presenilin 1 mice. *J. Neurosci.* 32, 17321–17331. doi: 10.1523/JNEUROSCI.1569-12.2012

Yamasaki, R., Lu, H., Butovsky, O., Ohno, N., Rietsch, A. M., Cialic, R., et al. (2014). Differential roles of microglia and monocytes in the inflamed central nervous system. *J. Exp. Med.* 211, 1533–1549. doi: 10.1084/jem.20132477

Yao, Y., Li, J., Niu, Y., Yu, J. Q., Yan, L., Miao, Z. H., et al. (2015). Resveratrol inhibits oligomeric Abeta-induced microglial activation via NADPH oxidase. *Mol. Med. Rep.* 12, 6133–6139. doi: 10.3892/mmr.2015.4199

Zhang, Q., Bian, G., Chen, P., Liu, L., Yu, C., Liu, F., et al. (2016). Aldose Reductase Regulates Microglia/Macrophages Polarization Through the cAMP Response Element-Binding Protein After Spinal Cord Injury in Mice. *Mol. Neurobiol.* 53, 662–676. doi: 10.1007/s12035-014-9035-8

Zhang, Q., Yuan, L., Zhang, Q., Gao, Y., Liu, G., Xiu, M., et al. (2015). Resveratrol attenuates hypoxia-induced neurotoxicity through inhibiting microglial activation. *Int. Immunopharmacol.* 28, 578–587. doi: 10.1016/j.intimp.2015.07.027

Zhao, S., Yang, J., Wang, L., Peng, S., Yin, J., Jia, L., et al. (2016). NF-kappaB Upregulates Type 5 Phosphodiesterase in N9 Microglial Cells: Inhibition by Sildenafil and Yonkenafil. *Mol. Neurobiol.* 53, 2647–2658. doi: 10.1007/s12035-015-9293-0

Zhao, W., Xie, W., Xiao, Q., Beers, D. R., and Appel, S. H. (2006). Protective effects of an anti-inflammatory cytokine, interleukin-4, on motoneuron toxicity induced by activated microglia. *J. Neurochem.* 99, 1176–1187.

4

A Combination of *Ex vivo* Diffusion MRI and Multiphoton to Study Microglia/Monocytes Alterations after Spinal Cord Injury

Harun N. Noristani[1,2†], Hassan Boukhaddaoui[1†], Guillaume Saint-Martin[2,3], Pauline Auzer[1], Rahima Sidiboulenouar[3], Nicolas Lonjon[2,4], Eric Alibert[3], Nicolas Tricaud[1], Christophe Goze-Bac[3], Christophe Coillot[3] and Florence E. Perrin[1,2*]

[1] Institut National de la Santé et de la Recherche Médicale, U1051, Montpellier, France, [2] University of Montpellier, Montpellier; Institut National de la Santé et de la Recherche Médicale, U1198, Montpellier; École Pratique des Hautes Études, Paris, France, [3] Charles Coulomb Laboratory, UMR 5221 Centre National de la Recherche Scientifique, Montpellier, France, [4] Centre Hospitalier Universitaire de Montpellier (CHRU), Gui de Chauliac Hospital, Montpellier, France

***Correspondence:**
Florence E. Perrin
florence.perrin@inserm.fr

[†] These authors have contributed equally to this work.

Central nervous system (CNS) injury has been observed to lead to microglia activation and monocytes infiltration at the lesion site. *Ex vivo* diffusion magnetic resonance imaging (diffusion MRI or DWI) allows detailed examination of CNS tissues, and recent advances in clearing procedures allow detailed imaging of fluorescent-labeled cells at high resolution. No study has yet combined *ex vivo* diffusion MRI and clearing procedures to establish a possible link between microglia/monocytes response and diffusion coefficient in the context of spinal cord injury (SCI). We carried out *ex vivo* MRI of the spinal cord at different time-points after spinal cord transection followed by tetrahydrofuran based clearing and examined the density and morphology of microglia/monocytes using two-photon microscopy. Quantitative analysis revealed an early marked increase in microglial/monocytes density that is associated with an increase in the extension of the lesion measured using diffusion MRI. Morphological examination of microglia/monocytes somata at the lesion site revealed a significant increase in their surface area and volume as early as 72 hours post-injury. Time-course analysis showed differential microglial/monocytes response rostral and caudal to the lesion site. Microglia/monocytes showed a decrease in reactivity over time caudal to the lesion site, but an increase was observed rostrally. Direct comparison of microglia/monocytes morphology, obtained through multiphoton, and the longitudinal apparent diffusion coefficient (ADC), measured with diffusion MRI, highlighted that axonal integrity does not correlate with the density of microglia/monocytes or their somata morphology. We emphasize that differential microglial/monocytes reactivity rostral and caudal to the lesion site may thus coincide, at least partially, with reported temporal differences in debris clearance. Our study demonstrates that the combination of *ex vivo* diffusion MRI and two-photon microscopy may be used to follow structural tissue alteration. Lesion extension coincides with microglia/monocytes density; however, a direct relationship between ADC and microglia/monocytes density and morphology was not observed. We highlighted a differential rostro-caudal microglia/monocytes reactivity that may correspond to a temporal difference in debris clearance and axonal integrity. Thus, potential therapeutic strategies targeting microglia/monocytes after SCI may need to be adjusted not only with the time after injury but also relative to the location to the lesion site.

Keywords: spinal cord injury, microglia/monocytes, *ex vivo* diffusion MRI, tissue clearing, two-photon

INTRODUCTION

Spinal cord injury (SCI) is a devastating neuropathology affecting over 2.5 million people worldwide (van den Berg et al., 2010). Depending on the anatomical level and the severity of the spinal cord lesion, clinical symptoms range from minor sensory/motor damage to complete quadriplegia.

In clinic, magnetic resonance imaging (MRI) is the only non-invasive method for examining the impact of the insult on the structure and function of human spinal cord (Wheeler-Kingshott et al., 2014). MRI is also well adapted for following the evolution of the lesion in pre-clinical animal models of SCI (Bonny et al., 2004; Denic et al., 2011). In particular, *ex vivo* MRI analysis provides high resolution images of the spinal cord, allowing accurate assessment of lesion-induced tissue alterations. Recently, we have shown that *ex vivo* ^{1}H-MRI (9.4T) closely correlates with histological examination of the injured spinal cord after different lesion severities (Noristani et al., 2015).

Diffusion weighted MRI (diffusion MRI, or DWI) reflects the local dynamics of water molecules in the tissue. The structure of tissues can be characterized by the capability of water to diffuse along preferential directions and can be quantitatively assessed using the apparent diffusion coefficient (ADC). DWI thus offers information on tissue integrity and structure that cannot be obtained by conventional ^{1}H-MRI. In particular, the longitudinal ADC (lADC), which represents the diffusivity along the rostro-caudal axis and reflects the integrity of white matter fibers, is often decreased in the presence of axonal injury (Song et al., 2003; Vedantam et al., 2014). In the spinal cord, diffusion MRI is often applied to evaluate myelin integrity (Bonny et al., 2004) but may also be applied to assess morphological alterations of cell populations, including glia. In addition, diffusion MRI has been used to examine the 3-dimensional (3D) structure and architecture of post-mortem brains for review, [see Bastiani and Roebroeck (2015)].

Numerous animal models have been developed to study SCI pathophysiology including spinal cord compression, contusion, ischemia and transection (Lee and Lee, 2013). Whilst these animal models partially recapitulate clinical symptoms, they have important limitations due to the high level of inter-individual differences in the severity of the lesion (Basso et al., 1996; Onifer et al., 2007). Although transection of the spinal cord is regarded as the most severe model of SCI, it has the advantage of minimizing the inter-individual differences in injury severity (M'Dahoma et al., 2014) and is more easily quantified using MRI (Wang et al., 2014). Because of its high reproducibility, transection of the spinal cord reduces the need for a large number of animals to obtain biologically robust results. The majority of studies using transection as SCI models have focused on rats (Basso et al., 1996; Antri et al., 2005; Onifer et al., 2007; M'Dahoma et al., 2014); however, transgenic mice offer advantages to better understand the pathophysiological mechanisms involved in SCI.

SCI pathophysiology includes damage to the blood-spinal cord barrier, monocytes infiltration at the lesion site and elevated immune response, all contributing to neuronal demise. In addition, SCI triggers the pronounced activation of glial cells, including microglia. Microglia, the resident immune cells of the central nervous system (CNS) are the first activated glial population observed after SCI (Tian et al., 2007) and contribute to monocytes-derived macrophages recruitment to the lesion site. Under physiological conditions, microglia display a ramified morphology with small somata and long/thin cellular processes that continuously scan their territorial domains (Kettenmann et al., 2011). Following SCI, microglia migrate toward the lesion site, where they acquire an amoeboid morphology with large somata and short/thick processes (Tian et al., 2007; Noristani et al., 2017). One means of studying microglia is to use CX3CR1^{eGFP} transgenic mice, which express enhanced green fluorescent protein (eGFP) downstream of the Cx3cr1 promoter, a chemokine receptor highly expressed in microglia, circulating monocytes and resident macrophages (Jung et al., 2000; Gautier et al., 2012; Wolf et al., 2013). Microglia and peripheral monocytes of common myelomonocytic origin display similar morphologies and express common surface receptors and signaling molecules (Schmitz et al., 2009; Kettenmann et al., 2011). Recent reports identified potential markers, including Ly6C, to distinguish between microglia and monocytes (Chiu et al., 2013; Butovsky et al., 2014; Gosselin et al., 2014; Bennett et al., 2016); however, to our knowledge, no transgenic mice expressing a fluorescent marker downstream of Ly6C have been generated.

Although the activation of microglia/monocytes after SCI have been acknowledged for almost a century, little is currently known about their density after injury and their longitudinal repartition along the spinal cord axis rostral and caudal to the lesion site (Schnell et al., 1999; Kigerl et al., 2006; Stirling and Yong, 2008). Earlier studies using semi-quantitative histology reported a time-dependent increase in microglia/monocytes density up to 7 days after dorsal spinal cord hemisection in mice (Stirling and Yong, 2008). Other histological study revealed a peak of microglia/monocyte reactivity in mice between 7

Abbreviations: CNS, Central nervous system; MRI, magnetic resonance imaging; 1H-MRI, proton MRI; diffusion weighted MRI (diffusion MRI); eGFP, enhanced green fluorescent protein; PBS, phosphate base saline; PFA, paraformaldehyde; SCI, spinal cord injury; TR, repetition time; TE, Echo Time; NE, echo number; AVG, average; FOV, field of view; ADC, apparent diffusion coefficient.

and 14 days post-injury after contusion of the spinal cord (Kigerl et al., 2006). More recent studies using quantitative flow cytometry have shown that the increased microglia/monocytes density observed within 2 days post-contusion injury in mice is subsequently reduced starting from 4 days post-SCI (Stirling and Yong, 2008). Contradictory findings have also been reported in rats after contusion SCI with a peak in microglia/monocyte density between 2 (Abdanipour et al., 2013) and 7 days post-injury (Beck et al., 2010).

To develop efficient therapies that target the inflammatory response after SCI, it is necessary to acquire precise knowledge of microglia/monocytes density, not only at acute and chronic stages post-injury but also at different distances from the lesion epicenter. Previous studies on microglia/monocyte density after SCI relied on histology combined with manual cell counting (Schnell et al., 1999; Kigerl et al., 2009; Adamczak et al., 2010), which provides only semi-quantitative data, at best. In addition, standard histological analyses require tissue sectioning, making 3D analysis of microglia/monocytes throughout the whole tissue virtually impossible. Clearing, a recent advancement in tissue processing that renders intact organs transparent, allows fast 3D analyses of the entire spinal cord (Erturk et al., 2012; Chung et al., 2013; Renier et al., 2014; Tomer et al., 2014; Yang et al., 2014).

To date, only one study has reported changes in microglia/monocytes density after spinal cord hemisection in mice using the clearing approach (Erturk et al., 2012). However, the authors analyzed only a single time-point (10 days after lesion) with no indications of microglia/monocytes density at either acute or more chronic stages post-injury. In addition, Erturk et al. (2012) mainly focused on the lesion epicenter and did not provide data regarding microglia/monocytes density at more distal locations (Erturk et al., 2012). Given the dynamic reactivity of microglia/monocytes, it is necessary to study their alterations in acute and chronic stages after SCI and at different distances both rostral and caudal to the lesion site. Finally, even if numerous studies have reported microglia/monocytes activation after SCI, none has quantified their morphological changes after injury.

Our aim was to examine detailed SCI-induced tissues and cellular alterations at different time-points and distances from the lesion site using (a) high resolution *ex vivo* diffusion MRI and (b) two-photon imaging of cleared spinal cords to evaluate 3D changes in microglia/monocytes density and morphology. Our specific objective was to identify a possible correlation between *ex vivo* diffusion MRI signals, which reflect the structure of tissues, and microglial/monocytes density/morphology. Since microglia are involved in debris clearance, we hypothesized that lesion size may be related, at least partially, to microglia reactivity. We thus first compared modifications in microglia/monocytes density and morphology to the extension of the lesion evaluated by DWI. We then compared the density and the morphology of microglia/monocytes at different distances on both sides of the lesion. Finally, we tried to determine whether or not axonal integrity, reflected by the lADC, correlates with microglia density and morphology. We found that microglial/monocytes density coincides with lesion extension; however, lADC does not seems to correlate with microglia/monocyte density and morphology. We also established that microglial/monocytes somata morphology is different rostral and caudal to the lesion epicenter. Our results constitute the first detailed 3D analysis of a cell populations in the spinal cord after lesion using a combination of *ex vivo* diffusion MRI and two-photon microscopy.

MATERIALS AND METHODS

Ethic Approval

Experimental procedures followed the European legislative, administrative and statutory measures for animal experimentation (86/609/EEC). The study was approved by the "Direction des Services Vétérinaires de l'Hérault" and the "Ministère de l'Education Nationale, de l'Enseignement Supérieur et de la Recherche, ethics committee N°36," France (authorization number 34118).

Animals and Spinal Cord Injury

Transgenic mice expressing enhanced green fluorescent protein (eGFP) in microglia/monocytes (CX3CR1$^{+/eGFP}$) (Jung et al., 2000) were obtained from Dr. Dan Littman, Howard Hughes Medical Institute, Skirball Institute, NYU Medical Centre, New York, USA and maintained on a C57BL/6 background (The Jackson Laboratory, Bar Harbor, ME, USA). Heterozygous eGFP$^{-/+}$ mice were used in the current study. All mice were housed in controlled conditions (hygrometry, temperature and 12-h light/dark cycle) with free access to food and water. Adult male mice (12 weeks of age) were anesthetized by inhalation of 1.5% isoflurane (Aerane, Baxter, Deerfield, IL, USA). The skin and muscles overlying the low thoracic segment of the rachis were cut, followed by a dorsal laminectomy of the thoracic 9 (T9) vertebra. Meninges were incised and transection of the spinal cord was carried out under a microscope using a micro-scalpel (FST, Heidelberg, Germany). Lesions were made at T9 level to obtain complete paraplegia whilst preserving full respiratory function. Following lesion, muscles and skin were sutured and animals were left to recover on a heated surface (not exceeding 38°C). Bladders were emptied manually twice daily and bodyweight was measured throughout the study period. Three time-points were chosen to reveal microglia/monocytes changes both at acute (72 hours) and chronic (4 and 6 weeks) stages after severe spinal cord lesion. Non-injured group served as control ($n = 4$ for each group).

Tissue Processing

Mice were deeply anesthetized via intraperitoneal injection of tribromoethanol (500 mg/kg) followed by transcardial perfusion using cold 0.1 M phosphate buffer saline (PBS) at pH 7.2 and 4% paraformaldehyde (PFA, Sigma Aldrich, Saint Louis, USA). The entire spinal cords were then dissected and post-fixed in the 4% PFA for an additional 2 h.

Ex vivo Diffusion Weighted Imaging

Spinal cords were positioned in a 5-mm-diameter glass tube filled with 0.1 M PBS surrounded by a custom-made ribbon solenoid coil (40 mm in length, 8 mm outer diameter and

4 turns, **Supplementary Figure 1K**) (Coillot et al., 2016) and imaged using 9.4 Tesla apparatus (Agilent Varian 9.4/160/ASR, Santa Clara, California, USA) associated with VnmrJ imaging acquisition system (Agilent, Palo Alto, California, USA). The use of the custom-made ribbon solenoid coil enhanced signal-to-noise ratio (SNR) and, drastically reduced acquisition time. Specifically, for this experiment, SNR was increased by 7 compared to a regular 43 mm quadrature volumic coil. We first acquired high resolution T2 weighed ^{1}H-MRI using a spin echo sequence to obtain MR images without diffusion-weighting (diffusion gradient: G = 0 G.cm^{-1}). The following acquisition parameters were used: delta = 6.88 ms, G = 0 G/cm^{-1}, separation = 15.05 ms, (TR) repetition time = 1,580 ms, (TE) echo time = 30.55 ms, AVG = 30, FOV = 10 × 10 mm, slices = 36, thickness = 1 mm without gap and acquisition matrix = 128 × 128. Scanning time: approximately 90 min. Diffusion-weighted MRI sequence was then used to acquire DWI and to calculate the ADC. ADC is a quantitative measurement of local water diffusion (mm^2.s^{-1}) on a given region and direction which is sensitive to the local structure and anisotropy of tissues. ADC results from the combination of acquisitions with (S at $b = 500$) and without (S0 at $b = 0$) diffusion gradient. To acquire axial images, the sensitivity of diffusion MRI was preliminary evaluated in three directions including the longitudinal axis of the spinal cord. Longitudinal DWI offered better signal-to-noise ratio and image contrast to discriminate between the intact and the damaged regions of the spinal cord. We thus acquired DWI only on the longitudinal axis with the following parameters: magnetic field gradient G = 20 G.cm^{-1} during 6.88 ms, separation = 15.05 ms; (TR) repetition time = 1,580 ms, (TE) echo time = 30.55 ms, AVG = 30, FOV = 10 × 10 mm, slices = 36, thickness = 1 mm without gap and acquisition matrix = 128 × 128. Scanning time: approximately 180 min. Diffusion data were processed by using a MATLAB-based in-house toolbox. All MRI visualization and segmentation were done using Myrian software (Intrasense, Montpellier, France); intact (entire spinal cord, white and gray matters) and damaged tissues were manually surrounded (**Figures 1B–D** and **Supplementary Figures 1A–J**).

Tissue Clearing and Two-Photon Image Acquisition

After diffusion MRI acquisition, spinal cords were first rinsed in 0.1 M PBS and clarified using the 3-dimensional imaging of solvent cleared organs (3DISCO) procedure, as previously described (Erturk et al., 2012). Briefly, spinal cords were incubated in 50, 70, and 80% tetrahydrofuran (THF, Sigma Aldrich, Saint Louis, USA) followed by three incubations in 100% THF (30 min each). Spinal cords were then placed in dichloromethane (Sigma Aldrich, Saint Louis, USA) for 30 min and finally in dibenzyl ether (DBE, Sigma Aldrich, Saint Louis, USA) for 20–30 min, until the samples became transparent (**Figure 2**). All incubation steps were done in the dark; spinal cords were placed in glass vials on a rotator. Samples were then mounted on a glass slide in DBE and coversliped, then immediately imaged using a two-photon scanning microscope (Zeiss LSM 7MP) equipped with a femtosecond pulsed Ti:Sapphire laser (Ultra II, Coherent) at 950 nm. We scanned at a 1,024 × 1,024 pixel resolution and 5 μm z steps; full 3D scan took 20–30 min.

Microglial/Monocytes Quantification

To quantify microglia/monocytes density (numerical density (N_V), number (#)/mm^3) throughout the entire thickness of spinal cord, we chose 3 different zones located at different distances from the edge of the lesion site: 0–500 μm immediately adjacent to the injury site as well as 500-1,000 and 4,000–4,500 μm away from the lesion epicenter, both rostral and caudal to the injury site (**Figure 3**). For non-injured controls, we analyzed equivalent anatomical levels of the spinal cord. Tissue volumes and microglial/monocytes density were calculated using the 3D image processing software Imaris x64 7.2.2. (Bitplane AG, Zürich, Switzerland). Microglia/monocytes were converted into 3D objects for fully automated counting (**Supplementary Video 1**). To ensure accuracy of the counts, selected segments were rotated to different angles and assessed visually. Only a sub-population of microglia/monocytes with no overlapping processes were selected for morphological analysis of their somata. Microglial/monocytes somata morphology was measured in 190–300 cells per time-point and compared to those of the un-injured control. The original scan was also converted into 3D objects for automated morphological analysis. Given that microglial/monocyte activation is characterized by pronounced enlargement of their somata, morphological analysis was carried out using Imaris to determine somata surface area (μm^2) and volume (μm^3), as previously described (Rodriguez et al., 2015).

Statistical Analysis

Un-paired *t*-tests were used to compare differences between 2 groups. The Wilcoxon signed-rank test was used to compare ADC values between groups along an 8 mm segment centered on the lesion site. A paired-*t*-test was used to compare ADC values between groups in the rostral and caudal segments. Significance was defined as $p \leq 0.05$.

All data were analyzed using GraphPad Prism 4.0 (GraphPad Software, Inc., CA, USA). Data are shown as the mean ± standard error of the mean (SEM).

RESULTS

Ex vivo Diffusion MRI Allows Quantification of Lesion Extension and Volume

We acquired 36 axial diffusion MR images (1 mm thick) over a 3.6 cm segment centered on the lesion epicenter (**Figure 1A**). We then quantified the rostro-caudal extension of the lesion. Lesion segmentation was carried out manually by outlining the spared (**Figures 1B,D**, *green: total; blue: gray matter*) and injured (**Figures 1C,D**, *red*) tissues on axial images. The mean extension of the lesion at 72 hours was 4 ± 0.4 mm centered on the epicenter and decreased to 2.75 ± 0.25 and 3 ± 0 mm by 4 and 6 weeks, respectively, thus revealing a significant decrease in rostro-caudal extension of the lesion between 72 hours and 4 weeks post-injury, followed by a stabilization (**Figure 1E**). The mean lesion

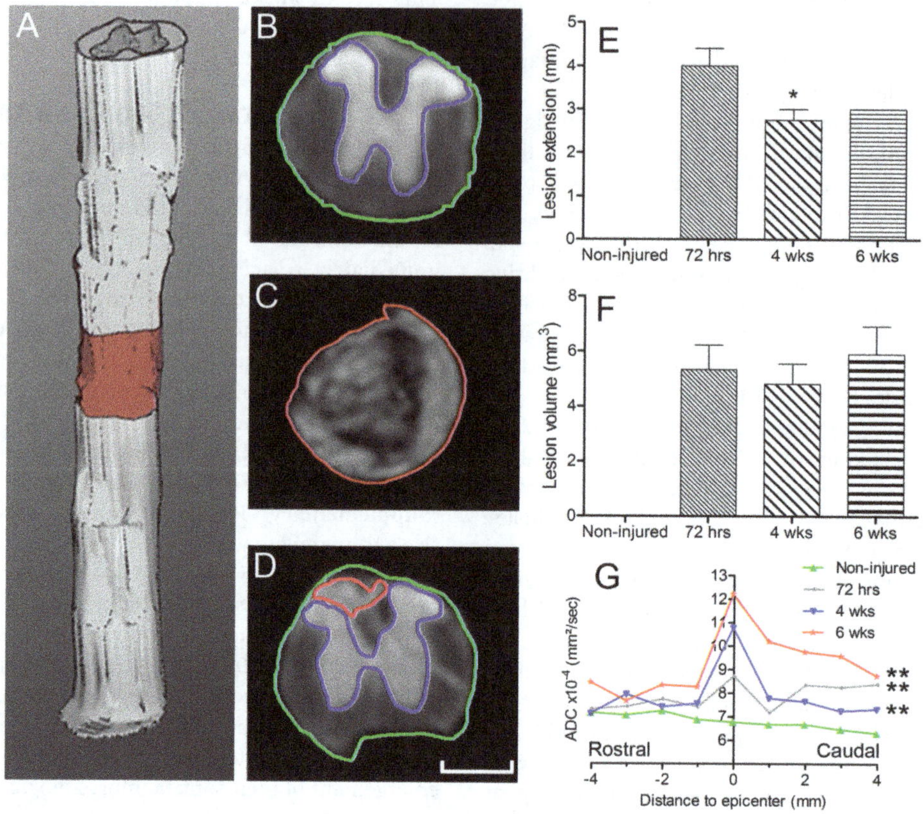

FIGURE 1 | *Ex vivo* diffusion ^{1}H-MRI assessments following SCI. 3D reconstruction of an injured spinal cord **(A)**, the red area represents lesion extension. Images of *ex vivo* diffusion MRI from mouse spinal cord rostral **(B)** within **(C)** and caudal **(D)** to the lesion epicenter. Note the excellent anatomical resolution of the spinal cord that clearly distinguishes the entire spinal cord (outlined in green in **B** and **D**), damaged spinal cord tissues (outlined in red in **C** and **D**) as well as the intact gray matter (outlined in blue in **B** and **D**). Bar graph displaying the evolution of the extension of the lesion at different stages after complete SCI **(E)**. Bar graph showing changes in the volume of the lesion at different time-points after injury **(F)**. Line graph displaying changes in apparent diffusion coefficients along the spinal cord at different stages after SCI **(G)**. Statistics: $^{*}P < 0.05$ and $^{***}P < 0.001$. **(E)**, 4 weeks compared to 72 hours post-lesion, un-paired *t*-test. **(G)**, All groups are compared to the non-injured control, Wilcoxon signed-rank test.

volume amounted to 5.3 ± 0.9, 4.8 ± 0.7, and $5.9 \pm 1\ \text{mm}^3$ at 72 hours, 4 and 6 weeks post-injury, respectively, and quantitative assessment showed no significant changes over time (**Figure 1F**).

Water Diffusion Modification Is Time-Dependent

We then quantified the diffusion of the water in the tissues using diffusion MRI and evaluated changes in ADC values. At the lesion site, no clear distinction between the gray and white matter was possible due to complete tissue damage (**Figure 1C**). ADC was measured on an 8 mm segment centered on the lesion site. Overall, non-injured spinal cords showed an ADC of $6.78 \times 10^{-4}\ \text{mm}^2/\text{s}$ (**Figure 1G**). The mean ADC value at the lesion epicenter reached 8.73, 10.78, and $12.22 \times 10^{-4}\ \text{mm}^2/\text{s}$ at 72 hours, 4 and 6 weeks, respectively (**Figures 1C,G**). Moreover, an overall increase in the ADC contiguous to the lesion site, both rostral and caudal, was observed from 72 hours up to 6 weeks post-injury (**Figure 1G**). For all post-injury time points, the ADC was higher in the caudal than in the rostral segments 4 mm away from the lesion site. Moreover, there was an increased ADC 6 weeks post-injury in the rostral segment, whereas the ADC in the caudal segment remained relatively stable after injury (**Figure 1G**). All injured groups displayed a significant increase in ADC compared to non-injured animals; however, no significant differences between post-injury time points were observed (**Figure 1G, Table 1**). A Wilcoxon signed-rank test showed a significant increase in ADC between 72 hours and 6 weeks post-injury (**Figure 1G, Table 1**) compared to non-injured animals. To provide a more in-depth analysis, we analyzed separately the rostral and caudal segments. A paired *t*-test revealed a significant increase in ADC 72 hours and 6 weeks post-injury in the caudal segment when compared to non-injured animals; conversely, the injury did not modify the ADC in the rostral segment (**Table 1**).

Together, these data show that, in contrast to the quantification of the extension and the volume of the lesion, the quantification of water diffusion allows identification of time-dependent modifications. Moreover, we highlight differences in water diffusion between segments located symmetrically rostral and caudal to the lesion site.

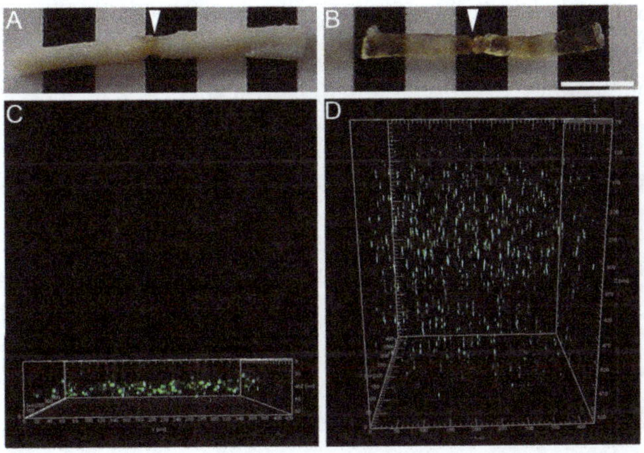

FIGURE 2 | Two-photon imaging of the spinal cord before and after clearing. Photographs showing an injured spinal cord (arrows) before **(A)** and after **(B)** clearing. Using two-photon microscopy, the spinal cord was imaged before and after clearing. Two-photon micrographs displaying eGFP-expressing microglia/monocytes before **(C)** and after **(D)** clearing. Note that, before clearing, <100 μm of the spinal cord's thickness could be imaged, while clearing allowed imaging of the entire thickness of the spinal cord. X axis: perpendicular to the sample; Y axis: longitudinal to the sample and Z axis represent the depth of imaging. Scale bars **(A,B)**: 5 mm.

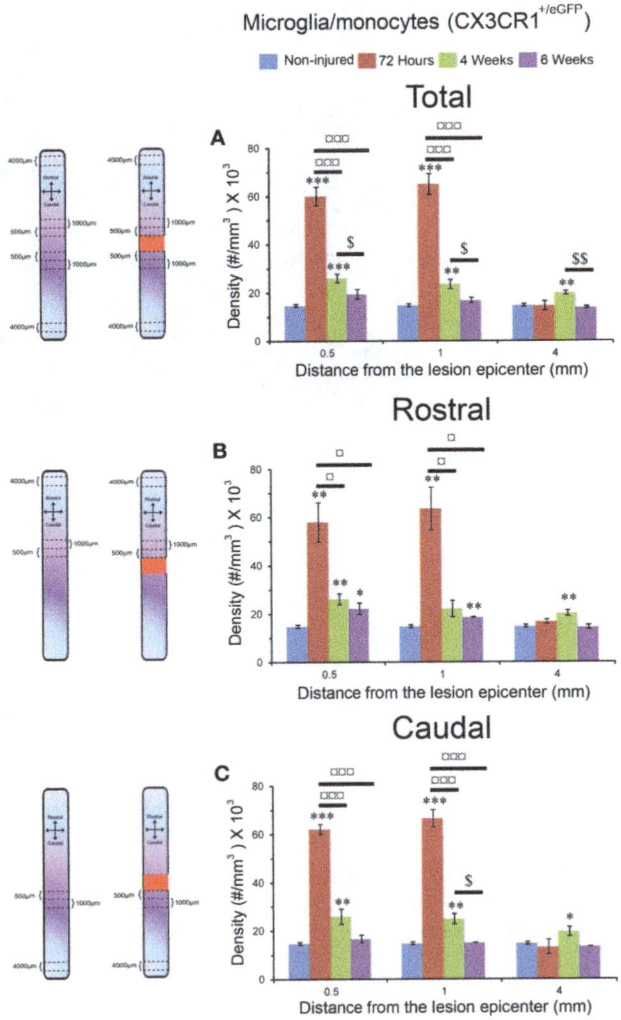

FIGURE 3 | Increased microglia/monocytes density early after SCI. Schematic drawing of longitudinal spinal cord from non-injured control and after transection illustrating the lesion site (red rectangle) and the different zones (dashed lines) where microglia/monocytes densities were measured. Bar graphs displaying SCI-induced changes in microglia/monocytes density at different time-points and distances from the lesion epicenter. A strong increase in microglia/monocytes density is observed at 72 hours post-lesion both rostral and caudal to the lesion site **(A–C)**. $^{*}P < 0.05$, $^{**}P < 0.01$, $^{***}P < 0.001$ compared to un-injured control, $^{□}P < 0.05$, $^{□□□}P < 0.001$ compared to 72 h post-lesion, $^{\$}P < 0.05$ compared to 4 weeks post-lesion group, un-paired *t*-test.

Increased Microglia/Monocytes Density after Complete SCI

We used tetrahydrofuran (THF)-based clearing to render the adult spinal cord transparent while preserving eGFP signal in microglia/monocytes (**Figure 2**). While un-cleared tissue can only be imaged at a depth of <100 μm using two-photon microscope (**Figures 2A,C**), clearing of the spinal cord permitted imaging throughout its entire thickness (**Figures 2B,D**).

Using two-photon image analysis, we determined microglia/monocytes density in samples that previously underwent *ex vivo* diffusion MRI at acute (72 hours) and chronic stages (4 and 6 weeks) after complete SCI and compared to that of un-injured controls. Microglial/monocytes density was evaluated in CX3CR1$^{+/eGFP}$ mice at distances of 0–500, 500–1,000, and 4,000–4,500 μm from the lesion site (**Figure 3**). The increase in microglia/monocytes density was particularly evident at acute compared to more chronic stages (**Figure 3**). In addition, as expected, areas adjacent to the lesion site displayed a greater increase in microglia/monocytes density than more distal regions (**Figure 3**). Quantitative analysis revealed significant increases in microglia/monocytes density at 72 hours and 4 weeks post-lesion compared to non-injured controls (**Figure 3A**). By 6 weeks post-injury, microglia/monocytes density decreased considerably, retuning to non-injured control level at 4 mm distal to the lesion site (**Figure 3A**). Overall, microglia/monocytes density was similarly elevated both rostral and caudal to the lesion site (**Figures 3B,C**).

Together, these data show (1) there is a greater increase in microglial/monocytes density contiguous to the lesion compared to more distal regions, (2) the highest microglial/monocytes density is observed at 72 hours post-injury, followed by a decrease at chronic stages after SCI, and (3) there is generally a similar increase in microglial/monocytes density after injury rostral and caudal to the lesion site.

Changes in Microglial/Monocytes Somata Morphology Are Different Rostral and Caudal to the Lesion Site

Microglia/monocytes activation is characterized by a pronounced modification of their morphology. We thus quantified the surface area (μm^2) and volume (μm^3) of the somata of at least

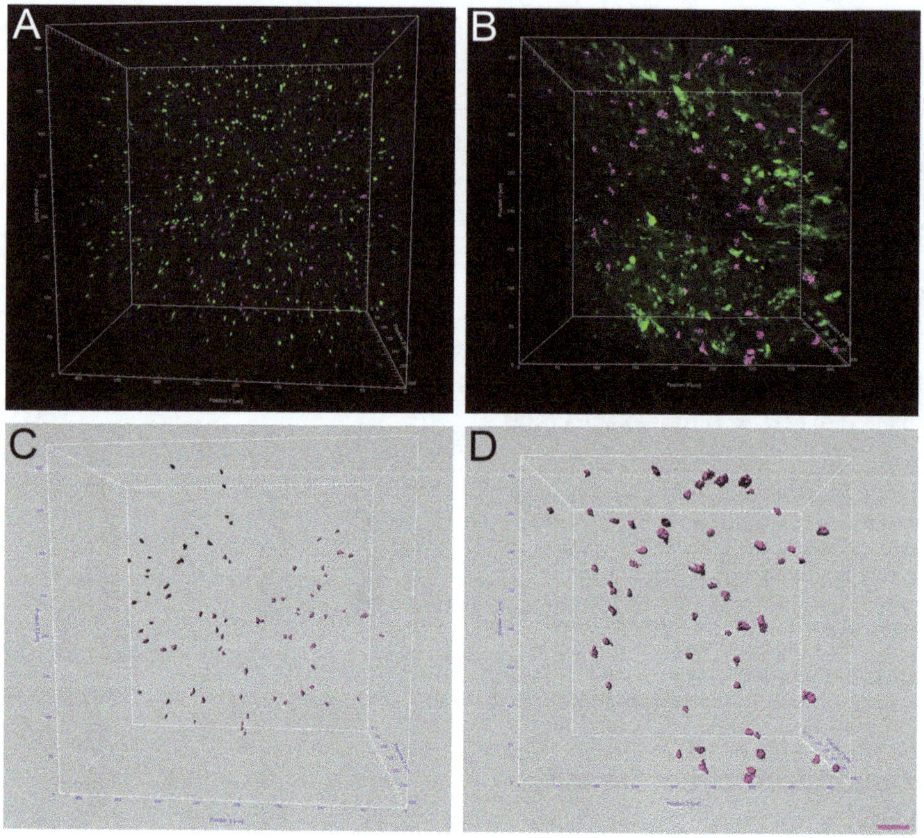

FIGURE 4 | Increased microglia/monocytes activation after SCI. Two-photon micrographs displaying representative eGFP-positive microglia used for morphological analysis **(A,B)**. A sub-population of microglia/monocytes somata with no overlapping was selected (pink objects in **C,D**) for morphological analysis from both non-injured control **(A,C)** and injured animals **(B,D)**. 3D reconstruction and Imaris-based quantification of microglia/monocytes somata morphology in CX3CR1$^{+/eGFP}$ mice **(C,D)**. Scale bars **(A–D)**: 50 μm.

190 individual cells per time-point. Only microglia/monocytes without overlapping somata with their neighboring cells were selected for morphological analysis (**Figure 4**, *pink objects*). Analyses were done at 500 μm rostral to the lesion site as well as 4 mm both rostral and caudal to the lesion epicenter (**Figure 5**). The increase in microglia/monocytes somata surface area and volume was particularly evident in the 500 μm segment rostral to the lesion than in more distant regions on both the rostral and caudal sides (**Figure 5**). Quantitative analysis of microglia/monocyte soma surface area and volume in proximity to the lesion site revealed a significant increase from 72 hours to 6 weeks post-injury (**Figures 5B,E**). Rostral to the lesion site, the size of microglia/monocytes somata displayed a time-dependent increase (**Figures 5A,D**), while caudal to the lesion site there was a continuous decrease in somata surface area and volume (**Figures 5C,F**). Thus, time course analysis of microglia/monocytes somata morphology revealed opposite responses rostral (**Figures 5A,D**) and caudal (**Figures 5C,F**) to the lesion site.

Together, these findings demonstrated that (1) microglia/monocytes display over a 5-fold increase in average somata size adjacent to the lesion site that remains elevated up to 6 weeks post-lesion, (2) microglia/monocytes rostral to the lesion site display a time-dependent increase in somata size, and (3) microglia/monocytes caudal to the lesion site display a time-dependent decrease in somata size. We thus highlight variation between segments located symmetrically rostral and caudal to the lesion site.

Microglial/Monocytes Density Coincides with Lesion Extension Following Complete SCI

We then investigated the potential link between injury-induced tissue re-organization and neuroinflammation in the injured spinal cord by examining putative correlation between *ex vivo* diffusion MRI and microglia/monocytes density. The increase in lesion extension, which was greatest at 72 hours post-injury amongst all the time points analyzed, coincided with the upsurge of microglia/monocytes density (**Figures 1E, 3A** and **Supplementary Figure 2**).

Lastly, we compared ADC values with the density and morphology of microglia/monocytes somata (**Supplementary**

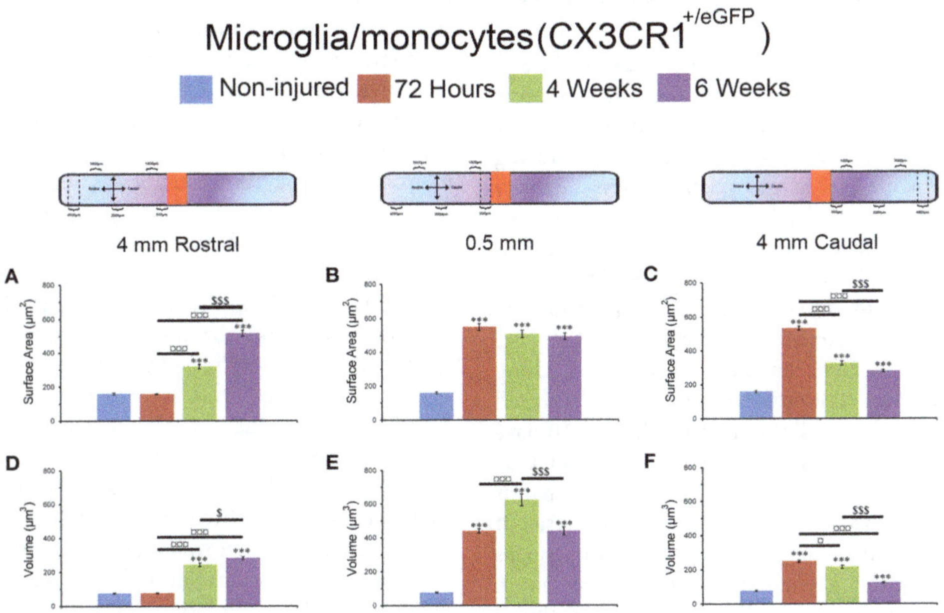

FIGURE 5 | Morphological alterations of microglia/monocytes after SCI. Schematic drawing of longitudinal spinal cord after transection illustrating the lesion site (red rectangle) and the different zones (dashed lines) where microglia/monocytes morphologies were measured. Bar graphs indicating SCI-induced alterations in microglial/monocytes somata surface area **(A–C)** and volume **(D–F)** at different time-points after lesion. A pronounced increase in microglial/monocytes somata surface area and volume was evident at 500 µm rostral to the lesion epicenter as early as 72 hours post-lesion that continued until 6 weeks post-lesion **(B,E)**. At 4 mm rostral to the lesion site, microglia/monocytes displayed a time-dependent increase starting at 4 weeks **(A,D)**, whereas 4 mm caudal to the lesion there was a time-dependent decrease in microglia/monocytes somata surface area and volume starting at 72 hours **(C,F)**. ***$P < 0.001$ compared to un-injured control, *$P < 0.05$, ***$P < 0.001$ compared to 72 hours post-lesion, $^{\$}P < 0.05$ and $^{\$\$\$}P < 0.001$ compared to 4 weeks post-lesion group, un-paired *t*-test.

TABLE 1 | Quantification of longitudinal ADC over time following SCI.

	72 hours vs. NI	4 weeks vs. NI	6 weeks vs. NI	72 hours vs. 4 weeks	72 hours vs. 6 weeks	4 vs. 6 weeks
Total: −4 to 4 mm (Wilcoxon)	**	**	**	ns	**	**
Rostral: −4 to 0 (paired *t*-test)	ns	ns	ns	ns	ns	ns
Caudal: 0 to +4 mm (paired *t*-test)	**	ns	**	ns	*	***

*Comparison between injured animals at different time-points post-injury and non-injured animals. The Wilcoxon signed-rank test was used to compare ADC values between groups along an 8 mm segment centered on the lesion site. "Total" represents the entire segment of the spinal cord (**Figure 1G**; −4 to +4 mm). A paired-t-test was used to compare ADC values between groups in the rostral and caudal segments. "Rostral" and "caudal" refer to quantifications on each side of the lesion (**Figure 1G**; rostral: −4 to lesion; caudal: +4 mm to lesion). Percentages represent the comparison with the value from un-injured control group. NI, non-injured, ns, non-significant. *P < 0.05 and **P < 0.01, un-paired t-test.*

Figure 2). Rostral to the lesion site, the ADC at all time-points post-injury was similar to that of the non-injured control (**Figure 1G**). At the lesion site, ADC increased in a time-dependent manner (**Figure 1G**). All injured groups, except at 4 weeks post-injury (**Table 1**), displayed a higher ADC caudal to the lesion than the non-injured control. Unlike ADC, microglia/monocytes somata showed changes in surface area and volume both rostral and caudal to the epicenter (**Figures 1G, 5** and **Supplementary Figure 2**). Thus, ADC does not seem to be correlated with microglia/monocytes somata morphology.

DISCUSSION

In the current study we performed a transection of the spinal cord in transgenic mice that express eGFP in microglia/monocytes ($CX3CR1^{+/eGFP}$). We then carried out *ex vivo* diffusion MRI analyses of the spinal cord at acute (72 hours) and chronic (4 and 6 weeks) stages after the lesion, followed by tetrahydrofuran-based clearing and quantitative assessment of microglia/monocytes density and somata morphology using two-photon microscopy. Diffusion MRI offers better contrast than T2 weighted images allowing a more accurate identification of damaged tissues. Our findings suggest an early increase in the extension of the lesion that is significantly reduced by 4 weeks post-injury. Interestingly, the increase in lesion extension positively coincides with an increase in microglia/monocytes density. We also observe differences in microglia/monocytes somata morphology rostral and caudal to the lesion site that is compatible with cell debris and/or myelin clearance. This is the first study that combines *ex vivo* diffusion MRI with two-photon microscopy to document spatiotemporal changes in microglia/monocytes after severe SCI.

Microglia/Monocytes Density after Severe SCI

Despite the established presence of neuroinflammation in SCI pathophysiology, only a few studies have investigated post-injury microglia/monocytes density in mice, and findings are contradictory (Schnell et al., 1999; Kigerl et al., 2006; Stirling and Yong, 2008). A peak increase in microglia/monocytes density had been shown between 7 and 14 days post-injury (Schnell et al., 1999; Kigerl et al., 2006) but has also been reported as early as 2 days post-lesion (Stirling and Yong, 2008). In addition to the different techniques used to quantify microglia/monocyte density, differences in mouse strains may also account for these discrepancies (Basso et al., 2006; Lapointe et al., 2006). Using tissue clearing, Erturk and colleagues more recently reported a pronounced increase in microglia/monocytes density 10 days after spinal cord hemisection in mice (Erturk et al., 2012). Our quantitative analysis in severely injured spinal cords expands previous reports and provides a comprehensive analysis of microglia/monocytes density not only at acute and chronic stages after SCI but also at different distances from the lesion epicenter. Specifically, we observed that microglia/monocytes density is increased at 72 hours post-injury, then significantly reduced by 4 and 6 weeks with no major differences between the regions rostral and caudal to the lesion site. Although the pronounced increase in microglia/monocytes density at 72 hours post-injury may be attributed to infiltrating monocytes, CNS resident microglia can proliferate in the absence of peripheral monocytes (Elmore et al., 2014). Recent molecular study from our laboratory also confirmed that microglia are primarily involved in proliferation at 72 hours post-lesion (Noristani et al., 2017). In fact, resident microglia display greater proliferation compared to infiltrating monocytes after SCI (Greenhalgh and David, 2014). The increase in microglia/monocyte density at 72 hours occurred concomitantly with the greatest lesion extension observed by diffusion MRI. Modifications in diffusion MRI represent changes in the displacement of water molecules within different tissue compartments of the spinal cord. Thus, the positive association between microglia/monocytes density and lesion extension most likely corresponds to the early vasogenic edema resulting from plasma leakage and concomitant monocyte infiltration/microglia proliferation. Given that CX3CR1 is expressed both in infiltrating monocytes and resident microglia, in the current study, we cannot distinguish the exact proportion of these cells after SCI.

SCI Induces Pronounced Alterations in Microglia/Monocytes Morphology

Although numerous studies have reported microglia/monocytes activation after injury (David and Kroner, 2011), no study to our knowledge has carried out quantitative analysis of injury-induced alteration of microglia/monocytes morphology. The most notable morphological alterations include a more than 3-fold increase in somata surface area and a more than 6-fold increase in somata volume that is most evident adjacent to the lesion site. The increase in somata volume induced by SCI is considerably higher than that reported in microglia following physiological stimulation, such as voluntary wheel running (Rodriguez et al., 2015). Interestingly, microglial/monocytes somata morphology distal to the lesion epicenter showed a clear difference in the regions rostral and caudal to the injury site (see **Figure 6**). Rostral to the lesion site, microglia/monocytes displayed a time-dependent increase in their reactivity that continued up to 6 weeks post-injury. In contrast, the greatest microglia/monocytes reactivity was observed caudal to the lesion site at 72 hours and decreased progressively between 4 and 6 weeks post-lesion. Measurements of ADC rostral and caudal to the lesion site also showed strong differences. Specifically, the ADC rostral to the lesion remained similar to that of un-injured controls throughout the 6 weeks following spinal cord trauma. In contrast, the ADC caudal to the lesion was significantly higher in all injured groups than the non-injured control. In the spinal cord, water diffuses in the white matter along the fibrous myelinated axons, which are orientated in a rostro-caudal direction. Diffusion MRI parameters, such as ADC are very sensitive to the changes in axonal integrity that occur during demyelination and inflammation (Stroman et al., 2014). Thus, an elevated ADC caudal to the lesion site might reflect demyelination. Indeed, even though limited and/or inadequate re-myelination may occur caudal to the lesion site after incomplete SCI (Alizadeh et al., 2015), this does not occur after a transection of the spinal cord. Microglia are predominantly involved in phagocytosis of damaged myelin sheaths and clearance of debris of axons caudal to the injury site that undergo Wallerian degeneration. The time-dependent decrease in microglia/monocytes reactivity caudal to the lesion site might thus reflect reduced myelin/debris clearance that is almost completed by 6 weeks post-injury. Rostral to the lesion site, the time-dependent augmentation in microglia/monocytes

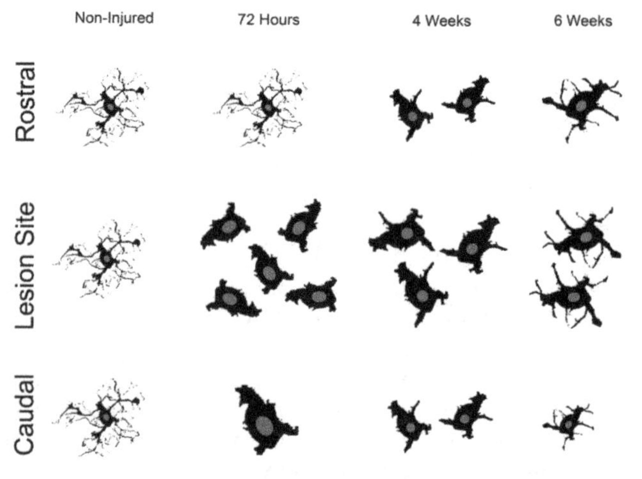

FIGURE 6 | Schematic cartoon illustrating the overall microglial/monocytes response after SCI rostral and caudal to the lesion epicenter. Rostral to the lesion site, microglia/monocytes undergo gradual activation that continues up to 6 weeks post-lesion. Adjacent to the lesion site, there is a pronounced increase in microglia/monocytes density and reactivity. Subsequently, microglia/monocytes density is reduced adjacent to the lesion site; however, their increased reactivity is sustained at more chronic stages after injury. Caudal to the lesion site, pronounced microglia/monocytes reactivity is evident early after lesion and is then reduced at more chronic stages.

reactivity up to 6 weeks post-injury may correspond to a dying-back phenomenon and/or abortive regeneration. Indeed, while the distal segment of a cut axon undergoes Wallerian degeneration, the proximal segment dies back over a period of few days or weeks. At the tip of the axon rostral to the lesion site, "retraction balls" form and are physically disconnected from the axon. Moreover, the edge of the cut axon presents a structure that resembles a growth cone but is "dystrophic" (Steward, 2014), suggesting that there is a persistent regeneration attempt by the injured axon. However, since injured axons do not regrow to their targets, this regenerative process had been named "abortive regeneration" by Ramón y Cajal (1907). We thus hypothesize that the activated microglia/monocytes we observed rostral to the lesion site at 4 and 6 weeks post-lesion correspond to a delayed clearance of debris resulting from dying back and/or abortive regeneration. In addition, we cannot exclude the possibility that there may also be a greater infiltration of monocytes from the periphery caudal to the lesion site compared to rostral.

In this study we show that the greatest lesion extension observed following spinal cord transection, quantified using *ex vivo* diffusion MRI, occurs at 72 hours post-injury and coincides with changes in microglia/monocytes density but not with somata morphology. Using cleared spinal cords and two-photon imaging we also observed differences over time in microglia/monocytes somata morphology which, combined with diffusion MRI results, is compatible with time-dependent phagocytosis of debris by microglia/monocytes rostral and caudal to the lesion site.

CONCLUSION

Our study confirms that the combination of *ex vivo* diffusion MRI and two-photon microscopy may be used effectively to follow structural tissue alterations and their putative relation to a given cell population after CNS lesion. However, no direct correlation was found between microglia/monocytes morphology and ADC that may results from the different resolution scales of the two methods. Analysis with the two-photon microscopy highlighted that differential microglia/monocytes reactivity caudal and rostral to the lesion may correspond to temporal differences in clearing processes and/or remaining of non-damaged axons. Our study points out the necessity of adjusting therapeutic strategies targeting microglia/monocytes after SCI to time post-injury and location of the lesion site.

AUTHOR CONTRIBUTIONS

HN conceptualized the research, participated in the design of the study, performed all experiments, analyzed the data and contributed to the writing of the manuscript; HB participated in the design and analysis of the two-photon study; GS participated in MRI acquisition and analysis; PA participated in spinal cord clarification and in two-photon acquisition and analysis; RS participated in the design of the MRI coil; NL participated in SCI experiments; EA participated in MRI acquisition; NT participated in two-photon experiments; CG participated in MRI acquisition and analysis; CC participated in the design of the MRI coil and FP conceptualized the research, designed the project, participated in the analysis and interpretation of data, drafting the work and final approval. All authors read and approved the final manuscript.

FUNDING

This work was supported by the patient organizations "Verticale" and "Demain Debout Aquitaine" [to FP, HN, and GS] and [to FP, HN, and PA], respectively, a European Research Council grant (FP7-IDEAS-ERC 311610 to NT) as well as by the LabeX NUMEV [to GS]. Funding bodies had no role in the design of the study, analysis, and interpretation of data and in writing the manuscript.

ACKNOWLEDGMENTS

We thank Alain Privat and Sylvain Bartolami for their constructive discussion. We also thank Anthony Ciston for correction of the English text.

SUPPLEMENTARY MATERIAL

Supplementary Figure 1 | *Ex vivo* MRI assessments following SCI. *Ex vivo* T2 weighted images (**B**, **D**, **F**, **H**, and **J**) and diffusion MRI (**A**, **C**, **E**, **G**, and **I**) from the same mouse spinal cord rostral **(A–D)** within **(E,F)** and caudal **(G–J)** to the lesion epicenter **(E–F)**. Panels **(C,D)** correspond to annotated images of **(A,B)**; **(I,J)** correspond to annotated images of **(G,H)**. Entire spinal cord (surrounded in green in **C**,**D** and **I**,**J**), damaged spinal cord tissues (surrounded in red in **E**, **F**, and **I**) and intact gray matter (surrounded in blue in **C**, **D** and **I**, **J**). Note that the superior contrast of DWI as compared to T2 weighted images allows better identification of damaged tissues **(G–J)**. Photograph of the custom-made ribbon solenoid coil used for *ex vivo* diffusion MRI acquisition **(F)**.

Supplementary Figure 2 | Bar graph representations of Tables 2A–D.

Supplementary Video 1 | A cleared spinal cord of an un-injured CX3CR1$^{+/eGFP}$ mouse imaged with two-photon microscopy to assess microglia/monocytes density. Clearing of the spinal cord substantially improves the depth of two-photon imaging. For fully automated counting of microglia/monocytes, scans were converted into 3D objects. The animation was created using Imaris.

REFERENCES

Abdanipour, A., Tiraihi, T., Taheri, T., and Kazemi, H. (2013). Microglial activation in rat experimental spinal cord injury model. *Iran. Biomed. J.* 17, 214–220. doi: 10.6091/ibj.1213.2013

Adamczak, J. M., Farr, T. D., Seehafer, J. U., Kalthoff, D., and Hoehn, M. (2010). High field BOLD response to forepaw stimulation in the mouse. *Neuroimage* 51, 704–712. doi: 10.1016/j.neuroimage.2010.02.083

Alizadeh, A., Dyck, S. M., and Karimi-Abdolrezaee, S. (2015). Myelin damage and repair in pathologic CNS: challenges and prospects. *Front. Mol. Neurosci.* 8:35. doi: 10.3389/fnmol.2015.00035

Antri, M., Barthe, J. Y., Mouffle, C., and Orsal, D. (2005). Long-lasting recovery of locomotor function in chronic spinal rat following chronic combined pharmacological stimulation of serotonergic receptors with 8-OHDPAT and quipazine. *Neurosci. Lett.* 384, 162–167. doi: 10.1016/j.neulet.2005.04.062

Basso, D. M., Beattie, M. S., and Bresnahan, J. C. (1996). Graded histological and locomotor outcomes after spinal cord contusion using the NYU weight-drop device versus transection. *Exp. Neurol.* 139, 244–256. doi: 10.1006/exnr.1996.0098

Basso, D. M., Fisher, L. C., Anderson, A. J., Jakeman, L. B., McTigue, D. M., and Popovich, P. G. (2006). Basso mouse scale for locomotion detects differences in recovery after spinal cord injury in five common mouse strains. *J. Neurotrauma* 23, 635–659. doi: 10.1089/neu.2006.23.635

Bastiani, M., and Roebroeck, A. (2015). Unraveling the multiscale structural organization and connectivity of the human brain: the role of diffusion MRI. *Front. Neuroanat.* 9:77. doi: 10.3389/fnana.2015.00077

Beck, K. D., Nguyen, H. X., Galvan, M. D., Salazar, D. L., Woodruff, T. M., and Anderson, A. J. (2010). Quantitative analysis of cellular inflammation after traumatic spinal cord injury: evidence for a multiphasic inflammatory response in the acute to chronic environment. *Brain* 133(Pt. 2), 433–447. doi: 10.1093/brain/awp322

Bennett, M. L., Bennett, F. C., Liddelow, S. A., Ajami, B., Zamanian, J. L., Fernhoff, N. B., et al. (2016). New tools for studying microglia in the mouse and human CNS. *Proc. Natl. Acad. Sci. U.S.A.* 113, E1738–E1746. doi: 10.1073/pnas.1525528113

Bonny, J. M., Gaviria, M., Donnat, J. P., Jean, B., Privat, A., and Renou, J. P. (2004). Nuclear magnetic resonance microimaging of mouse spinal cord *in vivo*. *Neurobiol. Dis.* 15, 474–482. doi: 10.1016/j.nbd.2003.1 1.026

Butovsky, O., Jedrychowski, M. P., Moore, C. S., Cialic, R., Lanser, A. J., Gabriely, G., et al. (2014). Identification of a unique TGF-beta-dependent molecular and functional signature in microglia. *Nat. Neurosci.* 17, 131–143. doi: 10.1038/nn.3599

Chiu, I. M., Morimoto, E. T., Goodarzi, H., Liao, J. T., O'Keeffe, S., Phatnani, H. P., et al. (2013). A neurodegeneration-specific gene-expression signature of acutely isolated microglia from an amyotrophic lateral sclerosis mouse model. *Cell Rep.* 4, 385–401. doi: 10.1016/j.celrep.2013.06.018

Chung, K., Wallace, J., Kim, S. Y., Kalyanasundaram, S., Andalman, A. S., Davidson, T. J., et al. (2013). Structural and molecular interrogation of intact biological systems. *Nature* 497, 332–337. doi: 10.1038/nature 12107

Coillot, C., Sidiboulenouar, R., Nativel, E., Zanca, M., Alibert, E., and Saint Martin, G. (2016). Signal modeling of a MRI ribbon solenoid coil dedicated to spinal cord injuries investigations. *J. Sens. Sens. Sys.* 5, 137–145. doi: 10.5194/jsss-5-137-2016

David, S., and Kroner, A. (2011). Repertoire of microglial and macrophage responses after spinal cord injury. *Nat. Rev. Neurosci.* 12, 388–399. doi: 10.1038/nrn3053

Denic, A., Macura, S. I., Mishra, P., Gamez, J. D., Rodriguez, M., and Pirko, I. (2011). MRI in rodent models of brain disorders. *Neurotherapeutics* 8, 3–18. doi: 10.1007/s13311-010-0002-4

Elmore, M. R., Najafi, A. R., Koike, M. A., Dagher, N. N., Spangenberg, E. E., Rice, R. A., et al. (2014). Colony-stimulating factor 1 receptor signaling is necessary for microglia viability, unmasking a microglia progenitor cell in the adult brain. *Neuron* 82, 380–397. doi: 10.1016/j.neuron.2014.02.040

Erturk, A., Mauch, C. P., Hellal, F., Forstner, F., Keck, T., Becker, K., et al. (2012). Three-dimensional imaging of the unsectioned adult spinal cord to assess axon regeneration and glial responses after injury. *Nat. Med.* 18, 166–171. doi: 10.1038/nm.2600

Gautier, E. L., Shay, T., Miller, J., Greter, M., Jakubzick, C., Ivanov, S., et al. (2012). Gene-expression profiles and transcriptional regulatory pathways that underlie the identity and diversity of mouse tissue macrophages. *Nat. Immunol.* 13, 1118–1128. doi: 10.1038/ni.2419

Gosselin, D., Link, V. M., Romanoski, C. E., Fonseca, G. J., Eichenfield, D. Z., Spann, N. J., et al. (2014). Environment drives selection and function of enhancers controlling tissue-specific macrophage identities. *Cell* 159, 1327–1340. doi: 10.1016/j.cell.2014.11.023

Greenhalgh, A. D., and David, S. (2014). Differences in the phagocytic response of microglia and peripheral macrophages after spinal cord injury and its effects on cell death. *J. Neurosci.* 34, 6316–6322. doi: 10.1523/JNEUROSCI.4912-13.2014

Jung, S., Aliberti, J., Graemmel, P., Sunshine, M. J., Kreutzberg, G. W., Sher, A., et al. (2000). Analysis of fractalkine receptor CX(3)CR1 function by targeted deletion and green fluorescent protein reporter gene insertion. *Mol. Cell. Biol.* 20, 4106–4114. doi: 10.1128/MCB.20.11.4106-4114.2000

Kettenmann, H., Hanisch, U. K., Noda, M., and Verkhratsky, A. (2011). Physiology of microglia. *Physiol. Rev.* 91, 461–553. doi: 10.1152/physrev.00011.2010

Kigerl, K. A., Gensel, J. C., Ankeny, D. P., Alexander, J. K., Donnelly, D. J., and Popovich, P. G. (2009). Identification of two distinct macrophage subsets with divergent effects causing either neurotoxicity or regeneration in the injured mouse spinal cord. *J. Neurosci.* 29, 13435–13444. doi: 10.1523/JNEUROSCI.3257-09.2009

Kigerl, K. A., McGaughy, V. M., and Popovich, P. G. (2006). Comparative analysis of lesion development and intraspinal inflammation in four strains of mice following spinal contusion injury. *J. Comp. Neurol.* 494, 578–594. doi: 10.1002/cne.20827

Lapointe, N. P., Ung, R. V., Bergeron, M., Cote, M., and Guertin, P. A. (2006). Strain-dependent recovery of spontaneous hindlimb movement in spinal cord transected mice (CD1, C57BL/6, BALB/c). *Behav. Neurosci.* 120, 826–834. doi: 10.1037/0735-7044.120.4.826

Lee, D. H., and Lee, J. K. (2013). Animal models of axon regeneration after spinal cord injury. *Neurosci. Bull.* 29, 436–444. doi: 10.1007/s12264-013-1365-4

M'Dahoma, S., Bourgoin, S., Kayser, V., Barthelemy, S., Chevarin, C., Chali, F., et al. (2014). Spinal cord transection-induced allodynia in rats-behavioral, physiopathological and pharmacological characterization. *PLoS ONE* 9:e102027. doi: 10.1371/journal.pone.0102027

Noristani, H. N., Gerber, Y. N., Sabourin, J.-C., Le Corre, M., Lonjon, N., Mestre-Frances, N., et al. (2017). RNA-Seq analysis of microglia reveals time-dependent activation of specific genetic programs following spinal cord injury. *Front. Mol. Neurosci.* 10:90. doi: 10.3389/fnmol.2017.00090

Noristani, H. N., Lonjon, N., Cardoso, M., Le Corre, M., Chan-Seng, E., Captier, G., et al. (2015). Correlation of *in vivo* and *ex vivo* (1)H-MRI with histology in two severities of mouse spinal cord injury. *Front. Neuroanat.* 9:24. doi: 10.3389/fnana.2015.00024

Onifer, S. M., Rabchevsky, A. G., and Scheff, S. W. (2007). Rat models of traumatic spinal cord injury to assess motor recovery. *ILAR J.* 48, 385–395. doi: 10.1093/ilar.48.4.385

Ramón y Cajal, S. R. (1907). *Regeneración de los Nervios*. [Translation and edited by J. Bresler (1908) Studien über Nervenregeneration, Johann Ambrosius Barth].

Renier, N., Wu, Z., Simon, D. J., Yang, J., Ariel, P., and Tessier-Lavigne, M. (2014). iDISCO: a simple, rapid method to immunolabel large tissue samples for volume imaging. *Cell* 159, 896–910. doi: 10.1016/j.cell.2014.10.010

Rodriguez, J. J., Noristani, H. N., and Verkhratsky, A. (2015). Microglial response to Alzheimer's disease is differentially modulated by voluntary wheel running and enriched environments. *Brain Struct. Funct.* 220, 941–953. doi: 10.1007/s00429-013-0693-5

Schmitz, G., Leuthauser-Jaschinski, K., and Orso, E. (2009). Are circulating monocytes as microglia orthologues appropriate biomarker targets for neuronal diseases? *Cent. Nerv. Syst. Agents Med. Chem.* 9, 307–330. doi: 10.2174/187152409789630424

Schnell, L., Fearn, S., Klassen, H., Schwab, M. E., and Perry, V. H. (1999). Acute inflammatory responses to mechanical lesions in the CNS: differences between brain and spinal cord. *Eur. J. Neurosci.* 11, 3648–3658. doi: 10.1046/j.1460-9568.1999.00792.x

Song, S. K., Sun, S. W., Ju, W. K., Lin, S. J., Cross, A. H., and Neufeld, A. H. (2003). Diffusion tensor imaging detects and differentiates axon and myelin degeneration in mouse optic nerve after retinal ischemia. *Neuroimage* 20, 1714–1722. doi: 10.1016/j.neuroimage.2003.07.005

Steward, O. (2014). *Neural Repair and Rehabilitation*. Minneapolis, MN: United Council for Neurologic Subspecialties.

Stirling, D. P., and Yong, V. W. (2008). Dynamics of the inflammatory response after murine spinal cord injury revealed by flow cytometry. *J. Neurosci. Res.* 86, 1944–1958. doi: 10.1002/jnr.21659

Stroman, P. W., Wheeler-Kingshott, C., Bacon, M., Schwab, J. M., Bosma, R., Brooks, J., et al. (2014). The current state-of-the-art of spinal cord imaging: methods. *Neuroimage* 84, 1070–1081. doi: 10.1016/j.neuroimage.2013.04.124

Tian, D. S., Dong, Q., Pan, D. J., He, Y., Yu, Z. Y., Xie, M. J., et al. (2007). Attenuation of astrogliosis by suppressing of microglial proliferation with the cell cycle inhibitor olomoucine in rat spinal cord injury model. *Brain Res.* 1154, 206–214. doi: 10.1016/j.brainres.2007.04.005

Tomer, R., Ye, L., Hsueh, B., and Deisseroth, K. (2014). Advanced CLARITY for rapid and high-resolution imaging of intact tissues. *Nat. Protoc.* 9, 1682–1697. doi: 10.1038/nprot.2014.123

van den Berg, M. E., Castellote, J. M., Mahillo-Fernandez, I., and de Pedro-Cuesta, J. (2010). Incidence of spinal cord injury worldwide: a systematic review. *Neuroepidemiology* 34, 184–192. discussion: 192. doi: 10.1159/000279335

Vedantam, A., Jirjis, M. B., Schmit, B. D., Wang, M. C., Ulmer, J. L., and Kurpad, S. N. (2014). Diffusion tensor imaging of the spinal cord: insights from animal and human studies. *Neurosurgery* 74, 1–8. discussion: 8; quiz: 8. doi: 10.1227/neu.0000000000000171

Wang, F., Huang, S. L., He, X. J., and Li, X. H. (2014). Determination of the ideal rat model for spinal cord injury by diffusion tensor imaging. *Neuroreport* 25, 1386–1392. doi: 10.1097/WNR.0000000000000278

Wheeler-Kingshott, C. A., Stroman, P. W., Schwab, J. M., Bacon, M., Bosma, R., Brooks, J., et al. (2014). The current state-of-the-art of spinal cord imaging: applications. *Neuroimage* 84, 1082–1093. doi: 10.1016/j.neuroimage.2013.07.014

Wolf, Y., Yona, S., Kim, K. W., and Jung, S. (2013). Microglia, seen from the CX3CR1 angle. *Front. Cell. Neurosci.* 7:26. doi: 10.3389/fncel.2013.00026

Yang, B., Treweek, J. B., Kulkarni, R. P., Deverman, B. E., Chen, C. K., Lubeck, E., et al. (2014). Single-cell phenotyping within transparent intact tissue through whole-body clearing. *Cell* 158, 945–958. doi: 10.1016/j.cell.2014.07.017

5

Recent Advances in the Study of Bipolar/Rod-Shaped Microglia and their Roles in Neurodegeneration

Ngan Pan Bennett Au [1] ***and Chi Him Eddie Ma*** [1,2,3]*

[1]Department of Biomedical Sciences, City University of Hong Kong, Kowloon Tong, Hong Kong, [2]Centre for Biosystems, Neuroscience, and Nanotechnology, City University of Hong Kong, Kowloon Tong, Hong Kong, [3]State Key Laboratory in Marine Pollution, City University of Hong Kong, Kowloon Tong, Hong Kong

***Correspondence:**
Chi Him Eddie Ma
eddiema@cityu.edu.hk

Microglia are the resident immune cells of the central nervous system (CNS) and they contribute to primary inflammatory responses following CNS injuries. The morphology of microglia is closely associated with their functional activities. Most previous research efforts have attempted to delineate the role of ramified and amoeboid microglia in the pathogenesis of neurodegenerative diseases. In addition to ramified and amoeboid microglia, bipolar/rod-shaped microglia were first described by Franz Nissl in 1899 and their presence in the brain was closely associated with the pathology of infectious diseases and sleeping disorders. However, studies relating to bipolar/rod-shaped microglia are very limited, largely due to the lack of appropriate *in vitro* and *in vivo* experimental models. Recent studies have reported the formation of bipolar/rod-shaped microglia trains in *in vivo* models of CNS injury, including diffuse brain injury, focal transient ischemia, optic nerve transection and laser-induced ocular hypertension (OHT). These bipolar/rod-shaped microglia formed end-to-end alignments in close proximity to the adjacent injured axons, but they showed no interactions with blood vessels or other types of glial cell. Recent studies have also reported on a highly reproducible *in vitro* culture model system to enrich bipolar/rod-shaped microglia that acts as a powerful tool with which to characterize this form of microglia. The molecular aspects of bipolar/rod-shaped microglia are of great interest in the field of CNS repair. This review article focuses on studies relating to the morphology and transformation of microglia into the bipolar/rod-shaped form, along with the differential gene expression and spatial distribution of bipolar/rod-shaped microglia in normal and pathological CNSs. The spatial arrangement of bipolar/rod-shaped microglia is crucial in the reorganization and remodeling of neuronal and synaptic circuitry following CNS injuries. Finally, we discuss the potential neuroprotective roles of bipolar/rod-shaped microglia, and the possibility of transforming ramified/amoeboid microglia into bipolar/rod-shaped microglia. This will be of considerable clinical benefit in the development of novel therapeutic strategies for treating various neurodegenerative diseases and promoting CNS repair after injury.

Keywords: bipolar/rod-shaped microglia, amoeboid microglia, ramified microglia, neurodegenerative diseases, synapse

INTRODUCTION

Microglia are generally considered as phenotypically diverse immune cells which reside in the central nervous system (CNS). The morphological changes of microglia are closely associated with their function and the microenvironment in which they reside (Chamak and Mallat, 1991; Suzumura et al., 1991; Szabo and Gulya, 2013; Tam and Ma, 2014; Tam et al., 2016). Under normal physiological conditions, microglia adopt a "surveying" phenotype, referred to as "ramified microglia" with compact cell bodies and elongated branching processes (Hanisch and Kettenmann, 2007). Ramified microglia frequently extend and retract their highly motile processes so that they can actively sense and survey their microenvironment to detect subtle changes, but without disrupting the existing neuronal circuitry (Nimmerjahn et al., 2005). Ramified microglia in the immediate vicinity of micro-lesions respond rapidly and quickly transform into an active state, thus allowing them to migrate towards the site of injury (Davalos et al., 2005; Nimmerjahn et al., 2005). Ramified microglia first thicken, withdraw their processes, enlarge their cell bodies, and subsequently transform into an amoeboid morphology. Amoeboid microglia are regarded as "activated" microglia since they are responsible for antigen presentation, the production of an exhaustive list of inflammatory cytokines, chemokines and neurotrophic factors and are responsible for the removal of cellular debris by phagocytosis (Wyss-Coray and Mucke, 2002; Glass et al., 2010). Recent studies have also shown that amoeboid microglia are closely associated with neurological disorders such as brain injuries, Alzheimer's disease (AD), Parkinson's disease (PD) and Huntington's disease (HD) in which chronic neuroinflammation is usually observed (Glass et al., 2010; Krause and Müller, 2010; Smith et al., 2012). Amoeboid microglia are also detected in early and late stages of the onset of neurodegenerative diseases (Lynch, 2009). Studying the association of microglia with disease progression is therefore very attractive to neuroscientists, particularly in terms of neurodegeneration and neuroprotection.

Over the past few decades, most studies have focused upon the well-characterized ramified and amoeboid microglia, and studies of bipolar/rod-shaped microglia remain scarce due to the lack of a well-established *in vitro* culture system and a highly reproducible *in vivo* animal model with which to study this form of microglia. There is compelling evidence to suggest that bipolar/rod-shaped microglia play a pivotal role in CNS repair since they align end-to-end along with the damaged axons following traumatic brain injury (Ziebell et al., 2012; Taylor et al., 2014). Bipolar/rod-shaped microglia are also highly phagocytic and proliferative in nature (Ziebell et al., 2012; Tam and Ma, 2014), and are involved in the internalization of degenerating neurons following CNS injury (Yuan et al., 2015). Bipolar/rod-shaped microglia express a distinctive transcriptional profile in response to immunological stimuli such as lipopolysaccharides (LPS), and quickly transform into amoeboid microglia (Tam and Ma, 2014; Tam et al., 2016). This suggests that bipolar/rod-shaped microglia might be a transitional stage between the ramified and amoeboid microglia (Suzumura et al., 1990; Bohatschek et al., 2001; Jonas et al., 2012). A recent case study involving autopsy of over 160 patients showed that the presence of bipolar/rod-shaped microglia in the hippocampus and cerebral cortex was directly related to an AD cohort with aging and AD-related pathology such as dementia, and the formation of senile plaques and neurofibrillary tangles (NFTs; Bachstetter et al., 2015, 2017).

In this review article, we summarize our current understanding of bipolar/rod-shaped microglia based upon recent studies which have defined the role of this form of microglia in neurological diseases. We also discuss the potential neuroprotective role of bipolar/rod-shaped microglia in neurodegenerative diseases. Accumulating evidence suggests that the formation of bipolar/rod-shaped microglia might be potentially beneficial, not only in protecting the CNS neurons against progressive neuronal degeneration induced by chronic neuroinflammation, but also in helping with the reorganization of neuronal circuitry. This review aims to provide a more in-depth understanding of bipolar/rod-shaped microglia in order to provide new focus in the development of therapeutic strategies for neurodegenerative diseases.

THE DISCOVERY AND IDENTIFICATION OF BIPOLAR/ROD-SHAPED MICROGLIA

Bipolar/rod-shaped microglia were first identified as an activated form of microglia by Nissl (1899) more than a century ago. In this original study, Nissl examined glia cell morphology in cerebral cortices from patients who suffered from paralytic dementia, and he described this form of microglia as "strung-out, extremely slim with infinitely long processes". These bipolar/rod-shaped microglia extend their processes into pyramidal neuronal layers and are aligned with the growing tips of dendrites from nearby neurons (Nissl, 1899). Further studies showed that bipolar/rod-shaped microglia were also present in cerebral cortices in neurological disorders associated with typhus infections and syphilis, as well as sleeping disorders (Spielmeyer, 1922). The incidence of these neurological disorders was dramatically reduced, largely due to the discovery of penicillin. Thus, studies on this microglia subtype gradually reduced and researchers became unfamiliar with this form of microglia due to their rare occurrence in pathological brains (Graeber, 2010). This might account for our limited knowledge of bipolar/rod-shaped microglia, even though they were discovered more than a century ago.

Over the past two decades, bipolar/rod-shaped microglia were observed in several chronic neuropathological disorders, including viral encephalitis, lead encephalopathy and subacute sclerosing panencephalitis (SSPE). Patients with viral encephalitis exhibit microglial nodule formation in the brain which represents a hallmark pathological feature, regardless of the type and origin of the virus. This microglial nodule consists of a bundle of activated bipolar/rod-shaped microglia, reactive astrocytes, infiltrated macrophage and degenerating axons (Nelson et al., 2002). In a rat model of chronic lead (a heavy metal) intoxication, microglia were transformed into bipolar/rod-shaped with enlarged endoplasmic reticuli and a large quantity of cytoplasmic lipid inclusions after 9 months of continuous exposure to lead (Markov and Dimova, 1974). Autopsy of brains from SSPE patients further revealed that bipolar/rod-shaped microglia were the predominant form of microglia in the cortical area, as well as in the white matter (Wierzba-Bobrowicz et al., 2002; Boche et al., 2013). These studies collectively suggest that bipolar/rod-shaped microglia are often observed in various neuropathological disorders.

MORPHOLOGICAL DYNAMICS OF RAMIFIED, BIPOLAR/ROD-SHAPED AND AMOEBOID MICROGLIA

Bipolar/rod-shaped microglia are seldom observed in cultures owing to the small number of this microglia subtype in the overall microglia population (Suzumura et al., 1990; Bohatschek et al., 2001; Hoffmann et al., 2003; Szabo and Gulya, 2013). Primary microglia usually adopt an amoeboid morphology when cultured on non-coated surface (Suzumura et al., 1990; Kann et al., 2004). After treating with granulocyte-macrophage colony stimulating factor (GM-CSF), amoeboid microglia transformed into bipolar/rod-shaped microglia with elongated cell bodies and highly polarized processes following 5 days of incubation. The bipolar/rod-shaped microglia were highly proliferative compared to the amoeboid microglia (Suzumura et al., 1990).

Further study showed that the majority of microglia adopted ramified morphology when co-culturing on an astrocyte monolayer. The ramified microglia quickly transformed into bipolar/rod-shaped microglia within 3 h following the addition of rat brain lysate to the co-cultures, and these bipolar/rod-shaped microglia were gradually transformed into amoeboid microglia after 12 h of incubation. Interestingly, removal of brain lysate by washing off the culture medium induced a reverse transformation of amoeboid into bipolar/rod-shaped microglia within 24 h, and gradually transformed back into ramified microglia following 96 h of incubation without the brain lysate (Bohatschek et al., 2001).

One study showed that in rat hippocampal slice cultures, microglia adopted mixed and diverse morphological forms ranging from ramified, bipolar/rod-shaped to amoeboid 72 h following LPS challenge (Papageorgiou et al., 2016). Unlike other studies, the number of amoeboid microglia in hippocampal slice cultures remained unchanged after LPS stimulation (Gao et al., 2002; Qin L. et al., 2007). Also, the levels of pro-inflammatory cytokines such as interleukin 1 beta (IL-1β) and tumor necrosis factor α (TNFα) were significantly elevated, and the neuronal architecture remained largely intact without any detectable neuronal loss. In contrast, the number of amoeboid microglia was markedly increased when exposed to both LPS and interferon gamma (IFNγ), which demonstrated a significant neuronal loss (Papageorgiou et al., 2016). Transformation of bipolar/rod-shaped microglia into amoeboid microglia, and the induced neurotoxicity might involve the crosstalk between microglia and infiltrated leukocytes since IFNγ is mainly secreted by leukocytes but not by microglia (Papageorgiou et al., 2016).

Accumulating evidence suggests that morphological transformation of microglia involves the change in electrophysiological properties and intracellular calcium concentration ($[Ca^{2+}]i$) of the microglial cells. Astrocytes are known to produce macrophage colony stimulating factor (M-CSF), which induces the transformation of amoeboid microglia into a mix of ramified (vast majority) and bipolar/rod-shaped microglia (small number) within few hours along with voltage-gated sodium (Na^+) and outward potassium (K^+) current increase in the transformed microglia (Frei et al., 1992; Korotzer and Cotman, 1992; Liu et al., 1994; Sievers et al., 1994; Eder et al., 1998; Kann et al., 2004). Ramified and bipolar/rod-shaped microglia returned to amoeboid morphology after washing out the astrocyte-conditioned medium (ACM; Eder et al., 1998). Further experiments showed the involvement of chloride (Cl^-) channel in ramification of microglia. Cl^- channel blockers added to the ACM inhibited the transformation of microglia; however, blocking Na^+ and K^+ channels did not affect the ramification process (Eder et al., 1998). Ramification of microglia involves in membrane stretching (i.e., extension of processes) and cytoskeletal reorganization that might activate Cl^- channel. Stretching of microglial cell membrane under experimental condition was induced by a fine movement of recording patch pipette resulting in a current activation mediated mainly by Cl^- ions (Eder et al., 1998).

The change in $[Ca^{2+}]i$ serves as a signal transduction pathway to control various cellular events such as cell migration, proliferation, release of cytokines and morphological transformation of microglia (Möller, 2002; Farber and Kettenmann, 2006). Microglia express purinergic receptors and G protein-coupled receptor CD88 to regulate the $[Ca^{2+}]i$ of microglia (Farber and Kettenmann, 2006). Microglia irrespective of their morphology, including ramified and bipolar/rod-shaped microglia in ACM-treated microglia cultures, or amoeboid microglia on non-coated surface, showed a transient increase in $[Ca^{2+}]i$ in response to the agonists of purinergic receptor (i.e., ATP and UTP) and CD88 (i.e., Complement factor 5a, C5a), respectively (Möller et al., 2000; Kann et al., 2004). In contrast, LPS-induced activation of microglia resulted in a chronic increase in the basal $[Ca^{2+}]i$, and suppression of UTP- and C5a-evoked transient increase in $[Ca^{2+}]i$ (Hoffmann et al., 2003). The UTP- and C5a-evoked transient increase in $[Ca^{2+}]i$ was successfully restored with the suppression of LPS-induced elevation of $[Ca^{2+}]i$ by BAPTA and AG126 (Hoffmann et al., 2003; Kann et al., 2004). The LPS-induced production of pro-inflammatory cytokines TNFα and IL-6, and nitric oxide (NO) by activated microglia requires the elevation of $[Ca^{2+}]i$. The release of cytokine and NO were significantly reduced by the blockade of intracellular calcium release in LPS-treated microglia using BAPTA (Hoffmann et al., 2003). ACM-induced ramified and bipolar/rod-shaped microglia did not differ functionally from amoeboid microglia grown on non-coated surface. However, the LPS-stimulated microglia behave differently in regulating

$[Ca^{2+}]$ (Möller et al., 2000; Hoffmann et al., 2003; Kann et al., 2004).

CELL CULTURE MODEL SYSTEMS FOR STUDYING BIPOLAR/ROD-SHAPED MICROGLIA

The study of bipolar/rod-shaped microglia has been limited by the lack of *in vitro* and *in vivo* model systems with which to study this form of microglia. Unlike the case for bipolar/rod-shaped microglia, there are many well-defined cell culture systems available to purify ramified and amoeboid microglia, which provide us with a better understanding of the molecular and cellular properties of these microglia subtypes. In general, primary microglia cultured on a fibronectin-coated surface enrich ramified microglia, while microglia cultured on a laminin-coated surface enrich amoeboid microglia (Chamak and Mallat, 1991). Many studies have already taken advantage of this relatively simple culture system to examine how microglia respond to various factors such as ATP (Hide et al., 2000; Honda et al., 2001), LPS (Nakamura et al., 1999; Qin H. et al., 2007; Pannell et al., 2014), and cytokines (Merrill, 1991). Moreover, cell culture systems allow researchers to examine gene expression profiling (Duke et al., 2004; Horvath et al., 2008), along with cellular properties such as cell migration (Honda et al., 2001; Haynes et al., 2006), phagocytic activity (Townsend et al., 2005; Koizumi et al., 2007), electrophysiological properties (Eder et al., 1998) and intracellular calcium activity (Hoffmann et al., 2003; Kann et al., 2004) in different forms of microglia. In few studies, in which ramified and partially bipolar/rod-shaped microglia were induced within the same culture *in vitro*, the functional differences of these two distinct microglia phenotypes were not explored in detail (Eder et al., 1998; Möller et al., 2000; Kann et al., 2004).

Recently, we established a cost-effective and highly reproducible method with which to enrich bipolar/rod-shaped microglia *in vitro* (Tam and Ma, 2014; Tam et al., 2016) and thus study gene expression profiles and characterize morphological changes systemically. Primary microglia were isolated from postnatal mice and grown on a poly-D-lysine and laminin-coated surface with multiple scratches (**Figure 1**). Microglia actively migrated towards the scratched surface (Tam and Ma, 2014) where the laminin coating was scratched off (Tam et al., 2016) during the initial hours after cell seeding, and microglia colonized upon the laminin-free scratched surface developed elongated and bipolar processes, beginning from the first day *in vitro* (DIV; Tam and Ma, 2014; Tam et al., 2016). Bipolar/rod-shaped microglia with elongated processes quickly formed end-to-end alignments on the scratched poly-D-lysine and laminin-coated surface after 1 DIV (Tam and Ma, 2014). In contrast, although trains of bipolar/rod-shaped microglia could be formed on scratched surface pre-coated with poly-D-lysine only, these trains of bipolar/rod-shaped microglia failed to maintain and the microglia alignments disappeared after 3 DIV. This suggests that laminin is crucial in stabilizing the formation of microglia alignments since the trains of bipolar/rod-shaped microglia could be maintained for at least 6 DIV on the scratched poly-D-lysine and laminin-coated surface (Tam et al., 2016). In rats, bipolar/rod-shaped microglia aligned end-to-end at the injury site within 1 day of diffuse brain injury *in vivo* (Ziebell et al., 2012). In line with an *in vivo* study on human pathological brains (Wierzba-Bobrowicz et al., 2002), bipolar/rod-shaped microglia in culture showed high immunoreactivity to proliferating cell nuclear antigen (PCNA, a cell proliferation marker), indicating that they were highly proliferative. The gene expression of both M1 (i.e., *Tnf*, *Il-1b*, *Cd32* and *Cd86*) and M2 (i.e., *Il-10* and *Tgf-β*) markers was markedly reduced in bipolar/rod-shaped microglia at the time when trains of microglia were formed (i.e., 2 DIV). In contrast, amoeboid microglia are known to produce significantly higher levels of pro-inflammatory cytokines compared to bipolar/rod-shaped microglia (Tam and Ma, 2014). Amoeboid microglia colonized in the non-scratched area (i.e., laminin-coated surface), thus demonstrating their ability to digest the laminin coating (Stolzing et al., 2002; Tam et al., 2016) with the up-regulation of laminin-cleaving proteins, Adam9 and Ctss, compared to bipolar/rod-shaped microglia which colonized in the laminin-free scratched surface (Tam et al., 2016). In addition, bipolar/rod-shaped microglia were morphologically dynamic and could rapidly transform into amoeboid microglia within 30 min in response to LPS (i.e., a M1 stimulus). This involved the up-regulation of pro-inflammatory cytokines (*Il-1b* and *Tnf*) and activation of the Jak/Stat3 signaling pathway (Tam and Ma, 2014). Amoeboid microglia which had transformed from bipolar/rod-shaped microglia regained the ability to cleave laminin via the up-regulation of the laminin-cleaving proteins, Adam9 and Ctss, while their gene expression in LPS-treated amoeboid microglia-enriched cultures remained unchanged (Tam et al., 2016). Taken together, our recently established cell culture system successfully enriched bipolar/rod-shaped microglia forming end-to-end alignments *in vitro* (Tam and Ma, 2014; Tam et al., 2016) that resemble the spatial arrangement of trains of bipolar/rod-shaped microglia after CNS injury *in vivo* (Ziebell et al., 2012; Taylor et al., 2014; Yuan et al., 2015). However, bipolar/rod-shaped microglia formed after GM-CSF and brain lysate stimulation did not form end-to-end alignments (Suzumura et al., 1990; Bohatschek et al., 2001), which indicate that a physical scratched surface (perhaps mimicking the site of injury) is required for the end-to-end alignment formation.

BIPOLAR/ROD-SHAPED MICROGLIA IN BRAIN INJURY

Colonization and trains of bipolar/rod-shaped microglia are not normally observed in the naïve rat brain (Taylor et al., 2014), and are only occasionally found in the cerebral cortex and thalamus of rodent brain (Lawson et al., 1990; Taylor et al., 2014). Following midline fluid percussion injury (mFPI), an animal model of traumatic brain injury, ramified microglia which used to be evenly distributed throughout the cortical

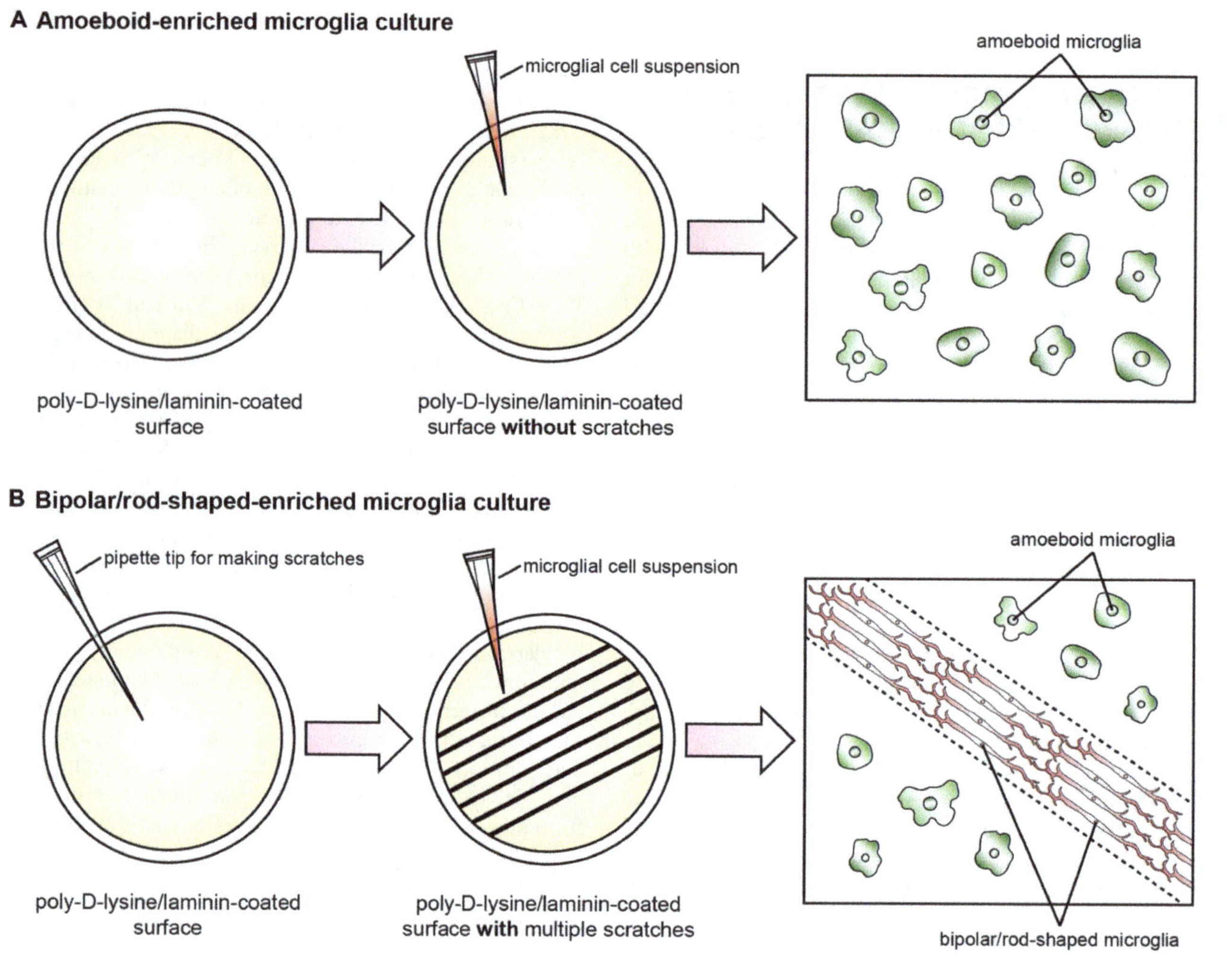

FIGURE 1 | Schematic diagram illustrating the cell culture model systems to enrich amoeboid and bipolar/rod-shaped microglia. Cerebral cortices dissected from postnatal mice were trypsinized and dissociated mechanically, and the cell suspension was plated onto a poly-D-lysine-coated culture flask. The microglia were then isolated from the mixed primary cortical cultures after 10–12 days by gently shaking. The purity of the microglia cultures prepared by this method was >99% (Tam and Ma, 2014; Tam et al., 2016). **(A)** The vast majority of primary microglia maintained an amoeboid-like morphology after culturing on a poly-D-lysine/laminin-coated surface without any physical scratches. **(B)** Multiple physical scratches generated by a P200 pipette tip removed the laminin coating, which created laminin-free zones between the non-scratched areas. The primary microglia actively migrated to the scratched area and formed trains of bipolar/rod-shaped microglia (red) in parallel with the direction of the scratches (dotted lines). By contrast, the microglia colonized in the non-scratched surfaces maintained amoeboid morphology (green) while the laminin coating was still intact.

area were activated and adopted a "rod-like" morphology. The cell bodies of these "rod-like" microglia were elongated and their primary processes projected toward the two ends, and formed trains of bipolar/rod-shaped microglia (Taylor et al., 2014). These bipolar/rod-shaped microglia appeared to be highly polarized in response to brain injury. In rats, the vast majority of bipolar/rod-shaped microglia started colonizing the primary somatosensory barrel field (S1BF) region in the cerebral cortex to form end-to-end alignments perpendicular to the dural surface across the cortical layers as early as 1-day post injury (dpi). An increased number of bipolar/rod-shaped microglia, with significant microglia alignments, were observed at 2 dpi, which became more prominent by 7 dpi (Ziebell et al., 2012). More importantly, these bipolar/rod-shaped microglia were phenotypically distinct from other forms of microglia (i.e., ramified and amoeboid microglia) with significant increase in cell length to width ratio, and reduced number and length of side branches (Taylor et al., 2014). Most of the bipolar/rod-shaped microglia exhibited high immunoreactivity to ED1 (a phagocytic marker), but only a few showed immunoreactivity to OX6 (a major histocompatibility complex (MHC) class II marker; Ziebell et al., 2012). This indicated that bipolar/rod-shaped microglia are highly phagocytic (Bauer et al., 1994; Cho et al., 2006). Interestingly, bipolar/rod-shaped microglia with high phagocytic activity were not involved in the clearance of myelin debris since no internalized myelin was observed within the bipolar/rod-shaped microglia. Furthermore, the aligned bipolar/rod-shaped microglia showed no direct contact with other glia cells such as oligodendrocytes and astrocytes after brain injury (Ziebell et al., 2012). The trains of bipolar/rod-shaped microglia aligned end-to-end along the injured axons, which was consistent with other studies (Nissl, 1899; Spielmeyer, 1922; Cho et al., 2006). Nevertheless, how these trains of bipolar/rod-shaped microglia are formed has yet to be elucidated, as does their functional role, particularly their association with neuronal processes.

BIPOLAR/ROD-SHAPED MICROGLIA IN ALZHEIMER'S DISEASE

AD is one of the most common neurodegenerative diseases and affects approximately 48 million people worldwide. Aberrant beta amyloid precursor protein (βAPP) metabolism and the subsequent increased deposition of β-amyloid peptides in senile plaques is the major pathological hallmark of AD (Selkoe, 2000). In the early stages of AD pathology, microglia recruited to the senile plaques show strong phagocytic activity and are able to internalize β-amyloid peptides via the class A scavenger receptor (Shaffer et al., 1995; Paresce et al., 1996, 1997). Microglia secrete proteolytic enzymes such as neprilysin, matrix metalloproteinase 9 (MMP-9), plasminogen and insulin-degrading enzyme (IDE), which are capable of degrading β-amyloid peptides (Leissring et al., 2003; Yan et al., 2006). Activated microglia are always detected in the senile plaque core of AD patients (Wegiel and Wisniewski, 1990; Dickson et al., 1993). In a mouse model of AD, the massive infiltration of bone marrow-derived microglia into the senile plaque core significantly disrupted β-amyloid aggregation and reduced the formation of senile plaques in the AD brain (Simard et al., 2006). Genetically modified mice with limited microglia recruitment to the senile plaques during the early onset of AD markedly elevated β-amyloid peptide levels and increased mortality in a transgenic mouse model of AD (El Khoury et al., 2007). These studies further demonstrate the neuroprotective roles of microglia within the early stages of AD pathogenesis. Nevertheless, microglia are known to secrete neurotoxic factors such as IL-1β, NO and TNFα following prolonged exposure to accumulated β-amyloid peptides (Dickson et al., 1993; Barger and Harmon, 1997; Hickman et al., 2008). These activated microglia also exert strong neurotoxicity to hippocampal neurons both *in vitro* (Giulian et al., 1996; Barger and Harmon, 1997) and *in vivo* (Giulian et al., 1995). In another study, the expression of β-amyloid-binding receptors and β-amyloid-degrading enzymes in the microglia of 14-month-old AD mice were markedly reduced as compared to age-matched wild type littermates; meanwhile, expression of the pro-inflammatory cytokines, IL-1β and TNFα, were elevated in microglia (Hickman et al., 2008). This suggests that the phagocytic activity of microglia is significantly impaired upon prolonged exposure to β-amyloid. Studies have also shown that β-amyloid peptides also stimulate astrocytes which greatly reduces the secretion of pro-inflammatory cytokines and NO from β-amyloid-treated microglia (von Bernhardi and Eugenín, 2004). The phagocytic capability of microglia to clear senile plaques was inhibited during co-culture with astrocytes (DeWitt et al., 1998). These findings account for the progressive deposition of β-amyloid peptides even though abundant microglia are present in senile plaques. The accumulation of β-amyloid plaques cause massive neuronal loss, resulting in subsequent cognitive impairments, as demonstrated in AD patients and animal models of AD (West et al., 1994; Casas et al., 2004; Oakley et al., 2006).

Another major pathological hallmark of AD is the deposition of NFTs, which are aggregates of a hyper-phosphorylated form of tau (Ballatore et al., 2007; Ittner and Götz, 2011). Under normal physiological conditions, the expression of tau appeared to be most abundant in axons with some expression in the dendrites (Ittner et al., 2010; Ittner and Götz, 2011). Tau binds to the axons to stabilize the microtubules and promote microtubule assembly (Weingarten et al., 1975; Kadavath et al., 2015), and regulate microtubule-dependent axonal transport via the modulation of motor proteins including dynein and kinesin (Dixit et al., 2008; Scholz and Mandelkow, 2014). Under the pathological condition of AD, however, tau becomes increasingly phosphorylated which causes tau to become detached from the microtubules (Ballatore et al., 2007). The increased level of unbound tau in the cytoplasm increases the likelihood of tau misfolding, resulting in the aggregation and fibril formation of tau (Ross and Poirier, 2004; Kuret et al., 2005a,b). In transgenic mice expressing human mutant tau (P301L), profound microglial activation was observed in the dentate gyrus with extensive degeneration of the axonal terminals. The degenerating axonal terminals, and their synapses, were wrapped by activated microglia. In parallel, a significant reduction of synapsin-I (a synaptic vesicle marker) and postsynaptic density protein 95 (PSD-95, a postsynaptic marker) immunoreactivity indicated a massive loss of synapses during disease progression (de Calignon et al., 2012).

Similar tau pathology was also observed in a transgenic mouse model expressing a different mutant form of human tau (P301S). Tau pathology began at 6-months of age in the P301S tau mutant mice and widespread neuronal loss was detected in these mutants by 8-months of age; microglial activation was detected as early as in the 4-month-old mice. The hippocampal neurons of 4-month-old mutant mice exhibited high levels of immunoreactivity to pro-inflammatory cytokine IL-1β. Administration of the immunosuppressant FK506 to these mutant mice markedly attenuated the inflammatory responses resulting in a significant reduction of activated microglia, tau pathology and neuronal loss (Yoshiyama et al., 2007). Microglia activation has also been commonly observed in transgenic animal models of AD expressing other forms of mutant tau (Ikeda et al., 2005; Zilka et al., 2009; Bhaskar et al., 2010).

Several lines of evidence suggest that chronic inflammation in the brain is likely to exacerbate the formation of NFT and disease-related pathology (Kitazawa et al., 2004; Maccioni et al., 2010). Following exposure to soluble βAPP, the levels of pro-inflammatory cytokine IL-1β was elevated in cultured primary microglia. Co-culturing the primary cortical neurons with βAPP-treated microglia resulted in a substantial increase in tau phosphorylation. However, co-culturing primary neurons with activated microglia pre-treated with an IL-1 receptor (IL-1R)-blocking antibody significantly reduced the phosphorylation of tau in neurons, suggesting that the elevated IL-1β level in activated microglia plays a pivotal role in augmenting tau phosphorylation (Li et al., 2003). In a transgenic mouse model of AD, the *in vivo* administration of LPS induced significant levels of inflammation throughout the cerebral cortex and hippocampus, as well as microglial activation and an increased level of IL-1β, thus resulting in increased tau phosphorylation while the level of β-amyloid remained unchanged (Kitazawa et al., 2005). The activity of Cdk5, a potent mediator of tau phosphorylation (Town et al., 2002), was also significantly elevated following LPS treatment (Kitazawa et al., 2005). In other studies, the selective blockade of IL-1β-mediated signaling pathways using IL-1R blocking antibodies (Kitazawa et al., 2011) or the Cdk5 inhibitor roscovitine (Kitazawa et al., 2005) markedly reduced tau phosphorylation via suppression of the tau kinase p25 activity.

Ablation of Cx3cr1 in mice results in increased microglial activation which exaggerates LPS-induced tau phosphorylation and tau pathology-related behavioral abnormalities including the loss of motor coordination, motor deficits and memory loss (Bhaskar et al., 2010). In contrast, the overexpression of Cx3cr1 in mice suppresses microglial activation and tau phosphorylation. Subsequent neuronal loss in the hippocampus was greatly reduced in mice overexpressing Cx3cr1 (Nash et al., 2013). Pre-treating primary cortical neurons with an IL-1R antagonist could also prevent neurons from the hyper-phosphorylation of tau following exposure to a conditioned medium derived from Cx3cr1-deficient microglia (Bhaskar et al., 2010). Collectively, these studies suggested that microglial activation contributes to the augmentation of tau phosphorylation and its subsequent pathogenesis and that IL-1β is one of the most important pro-inflammatory cytokines responsible for the induction of tau phosphorylation following microglial activation.

In AD patients, infiltrated microglia typically adopt amoeboid morphology (McGeer et al., 1988; Haga et al., 1989; Itagaki et al., 1989); similar findings have been demonstrated in mouse models of AD (Wegiel et al., 2003, 2004; Simard et al., 2006). Amoeboid microglia are mainly localized in the hippocampus and cerebral cortex, where β-amyloid aggregates are formed (Simard et al., 2006), and are responsible for the clearance of β-amyloid aggregates (Shaffer et al., 1995; Paresce et al., 1996). Interestingly, some of the activated microglia adopt an elongated, and highly polarized rod-like morphology, within or in close proximity to senile plaques in patients (Wierzba-Bobrowicz et al., 2002). Trains of bipolar/rod-shaped microglia were predominantly aligned end-to-end in the CA1 and CA2/3 regions of AD hippocampus (Bachstetter et al., 2015). The presence of a characteristic train of bipolar/rod-shaped microglia in an animal model of experimental diffuse traumatic brain injury demonstrated the potential key roles of bipolar/rod-shaped microglia in neuronal survival (Ziebell et al., 2012). Microglial were aligned parallel to damaged neuronal fibers but without physical contact (Bachstetter et al., 2015). In the cerebral cortex of patients with AD, a subset of microglia showed strong immunoreactivity to tau; this subset showed a rod-like morphology with elongated processes (Odawara et al., 1995). The presence of tau-positive bipolar/rod-shaped microglia remained unexplained but may have been due to the internalization of tau-positive degenerated axonal terminals, as significant synaptic loss was observed in the progression of tau pathology (de Calignon et al., 2012). Following the administration of LPS in mice, bipolar/rod-shaped microglia were observed in the cerebral cortex and hippocampus where the levels of phosphorylated tau remained high (Lee et al., 2010). Our early studies also showed that bipolar/rod-shaped microglia expressed a significantly lower level of IL-1β compared with amoeboid microglia (Tam and Ma, 2014). The presence of bipolar/rod-shaped microglia might attenuate the substantial increase in tau phosphorylation induced by microglial activation, and subsequent neuronal loss and functional abnormalities during the progression of AD. Taken together, these findings suggest that bipolar/rod-shaped microglia might be involved in the pathogenesis of AD, or even in the repair process during disease progression (Wierzba-Bobrowicz et al., 2002).

BIPOLAR/ROD-SHAPED MICROGLIA IN PARKINSON'S DISEASE

PD is the second most common neurodegenerative disorder after AD and affects approximately 10 million people worldwide (Dorsey et al., 2007; Delenclos et al., 2016). The cause of PD remains largely unknown since only about 5%–10% of PD patients are related to genetic mutations (Toulouse and Sullivan, 2008), and more than 90% of PD patients remain idiopathic. The pathological features of PD include the widespread loss of dopaminergic neurons in the substantia nigra, resulting in the loss of ascending axonal projections to the striatum. In fact, approximate 50% of dopaminergic neurons are lost and 80% of striatal dopamine is depleted by the time patients are diagnosed with PD (Toulouse and Sullivan, 2008; Long-Smith et al., 2009).

Accumulating evidence suggests that chronic inflammation plays an indispensable role in the degeneration of dopaminergic neurons. Activated microglia accumulate in the substantia nigra of PD patients, where significant neuronal death has been observed (McGeer et al., 1988; Hirsch et al., 1998; Ouchi et al., 2005, 2009; Gerhard et al., 2006). The accumulated microglia are mainly localized in the degenerating neurons. Many pro-inflammatory cytokines, including TNFα, IL-1β, IFNγ and IL-6, have been detected in the brain, as well as in the cerebrospinal fluid and blood plasma, of PD patients (Mogi et al., 1994a,b; Müller et al., 1998; Mount et al., 2007). The combined effects of pro-inflammatory cytokines, including TNFα, IL-1β and IFNγ, have been demonstrated to stimulate the production of NO in a microglia cell line BV-2 (Sheng et al., 2011). NO produced by microglia after treated with LPS and IFNγ induced significant neuronal loss as demonstrated in primary neuron-glia co-culture (Dawson et al., 1994) and in rat hippocampal slice cultures (Papageorgiou et al., 2016). In PD patients, accumulated microglia showed strong inducible NO synthase (iNOS), and cyclooxygenase-2 (Cox-2) immunoreactivity (Hunot et al., 1996; Knott et al., 2000). The elevated level of iNOS and NO production in microglia was associated with the progressive loss of dopaminergic neurons in culture (Le et al., 2001) and in an animal model of PD (Liberatore et al., 1999; Dehmer et al., 2000; Kokovay and Cunningham, 2005; Aquilano et al., 2008). Cox-2 mediates microglial activation and the subsequent secondary neuronal death of dopaminergic neurons since the inhibition of Cox-2 significantly reduced microglial activation and dopaminergic neuronal loss in an animal model of PD (Vijitruth et al., 2006). These studies demonstrated the causal relationship between the prolonged activation of microglia and the subsequent loss of dopaminergic neurons during the pathogenesis of PD.

The major cause for the activation of microglia resulting in prolonged inflammation in PD patients has remained elusive, but evidence suggests that factors released by dying neurons might be responsible (Long-Smith et al., 2009). Several factors released by injured neurons can trigger microglial activation, including α-synuclein aggregates (Zhang et al., 2005; Daniele et al., 2015; Kim et al., 2016), MMP-3 (Kim et al., 2005, 2007) and neuromelanin (Wilms et al., 2003). The presence of such factors in the microglial microenvironment not only induces activation of microglia, but also the secretion of neurotoxic factors which leads to further neuronal cell death during the progression of PD (Kim and Joh, 2006).

In the later stages of PD, bipolar/rod-shaped microglia have been found in close proximity to degenerating dopaminergic neurons in the substantia nigra of patient (McGeer et al., 1988). In a rat model of PD, 3 days after LPS infusion (an animal model to induce neuroinflammation and substantial loss of dopaminergic neurons in the substantia nigra), profound activation of microglia was found in the substantia nigra ipsilateral to the LPS infusion. At this early time point, most microglia adopted bipolar/rod-shaped morphology with enlarged cell bodies and elongated processes. One week after LPS infusion, bipolar/rod-shaped microglia were transformed into amoeboid microglia, and such activation of microglia persisted up to 8 weeks after LPS infusion. The transformation of bipolar/rod-shaped microglia into amoeboid microglia was correlated with significant neuronal loss during the later stages (i.e., 4–6 weeks after LPS infusion; Gao et al., 2002). Amoeboid microglia are known to secrete neurotoxic factors to induce neuronal cell death (Gao et al., 2003; Qin et al., 2004). Interestingly, bipolar/rod-shaped microglia were observed in the activated microglial population (CD11b-positive) 24 h after treatment with aggregated α-synuclein (a pathological hallmark of PD; Zhang et al., 2005). However, whether the existence of bipolar/rod-shaped microglia in PD brains is neuroprotective remains elusive.

BIPOLAR/ROD-SHAPED MICROGLIA IN HUNTINGTON'S DISEASE

HD refers to an inherited genetic disorder characterized by the substantial loss of neurons in medium-sized spiny neurons within the corpus striatum and cerebral cortex (Vonsattel et al., 1985; Vonsattel and DiFiglia, 1998). The classic hallmark of neuropathology in HD is neuronal loss with nuclear and cytoplasmic inclusion of mutant Huntingtin protein and polyglutamine in degenerating neurons (Davies et al., 1997). Several studies suggest that microglia activation shows strong correlation with the pathogenesis of HD (Singhrao et al., 1999; Sapp et al., 2001; Pavese et al., 2006; Björkqvist et al., 2008; Politis et al., 2011; Crotti et al., 2014). Amoeboid microglia were mostly observed throughout the whole corpus striatum as well as the frontal and parietal lobe of the cerebral cortex in HD patients (Sapp et al., 2001; Pavese et al., 2006). The number of microglia was increased within the area where substantial neuronal loss was also detected (Sapp et al., 2001). A recent inflammatory profiling study provided further support for the association between the number of microglia and HD progression. Elevated levels of pro-inflammatory cytokines (IL-1β and TNFα) were detected in the corpus striatum. The level of other inflammatory mediators, such as IL-6, IL-8 and MMP-9, was altered in HD patients with chronic inflammation (Silvestroni et al., 2009). This indicated that the overproduction of pro-inflammatory factors by activated microglia induced neurotoxicity in neurons, thus resulting in neuronal cell death.

In the corpus straitum of HD patients, where the majority of microglia adopted amoeboid morphology, bipolar/rod-shaped microglia have been found aligned along the dendrites of pyramidal neurons in less affected regions of the cerebral cortex as well as in the cerebellum where the dendrites of Purkinje cells and the axonal projections of granule cells were mainly found. The elongated processes of bipolar/rod-shaped microglia were in close contact with the neuronal soma and their adjacent axons (Sapp et al., 2001). Bipolar/rod-shaped microglia showed high immunoreactivity to thymosin β4 and CR3/43, which are both specific for reactive microglia (Graeber et al., 1994).

BIPOLAR/ROD-SHAPED MICROGLIA IN OTHER NEURODEGENERATIVE DISEASES

Glaucoma is a neurodegenerative disease characterized by the loss of retinal ganglion cells and subsequent axonal degeneration in the optic nerve (Quigley et al., 1981, 1988, 1989). As with AD and PD, the prolonged activation of microglia contributes, at least in part, to the pathology of glaucoma (Neufeld, 1999; Yuan and Neufeld, 2001; Bosco et al., 2008). In a mouse ocular hypertension (OHT) model of glaucoma, bipolar/rod-shaped microglia were observed in the OHT eyes, but not in the contralateral side which appeared to adopt a ramified morphology. The processes of bipolar/rod-shaped microglia were in close proximity to each other and aligned end-to-end in the retinal nerve fiber layer (NFL). Bipolar/rod-shaped microglia expressed high levels of phagocytic markers (CD68/ED-1 and MHC-II) but relatively low levels of M1 (CD86) and M2 (Ym1) markers (Ziebell et al., 2012; de Hoz et al., 2013). In contrast, low levels of MHC-II immunoreactivity were detected in ramified microglia in the non-injured eyes (de Hoz et al., 2013). This indicates that bipolar/rod-shaped microglia are immunophenotypically distinct from other forms of microglia.

In a rat model of optic nerve transection, bipolar/rod-shaped microglia aligned end-to-end almost exclusively in the ganglion cell layer (GCL) and NFL 7 days after injury. This phenomenon became more pronounced at day 14 and 21 after injury, and the bipolar/rod-shaped microglial alignments disappeared 6 weeks after injury. The bipolar/rod-shaped microglia aligned along the βIII-tubulin-positive neuronal fibers and exhibited strong phagocytic activity to actively internalize degenerating axons (Yuan et al., 2015). Following 10-min focal middle cerebral artery (MCA) ischemia in rats, bipolar/rod-shaped microglial alignments were mainly found in the cerebral cortex around the infarct after 48 and 72 h of reperfusion. However, a more severe injury caused by 120-min focal MCA ischemia induced the microglia to adopt an amoeboid-like phenotype (Zhan et al., 2008). Bipolar/rod-shaped microglia are in a close association with injured neuronal processes, suggesting that they might be involved in the maintenance of neuronal circuitry in the development of neurodegenerative diseases.

POSSIBLE INVOLVEMENT OF BIPOLAR/ROD-SHAPED MICROGLIA IN "SYNAPTIC STRIPPING"

There is a growing body of evidence regarding the bipolar/rod-shaped microglia aligned end-to-end in close proximity along injured axons at an early stage after CNS injury (Zhan et al., 2008; Ziebell et al., 2012; de Hoz et al., 2013; Taylor et al., 2014; Yuan et al., 2015). The trains of bipolar/rod-shaped microglia have prompted researchers to consider their involvement in the reorganization of neuronal circuitry following CNS injury.

The active removal of synaptic terminals by microglia was first observed in the facial nerve injury model by Blinzinger and Kreutzberg (1968), and is now referred to as "synaptic stripping". Following facial nerve transection in rats, microglia underwent rapid proliferation at the lesion site and migrated to the cell bodies of damaged motor neurons (Graeber et al., 1988) to remove the synaptic boutons from injured neurons (Blinzinger and Kreutzberg, 1968). Synaptic stripping usually takes place within the first few days after injury by interposing the fine microglial processes to the junction between pre-synaptic elements and the post-synaptic cell soma (Moran and Graeber, 2004). Synaptic stripping in the cortical region has also been observed during inflammation induced by heat-killed bacteria in rats. Upon microglial activation, the microglial processes wrap around the cell bodies of cortical neurons, and extend their processes to the axons. Electron microscopy imaging revealed that the synaptic terminals were lost while the microglial processes were in direct contact with the neuronal soma, further suggesting the potential role of microglia in the removal of dysfunctional synapses (Trapp et al., 2007).

Over the last decade, advances in *in vivo* two-photon imaging have enabled the direct visualization of interactions between fluorescently-labeled neurons and microglia in the living brain of genetically modified mice. The processes of ramified microglia made very brief, but direct, contact with the synaptic terminal once per hour. However, the interactions between microglial processes and pre-synaptic boutons were dramatically increased following transient cerebral ischemia. Such a prolonged microglia-synapse interaction usually resulted in the disappearance of pre-synaptic terminals. This suggests that microglia actively detect synaptic conditions, and are involved in synaptic stripping and the subsequent remodeling of neuronal circuitry (Wake et al., 2009).

The specific spatial arrangement of bipolar/rod-shaped microglia after injury indicates their strong association with damaged axons; however, whether this form of microglia is involved in synaptic stripping remains uncertain. Nevertheless, it is noteworthy to mention that microglia morphology varies significantly across different brain regions. In normal adult mouse brain, bipolar/rod-shaped microglia with elongated cell bodies and extremely long primary processes are mainly localized in axon-rich white matter regions including the corpus callosum (i.e., the largest white matter structure in the brain), the molecular layer of the cerebellum (which only consists of axonal projections from Purkinje cells) and the fimbria area in the hippocampus. Bipolar/rod-shaped microglia align in parallel to the adjacent axons (Lawson et al., 1990). The molecular determinants which direct the microglia to adopt a bipolar/rod-shaped phenotype in these brain regions remain poorly understood. However, it is plausible to reason that bipolar/rod-shaped microglia might participate in experience-dependent remodeling and the elimination of synapses, given that they are in such a close spatial association with axonal terminals and the dominance of bipolar/rod-shaped microglia within the axon-rich white matter region (Tremblay et al., 2010). More importantly, the structural removal of impaired synapses from injured axons might be essential to the entire neuronal circuitry in order to make room for the establishment of new connections. This might facilitate the injured nervous system to restore original function after damage (Hanisch and Kettenmann, 2007), but this will require further research.

FUTURE PERSPECTIVE: NEUROPROTECTIVE ROLES OF BIPOLAR/ROD-SHAPED MICROGLIA

Inflammation-mediated neurodegenerative diseases usually share convergent mechanisms to amplify the inflammatory responses which result in neurotoxicity and subsequent neuronal cell death. Sustained microglia activation is the pathological hallmark of many neurodegenerative diseases which involve the secretion of neurotoxic factors from microglia thus resulting in neuronal loss during the early stages of disease onset (Glass et al., 2010). Interestingly, the presence of bipolar/rod-shaped microglia in the affected region usually takes place at the initial phase of microglial activation before the disease advances from early to later stages. During the end stage of disease, bipolar/rod-shaped microglia can be found in the less affected regions while amoeboid microglia are predominantly seen in the affected regions. This implies that bipolar/rod-shaped microglia might induce neuroprotection and slow down the progression of disease.

Despite the fact that persistent microglial activation is harmful to neurons, as demonstrated in many neurodegenerative diseases, the transient activation of bipolar/rod-shaped microglia might be beneficial in CNS damage to facilitate post-injury neuronal repair mechanisms. Brain injury is known to induce the transient formation of trains of bipolar/rod-shaped microglia at the injury site during the initial phase of injury (Zhan et al., 2008; Ziebell et al., 2012; Taylor et al., 2014). Previous studies by ourselves, and others, have shown that this form of microglia is highly proliferative (Suzumura et al., 1991; Wierzba-Bobrowicz et al., 2002; Tam and Ma, 2014). Inhibition of microglia proliferation at the site of injury showed augmentation of brain damage in the cerebral cortex following ischemic insult in mice (Denes et al., 2007; Lalancette-Hébert et al., 2007). These studies collectively suggest that the initial activation of microglia, and the transient formation of highly proliferative bipolar/rod-shaped microglial alignments, might be essential for expanding the microglial milieu at the site of injury, and exert potential neuroprotection to limit secondary damage to the CNS. Further studies on inhibiting such proliferation and formation of bipolar/rod-shaped microglia alignments in response to diffuse brain injury (Ziebell et al., 2012; Taylor et al., 2014) will be required to elucidate the neuroprotective roles of bipolar/rod-shaped microglia in brain injury.

Bipolar/rod-shaped microglia expressed relatively lower levels of pro-inflammatory cytokines (TNFα and IL1-β) compared to amoeboid microglia (Tam and Ma, 2014). However, upon LPS stimulation, bipolar/rod-shaped microglia were quickly transformed into amoeboid microglia expressing high levels of pro-inflammatory cytokines within a very short period of time (Tam and Ma, 2014; Tam et al., 2016). These "transformed" amoeboid microglia also regained proteolytic properties to degrade laminin (Tam et al., 2016), an extracellular matrix protein which promotes axonal regeneration. Earlier, we stated that bipolar/rod-shaped microglia are usually present during the early phase of neurodegenerative diseases when inflammation is not prominent, while almost exclusively amoeboid microglia have been found in pathological brain at the very late stage of disease onset when neuroinflammation persisted. Further studies should focus on the possibility of bipolar/rod-shaped microglia being transformed into amoeboid microglia during disease progression in animal models. We strongly believe that by transforming the amoeboid microglia into more neuroprotective bipolar/rod-shaped microglia might offer a promising new therapeutic strategy for neurodegenerative diseases and disorders involving chronic neuroinflammation. Our previous study demonstrated that bipolar/rod-shaped microglia expressed high levels of anti-inflammatory cytokines such as IL-10 and TGF-β (Tam and Ma, 2014). IL-10 is known to inhibit the production of pro-inflammatory cytokines (Sawada et al., 1999). Transforming amoeboid microglia back into bipolar/rod-shaped microglia might be a possible strategy to reduce further damage to CNS neurons by minimizing the production of neurotoxic cytokines.

Accumulating evidence also suggests that the removal of dysfunctional synaptic terminals by microglia is of great importance for subsequent neuronal repair. Followed by facial nerve injury, the loss of synapses appeared to be one of the earliest responses brought about by microglial activation (Blinzinger and Kreutzberg, 1968; Moran and Graeber, 2004). This may be considered as a neuroprotective response since the removal of dysfunctional synapses prevented injured neurons from excitotoxicity leading to better neuronal survival (Wake et al., 2009; Kato et al., 2016). The preserved motor neurons then reactivate their intrinsic growth program to regrow injured axons, and to reconnect with the original target muscle for functional synapse formation (Wake et al., 2009; Perry and O'Connor, 2010). Recent investigations on microglia-neuron interactions using *in vivo* two-photon imaging and patch clamp methods further support the neuroprotective roles of microglia. Microglia actively migrate towards and enwrap the swollen axons induced by neuronal hyperactivity. Pharmacological blockade of microglial migration prevented microglia from physically contacting the swollen axons. The neurons eventually underwent apoptotic cell death due to excitotoxicity (Kato et al., 2016). After optic nerve transection, bipolar/rod-shaped microglia internalized the injured optic nerve fibers and the degenerating retinal ganglion cells (Yuan et al., 2015). The close association between bipolar/rod-shaped microglia and injured axonal fibers might be linked to the reorganization of neuronal circuitry, and subsequent neuronal regenerative processes. Chronic neuroinflammation usually results in significant neuronal loss. Therefore, by switching microglial morphology from amoeboid form to bipolar/rod-shaped microglia might help to actively remove the impaired synaptic clefts and injured axons, thus creating more favorable conditions for axonal regrowth and the re-establishment of new synaptic connections.

Collectively, an in-depth understanding of the spatial and temporal activation of bipolar/rod-shaped microglia, and their association with degenerating axons, would render them excellent candidates with which to devise new strategies for treating neurodegenerative diseases. The recent establishment of a cost-effective and highly reproducible *in vitro* cell culture system to enrich bipolar/rod-shaped microglia allows more comprehensive studies on their gene and secretory protein expression profiles (Tam and Ma, 2014; Tam et al., 2016). It would be of great interest to explore if bipolar/rod-shaped microglia could also secrete neurotrophic factors such as brain-derived neurotrophic factor (BDNF), nerve growth factor (NGF) and neurotrophin-3 (NT-3; Nakajima et al., 2001), which contribute to the promotion of neuronal survival following injury and neurodegeneration (Hanisch and Kettenmann, 2007). Further research is now required to elucidate the mechanisms underlying the regulation of transformation from bipolar/rod-shaped microglia into amoeboid microglia and how this morphological change can be reversed to the bipolar/rod-shaped or ramified microglia (**Figure 2**). More importantly,

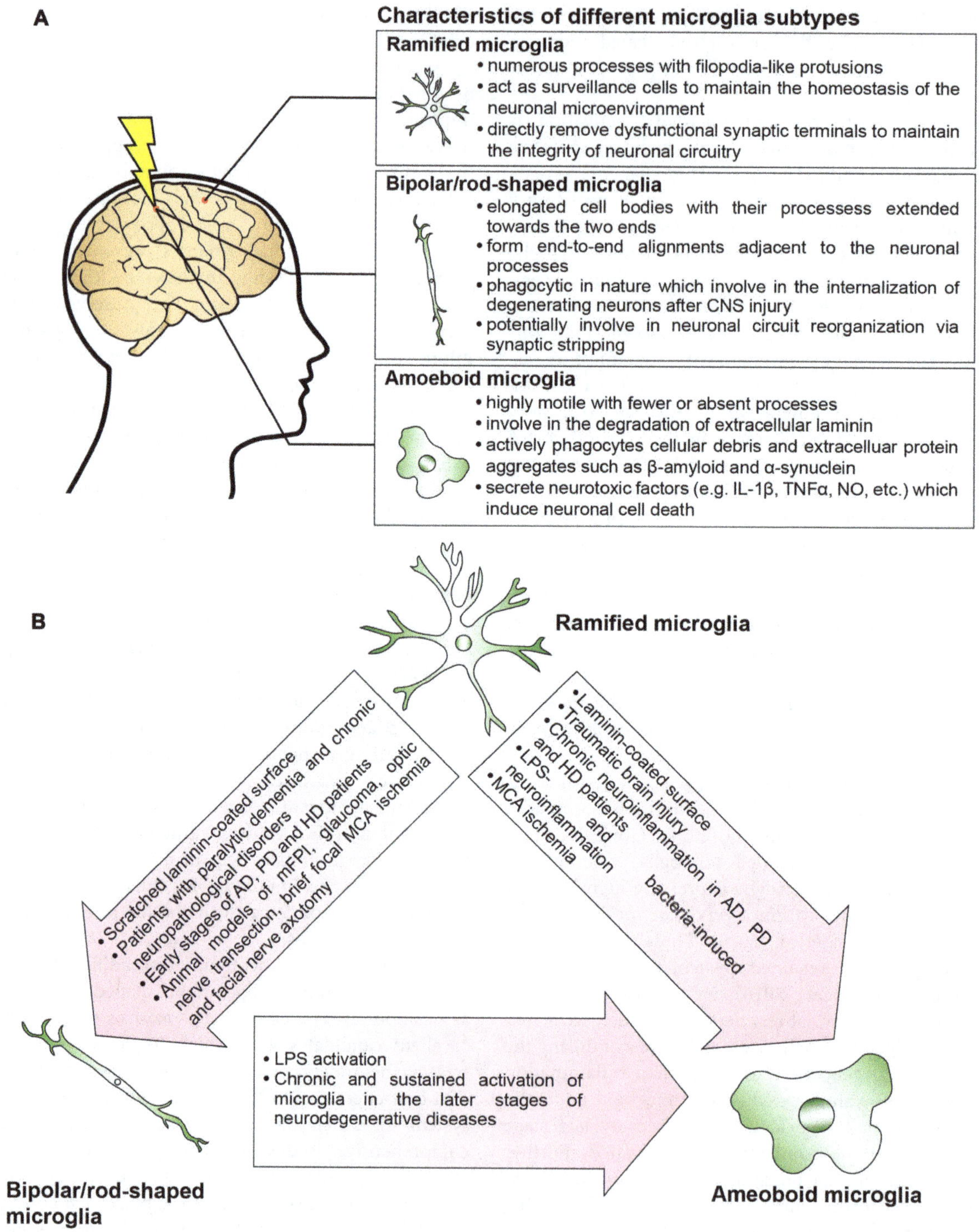

FIGURE 2 | Microglia are phenotypically dynamic. (A) The functional roles of microglia in normal or pathological central nervous system (CNS) are tightly associated with their morphological changes. Ramified microglia actively sense the subtle changes in CNS microenvironment. Bipolar/rod-shaped microglia form end-to-end alignments in close proximity to damaged neuronal fibers, suggesting that their functions are related to synaptic reorganization. Amoeboid microglia are extremely motile which actively migrate towards the injury site. They are highly phagocytic to internalize cellular debris and secrete neurotoxic factors which induce neuronal cell death. However, there are microglia subtypes that have yet not been fully characterized (i.e., hyper-ramified, bushy-like and spider-like microglia; Karperien et al., 2013; Ziebell et al., 2015). **(B)** In normal healthy CNS, most of the microglia are displayed as ramified microglia. In response to the change in the microenvironment, the ramified microglia undergo rapid transformation into bipolar/rod-shaped microglia or amoeboid microglia depending on the types of stimulus. Bipolar/rod-shaped microglia can quickly transform into amoeboid microglia in response to lipopolysaccharide (LPS) activation. The amoeboid microglia transformed from bipolar/rod-shaped microglia secrete pro-inflammatory cytokines and degrade extracellular laminin.

the development of new therapeutic interventions by switching the microglial phenotype from amoeboid to bipolar/rod-shaped microglia might shed new light on pathogenesis and identify targets for treating neurodegenerative diseases.

AUTHOR CONTRIBUTIONS

NPBA and CHEM discussed and formed the review focus. NPBA conducted the literature review and wrote the first draft of the manuscript under the supervision of CHEM. CHEM evaluated and revised the manuscript for final submission. All authors have made substantial and intellectual contributions to the current work and approved the final version for submission.

ACKNOWLEDGMENTS

This work is supported in part by The Health and Medical Research Fund (HMRF), Food and Health Bureau, Hong Kong Special Administrative Region Government (Ref. No: 12134101), GRF grants from the Research Grant Council of the Hong Kong Special Administrative Region Government (CityU 160813 and CityU 11100015), and City University of Hong Kong Seed Funding (7004587).

REFERENCES

Aquilano, K., Baldelli, S., Rotilio, G., and Ciriolo, M. R. (2008). Role of nitric oxide synthases in Parkinson's disease: a review on the antioxidant and anti-inflammatory activity of polyphenols. *Neurochem. Res.* 33, 2416–2426. doi: 10.1007/s11064-008-9697-6

Bachstetter, A. D., Ighodaro, E. T., Hassoun, Y., Aldeiri, D., Neltner, J. H., Patel, E., et al. (2017). Rod-shaped microglia morphology is associated with aging in 2 human autopsy series. *Neurobiol. Aging* 52, 98–105. doi: 10.1016/j.neurobiolaging.2016.12.028

Bachstetter, A. D., Van Eldik, L. J., Schmitt, F. A., Neltner, J. H., Ighodaro, E. T., Webster, S. J., et al. (2015). Disease-related microglia heterogeneity in the hippocampus of Alzheimer's disease, dementia with Lewy bodies and hippocampal sclerosis of aging. *Acta Neuropathol. Commun.* 3:32. doi: 10.1186/s40478-015-0209-z

Ballatore, C., Lee, V. M., and Trojanowski, J. Q. (2007). Tau-mediated neurodegeneration in Alzheimer's disease and related disorders. *Nat. Rev. Neurosci.* 8, 663–672. doi: 10.1038/nrn2194

Barger, S. W., and Harmon, A. D. (1997). Microglial activation by Alzheimer amyloid precursor protein and modulation by apolipoprotein E. *Nature* 388, 878–881. doi: 10.1038/42257

Bauer, J., Sminia, T., Wouterlood, F. G., and Dijkstra, C. D. (1994). Phagocytic activity of macrophages and microglial cells during the course of acute and chronic relapsing experimental autoimmune encephalomyelitis. *J. Neurosci. Res.* 38, 365–375. doi: 10.1002/jnr.490380402

Bhaskar, K., Konerth, M., Kokiko-Cochran, O. N., Cardona, A., Ransohoff, R. M., and Lamb, B. T. (2010). Regulation of tau pathology by the microglial fractalkine receptor. *Neuron* 68, 19–31. doi: 10.1016/j.neuron.2010.08.023

Björkqvist, M., Wild, E. J., Thiele, J., Silvestroni, A., Andre, R., Lahiri, N., et al. (2008). A novel pathogenic pathway of immune activation detectable before clinical onset in Huntington's disease. *J. Exp. Med.* 205, 1869–1877. doi: 10.1084/jem.20080178

Blinzinger, K., and Kreutzberg, G. (1968). Displacement of synaptic terminals from regenerating motoneurons by microglial cells. *Z. Zellforsch. Mikrosk. Anat.* 85, 145–157. doi: 10.1007/bf00325030

Boche, D., Perry, V. H., and Nicoll, J. A. (2013). Review: activation patterns of microglia and their identification in the human brain. *Neuropathol. Appl. Neurobiol.* 39, 3–18. doi: 10.1111/nan.12011

Bohatschek, M., Kloss, C. U., Kalla, R., and Raivich, G. (2001). *In vitro* model of microglial deramification: ramified microglia transform into amoeboid phagocytes following addition of brain cell membranes to microglia-astrocyte cocultures. *J. Neurosci. Res.* 64, 508–522. doi: 10.1002/jnr.1103

Bosco, A., Inman, D. M., Steele, M. R., Wu, G., Soto, I., Marsh-Armstrong, N., et al. (2008). Reduced retina microglial activation and improved optic nerve integrity with minocycline treatment in the DBA/2J mouse model of glaucoma. *Invest. Ophthalmol. Vis. Sci.* 49, 1437–1446. doi: 10.1167/iovs.07-1337

Casas, C., Sergeant, N., Itier, J. M., Blanchard, V., Wirths, O., van der Kolk, N., et al. (2004). Massive CA1/2 neuronal loss with intraneuronal and N-terminal truncated $A\beta_{42}$ accumulation in a novel Alzheimer transgenic model. *Am. J. Pathol.* 165, 1289–1300. doi: 10.1016/s0002-9440(10)63388-3

Chamak, B., and Mallat, M. (1991). Fibronectin and laminin regulate the *in vitro* differentiation of microglial cells. *Neuroscience* 45, 513–527. doi: 10.1016/0306-4522(91)90267-r

Cho, B. P., Song, D. Y., Sugama, S., Shin, D. H., Shimizu, Y., Kim, S. S., et al. (2006). Pathological dynamics of activated microglia following medial forebrain bundle transection. *Glia* 53, 92–102. doi: 10.1002/glia.20265

Crotti, A., Benner, C., Kerman, B. E., Gosselin, D., Lagier-Tourenne, C., Zuccato, C., et al. (2014). Mutant Huntingtin promotes autonomous microglia activation via myeloid lineage-determining factors. *Nat. Neurosci.* 17, 513–521. doi: 10.1038/nn.3668

Daniele, S. G., Béraud, D., Davenport, C., Cheng, K., Yin, H., and Maguire-Zeiss, K. A. (2015). Activation of MyD88-dependent TLR1/2 signaling by misfolded α-synuclein, a protein linked to neurodegenerative disorders. *Sci. Signal.* 8:ra45. doi: 10.1126/scisignal.2005965

Davalos, D., Grutzendler, J., Yang, G., Kim, J. V., Zuo, Y., Jung, S., et al. (2005). ATP mediates rapid microglial response to local brain injury *in vivo*. *Nat. Neurosci.* 8, 752–758. doi: 10.1038/nn1472

Davies, S. W., Turmaine, M., Cozens, B. A., DiFiglia, M., Sharp, A. H., Ross, C. A., et al. (1997). Formation of neuronal intranuclear inclusions underlies the neurological dysfunction in mice transgenic for the HD mutation. *Cell* 90, 537–548. doi: 10.1016/s0092-8674(00)80513-9

Dawson, V. L., Brahmbhatt, H. P., Mong, J. A., and Dawson, T. M. (1994). Expression of inducible nitric oxide synthase causes delayed neurotoxicity in primary mixed neuronal-glial cortical cultures. *Neuropharmacology* 33, 1425–1430. doi: 10.1016/0028-3908(94)90045-0

de Calignon, A., Polydoro, M., Suárez-Calvet, M., William, C., Adamowicz, D. H., Kopeikina, K. J., et al. (2012). Propagation of tau pathology in a model of early Alzheimer's disease. *Neuron* 73, 685–697. doi: 10.1016/j.neuron.2011.11.033

de Hoz, R., Gallego, B. I., Ramirez, A. I., Rojas, B., Salazar, J. J., Valiente-Soriano, F. J., et al. (2013). Rod-like microglia are restricted to eyes with laser-induced ocular hypertension but absent from the microglial changes in the contralateral untreated eye. *PLoS One* 8:e83733. doi: 10.1371/journal.pone.0083733

Dehmer, T., Lindenau, J., Haid, S., Dichgans, J., and Schulz, J. B. (2000). Deficiency of inducible nitric oxide synthase protects against MPTP toxicity *in vivo*. *J. Neurochem.* 74, 2213–2216. doi: 10.1046/j.1471-4159.2000.0742213.x

Delenclos, M., Jones, D. R., McLean, P. J., and Uitti, R. J. (2016). Biomarkers in Parkinson's disease: advances and strategies. *Parkinsonism Relat. Disord.* 22, S106–S110. doi: 10.1016/j.parkreldis.2015.09.048

Denes, A., Vidyasagar, R., Feng, J., Narvainen, J., McColl, B. W., Kauppinen, R. A., et al. (2007). Proliferating resident microglia after focal cerebral ischaemia in mice. *J. Cereb. Blood Flow Metab.* 27, 1941–1953. doi: 10.1038/sj.jcbfm.9600495

DeWitt, D. A., Perry, G., Cohen, M., Doller, C., and Silver, J. (1998). Astrocytes regulate microglial phagocytosis of senile plaque cores of Alzheimer's disease. *Exp. Neurol.* 149, 329–340. doi: 10.1006/exnr.1997.6738

Dickson, D. W., Lee, S. C., Mattiace, L. A., Yen, S. H., and Brosnan, C. (1993). Microglia and cytokines in neurological disease, with special reference to AIDS and Alzheimer's disease. *Glia* 7, 75–83. doi: 10.1002/glia.440070113

Dixit, R., Ross, J. L., Goldman, Y. E., and Holzbaur, E. L. (2008). Differential regulation of dynein and kinesin motor proteins by tau. *Science* 319, 1086–1089. doi: 10.1126/science.1152993

Dorsey, E. R., Constantinescu, R., Thompson, J. P., Biglan, K. M., Holloway, R. G., Kieburtz, K., et al. (2007). Projected number of people with Parkinson disease in the most populous nations, 2005 through 2030. *Neurology* 68, 384–386. doi: 10.1212/01.WNL.0000247740.47667.03

Duke, D. C., Moran, L. B., Turkheimer, F. E., Banati, R., and Graeber, M. B. (2004). Microglia in culture: what genes do they express? *Dev. Neurosci.* 26, 30–37. doi: 10.1159/000080709

Eder, C., Klee, R., and Heinemann, U. (1998). Involvement of stretch-activated Cl- channels in ramification of murine microglia. *J. Neurosci.* 18, 7127–7137.

El Khoury, J., Toft, M., Hickman, S. E., Means, T. K., Terada, K., Geula, C., et al. (2007). *Ccr2* deficiency impairs microglial accumulation and accelerates progression of Alzheimer-like disease. *Nat. Med.* 13, 432–438. doi: 10.1038/nm1555

Farber, K., and Kettenmann, H. (2006). Functional role of calcium signals for microglial function. *Glia* 54, 656–665. doi: 10.1002/glia.20412

Frei, K., Nohava, K., Malipiero, U. V., Schwerdel, C., and Fontana, A. (1992). Production of macrophage colony-stimulating factor by astrocytes and brain macrophages. *J. Neuroimmunol.* 40, 189–195. doi: 10.1016/0165-5728(92)90133-6

Gao, H. M., Hong, J. S., Zhang, W., and Liu, B. (2003). Synergistic dopaminergic neurotoxicity of the pesticide rotenone and inflammogen lipopolysaccharide: relevance to the etiology of Parkinson's disease. *J. Neurosci.* 23, 1228–1236.

Gao, H. M., Jiang, J., Wilson, B., Zhang, W., Hong, J. S., and Liu, B. (2002). Microglial activation-mediated delayed and progressive degeneration of rat nigral dopaminergic neurons: relevance to Parkinson's disease. *J. Neurochem.* 81, 1285–1297. doi: 10.1046/j.1471-4159.2002.00928.x

Gerhard, A., Pavese, N., Hotton, G., Turkheimer, F., Es, M., Hammers, A., et al. (2006). *In vivo* imaging of microglial activation with $[^{11}C](R)$-PK11195 PET in idiopathic Parkinson's disease. *Neurobiol. Dis.* 21, 404–412. doi: 10.1016/j.nbd.2005.08.002

Giulian, D., Haverkamp, L. J., Li, J., Karshin, W. L., Yu, J., Tom, D., et al. (1995). Senile plaques stimulate microglia to release a neurotoxin found in Alzheimer brain. *Neurochem. Int.* 27, 119–137. doi: 10.1016/0197-0186(95)00067-i

Giulian, D., Haverkamp, L. J., Yu, J. H., Karshin, W., Tom, D., Li, J., et al. (1996). Specific domains of β-amyloid from Alzheimer plaque elicit neuron killing in human microglia. *J. Neurosci.* 16, 6021–6037.

Glass, C. K., Saijo, K., Winner, B., Marchetto, M. C., and Gage, F. H. (2010). Mechanisms underlying inflammation in neurodegeneration. *Cell* 140, 918–934. doi: 10.1016/j.cell.2010.02.016

Graeber, M. B. (2010). Changing face of microglia. *Science* 330, 783–788. doi: 10.1126/science.1190929

Graeber, M. B., Bise, K., and Mehraein, P. (1994). CR3/43, a marker for activated human microglia: application to diagnostic neuropathology. *Neuropathol. Appl. Neurobiol.* 20, 406–408. doi: 10.1111/j.1365-2990.1994.tb00987.x

Graeber, M. B., Tetzlaff, W., Streit, W. J., and Kreutzberg, G. W. (1988). Microglial cells but not astrocytes undergo mitosis following rat facial nerve axotomy. *Neurosci. Lett.* 85, 317–321. doi: 10.1016/0304-3940(88)90585-x

Haga, S., Akai, K., and Ishii, T. (1989). Demonstration of microglial cells in and around senile (neuritic) plaques in the Alzheimer brain. An immunohistochemical study using a novel monoclonal antibody. *Acta Neuropathol.* 77, 569–575. doi: 10.1007/bf00687883

Hanisch, U. K., and Kettenmann, H. (2007). Microglia: active sensor and versatile effector cells in the normal and pathologic brain. *Nat. Neurosci.* 10, 1387–1394. doi: 10.1038/nn1997

Haynes, S. E., Hollopeter, G., Yang, G., Kurpius, D., Dailey, M. E., Gan, W. B., et al. (2006). The P2Y12 receptor regulates microglial activation by extracellular nucleotides. *Nat. Neurosci.* 9, 1512–1519. doi: 10.1038/nn1805

Hickman, S. E., Allison, E. K., and El Khoury, J. (2008). Microglial dysfunction and defective β-amyloid clearance pathways in aging Alzheimer's disease mice. *J. Neurosci.* 28, 8354–8360. doi: 10.1523/JNEUROSCI.0616-08.2008

Hide, I., Tanaka, M., Inoue, A., Nakajima, K., Kohsaka, S., Inoue, K., et al. (2000). Extracellular ATP triggers tumor necrosis factor-α release from rat microglia. *J. Neurochem.* 75, 965–972. doi: 10.1046/j.1471-4159.2000.0750965.x

Hirsch, E. C., Hunot, S., Damier, P., and Faucheux, B. (1998). Glial cells and inflammation in Parkinson's disease: a role in neurodegeneration? *Ann. Neurol.* 44, S115–S120. doi: 10.1002/ana.410440717

Hoffmann, A., Kann, O., Ohlemeyer, C., Hanisch, U. K., and Kettenmann, H. (2003). Elevation of basal intracellular calcium as a central element in the activation of brain macrophages (microglia): suppression of receptor-evoked calcium signaling and control of release function. *J. Neurosci.* 23, 4410–4419.

Honda, S., Sasaki, Y., Ohsawa, K., Imai, Y., Nakamura, Y., Inoue, K., et al. (2001). Extracellular ATP or ADP induce chemotaxis of cultured microglia through Gi/o-coupled P2Y receptors. *J. Neurosci.* 21, 1975–1982.

Horvath, R. J., Nutile-McMenemy, N., Alkaitis, M. S., and Deleo, J. A. (2008). Differential migration, LPS-induced cytokine, chemokine, and NO expression in immortalized BV-2 and HAPI cell lines and primary microglial cultures. *J. Neurochem.* 107, 557–569. doi: 10.1111/j.1471-4159.2008.05633.x

Hunot, S., Boissiere, F., Faucheux, B., Brugg, B., Mouatt-Prigent, A., Agid, Y., et al. (1996). Nitric oxide synthase and neuronal vulnerability in Parkinson's disease. *Neuroscience* 72, 355–363. doi: 10.1016/0306-4522(95)00578-1

Ikeda, M., Shoji, M., Kawarai, T., Kawarabayashi, T., Matsubara, E., Murakami, T., et al. (2005). Accumulation of filamentous tau in the cerebral cortex of human tau R406W transgenic mice. *Am. J. Pathol.* 166, 521–531. doi: 10.1016/s0002-9440(10)62274-2

Itagaki, S., McGeer, P. L., Akiyama, H., Zhu, S., and Selkoe, D. (1989). Relationship of microglia and astrocytes to amyloid deposits of Alzheimer disease. *J. Neuroimmunol.* 24, 173–182. doi: 10.1016/0165-5728(89)90115-x

Ittner, L. M., and Götz, J. (2011). Amyloid-β and tau—a toxic *pas de deux* in Alzheimer's disease. *Nat. Rev. Neurosci.* 12, 65–72. doi: 10.1038/nrn2967

Ittner, L. M., Ke, Y. D., Delerue, F., Bi, M., Gladbach, A., van Eersel, J., et al. (2010). Dendritic function of tau mediates amyloid-β toxicity in Alzheimer's disease mouse models. *Cell* 142, 387–397. doi: 10.1016/j.cell.2010.06.036

Jonas, R. A., Yuan, T. F., Liang, Y. X., Jonas, J. B., Tay, D. K., and Ellis-Behnke, R. G. (2012). The spider effect: morphological and orienting classification of microglia in response to stimuli *in vivo*. *PLoS One* 7:e30763. doi: 10.1371/journal.pone.0030763

Kadavath, H., Hofele, R. V., Biernat, J., Kumar, S., Tepper, K., Urlaub, H., et al. (2015). Tau stabilizes microtubules by binding at the interface between tubulin heterodimers. *Proc. Natl. Acad. Sci. U S A* 112, 7501–7506. doi: 10.1073/pnas.1504081112

Kann, O., Hoffmann, A., Schumann, R. R., Weber, J. R., Kettenmann, H., and Hanisch, U. K. (2004). The tyrosine kinase inhibitor AG126 restores receptor signaling and blocks release functions in activated microglia (brain macrophages) by preventing a chronic rise in the intracellular calcium level. *J. Neurochem.* 90, 513–525. doi: 10.1111/j.1471-4159.2004.02534.x

Karperien, A., Ahammer, H., and Jelinek, H. F. (2013). Quantitating the subtleties of microglial morphology with fractal analysis. *Front. Cell. Neurosci.* 7:3. doi: 10.3389/fncel.2013.00003

Kato, G., Inada, H., Wake, H., Akiyoshi, R., Miyamoto, A., Eto, K., et al. (2016). Microglial contact prevents excess depolarization and rescues neurons from excitotoxicity. *eNeuro* 3:ENEURO.0004-16.2016. doi: 10.1523/ENEURO.0004-16.2016

Kim, C., Lee, H. J., Masliah, E., and Lee, S. J. (2016). Non-cell-autonomous Neurotoxicity of α-synuclein Through Microglial Toll-like Receptor 2. *Exp. Neurobiol.* 25, 113–119. doi: 10.5607/en.2016.25.3.113

Kim, Y. S., and Joh, T. H. (2006). Microglia, major player in the brain inflammation: their roles in the pathogenesis of Parkinson's disease. *Exp. Mol. Med.* 38, 333–347. doi: 10.1038/emm.2006.40

Kim, Y. S., Choi, D. H., Block, M. L., Lorenzl, S., Yang, L., Kim, Y. J., et al. (2007). A pivotal role of matrix metalloproteinase-3 activity in dopaminergic neuronal degeneration via microglial activation. *FASEB J.* 21, 179–187. doi: 10.1096/fj.06-5865com

Kim, Y. S., Kim, S. S., Cho, J. J., Choi, D. H., Hwang, O., Shin, D. H., et al. (2005). Matrix metalloproteinase-3: a novel signaling proteinase from apoptotic neuronal cells that activates microglia. *J. Neurosci.* 25, 3701–3711. doi: 10.1523/JNEUROSCI.4346-04.2005

Kitazawa, M., Cheng, D., Tsukamoto, M. R., Koike, M. A., Wes, P. D., Vasilevko, V., et al. (2011). Blocking IL-1 signaling rescues cognition, attenuates tau pathology and restores neuronal β-catenin pathway function in an Alzheimer's disease model. *J. Immunol.* 187, 6539–6549. doi: 10.4049/jimmunol.1100620

Kitazawa, M., Oddo, S., Yamasaki, T. R., Green, K. N., and LaFerla, F. M. (2005). Lipopolysaccharide-induced inflammation exacerbates tau pathology by a cyclin-dependent kinase 5-mediated pathway in a transgenic model of Alzheimer's disease. *J. Neurosci.* 25, 8843–8853. doi: 10.1523/JNEUROSCI.2868-05.2005

Kitazawa, M., Yamasaki, T. R., and LaFerla, F. M. (2004). Microglia as a potential bridge between the amyloid β-peptide and tau. *Ann. N Y Acad. Sci.* 1035, 85–103. doi: 10.1196/annals.1332.006

Knott, C., Stern, G., and Wilkin, G. P. (2000). Inflammatory regulators in Parkinson's disease: iNOS, lipocortin-1 and cyclooxygenases-1 and -2. *Mol. Cell. Neurosci.* 16, 724–739. doi: 10.1006/mcne.2000.0914

Koizumi, S., Shigemoto-Mogami, Y., Nasu-Tada, K., Shinozaki, Y., Ohsawa, K., Tsuda, M., et al. (2007). UDP acting at P2Y6 receptors is a mediator of microglial phagocytosis. *Nature* 446, 1091–1095. doi: 10.1038/nature05704

Kokovay, E., and Cunningham, L. A. (2005). Bone marrow-derived microglia contribute to the neuroinflammatory response and express iNOS in the MPTP mouse model of Parkinson's disease. *Neurobiol. Dis.* 19, 471–478. doi: 10.1016/j.nbd.2005.01.023

Korotzer, A. R., and Cotman, C. W. (1992). Voltage-gated currents expressed by rat microglia in culture. *Glia* 6, 81–88. doi: 10.1002/glia.440060202

Krause, D. L., and Müller, N. (2010). Neuroinflammation, microglia and implications for anti-inflammatory treatment in Alzheimer's disease. *Int. J. Alzheimers Dis.* 2010:732806. doi: 10.4061/2010/732806

Kuret, J., Chirita, C. N., Congdon, E. E., Kannanayakal, T., Li, G., Necula, M., et al. (2005a). Pathways of tau fibrillization. *Biochim. Biophys. Acta* 1739, 167–178. doi: 10.1016/j.bbadis.2004.06.016

Kuret, J., Congdon, E. E., Li, G., Yin, H., Yu, X., and Zhong, Q. (2005b). Evaluating triggers and enhancers of tau fibrillization. *Microsc. Res. Tech.* 67, 141–155. doi: 10.1002/jemt.20187

Lalancette-Hébert, M., Gowing, G., Simard, A., Weng, Y. C., and Kriz, J. (2007). Selective ablation of proliferating microglial cells exacerbates ischemic injury in the brain. *J. Neurosci.* 27, 2596–2605. doi: 10.1523/JNEUROSCI.5360-06.2007

Lawson, L. J., Perry, V. H., Dri, P., and Gordon, S. (1990). Heterogeneity in the distribution and morphology of microglia in the normal adult mouse brain. *Neuroscience* 39, 151–170. doi: 10.1016/0306-4522(90)90229-w

Le, W., Rowe, D., Xie, W., Ortiz, I., He, Y., and Appel, S. H. (2001). Microglial activation and dopaminergic cell injury: an *in vitro* model relevant to Parkinson's disease. *J. Neurosci.* 21, 8447–8455.

Lee, D. C., Rizer, J., Selenica, M. L., Reid, P., Kraft, C., Johnson, A., et al. (2010). LPS- induced inflammation exacerbates phospho-tau pathology in rTg4510 mice. *J. Neuroinflammation* 7:56. doi: 10.1186/1742-2094-7-56

Leissring, M. A., Farris, W., Chang, A. Y., Walsh, D. M., Wu, X., Sun, X., et al. (2003). Enhanced proteolysis of β-amyloid in APP transgenic mice prevents plaque formation, secondary pathology, and premature death. *Neuron* 40, 1087–1093. doi: 10.1016/s0896-6273(03)00787-6

Li, Y., Liu, L., Barger, S. W., and Griffin, W. S. (2003). Interleukin-1 mediates pathological effects of microglia on tau phosphorylation and on synaptophysin synthesis in cortical neurons through a p38-MAPK pathway. *J. Neurosci.* 23, 1605–1611.

Liberatore, G. T., Jackson-Lewis, V., Vukosavic, S., Mandir, A. S., Vila, M., McAuliffe, W. G., et al. (1999). Inducible nitric oxide synthase stimulates dopaminergic neurodegeneration in the MPTP model of Parkinson disease. *Nat. Med.* 5, 1403–1409. doi: 10.1038/70978

Liu, W., Brosnan, C. F., Dickson, D. W., and Lee, S. C. (1994). Macrophage colony-stimulating factor mediates astrocyte-induced microglial ramification in human fetal central nervous system culture. *Am. J. Pathol.* 145, 48–53.

Long-Smith, C. M., Sullivan, A. M., and Nolan, Y. M. (2009). The influence of microglia on the pathogenesis of Parkinson's disease. *Prog. Neurobiol.* 89, 277–287. doi: 10.1016/j.pneurobio.2009.08.001

Lynch, M. A. (2009). The multifaceted profile of activated microglia. *Mol. Neurobiol.* 40, 139–156. doi: 10.1007/s12035-009-8077-9

Maccioni, R. B., Farías, G., Morales, I., and Navarrete, L. (2010). The revitalized tau hypothesis on Alzheimer's disease. *Arch. Med. Res.* 41, 226–231. doi: 10.1016/j.arcmed.2010.03.007

Markov, D. V., and Dimova, R. N. (1974). Ultrastructural alterations of rat brain microglial cells and pericytes after chronic lead poisoning. *Acta Neuropathol.* 28, 25–35. doi: 10.1007/bf00687515

McGeer, P. L., Itagaki, S., Boyes, B. E., and McGeer, E. G. (1988). Reactive microglia are positive for HLA-DR in the substantia nigra of Parkinson's and Alzheimer's disease brains. *Neurology* 38, 1285–1291. doi: 10.1212/wnl.38.8.1285

Merrill, J. E. (1991). Effects of interleukin-1 and tumor necrosis factor-α on astrocytes, microglia, oligodendrocytes, and glial precursors *in vitro*. *Dev. Neurosci.* 13, 130–137. doi: 10.1159/000112150

Mogi, M., Harada, M., Kondo, T., Riederer, P., Inagaki, H., Minami, M., et al. (1994a). Interleukin-1β, interleukin-6, epidermal growth factor and transforming growth factor-α are elevated in the brain from parkinsonian patients. *Neurosci. Lett.* 180, 147–150. doi: 10.1016/0304-3940(94)90508-8

Mogi, M., Harada, M., Riederer, P., Narabayashi, H., Fujita, K., and Nagatsu, T. (1994b). Tumor necrosis factor-α (TNF-α) increases both in the brain and in the cerebrospinal fluid from parkinsonian patients. *Neurosci. Lett.* 165, 208–210. doi: 10.1016/0304-3940(94)90746-3

Möller, T. (2002). Calcium signaling in microglial cells. *Glia* 40, 184–194. doi: 10.1002/glia.10152

Möller, T., Kann, O., Verkhratsky, A., and Kettenmann, H. (2000). Activation of mouse microglial cells affects P2 receptor signaling. *Brain Res.* 853, 49–59. doi: 10.1016/s0006-8993(99)02244-1

Moran, L. B., and Graeber, M. B. (2004). The facial nerve axotomy model. *Brain Res. Rev.* 44, 154–178. doi: 10.1016/j.brainresrev.2003.11.004

Mount, M. P., Lira, A., Grimes, D., Smith, P. D., Faucher, S., Slack, R., et al. (2007). Involvement of interferon-γ in microglial-mediated loss of dopaminergic neurons. *J. Neurosci.* 27, 3328–3337. doi: 10.1523/JNEUROSCI.5321-06.2007

Müller, T., Blum-Degen, D., Przuntek, H., and Kuhn, W. (1998). Interleukin-6 levels in cerebrospinal fluid inversely correlate to severity of Parkinson's disease. *Acta Neurol. Scand.* 98, 142–144. doi: 10.1111/j.1600-0404.1998.tb01736.x

Nakajima, K., Honda, S., Tohyama, Y., Imai, Y., Kohsaka, S., and Kurihara, T. (2001). Neurotrophin secretion from cultured microglia. *J. Neurosci. Res.* 65, 322–331. doi: 10.1002/jnr.1157

Nakamura, Y., Si, Q. S., and Kataoka, K. (1999). Lipopolysaccharide-induced microglial activation in culture: temporal profiles of morphological change and release of cytokines and nitric oxide. *Neurosci. Res.* 35, 95–100. doi: 10.1016/s0168-0102(99)00071-1

Nash, K. R., Lee, D. C., Hunt, J. B. Jr., Morganti, J. M., Selenica, M. L., Moran, P., et al. (2013). Fractalkine overexpression suppresses tau pathology in a mouse model of tauopathy. *Neurobiol. Aging* 34, 1540–1548. doi: 10.1016/j.neurobiolaging.2012.12.011

Nelson, P. T., Soma, L. A., and Lavi, E. (2002). Microglia in diseases of the central nervous system. *Ann. Med.* 34, 491–500. doi: 10.1080/078538902321117698

Neufeld, A. H. (1999). Microglia in the optic nerve head and the region of parapapillary chorioretinal atrophy in glaucoma. *Arch. Ophthalmol.* 117, 1050–1056. doi: 10.1001/archopht.117.8.1050

Nimmerjahn, A., Kirchhoff, F., and Helmchen, F. (2005). Resting microglial cells are highly dynamic surveillants of brain parenchyma *in vivo*. *Science* 308, 1314–1318. doi: 10.1126/science.1110647

Nissl, F. (1899). Über einige Beziehungen zwischen Nervenzellerkrankungen und gliösen Erscheinungen bei verschiedenen Psychosen. *Arch. Psychiatr.* 32, 656–676.

Oakley, H., Cole, S. L., Logan, S., Maus, E., Shao, P., Craft, J., et al. (2006). Intraneuronal β-amyloid aggregates, neurodegeneration and neuron loss in transgenic mice with five familial Alzheimer's disease mutations: potential factors in amyloid plaque formation. *J. Neurosci.* 26, 10129–10140. doi: 10.1523/JNEUROSCI.1202-06.2006

Odawara, T., Iseki, E., Kosaka, K., Akiyama, H., Ikeda, K., and Yamamoto, T. (1995). Investigation of tau-2 positive microglia-like cells in the subcortical nuclei of human neurodegenerative disorders. *Neurosci. Lett.* 192, 145–148. doi: 10.1016/0304-3940(95)11595-n

Ouchi, Y., Yagi, S., Yokokura, M., and Sakamoto, M. (2009). Neuroinflammation in the living brain of Parkinson's disease. *Parkinsonism Relat. Disord.* 15, S200–S204. doi: 10.1016/s1353-8020(09)70814-4

Ouchi, Y., Yoshikawa, E., Sekine, Y., Futatsubashi, M., Kanno, T., Ogusu, T., et al. (2005). Microglial activation and dopamine terminal loss in early Parkinson's disease. *Ann. Neurol.* 57, 168–175. doi: 10.1002/ana.20338

Pannell, M., Szulzewsky, F., Matyash, V., Wolf, S. A., and Kettenmann, H. (2014). The subpopulation of microglia sensitive to neurotransmitters/neurohormones is modulated by stimulation with LPS, interferon-γ and IL-4. *Glia* 62, 667–679. doi: 10.1002/glia.22633

Papageorgiou, I. E., Lewen, A., Galow, L. V., Cesetti, T., Scheffel, J., Regen, T., et al. (2016). TLR4-activated microglia require IFN-γ to induce severe neuronal dysfunction and death *in situ*. *Proc. Natl. Acad. Sci. U S A* 113, 212–217. doi: 10.1073/pnas.1513853113

Paresce, D. M., Chung, H., and Maxfield, F. R. (1997). Slow degradation of aggregates of the Alzheimer's disease amyloid β-protein by microglial cells. *J. Biol. Chem.* 272, 29390–29397. doi: 10.1074/jbc.272.46.29390

Paresce, D. M., Ghosh, R. N., and Maxfield, F. R. (1996). Microglial cells internalize aggregates of the Alzheimer's disease amyloid β-protein via a scavenger receptor. *Neuron* 17, 553–565. doi: 10.1016/s0896-6273(00)80187-7

Pavese, N., Gerhard, A., Tai, Y. F., Ho, A. K., Turkheimer, F., Barker, R. A., et al. (2006). Microglial activation correlates with severity in Huntington disease: a clinical and PET study. *Neurology* 66, 1638–1643. doi: 10.1212/01.wnl.0000222734.56412.17

Perry, V. H., and O'Connor, V. (2010). The role of microglia in synaptic stripping and synaptic degeneration: a revised perspective. *ASN Neuro* 2:e00047. doi: 10.1042/An20100024

Politis, M., Pavese, N., Tai, Y. F., Kiferle, L., Mason, S. L., Brooks, D. J., et al. (2011). Microglial activation in regions related to cognitive function predicts disease onset in Huntington's disease: a multimodal imaging study. *Hum. Brain Mapp.* 32, 258–270. doi: 10.1002/hbm.21008

Qin, H., Roberts, K. L., Niyongere, S. A., Cong, Y., Elson, C. O., and Benveniste, E. N. (2007). Molecular mechanism of lipopolysaccharide-induced SOCS-3 gene expression in macrophages and microglia. *J. Immunol.* 179, 5966–5976. doi: 10.4049/jimmunol.179.9.5966

Qin, L., Wu, X., Block, M. L., Liu, Y., Breese, G. R., Hong, J. S., et al. (2007). Systemic LPS causes chronic neuroinflammation and progressive neurodegeneration. *Glia* 55, 453–462. doi: 10.1002/glia.20467

Qin, L., Liu, Y., Wang, T., Wei, S. J., Block, M. L., Wilson, B., et al. (2004). NADPH oxidase mediates lipopolysaccharide-induced neurotoxicity and proinflammatory gene expression in activated microglia. *J. Biol. Chem.* 279, 1415–1421. doi: 10.1074/jbc.M307657200

Quigley, H. A., Addicks, E. M., Green, W. R., and Maumenee, A. E. (1981). Optic nerve damage in human glaucoma. II. The site of injury and susceptibility to damage. *Arch. Ophthalmol.* 99, 635–649. doi: 10.1001/archopht.1981.03930010635009

Quigley, H. A., Dunkelberger, G. R., and Green, W. R. (1988). Chronic human glaucoma causing selectively greater loss of large optic nerve fibers. *Ophthalmology* 95, 357–363. doi: 10.1016/s0161-6420(88)33176-3

Quigley, H. A., Dunkelberger, G. R., and Green, W. R. (1989). Retinal ganglion cell atrophy correlated with automated perimetry in human eyes with glaucoma. *Am. J. Ophthalmol.* 107, 453–464. doi: 10.1016/0002-9394(89)90488-1

Ross, C. A., and Poirier, M. A. (2004). Protein aggregation and neurodegenerative disease. *Nat. Med.* 10, S10–S17. doi: 10.1038/nm1066

Sapp, E., Kegel, K. B., Aronin, N., Hashikawa, T., Uchiyama, Y., Tohyama, K., et al. (2001). Early and progressive accumulation of reactive microglia in the Huntington disease brain. *J. Neuropathol. Exp. Neurol.* 60, 161–172. doi: 10.1093/jnen/60.2.161

Sawada, M., Suzumura, A., Hosoya, H., Marunouchi, T., and Nagatsu, T. (1999). Interleukin-10 inhibits both production of cytokines and expression of cytokine receptors in microglia. *J. Neurochem.* 72, 1466–1471. doi: 10.1046/j.1471-4159.1999.721466.x

Scholz, T., and Mandelkow, E. (2014). Transport and diffusion of Tau protein in neurons. *Cell. Mol. Life Sci.* 71, 3139–3150. doi: 10.1007/s00018-014-1610-7

Selkoe, D. J. (2000). The origins of Alzheimer disease: a is for amyloid. *JAMA* 283, 1615–1617. doi: 10.1001/jama.283.12.1615

Shaffer, L. M., Dority, M. D., Gupta-Bansal, R., Frederickson, R. C., Younkin, S. G., and Brunden, K. R. (1995). Amyloid β protein (Aβ) removal by neuroglial cells in culture. *Neurobiol. Aging* 16, 737–745. doi: 10.1016/0197-4580(95)00055-J

Sheng, W., Zong, Y., Mohammad, A., Ajit, D., Cui, J., Han, D., et al. (2011). Pro-inflammatory cytokines and lipopolysaccharide induce changes in cell morphology and upregulation of ERK1/2, iNOS and sPLA$_2$-IIA expression in astrocytes and microglia. *J. Neuroinflammation* 8:121. doi: 10.1186/1742-2094-8-121

Sievers, J., Schmidtmayer, J., and Parwaresch, R. (1994). Blood monocytes and spleen macrophages differentiate into microglia-like cells when cultured on astrocytes. *Ann. Anat.* 176, 45–51. doi: 10.1016/s0940-9602(11)80414-0

Silvestroni, A., Faull, R. L., Strand, A. D., and Möller, T. (2009). Distinct neuroinflammatory profile in post-mortem human Huntington's disease. *Neuroreport* 20, 1098–1103. doi: 10.1097/WNR.0b013e32832e34ee

Simard, A. R., Soulet, D., Gowing, G., Julien, J. P., and Rivest, S. (2006). Bone marrow-derived microglia play a critical role in restricting senile plaque formation in Alzheimer's disease. *Neuron* 49, 489–502. doi: 10.1016/j.neuron.2006.01.022

Singhrao, S. K., Neal, J. W., Morgan, B. P., and Gasque, P. (1999). Increased complement biosynthesis by microglia and complement activation on neurons in Huntington's disease. *Exp. Neurol.* 159, 362–376. doi: 10.1006/exnr.1999.7170

Smith, J. A., Das, A., Ray, S. K., and Banik, N. L. (2012). Role of pro-inflammatory cytokines released from microglia in neurodegenerative diseases. *Brain Res. Bull.* 87, 10–20. doi: 10.1016/j.brainresbull.2011.10.004

Spielmeyer, W. (1922). *Histopathologie des Nervensystems.* Berlin: J. Springer.

Stolzing, A., Wengner, A., and Grune, T. (2002). Degradation of oxidized extracellular proteins by microglia. *Arch. Biochem. Biophys.* 400, 171–179. doi: 10.1016/s0003-9861(02)00003-6

Suzumura, A., Marunouchi, T., and Yamamoto, H. (1991). Morphological transformation of microglia *in vitro*. *Brain Res.* 545, 301–306. doi: 10.1016/0006-8993(91)91302-h

Suzumura, A., Sawada, M., Yamamoto, H., and Marunouchi, T. (1990). Effects of colony stimulating factors on isolated microglia *in vitro*. *J. Neuroimmunol.* 30, 111–120. doi: 10.1016/0165-5728(90)90094-4

Szabo, M., and Gulya, K. (2013). Development of the microglial phenotype in culture. *Neuroscience* 241, 280–295. doi: 10.1016/j.neuroscience.2013.03.033

Tam, W. Y., and Ma, C. H. (2014). Bipolar/rod-shaped microglia are proliferating microglia with distinct M1/M2 phenotypes. *Sci. Rep.* 4:7279. doi: 10.1038/srep07279

Tam, W. Y., Au, N. P., and Ma, C. H. (2016). The association between laminin and microglial morphology *in vitro*. *Sci. Rep.* 6:28580. doi: 10.1038/srep28580

Taylor, S. E., Morganti-Kossmann, C., Lifshitz, J., and Ziebell, J. M. (2014). Rod microglia: a morphological definition. *PLoS One* 9:e97096. doi: 10.1371/journal.pone.0097096

Toulouse, A., and Sullivan, A. M. (2008). Progress in Parkinson's disease-where do we stand? *Prog. Neurobiol.* 85, 376–392. doi: 10.1016/j.pneurobio.2008.05.003

Town, T., Zolton, J., Shaffner, R., Schnell, B., Crescentini, R., Wu, Y., et al. (2002). p35/Cdk5 pathway mediates soluble amyloid-β peptide-induced tau phosphorylation *in vitro*. *J. Neurosci. Res.* 69, 362–372. doi: 10.1002/jnr.10299

Townsend, K. P., Town, T., Mori, T., Lue, L. F., Shytle, D., Sanberg, P. R., et al. (2005). CD40 signaling regulates innate and adaptive activation of microglia in response to amyloid β-peptide. *Eur. J. Immunol.* 35, 901–910. doi: 10.1002/eji.200425585

Trapp, B. D., Wujek, J. R., Criste, G. A., Jalabi, W., Yin, X., Kidd, G. J., et al. (2007). Evidence for synaptic stripping by cortical microglia. *Glia* 55, 360–368. doi: 10.1002/glia.20462

Tremblay, M. E., Lowery, R. L., and Majewska, A. K. (2010). Microglial interactions with synapses are modulated by visual experience. *PLoS Biol.* 8:e1000527. doi: 10.1371/journal.pbio.1000527

Vijitruth, R., Liu, M., Choi, D. Y., Nguyen, X. V., Hunter, R. L., and Bing, G. (2006). Cyclooxygenase-2 mediates microglial activation and secondary dopaminergic cell death in the mouse MPTP model of Parkinson's disease. *J. Neuroinflammation* 3:6. doi: 10.1186/1742-2094-3-6

von Bernhardi, R., and Eugenín, J. (2004). Microglial reactivity to β-amyloid is modulated by astrocytes and proinflammatory factors. *Brain Res.* 1025, 186–193. doi: 10.1016/j.brainres.2004.07.084

Vonsattel, J. P., and DiFiglia, M. (1998). Huntington disease. *J. Neuropathol. Exp. Neurol.* 57, 369–384. doi: 10.1097/00005072-199805000-00001

Vonsattel, J. P., Myers, R. H., Stevens, T. J., Ferrante, R. J., Bird, E. D., and Richardson, E. P. Jr., et al. (1985). Neuropathological classification of Huntington's disease. *J. Neuropathol. Exp. Neurol.* 44, 559–577. doi: 10.1097/00005072-198511000-00003

Wake, H., Moorhouse, A. J., Jinno, S., Kohsaka, S., and Nabekura, J. (2009). Resting microglia directly monitor the functional state of synapses *in vivo* and determine the fate of ischemic terminals. *J. Neurosci.* 29, 3974–3980. doi: 10.1523/JNEUROSCI.4363-08.2009

Wegiel, J., and Wisniewski, H. M. (1990). The complex of microglial cells and amyloid star in three-dimensional reconstruction. *Acta Neuropathol.* 81, 116–124. doi: 10.1007/BF00334499

Wegiel, J., Imaki, H., Wang, K. C., Wegiel, J., and Rubenstein, R. (2004). Cells of monocyte/microglial lineage are involved in both microvessel amyloidosis and fibrillar plaque formation in APPsw tg mice. *Brain Res.* 1022, 19–29. doi: 10.1016/j.brainres.2004.06.058

Wegiel, J., Imaki, H., Wang, K. C., Wegiel, J., Wronska, A., Osuchowski, M., et al. (2003). Origin and turnover of microglial cells in fibrillar plaques of APPsw transgenic mice. *Acta Neuropathol.* 105, 393–402. doi: 10.1007/s00401-002-0660-3

Weingarten, M. D., Lockwood, A. H., Hwo, S. Y., and Kirschner, M. W. (1975). A protein factor essential for microtubule assembly. *Proc. Natl. Acad. Sci. U S A* 72, 1858–1862. doi: 10.1073/pnas.72.5.1858

West, M. J., Coleman, P. D., Flood, D. G., and Troncoso, J. C. (1994). Differences in the pattern of hippocampal neuronal loss in normal ageing and Alzheimer's disease. *Lancet* 344, 769–772. doi: 10.1016/s0140-6736(94)92338-8

Wierzba-Bobrowicz, T., Gwiazda, E., Kosno-Kruszewska, E., Lewandowska, E., Lechowicz, W., Bertrand, E., et al. (2002). Morphological analysis of active microglia–rod and ramified microglia in human brains affected by some neurological diseases (SSPE, Alzheimer's disease and Wilson's disease). *Folia Neuropathol.* 40, 125–131.

Wilms, H., Rosenstiel, P., Sievers, J., Deuschl, G., Zecca, L., and Lucius, R. (2003). Activation of microglia by human neuromelanin is NF-kappaB dependent and involves p38 mitogen-activated protein kinase: implications for Parkinson's disease. *FASEB J.* 17, 500–502. doi: 10.1096/fj.02-0314fje

Wyss-Coray, T., and Mucke, L. (2002). Inflammation in neurodegenerative disease–a double-edged sword. *Neuron* 35, 419–432. doi: 10.1016/s0896-6273(02)00794-8

Yan, P., Hu, X., Song, H., Yin, K., Bateman, R. J., Cirrito, J. R., et al. (2006). Matrix metalloproteinase-9 degrades amyloid-β fibrils *in vitro* and compact plaques *in situ*. *J. Biol. Chem.* 281, 24566–24574. doi: 10.1074/jbc.M602440200

Yoshiyama, Y., Higuchi, M., Zhang, B., Huang, S. M., Iwata, N., Saido, T. C., et al. (2007). Synapse loss and microglial activation precede tangles in a P301S tauopathy mouse model. *Neuron* 53, 337–351. doi: 10.1016/j.neuron.2007.01.010

Yuan, L., and Neufeld, A. H. (2001). Activated microglia in the human glaucomatous optic nerve head. *J. Neurosci. Res.* 64, 523–532. doi: 10.1002/jnr.1104

Yuan, T. F., Liang, Y. X., Peng, B., Lin, B., and So, K. F. (2015). Local proliferation is the main source of rod microglia after optic nerve transection. *Sci. Rep.* 5:10788. doi: 10.1038/srep10788

Zhan, X., Kim, C., and Sharp, F. R. (2008). Very brief focal ischemia simulating transient ischemic attacks (TIAs) can injure brain and induce Hsp70 protein. *Brain Res.* 1234, 183–197. doi: 10.1016/j.brainres.2008.07.094

Zhang, W., Wang, T., Pei, Z., Miller, D. S., Wu, X., Block, M. L., et al. (2005). Aggregated α-synuclein activates microglia: a process leading to disease progression in Parkinson's disease. *FASEB J.* 19, 533–542. doi: 10.1096/fj.04-2751com

Ziebell, J. M., Adelson, P. D., and Lifshitz, J. (2015). Microglia: dismantling and rebuilding circuits after acute neurological injury. *Metab. Brain Dis.* 30, 393–400. doi: 10.1007/s11011-014-9539-y

Ziebell, J. M., Taylor, S. E., Cao, T., Harrison, J. L., and Lifshitz, J. (2012). Rod microglia: elongation, alignment, and coupling to form trains across the somatosensory cortex after experimental diffuse brain injury. *J. Neuroinflammation* 9:247. doi: 10.1186/1742-2094-9-247

Zilka, N., Stozicka, Z., Kovac, A., Pilipcinec, E., Bugos, O., and Novak, M. (2009). Human misfolded truncated tau protein promotes activation of microglia and leukocyte infiltration in the transgenic rat model of tauopathy. *J. Neuroimmunol.* 209, 16–25. doi: 10.1016/j.jneuroim.2009.01.013

6

Aging Microglia—Phenotypes, Functions and Implications for Age-Related Neurodegenerative Diseases

Björn Spittau[1,2]*

[1]Department of Molecular Embryology, Faculty of Medicine, Institute for Anatomy and Cell Biology, University of Freiburg, Freiburg, Germany, [2]Institute of Anatomy, University of Rostock, Rostock, Germany

***Correspondence:**
Björn Spittau
bjoern.spittau@anat.uni-freiburg.de*

Aging of the central nervous system (CNS) is one of the major risk factors for the development of neurodegenerative pathologies such as Parkinson's disease (PD) and Alzheimer's disease (AD). The molecular mechanisms underlying the onset of AD and especially PD are not well understood. However, neuroinflammatory responses mediated by microglia as the resident immune cells of the CNS have been reported for both diseases. The unique nature and developmental origin of microglia causing microglial self-renewal and telomere shortening led to the hypothesis that these CNS-specific innate immune cells become senescent. Age-dependent and senescence-driven impairments of microglia functions and responses have been suggested to play essential roles during onset and progression of neurodegenerative diseases. This review article summarizes the current knowledge of microglia phenotypes and functions in the aging CNS and further discusses the implications of these age-dependent microglia changes for the development and progression of AD and PD as the most common neurodegenerative diseases.

Keywords: aging, microglia, neurodegeneration, Alzheimer's disease (AD), Parkinson's disease (PD)

INTRODUCTION

Microglia are the resident immune cells of the central nervous system (CNS) and are involved in a multifaceted range of physiological as well as pathophysiological functions (Prinz and Priller, 2014). Recent scientific efforts have resulted in the elucidation of the developmental origin, the molecular signature and the versatile functions of these macrophage-like glia cells and gained insight into their nature. Especially, the developmental origin of microglia and the associated phenomenon that these CNS-specific immune cells underlie a self-propelling regeneration causing telomere shortening has resulted in the hypothesis that microglia age, develop age-dependent cellular dystrophy and become senescent (Streit, 2006). Microglial senescence has been linked to functional changes that are high likely to contribute to an age-dependent increase of microglia-mediated neuroinflammatory responses, which are believed to further threaten aged neurons and, thus, drive the progression of age-related neurodegenerative pathologies, such as Alzheimer's disease (AD) and Parkinson's disease (PD). This review article summarizes the current knowledge of functional and phenotypic properties of aged microglia and highlights the contribution of aged microglia to the development and progression of AD and PD.

MICROGLIA ORIGIN

The origin of microglia has long been debated and initial studies suggested that microglia differ substantially from perivascular and meningeal macrophages, which were described to derive from blood-borne monocytes and are constantly replenished (Hickey and Kimura, 1988; Bechmann et al., 2001). Recent reports have demonstrated that both, CNS-specific macrophages and microglia do not develop from circulating monocytes. CNS macrophages including perivascular macrophages, meningeal macrophages and to a lesser extent choroid plexus macrophages arise from hematopoietic precursors during embryonic development in a PU.1-dependent manner and further establish stable cell populations that do not experience turnover and replacement from bone-marrow-derived cells (Goldmann et al., 2016). The developmental origin of microglia has been revealed by elegant fate-mapping experiments, which clearly demonstrated that PU.1 and Irf8-dependent pathways are crucial for microglial embryonic development (Kierdorf et al., 2013). Moreover, this development from yolk sac progenitors is independent of IL-34. However, microglia migration towards and population of the CNS parenchyma relies on neuronal expression and secretion of IL-34, which serves as the most potent homing factor for microglia precursors (Greter et al., 2012). In order to sense IL-34, the microglial expression of colony stimulating factor-1 receptor (CSF1R) is required. Interestingly, the presence of CSF1 itself is not necessary for proper microglia development and colonization of the CNS (Ginhoux et al., 2010). The development of sophisticated methods to immediately isolate microglia and to further analyze their respective gene expression patterns have resulted in the observation that microglia display a unique microglia transcriptome demonstrating that microglia are distinct from other macrophage populations (Beutner et al., 2013). The establishment of this microglia-specific gene expression profile in mice is restricted to the first postnatal weeks and includes distinct microglia genes such as *Olfml3*, *Tmem119*, *Hexb* and *Fcrls*, which indicate microglia maturation (Bennett et al., 2016). Butovsky et al. (2014) have demonstrated that this maturation is dependent on the presence of Transforming growth factor beta 1 (TGFβ1). Using an elegant transgenic mice approach to overcome the lethal inflammatory phenotype of TGFβ1 mutant mice, this seminal study demonstrated that lack of TGFβ1 in the CNS results in decreased microglia numbers and loss of the microglia-specific gene expression signature. However, the molecular mechanisms of microglia maturation are likely to be more complicated and may not entirely rely on CNS-specific mediators. Recently, the contribution of gut microbiota has been demonstrated to regulate microglia maturation and functions in the CNS (Erny et al., 2015).

Upon establishment of the blood-brain-barrier (BBB), microglia undergo a constant self-renewal in order to maintain their population and it has been shown that no progenitor recruitment from blood circulation is contributing to this maintenance of microglia numbers throughout the lifetime (Ajami et al., 2007). Next to proliferation, microglial apoptosis contributes to maintaining the turnover of microglia in the adult CNS (Askew et al., 2017). A challenging central question is whether microglial self-renewal is the result of asymmetric cell division of microglial precursors in the CNS. Using selective CSF1R inhibitors, Elmore et al. (2014) were able to show that microglia could be effectively depleted (90% depletion) from the CNS. Surprisingly, a complete repopulation was observed and was mediated through a proliferation of nestin-positive precursors, which finally differentiated into microglia (Elmore et al., 2014). These results suggest that the microglia turnover in the adult CNS is mediated from a yet unknown precursor cell population or even from a not yet located stem cell niche. It will be of utmost interest to further characterize the endogenous microglia replenishment in the healthy and diseased CNS.

MICROGLIA ACTIVATION

The paradigm that microglia retain a resting state under non-pathological conditions and only react to endogenous and exogenous inflammatory stimuli has been critically evaluated by Nimmerjahn et al. (2005). Using 2-photon imaging, the authors have shown that microglia are constantly surveying their microenvironment in order to rapidly react and migrate towards impairments such as neuron death, BBB leakage or extracellular ATP accumulation (Nimmerjahn et al., 2005). This observation led to the conclusion that microglia might have important functions under physiological conditions. Recent reports have contributed to broaden our understanding that microglia capacities in the CNS include several essential features such as synaptic pruning (Stevens et al., 2007; Paolicelli et al., 2011; Hoshiko et al., 2012; Schafer et al., 2012), influencing functions of activated and/or over-activated neurons (Panatier and Robitaille, 2012), supporting cortical neuron survival (Ueno et al., 2013), shaping axonal projections (Pont-Lezica et al., 2014; Squarzoni et al., 2014), synapse formation during learning in the adult CNS (Parkhurst et al., 2013) as well as maintenance of synaptic functions in the mature retina (Wang et al., 2016). Although many of the abovementioned functions are mediated during the embryonic and postnatal development of the CNS, microglia support neuronal circuits and, thus, important neurological CNS functions throughout adulthood and aging.

Under pathological conditions microglia rapidly change their morphology and adopt activation states in order to adequately react to the activation-causing stimuli. Microglia proliferation has been reported after traumatic CNS injuries (Streit et al., 1999) and degenerative pathologies including optic nerve lesion (Wohl et al., 2010), AD (Kamphuis et al., 2012), prion disease (Gómez-Nicola et al., 2013), PD (Machado et al., 2016) or ischemia (Li et al., 2013).

Based on the nature of distinct microglia stimuli, pathogen-associated molecular patterns (PAMPs) and danger-associated molecular patterns (DAMPs) have been categorized and are detected by microglial receptors including Toll-like receptors (TLRs), NOD-like receptors (NLRs), RIG-like receptors (RLRs), AIM2-like receptors (ALRs) as well as C-type lectins

(Kigerl et al., 2014). In analogy to macrophages, which display remarkable plasticities in response to distinct environmental triggers (Mosser and Edwards, 2008), microglia activation has been subdivided into M1-like and M2-like activation states (Prinz and Priller, 2014). Although M1- and M2-like microglia polarization can be sufficiently induced *in vitro* by using Th1 cytokines such as IFNγ (Zhou et al., 2015) and Th2 cytokines such as IL4 (Zhou et al., 2012), these distinct activation patterns do not seem to be applicable *in vivo* (Ransohoff, 2016). Moreover, macrophage activation patterns classified as M1 and M2 further needs thorough revision due to increasing knowledge about distinct macrophage stimuli (Martinez and Gordon, 2014). With regard to their unique molecular signatures, resident microglia have to be distinguished from infiltrating monocytes/macrophages in terms of gene expression patterns, surface receptors and functions, respectively. Especially under pathological conditions microglia and macrophages display distinct functional properties. Infiltrating monocytes are able to contribute to the resident microglia pool during experimental autoimmune encephalomyelitis (EAE) and have been demonstrated to trigger EAE progression in this context (Ajami et al., 2011). Moreover, T-cell mediated macrophage activation seems to be essential for inflammatory demyelination processes observed during EAE (Yamasaki et al., 2014). Similar observations for monocyte/macrophage contribution to neuroinflammation and subsequent neurodegeneration has been reported for generalized seizures an animal model for epilepsy (Varvel et al., 2016). Of note, inflammatory M1 macrophages entering the aged brain due to BBB impairments have been demonstrated to negatively regulate synaptic functions and LTP formation in the hippocampus (Costello et al., 2016).

Recently identified microglia-specific genes such as *Tmem119* (Bennett et al., 2016) or *Fcrls* (Butovsky et al., 2014) and/or sophisticated microglia isolation protocols (de Haas et al., 2007) can be used in order to identify region-specific microglial differences. Differences in microglial surface receptor expressions (de Haas et al., 2008) and gene expression patterns (Doorn et al., 2015) have been reported and suggest the existence of different functional distinct microglia subpopulations in the CNS. This microglial diversity may be responsible for regionally localized homeostatic functions and might further underlie region-specific sensitivities to microglial dysregulation and involvement in age-related neurodegenerative processes (Grabert et al., 2016).

AGING MICROGLIA: PRIMING, FUNCTIONS AND PHENOTYPES

In healthy rodents, microglia make up 5%–12% of all CNS-specific cells. However, the distribution is diverse and some brain areas display higher densities of microglia (Lawson et al., 1990). Interestingly, the nigrostriatal system including substantia nigra (SN) and the caudate putamen (CPu) show significantly higher microglia densities than adjacent brain regions (Sharaf et al., 2013). Similar observations have been made in humans where microglia represent 0.5%–16.6% of all cells in the brain parenchyma. Moreover, the numbers of microglia in the white matter are higher compared to gray matter (Mittelbronn et al., 2001). Several studies have tried to address the age-related changes in microglia numbers in different species with diverse results. Whereas no obvious changes in Iba1$^+$ microglia numbers have been observed in the aged rat hippocampus (VanGuilder et al., 2011), reductions in microglia numbers were detected in the aged nigrostriatal system and cerebral cortex (Sharaf et al., 2013). However, in aged rhesus monkeys (25–35 years) the numbers of microglia increased and the cells displayed heterogeneous intracellular inclusions indicative of increased phagocytosis and reduced capacity to digest engulfed particles (Peters et al., 1991). Dystrophic changes in microglia have been detected in aged individuals and were much more prevalent in older subjects (68-year-old) than in the younger ones (38-year-old; Streit et al., 2004). Interestingly, it has been described that dystrophic or senescent microglia might undergo age-dependent degeneration and are believed to lose their neuroprotective functions, thereby, contributing to the age-dependent onset of sporadic AD (sAD; Streit et al., 2009). Altered microglia morphology and reduced arborization have been reported in the human brain during aging and in AD patients (Davies et al., 2016). It remains unclear whether the observed morphological changes are signs of microglia degeneration and a recent study suggests that the reported microglia dystrophy might reflect age-related cytoskeleton alterations (Tischer et al., 2016). Interestingly, direct Tau uptake by microglia has been reported (Bolós et al., 2016) and is enhanced by anti-tau antibodies in an Fc-receptor-dependent manner (Luo et al., 2015). Moreover, hyperphosphorylated Tau was detectable in aged common marmoset brains and was present in dystrophic microglia suggesting that clearance of pathological protein aggregates might foster microglia dystrophy (Rodriguez-Callejas et al., 2016).

Due to the unique nature of microglia and especially due to their self-renewal capacity, a telomere shortening was hypothesized during aging of microglia. Whereas cells with high proliferative potential, such as stem cells or cancer cells have increased telomerase activity in order to maintain telomere length, somatic cells with limited replication potential possess less telomerase activity (Satyanarayana et al., 2004; Blasco, 2007). Indeed, telomere shortening has been reported in cultured microglia (Flanary and Streit, 2004) and was associated with dementia in human AD brain samples (Flanary et al., 2007). However, it seems that mouse microglia do not develop dystrophy and telomere shortening under normal conditions due to the limited lifespan of mice. Transgenic approaches, such as the Ercc1 mutant mice, a DNA repair-deficient mouse model that displays features of accelerated aging in multiple tissues including the CNS have contributed to the understanding how aging might affect microglia functions. In Ercc1 mutant mice, microglia display hallmark features of priming and increased responses to systemic lipopolysaccharide (LPS) exposure as reflected by cytokine expression and phagocytosis (Raj et al., 2014). Mice lacking the telomerase RNA component (TERC) are characterized by an accelerated aging phenotype associated with enhanced microglia activation in response to LPS and a subsequent immune cell infiltration upon BBB dysregulation (Raj et al., 2015). These results indicate that microglial aging result in functional impairments and increased microglia activation, which is probably involved in the onset and/or progression of neurodegeneration.

Age-dependent microglia activation has been described in aged rodents (Perry et al., 1993), rats (Ogura et al., 1994), humans (Streit and Sparks, 1997) as well as non-human primates (Sheffield and Berman, 1998). Hallmarks of age-dependent microglia activation are increased expression of MHCII (Henry et al., 2009; VanGuilder et al., 2011), CD68 (Wong et al., 2005; Griffin et al., 2006) as well as increased levels of TLRs (Letiembre et al., 2007). Aged microglia have been characterized by the presence of lipofuscin inclusions, reduced processes complexity and increased expression pro-inflammatory (TNFα, IL1β, IL6) and anti-inflammatory (IL10, TGFβ1) cytokines. After LPS challenge aged microglia exhibit increased expression of TNFα, IL1β, IL6 and IL10 (Sierra et al., 2007). Furthermore, increased expression of macrophage inflammatory protein (MIP)1α, MIP1β and RANTES in different brain regions of aged mice have been detected (Felzien et al., 2001). In general, the reactivity of microglia upon stimulation seems to be increased during aging, which is further reflected by enhanced microglia activation in aged mice after injection of activating cytokines IL1β and IL12 to the hippocampus (Lee et al., 2013). This phenomenon has been described as microglia priming and TLR2, TLR3 and TLR4 seem to be essential to prime microglia but not astrocytes for ATP-dependent interleukin-1β release (Facci et al., 2014). Microglia priming induces a highly conserved transcriptional signature with aging- and disease-specific aspects (Holtman et al., 2015), which is dependent on High mobility group box 1 (HMGB1). HMGB1 mediates the neuroinflammatory priming in the aged CNS and inhibition of HMGB1 functions appears to desensitize aged microglia to an immune challenge, thus preventing exaggerated behavioral and neuroinflammatory responses following microglia stimulation (Fonken et al., 2016).

Expression levels of the complement genes, C3 and complement factor B (CFB), both of which being previously associated with age-related macular degeneration (AMD), increased during aging suggesting that senescent retinal microglia may contribute to complement dysregulation during disease pathogenesis and progression (Ma et al., 2013). Although these studies suggest an inflammatory microglia phenotype in aged mice, RNA sequencing revealed that aged microglia display decreased expression of genes associated with endogenous ligand recognition and upregulated genes associated with microbe recognition and host defense. Most interestingly, aged microglia presented increased expression of genes related to neuroprotection and neurorestoration (Hickman et al., 2013).

Among the functional impairments of aged microglia, a reduced capacity to engulf amyloid-β fibrils (Floden and Combs, 2011) and reduced chemotaxis, process motility and migration towards laser-induced injury and extracellular ATP (Damani et al., 2011) have been described. Moreover, cultured microglia from aged mice show a stronger reaction upon ATP-triggered activation, which is characterized by increased nitric oxide (NO) and TNFα release (Lai et al., 2013). Recently, it has been reported that myelin pieces are gradually released from aging myelin sheaths and are subsequently cleared by microglia. This myelin fragmentation increased with age and led to the formation of insoluble, lipofuscin-like lysosomal inclusions in microglia contributing to microglial senescence and immune dysfunctions in aging mice (Safaiyan et al., 2016). Age-dependent microglia dysfunctions might be further enhanced by loss of endogenous regulation of microglia functions and activation states. TGFβ1 has been demonstrated to promote quiescence of microglia *in vitro* (Spittau et al., 2013) and *in vivo* (Butovsky et al., 2014) and is a promising candidate to regulate microglia activation states. Moreover, TGFβ1 inhibits IFNγ-induced microglia activation and degeneration of midbrain dopaminergic (mDA) neurons (Zhou et al., 2015) and induces microglia-mediated engulfment of apoptotic cells via induction of microglial Mfge8 expression (Spittau et al., 2015). Age-dependent impairment of TGFβ1 signaling was lately described to reduce the protective functions of microglia promoting cytotoxic activation and potentiating microglia-mediated neurodegeneration (Tichauer et al., 2014).

Although most of the abovementioned studies have been performed in rodents, recent studies indicate that microglia priming and age-dependent microglia activation is also detectable in the human CNS. *In vivo* imaging using (R)-[(11)C]PK11195 and positron emission tomography revealed that activated microglia appear in several cortical and subcortical areas during healthy aging (Schuitemaker et al., 2012). Further, glial-specific genes shift their regional expression patterns during aging and especially microglia-specific genes globally display increased expression during aging (Soreq et al., 2017). Taken together, priming of microglia and age-related changes in microglia functions and activations are likely to be involved in the development and progression of neurodegenerative diseases such as AD and PD.

AGING AND AD AND PD

The most frequent neurodegenerative diseases are AD and PD, both of which sharing a common risk factor namely aging. AD is characterized by progressive cognitive impairments and behavioral disturbances. Neuropathological hallmarks such as neuron death, dystrophic neurites, synapse loss, amyloid plaques and neurofibrillary tangles are accompanied by reactive gliosis (Serrano-Pozo et al., 2011). Basically, AD can be categorized into two distinct subtypes: sAD and familial AD (fAD). Whereas sAD represent a polygenic disorder, fAD is linked to mutations and polymorphisms in genes such as Amyloid precursor protein (APP), Presenilin 1 (PSEN1) or Presenilin 2 (PSEN2) and account for 5%–10% of all AD cases (Bagyinszky et al., 2014). PD is characterized by the progressive loss of mDA neurons in the SN pars compacta and the subsequent reduction in dopamine levels in the basal ganglia, which results in classical movement disturbances such as akinesia, rigidity and tremor. Similar to

AD, PD cases can be divided into sporadic PD (sPD) and familial PD (fPD), the latter of which represents approximately 20%–25% of all PD cases. A common hallmark of sPD and fPD is the presence of intracellular inclusions termed Lewy bodies (Goedert, 2001; Jellinger, 2001). α-Synuclein (αSyn) has been identified as a major component of Lewy bodies in sporadic and familial cases and is believed to be the central player in PD etiology (Spillantini et al., 1998). Activated microglia have been described in both pathologies (McGeer et al., 1988) and microglia-mediated neuroinflammatory responses are believed to contribute to disease onset, severity and progression of AD (Heneka et al., 2015) and PD (Block et al., 2007).

In AD mouse models, microglia seem to build up a barrier that prevents neurotoxic effects of proto fibrillar Amyloid-β (Aβ) hotspots around amyloid plaques (Condello et al., 2015). Furthermore, microglia phagocytose Aβ in order to promote clearance of Aβ plaques. Aged microglia display reduced Aβ phagocytosis (Floden and Combs, 2011) and recently it has been demonstrated that Aβ engulfment by aged microglia results in Aβ redistribution rather than in a biophysical degradation of the protein aggregates (Njie et al., 2012). Interestingly, young microglia have been recently demonstrated to restore the amyloid clearance of aged microglia in an elegant *ex vivo* organotypic brain slice co-culturing approach (Daria et al., 2017). In transgenic APP23 mice, exacerbated age-dependent microglia activation and disturbances in microglial cytoskeletal regulations have been described which are high likely to contribute to further neurodegeneration (Janssen et al., 2016). Next to the deteriorated response of aged and primed microglia, complement factor C3 secreted from reactive astrocytes has been reported to interact with the microglial C3a receptor (C3aR) thereby mediating Aβ pathology and neuroinflammation in AD mouse models (Lian et al., 2016). However, lack of C3aR in APP transgenic mice results in decreased, rather than increased, Aβ deposition and C3aR-deficient microglia are more effective in degrading extracellular Aβ (Czirr et al., 2017). Although increased microglia responses as well as impairments of microglia-mediated clearance of Aβ seem to promote the progression of AD, the role of microglia contribution to AD pathology remains unclear. Interestingly, the ablation of microglia in APP transgenic mouse strains crossed with CD11b-HSVTK mice, in which nearly complete depletion of microglia was achieved after ganciclovir application, neither Aβ plaque formation nor amyloid-associated neuron dystrophy was depended on the presence of microglia (Grathwohl et al., 2009). Further studies will be essential in order to broaden our understanding of how microglia contribute to disease onset and progression and a special focus should be given on the role of aged microglia to elucidate the impact of aging on microglial functions in AD.

In PD, marked microglia reactions in the human SN have been observed, which are associated with extraneuronal neuromelanin deposits (Beach et al., 2007). Furthermore, human neuromelanin is able to induce microglia-mediated neuroinflammation and neurodegeneration in rats (Zecca et al., 2008) indicating that the release of neuromelanin from degenerating mDA neurons is a potent trigger for microglia activation. In rodents, toxin-based models, such as 1-methyl-4-phenyl-1,2,3,6-tetrahydropyridine (MPTP) are

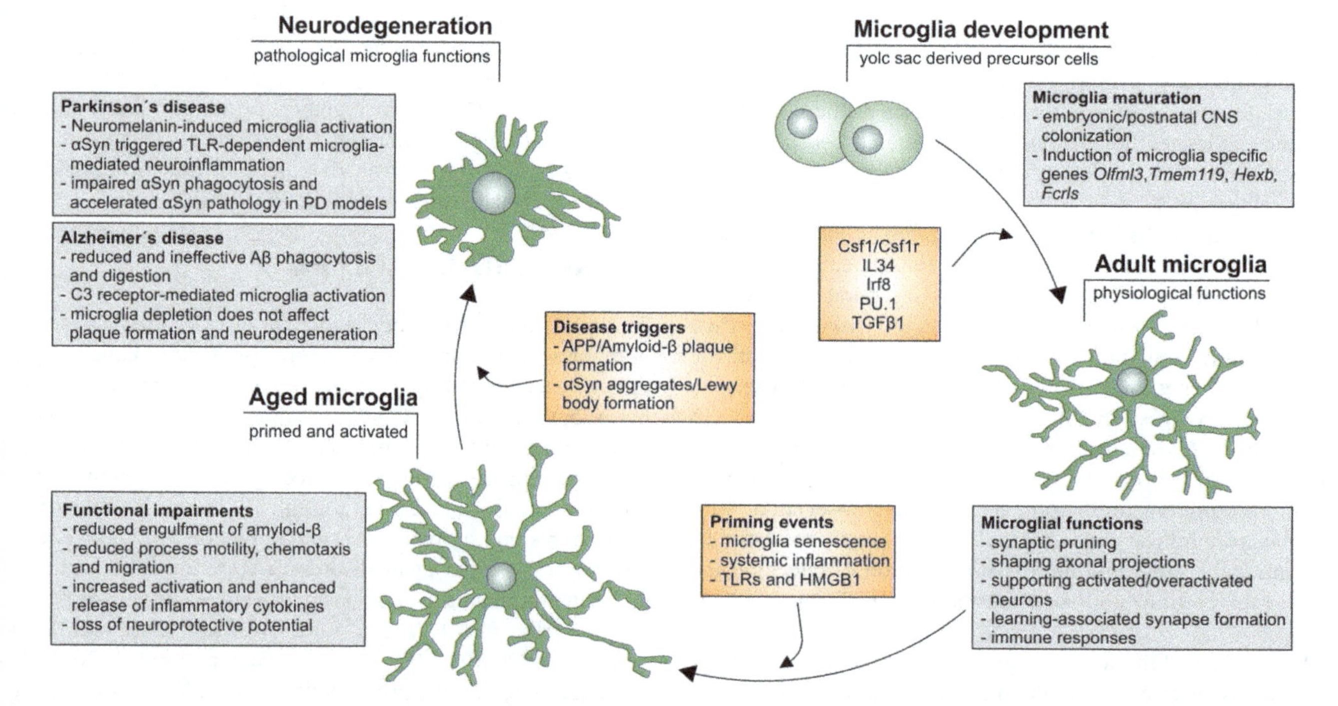

FIGURE 1 | Microglia life cycle. Schematic summary of microglial development, maturation as well as aging and the functional changes influencing onset, severity and progression of neurodegeneration in Alzheimer's disease (AD) and Parkinson's disease (PD).

employed to understand the contribution of microglia to onset and progression of mDA neuron degeneration (Machado et al., 2016). Although the contribution of microglia-mediated neuroinflammation has been clearly demonstrated (Block et al., 2007; Machado et al., 2016), the impact of aging is often ignored in these studies. Interestingly, microglia priming increases the response to the herbicide paraquat and, thus resulting in increased mDA neurodegeneration (Purisai et al., 2007) and aged monkeys display stronger and persistent microglia reactivity after MPTP application indicating microglial involvement in age-dependent degeneration of mDA neurons (Kanaan et al., 2008). It is high likely that age-dependent microglia priming involves epigenetic modifications as reported by Tang et al. (2014). The authors demonstrated that histone H3K27me3 demethylase Jumonji domain containing 3 (Jmjd3) is essential for M2-like microglia activation. Inhibition of Jmjd3 resulted in exacerbation of MPTP-induced mDA degeneration and aged mice displayed reduced Jmjd3 expression and increased H3K27me3 suggesting an age-dependent switch in microglia activation phenotypes (Tang et al., 2014). The effect of aging on the severity of MPTP-induced neurodegeneration is further supported by a study using Senescence-accelerated mouse prone 8 (SAMP8), a mouse line with early onset of senility which presents increased microglia activation and increased neurodegeneration after MPTP intoxication (Liu et al., 2010). Next to toxin-based models for PD, αSyn transgenic mice are often used to understand how αSyn aggregates contribute to neuroinflammation and neurodegeneration in PD. Non-aggregated αSyn is able to trigger TLR-mediated immune responses of microglia, a phenomenon that might contribute to the onset of sporadic and/or familial αSyn-related PD forms (Roodveldt et al., 2013). Notably, telomere shortening has been shown to accelerate αSyn pathology, which is linked to limited microglia function in the brainstem (Scheffold et al., 2016). This observation might be explained by age-dependent microglia deficits. Indeed, isolated microglia from adult mice display phagocytosis impairment of free and exosome-associated αSyn oligomers associated with enhanced TNFα secretion (Bliederhaeuser et al., 2016). Taken together, the contribution of aged microglia to the progressive nature of PD is most likely and the fact that the nigrostriatal system displays a high density of microglia (Sharaf et al., 2013) further supports the hypothesis that microglia are involved in PD pathogenesis. However, the molecular and functional changes of aged microglia are only partially understood and their contribution to neurodegeneration and neuroinflammation in aged individuals need to be further addressed in future studies.

CONCLUSION

Aging has been clearly demonstrated to affect microglia functions and activation states *in vitro* and *in vivo* and it further appears that the unique nature of microglia contributes to their age-dependent functional impairment. Moreover, the onset, severity and progression of neurodegenerative diseases such as AD and PD are influenced by aging and aging-associated changes in microglia functions (**Figure 1**). However, it is not clear whether aged microglia are responsible for the exacerbation of neurodegeneration in aged individuals or whether aged neurons itself are more prone to degenerative cues. Furthermore, the contribution of systemic age-dependent changes, such as obesity and metabolic diseases like diabetes, are likely to affect microglia and neuroinflammatory responses. Overall, the effect of aging on microglia needs to be further analyzed in order to better understand the molecular mechanisms underlying age-related changes in microglia phenotypes and functions.

AUTHOR CONTRIBUTIONS

BS wrote the manuscript.

FUNDING

This work was funded by grants from the Deutsche Forschungsgemeinschaft (DFG, SP 1555/2-1).

REFERENCES

Ajami, B., Bennett, J. L., Krieger, C., Tetzlaff, W., and Rossi, F. M. V. (2007). Local self-renewal can sustain CNS microglia maintenance and function throughout adult life. *Nat. Neurosci.* 10, 1538–1543. doi: 10.1038/nn2014

Ajami, B., Bennett, J. L., Krieger, C., McNagny, K. M., and Rossi, F. M. V. (2011). Infiltrating monocytes trigger EAE progression, but do not contribute to the resident microglia pool. *Nat. Neurosci.* 14, 1142–1149. doi: 10.1038/nn.2887

Askew, K., Li, K., Olmos-Alonso, A., Garcia-Moreno, F., Liang, Y., Richardson, P., et al. (2017). Coupled proliferation and apoptosis maintain the rapid turnover of microglia in the adult brain. *Cell Rep.* 18, 391–405. doi: 10.1016/j.celrep.2016.12.041

Bagyinszky, E., Youn, Y. C., An, S. S. A., and Kim, S. (2014). The genetics of Alzheimer's disease. *Clin. Interv. Aging* 9, 535–551. doi: 10.2147/CIA.S51571

Beach, T. G., Sue, L. I., Walker, D. G., Lue, L. F., Connor, D. J., Caviness, J. N., et al. (2007). Marked microglial reaction in normal aging human substantia nigra: correlation with extraneuronal neuromelanin pigment deposits. *Acta Neuropathol.* 114, 419–424. doi: 10.1007/s00401-007-0250-5

Bechmann, I., Priller, J., Kovac, A., Böntert, M., Wehner, T., Klett, F. F., et al. (2001). Immune surveillance of mouse brain perivascular spaces by blood-borne macrophages. *Eur. J. Neurosci.* 14, 1651–1658. doi: 10.1046/j.0953-816x.2001.01793.x

Bennett, M. L., Bennett, F. C., Liddelow, S. A., Ajami, B., Zamanian, J. L., Fernhoff, N. B., et al. (2016). New tools for studying microglia in the mouse and human CNS. *Proc. Natl. Acad. Sci. U S A* 113, E1738–E1746. doi: 10.1073/pnas.1525528113

Beutner, C., Linnartz-Gerlach, B., Schmidt, S. V., Beyer, M., Mallmann, M. R., Staratschek-Jox, A., et al. (2013). Unique transcriptome signature of mouse microglia. *Glia* 61, 1429–1442. doi: 10.1002/glia.22524

Blasco, M. A. (2007). Telomere length, stem cells and aging. *Nat. Chem. Biol.* 3, 640–649. doi: 10.1038/nchembio.2007.38

Bliederhaeuser, C., Grozdanov, V., Speidel, A., Zondler, L., Ruf, W. P., Bayer, H., et al. (2016). Age-dependent defects of alpha-synuclein oligomer uptake in microglia and monocytes. *Acta Neuropathol.* 131, 379–391. doi: 10.1007/s00401-015-1504-2

Block, M. L., Zecca, L., and Hong, J.-S. (2007). Microglia-mediated neurotoxicity: uncovering the molecular mechanisms. *Nat. Rev. Neurosci.* 8, 57–69. doi: 10.1038/nrn2038

Bolós, M., Llorens-Martín, M., Jurado-Arjona, J., Hernández, F., Rábano, A., and Avila, J. (2016). Direct evidence of internalization of tau by microglia *in vitro* and *in vivo*. *J. Alzheimers Dis.* 50, 77–87. doi: 10.3233/JAD-150704

Butovsky, O., Jedrychowski, M. P., Moore, C. S., Cialic, R., Lanser, A. J., Gabriely, G., et al. (2014). Identification of a unique TGF-β-dependent molecular and functional signature in microglia. *Nat. Neurosci.* 17, 131–143. doi: 10.1038/nn.3599

Condello, C., Yuan, P., Schain, A., and Grutzendler, J. (2015). Microglia constitute a barrier that prevents neurotoxic protofibrillar Aβ42 hotspots around plaques. *Nat. Commun.* 6:6176. doi: 10.1038/ncomms7176

Costello, D. A., Keenan, K., McManus, R. M., Falvey, A., and Lynch, M. A. (2016). The age-related neuroinflammatory environment promotes macrophage activation, which negatively impacts synaptic function. *Neurobiol. Aging* 43, 140–148. doi: 10.1016/j.neurobiolaging.2016.04.001

Czirr, E., Castello, N. A., Mosher, K. I., Castellano, J. M., Hinkson, I. V., Lucin, K. M., et al. (2017). Microglial complement receptor 3 regulates brain Aβ levels through secreted proteolytic activity. *J. Exp. Med.* 214, 1081–1092. doi: 10.1084/jem.20162011

Damani, M. R., Zhao, L., Fontainhas, A. M., Amaral, J., Fariss, R. N., and Wong, W. T. (2011). Age-related alterations in the dynamic behavior of microglia. *Aging Cell* 10, 263–276. doi: 10.1111/j.1474-9726.2010.00660.x

Daria, A., Colombo, A., Llovera, G., Hampel, H., Willem, M., Liesz, A., et al. (2017). Young microglia restore amyloid plaque clearance of aged microglia. *EMBO J.* 35, 583–603. doi: 10.15252/embj.201694591

Davies, D. S., Ma, J., Jegathees, T., and Goldsbury, C. (2016). Microglia show altered morphology and reduced arborization in human brain during aging and Alzheimer's disease. *Brain Pathol.* doi: 10.1111/bpa.12456 [Epub ahead of print].

de Haas, A. H., Boddeke, H. W. G. M., and Biber, K. (2008). Region-specific expression of immunoregulatory proteins on microglia in the healthy CNS. *Glia* 56, 888–894. doi: 10.1002/glia.20663

de Haas, A. H., Boddeke, H. W. G. M., Brouwer, N., and Biber, K. (2007). Optimized isolation enables *ex vivo* analysis of microglia from various central nervous system regions. *Glia* 55, 1374–1384. doi: 10.1002/glia.20554

Doorn, K. J., Brevé, J. J. P., Drukarch, B., Boddeke, H. W., Huitinga, I., Lucassen, P. J., et al. (2015). Brain region-specific gene expression profiles in freshly isolated rat microglia. *Front. Cell. Neurosci.* 9:84. doi: 10.3389/fncel.2015.00084

Elmore, M. R. P., Najafi, A. R., Koike, M. A., Dagher, N. N., Spangenberg, E. E., Rice, R. A., et al. (2014). Colony-stimulating factor 1 receptor signaling is necessary for microglia viability, unmasking a microglia progenitor cell in the adult brain. *Neuron* 82, 380–397. doi: 10.1016/j.neuron.2014.02.040

Erny, D., Hrabě de Angelis, A. L., Jaitin, D., Wieghofer, P., Staszewski, O., David, E., et al. (2015). Host microbiota constantly control maturation and function of microglia in the CNS. *Nat. Neurosci.* 18, 965–977. doi: 10.1038/nn.4030

Facci, L., Barbierato, M., Marinelli, C., Argentini, C., Skaper, S. D., and Giusti, P. (2014). Toll-like receptors 2, -3 and -4 prime microglia but not astrocytes across central nervous system regions for ATP-dependent interleukin-1β release. *Sci. Rep.* 4:6824. doi: 10.1038/srep06824

Felzien, L. K., McDonald, J. T., Gleason, S. M., Berman, N. E., and Klein, R. M. (2001). Increased chemokine gene expression during aging in the murine brain. *Brain Res.* 890, 137–146. doi: 10.1016/s0006-8993(00)03090-0

Flanary, B. E., Sammons, N. W., Nguyen, C., Walker, D., and Streit, W. J. (2007). Evidence that aging and amyloid promote microglial cell senescence. *Rejuvenation Res.* 10, 61–74. doi: 10.1089/rej.2006.9096

Flanary, B. E., and Streit, W. J. (2004). Progressive telomere shortening occurs in cultured rat microglia, but not astrocytes. *Glia* 45, 75–88. doi: 10.1002/glia.10301

Floden, A. M., and Combs, C. K. (2011). Microglia demonstrate age-dependent interaction with amyloid-β fibrils. *J. Alzheimers Dis.* 25, 279–293. doi: 10.3233/JAD-2011-101014

Fonken, L. K., Frank, M. G., Kitt, M. M., D'Angelo, H. M., Norden, D. M., Weber, M. D., et al. (2016). The alarmin HMGB1 mediates age-induced neuroinflammatory priming. *J. Neurosci.* 36, 7946–7956. doi: 10.1523/JNEUROSCI.1161-16.2016

Ginhoux, F., Greter, M., Leboeuf, M., Nandi, S., See, P., Gokhan, S., et al. (2010). Fate mapping analysis reveals that adult microglia derive from primitive macrophages. *Science* 330, 841–845. doi: 10.1126/science.1194637

Goedert, M. (2001). Alpha-synuclein and neurodegenerative diseases. *Nat. Rev. Neurosci.* 2, 492–501. doi: 10.1038/35081564

Goldmann, T., Wieghofer, P., Jordão, M. J. C., Prutek, F., Hagemeyer, N., Frenzel, K., et al. (2016). Origin, fate and dynamics of macrophages at central nervous system interfaces. *Nat. Immunol.* 17, 797–805. doi: 10.1038/ni.3423

Gómez-Nicola, D., Fransen, N. L., Suzzi, S., and Perry, V. H. (2013). Regulation of microglial proliferation during chronic neurodegeneration. *J. Neurosci.* 33, 2481–2493. doi: 10.1523/JNEUROSCI.4440-12.2013

Grabert, K., Michoel, T., Karavolos, M. H., Clohisey, S., Baillie, J. K., Stevens, M. P., et al. (2016). Microglial brain region-dependent diversity and selective regional sensitivities to aging. *Nat. Neurosci.* 19, 504–516. doi: 10.1038/nn.4222

Grathwohl, S. A., Kälin, R. E., Bolmont, T., Prokop, S., Winkelmann, G., Kaeser, S. A., et al. (2009). Formation and maintenance of Alzheimer's disease β-amyloid plaques in the absence of microglia. *Nat. Neurosci.* 12, 1361–1363. doi: 10.1038/nn.2432

Greter, M., Lelios, I., Pelczar, P., Hoeffel, G., Price, J., Leboeuf, M., et al. (2012). Stroma-derived interleukin-34 controls the development and maintenance of langerhans cells and the maintenance of microglia. *Immunity* 37, 1050–1060. doi: 10.1016/j.immuni.2012.11.001

Griffin, R., Nally, R., Nolan, Y., McCartney, Y., Linden, J., and Lynch, M. A. (2006). The age-related attenuation in long-term potentiation is associated with microglial activation. *J. Neurochem.* 99, 1263–1272. doi: 10.1111/j.1471-4159.2006.04165.x

Heneka, M. T., Carson, M. J., El Khoury, J., Landreth, G. E., Brosseron, F., Feinstein, D. L., et al. (2015). Neuroinflammation in Alzheimer's disease. *Lancet Neurol.* 14, 388–405. doi: 10.1016/S1474-4422(15)70016-5

Henry, C. J., Huang, Y., Wynne, A. M., and Godbout, J. P. (2009). Peripheral lipopolysaccharide (LPS) challenge promotes microglial hyperactivity in aged mice that is associated with exaggerated induction of both pro-inflammatory IL-1β and anti-inflammatory IL-10 cytokines. *Brain Behav. Immun.* 23, 309–317. doi: 10.1016/j.bbi.2008.09.002

Hickey, W. F., and Kimura, H. (1988). Perivascular microglial cells of the CNS are bone marrow-derived and present antigen *in vivo*. *Science* 239, 290–292. doi: 10.1126/science.3276004

Hickman, S. E., Kingery, N. D., Ohsumi, T. K., Borowsky, M. L., Wang, L.-C., Means, T. K., et al. (2013). The microglial sensome revealed by direct RNA sequencing. *Nat. Neurosci.* 16, 1896–1905. doi: 10.1038/nn.3554

Holtman, I. R., Raj, D. D., Miller, J. A., Schaafsma, W., Yin, Z., Brouwer, N., et al. (2015). Induction of a common microglia gene expression signature by aging and neurodegenerative conditions: a co-expression meta-analysis. *Acta Neuropathol. Commun.* 3:31. doi: 10.1186/s40478-015-0203-5

Hoshiko, M., Arnoux, I., Avignone, E., Yamamoto, N., and Audinat, E. (2012). Deficiency of the microglial receptor CX3CR1 impairs postnatal functional development of thalamocortical synapses in the barrel cortex. *J. Neurosci.* 32, 15106–15111. doi: 10.1523/JNEUROSCI.1167-12.2012

Janssen, L., Dubbelaar, M. L., Holtman, I. R., de Boer-Bergsma, J., Eggen, B. J. L., Boddeke, H. W. G. M., et al. (2016). Aging, microglia and cytoskeletal regulation are key factors in the pathological evolution of the APP23 mouse model for Alzheimer's disease. *Biochim. Biophys. Acta* 1863, 395–405. doi: 10.1016/j.bbadis.2016.11.014

Jellinger, K. A. (2001). The pathology of Parkinson's disease. *Adv. Neurol.* 86, 55–72.

Kamphuis, W., Orre, M., Kooijman, L., Dahmen, M., and Hol, E. M. (2012). Differential cell proliferation in the cortex of the APPswePS1dE9 Alzheimer's disease mouse model. *Glia* 60, 615–629. doi: 10.1002/glia.22295

Kanaan, N. M., Kordower, J. H., and Collier, T. J. (2008). Age and region-specific responses of microglia, but not astrocytes, suggest a role in selective vulnerability of dopamine neurons after 1-methyl-4-phenyl-1,2,3,6-tetrahydropyridine exposure in monkeys. *Glia* 56, 1199–1214. doi: 10.1002/glia.20690

Kierdorf, K., Erny, D., Goldmann, T., Sander, V., Schulz, C., Perdiguero, E. G., et al. (2013). Microglia emerge from erythromyeloid precursors via Pu.1- and Irf8-dependent pathways. *Nat. Neurosci.* 16, 273–280. doi: 10.1038/nn.3318

Kigerl, K. A., de Rivero Vaccari, J. P., Dietrich, W. D., Popovich, P. G., and Keane, R. W. (2014). Pattern recognition receptors and central nervous system repair. *Exp. Neurol.* 258, 5–16. doi: 10.1016/j.expneurol.2014.01.001

Lai, A. Y., Dibal, C. D., Armitage, G. A., Winship, I. R., and Todd, K. G. (2013). Distinct activation profiles in microglia of different ages: a systematic study in isolated embryonic to aged microglial cultures. *Neuroscience* 254, 185–195. doi: 10.1016/j.neuroscience.2013.09.010

Lawson, L. J., Perry, V. H., Dri, P., and Gordon, S. (1990). Heterogeneity in the distribution and morphology of microglia in the normal adult mouse brain. *Neuroscience* 39, 151–170. doi: 10.1016/0306-4522(90)90229-w

Lee, D. C., Ruiz, C. R., Lebson, L., Selenica, M.-L. B., Rizer, J., Hunt, J. B. Jr., et al. (2013). Aging enhances classical activation but mitigates alternative activation in the central nervous system. *Neurobiol. Aging* 34, 1610–1620. doi: 10.1016/j.neurobiolaging.2012.12.014

Letiembre, M., Hao, W., Liu, Y., Walter, S., Mihaljevic, I., Rivest, S., et al. (2007). Innate immune receptor expression in normal brain aging. *Neuroscience* 146, 248–254. doi: 10.1016/j.neuroscience.2007.01.004

Li, T., Pang, S., Yu, Y., Wu, X., Guo, J., and Zhang, S. (2013). Proliferation of parenchymal microglia is the main source of microgliosis after ischaemic stroke. *Brain* 136, 3578–3588. doi: 10.1093/brain/awt287

Lian, H., Litvinchuk, A., Chiang, A. C.-A., Aithmitti, N., Jankowsky, J. L., and Zheng, H. (2016). Astrocyte-microglia cross talk through complement activation modulates amyloid pathology in mouse models of Alzheimer's disease. *J. Neurosci.* 36, 577–589. doi: 10.1523/JNEUROSCI.2117-15.2016

Liu, J., Wang, M.-W., Gu, P., Ma, Q.-Y., Wang, Y.-Y., Geng, Y., et al. (2010). Microglial activation and age-related dopaminergic neurodegeneration in MPTP-treated SAMP8 mice. *Brain Res.* 1345, 213–220. doi: 10.1016/j.brainres.2010.05.043

Luo, W., Liu, W., Hu, X., Hanna, M., Caravaca, A., and Paul, S. M. (2015). Microglial internalization and degradation of pathological tau is enhanced by an anti-tau monoclonal antibody. *Sci. Rep.* 5:11161. doi: 10.1038/srep11161

Ma, W., Cojocaru, R., Gotoh, N., Gieser, L., Villasmil, R., Cogliati, T., et al. (2013). Gene expression changes in aging retinal microglia: relationship to microglial support functions and regulation of activation. *Neurobiol. Aging* 34, 2310–2321. doi: 10.1016/j.neurobiolaging.2013.03.022

Machado, V., Zöller, T., Attaai, A., and Spittau, B. (2016). Microglia-mediated neuroinflammation and neurotrophic factor-induced protection in the MPTP mouse model of Parkinson's disease-lessons from transgenic mice. *Int. J. Mol. Sci.* 17:E151. doi: 10.3390/ijms17020151

Martinez, F. O., and Gordon, S. (2014). The M1 and M2 paradigm of macrophage activation: time for reassessment. *F1000Prime Rep.* 6:13. doi: 10.12703/P6-13

McGeer, P. L., Itagaki, S., Boyes, B. E., and McGeer, E. G. (1988). Reactive microglia are positive for HLA-DR in the substantia nigra of Parkinson's and Alzheimer's disease brains. *Neurology* 38, 1285–1291. doi: 10.1212/WNL.38.8.1285

Mittelbronn, M., Dietz, K., Schluesener, H. J., and Meyermann, R. (2001). Local distribution of microglia in the normal adult human central nervous system differs by up to one order of magnitude. *Acta Neuropathol.* 101, 249–255.

Mosser, D. M., and Edwards, J. P. (2008). Exploring the full spectrum of macrophage activation. *Nat. Rev. Immunol.* 8, 958–969. doi: 10.1038/nri2448

Nimmerjahn, A., Kirchhoff, F., and Helmchen, F. (2005). Resting microglial cells are highly dynamic surveillants of brain parenchyma *in vivo*. *Science* 308, 1314–1318. doi: 10.1126/science.1110647

Njie, E. G., Boelen, E., Stassen, F. R., Steinbusch, H. W. M., Borchelt, D. R., and Streit, W. J. (2012). *Ex vivo* cultures of microglia from young and aged rodent brain reveal age-related changes in microglial function. *Neurobiol. Aging* 33, 195.e1–195.e12. doi: 10.1016/j.neurobiolaging.2010.05.008

Ogura, K., Ogawa, M., and Yoshida, M. (1994). Effects of ageing on microglia in the normal rat brain: immunohistochemical observations. *Neuroreport* 5, 1224–1226. doi: 10.1097/00001756-199406020-00016

Panatier, A., and Robitaille, R. (2012). The soothing touch: microglial contact influences neuronal excitability. *Dev. Cell* 23, 1125–1126. doi: 10.1016/j.devcel.2012.11.015

Paolicelli, R. C., Bolasco, G., Pagani, F., Maggi, L., Scianni, M., Panzanelli, P., et al. (2011). Synaptic pruning by microglia is necessary for normal brain development. *Science* 333, 1456–1458. doi: 10.1126/science.1202529

Parkhurst, C. N., Yang, G., Ninan, I., Savas, J. N., Yates, J. R. III., Lafaille, J. J., et al. (2013). Microglia promote learning-dependent synapse formation through brain-derived neurotrophic factor. *Cell* 155, 1596–1609. doi: 10.1016/j.cell.2013.11.030

Perry, V. H., Matyszak, M. K., and Fearn, S. (1993). Altered antigen expression of microglia in the aged rodent CNS. *Glia* 7, 60–67. doi: 10.1002/glia.440070111

Peters, A., Josephson, K., and Vincent, S. L. (1991). Effects of aging on the neuroglial cells and pericytes within area 17 of the rhesus monkey cerebral cortex. *Anat. Rec.* 229, 384–398. doi: 10.1002/ar.1092290311

Pont-Lezica, L., Beumer, W., Colasse, S., Drexhage, H., Versnel, M., and Bessis, A. (2014). Microglia shape corpus callosum axon tract fasciculation: functional impact of prenatal inflammation. *Eur. J. Neurosci.* 39, 1551–1557. doi: 10.1111/ejn.12508

Prinz, M., and Priller, J. (2014). Microglia and brain macrophages in the molecular age: from origin to neuropsychiatric disease. *Nat. Rev. Neurosci.* 15, 300–312. doi: 10.1038/nrn3722

Purisai, M. G., McCormack, A. L., Cumine, S., Li, J., Isla, M. Z., and Di Monte, D. A. (2007). Microglial activation as a priming event leading to paraquat-induced dopaminergic cell degeneration. *Neurobiol. Dis.* 25, 392–400. doi: 10.1016/j.nbd.2006.10.008

Raj, D. D. A., Jaarsma, D., Holtman, I. R., Olah, M., Ferreira, F. M., Schaafsma, W., et al. (2014). Priming of microglia in a DNA-repair deficient model of accelerated aging. *Neurobiol. Aging* 35, 2147–2160. doi: 10.1016/j.neurobiolaging.2014.03.025

Raj, D. D. A., Moser, J., van der Pol, S. M. A., van Os, R. P., Holtman, I. R., Brouwer, N., et al. (2015). Enhanced microglial pro-inflammatory response to lipopolysaccharide correlates with brain infiltration and blood-brain barrier dysregulation in a mouse model of telomere shortening. *Aging Cell* 14, 1003–1013. doi: 10.1111/acel.12370

Ransohoff, R. M. (2016). A polarizing question: do M1 and M2 microglia exist? *Nat. Neurosci.* 19, 987–991. doi: 10.1038/nn.4338

Rodriguez-Callejas, J. D., Fuchs, E., and Perez-Cruz, C. (2016). Evidence of tau hyperphosphorylation and dystrophic microglia in the common marmoset. *Front. Aging Neurosci.* 8:315. doi: 10.3389/fnagi.2016.00315

Roodveldt, C., Labrador-Garrido, A., Gonzalez-Rey, E., Lachaud, C. C., Guilliams, T., Fernandez-Montesinos, R., et al. (2013). Preconditioning of microglia by α-synuclein strongly affects the response induced by toll-like receptor (TLR) stimulation. *PLoS One* 8:e79160. doi: 10.1371/journal.pone.0079160

Safaiyan, S., Kannaiyan, N., Snaidero, N., Brioschi, S., Biber, K., Yona, S., et al. (2016). Age-related myelin degradation burdens the clearance function of microglia during aging. *Nat. Neurosci.* 19, 995–998. doi: 10.1038/nn.4325

Satyanarayana, A., Manns, M. P., and Rudolph, K. L. (2004). Telomeres and telomerase: a dual role in hepatocarcinogenesis. *Hepatology* 40, 276–283. doi: 10.1002/hep.20308

Schafer, D. P., Lehrman, E. K., Kautzman, A. G., Koyama, R., Mardinly, A. R., Yamasaki, R., et al. (2012). Microglia sculpt postnatal neural circuits in an activity and complement-dependent manner. *Neuron* 74, 691–705. doi: 10.1016/j.neuron.2012.03.026

Scheffold, A., Holtman, I. R., Dieni, S., Brouwer, N., Katz, S.-F., Jebaraj, B. M. C., et al. (2016). Telomere shortening leads to an acceleration of synucleinopathy and impaired microglia response in a genetic mouse model. *Acta Neuropathol. Commun.* 4:87. doi: 10.1186/s40478-016-0364-x

Schuitemaker, A., van der Doef, T. F., Boellaard, R., van der Flier, W. M., Yaqub, M., Windhorst, A. D., et al. (2012). Microglial activation in healthy aging. *Neurobiol. Aging* 33, 1067–1072. doi: 10.1016/j.neurobiolaging.2010.09.016

Serrano-Pozo, A., Frosch, M. P., Masliah, E., and Hyman, B. T. (2011). Neuropathological alterations in Alzheimer disease. *Cold Spring Harb. Perspect. Med.* 1:a006189. doi: 10.1101/cshperspect.a006189

Sharaf, A., Krieglstein, K., and Spittau, B. (2013). Distribution of microglia in the postnatal murine nigrostriatal system. *Cell Tissue Res.* 351, 373–382. doi: 10.1007/s00441-012-1537-y

Sheffield, L. G., and Berman, N. E. (1998). Microglial expression of MHC class II increases in normal aging of nonhuman primates. *Neurobiol. Aging* 19, 47–55. doi: 10.1016/s0197-4580(97)00168-1

Sierra, A., Gottfried-Blackmore, A. C., McEwen, B. S., and Bulloch, K. (2007). Microglia derived from aging mice exhibit an altered inflammatory profile. *Glia* 55, 412–424. doi: 10.1002/glia.20468

Soreq, L., UK Brain Expression Consortium, North American Brain Expression Consortium, Rose, J., Soreq, E., Hardy, J., et al. (2017). Major shifts in glial regional identity are a transcriptional hallmark of human brain aging. *Cell Rep.* 18, 557–570. doi: 10.1016/j.celrep.2016.12.011

Spillantini, M. G., Crowther, R. A., Jakes, R., Hasegawa, M., and Goedert, M. (1998). α-Synuclein in filamentous inclusions of Lewy bodies from Parkinson's disease and dementia with lewy bodies. *Proc. Natl. Acad. Sci. U S A* 95, 6469–6473. doi: 10.1073/pnas.95.11.6469

Spittau, B., Rilka, J., Steinfath, E., Zöller, T., and Krieglstein, K. (2015). TGFβ1 increases microglia-mediated engulfment of apoptotic cells via upregulation of the milk fat globule-EGF factor 8. *Glia* 63, 142–153. doi: 10.1002/glia.22740

Spittau, B., Wullkopf, L., Zhou, X., Rilka, J., Pfeifer, D., and Krieglstein, K. (2013). Endogenous transforming growth factor-beta promotes quiescence of primary microglia *in vitro*. *Glia* 61, 287–300. doi: 10.1002/glia.22435

Squarzoni, P., Oller, G., Hoeffel, G., Pont-Lezica, L., Rostaing, P., Low, D., et al. (2014). Microglia modulate wiring of the embryonic forebrain. *Cell Rep.* 8, 1271–1279. doi: 10.1016/j.celrep.2014.07.042

Stevens, B., Allen, N. J., Vazquez, L. E., Howell, G. R., Christopherson, K. S., Nouri, N., et al. (2007). The classical complement cascade mediates CNS synapse elimination. *Cell* 131, 1164–1178. doi: 10.1016/j.cell.2007.10.036

Streit, W. J. (2006). Microglial senescence: does the brain's immune system have an expiration date? *Trends Neurosci.* 29, 506–510. doi: 10.1016/j.tins.2006.07.001

Streit, W. J., Braak, H., Xue, Q.-S., and Bechmann, I. (2009). Dystrophic (senescent) rather than activated microglial cells are associated with tau pathology and likely precede neurodegeneration in Alzheimer's disease. *Acta Neuropathol.* 118, 475–485. doi: 10.1007/s00401-009-0556-6

Streit, W. J., Sammons, N. W., Kuhns, A. J., and Sparks, D. L. (2004). Dystrophic microglia in the aging human brain. *Glia* 45, 208–212. doi: 10.1002/glia.10319

Streit, W. J., and Sparks, D. L. (1997). Activation of microglia in the brains of humans with heart disease and hypercholesterolemic rabbits. *J. Mol. Med.* 75, 130–138. doi: 10.1007/s001090050097

Streit, W. J., Walter, S. A., and Pennell, N. A. (1999). Reactive microgliosis. *Prog. Neurobiol.* 57, 563–581. doi: 10.1016/s0301-0082(98)00069-0

Tang, Y., Li, T., Li, J., Yang, J., Liu, H., Zhang, X. J., et al. (2014). Jmjd3 is essential for the epigenetic modulation of microglia phenotypes in the immune pathogenesis of Parkinson's disease. *Cell Death Differ.* 21, 369–380. doi: 10.1038/cdd.2013.159

Tichauer, J. E., Flores, B., Soler, B., Eugenín-von Bernhardi, L., Ramírez, G., and von Bernhardi, R. (2014). Age-dependent changes on TGFβ1 Smad3 pathway modify the pattern of microglial cell activation. *Brain Behav. Immun.* 37, 187–196. doi: 10.1016/j.bbi.2013.12.018

Tischer, J., Krueger, M., Mueller, W., Staszewski, O., Prinz, M., Streit, W. J., et al. (2016). Inhomogeneous distribution of Iba-1 characterizes microglial pathology in Alzheimer's disease. *Glia* 64, 1562–1572. doi: 10.1002/glia.23024

Ueno, M., Fujita, Y., Tanaka, T., Nakamura, Y., Kikuta, J., Ishii, M., et al. (2013). Layer V cortical neurons require microglial support for survival during postnatal development. *Nat. Neurosci.* 16, 543–551. doi: 10.1038/nn.3358

VanGuilder, H. D., Bixler, G. V., Brucklacher, R. M., Farley, J. A., Yan, H., Warrington, J. P., et al. (2011). Concurrent hippocampal induction of MHC II pathway components and glial activation with advanced aging is not correlated with cognitive impairment. *J. Neuroinflammation* 8:138. doi: 10.1186/1742-2094-8-138

Varvel, N. H., Neher, J. J., Bosch, A., Wang, W., Ransohoff, R. M., Miller, R. J., et al. (2016). Infiltrating monocytes promote brain inflammation and exacerbate neuronal damage after status epilepticus. *Proc. Natl. Acad. Sci. U S A* 113, E5665–E5674. doi: 10.1073/pnas.1604263113

Wang, X., Zhao, L., Zhang, J., Fariss, R. N., Ma, W., Kretschmer, F., et al. (2016). Requirement for microglia for the maintenance of synaptic function and integrity in the mature retina. *J. Neurosci.* 36, 2827–2842. doi: 10.1523/JNEUROSCI.3575-15.2016

Wohl, S. G., Schmeer, C. W., Witte, O. W., and Isenmann, S. (2010). Proliferative response of microglia and macrophages in the adult mouse eye after optic nerve lesion. *Invest. Ophthalmol. Vis. Sci.* 51, 2686–2696. doi: 10.1167/iovs.09-4537

Wong, A. M., Patel, N. V., Patel, N. K., Wei, M., Morgan, T. E., de Beer, M. C., et al. (2005). Macrosialin increases during normal brain aging are attenuated by caloric restriction. *Neurosci. Lett.* 390, 76–80. doi: 10.1016/j.neulet.2005.07.058

Yamasaki, R., Lu, H., Butovsky, O., Ohno, N., Rietsch, A. M., Cialic, R., et al. (2014). Differential roles of microglia and monocytes in the inflamed central nervous system. *J. Exp. Med.* 211, 1533–1549. doi: 10.1084/jem.20132477

Zecca, L., Wilms, H., Geick, S., Claasen, J.-H., Brandenburg, L.-O., Holzknecht, C., et al. (2008). Human neuromelanin induces neuroinflammation and neurodegeneration in the rat substantia nigra: implications for Parkinson's disease. *Acta Neuropathol.* 116, 47–55. doi: 10.1007/s00401-008-0361-7

Zhou, X., Spittau, B., and Krieglstein, K. (2012). TGFβ signalling plays an important role in IL4-induced alternative activation of microglia. *J. Neuroinflammation* 9:210. doi: 10.1186/1742-2094-9-210

Zhou, X., Zöller, T., Krieglstein, K., and Spittau, B. (2015). TGFβ1 inhibits IFNγ-mediated microglia activation and protects mDA neurons from IFNγ-driven neurotoxicity. *J. Neurochem.* 134, 125–134. doi: 10.1111/jnc.13111

7

Nutritional and Pharmacological Strategies to Regulate Microglial Polarization in Cognitive Aging and Alzheimer's Disease

*Emiliano Peña-Altamira *, Sabrina Petralla, Francesca Massenzio, Marco Virgili, Maria L. Bolognesi and Barbara Monti*

Department of Pharmacy and Biotechnology, University of Bologna, Bologna, Italy

***Correspondence:**
Emiliano Peña-Altamira
luis.penaaltamira3@unibo.it

The study of microglia, the immune cells of the brain, has experienced a renaissance after the discovery of microglia polarization. In fact, the concept that activated microglia can shift into the M1 pro-inflammatory or M2 neuroprotective phenotypes, depending on brain microenvironment, has completely changed the understanding of microglia in brain aging and neurodegenerative diseases. Microglia polarization is particularly important in aging since an increased inflammatory status of body compartments, including the brain, has been reported in elderly people. In addition, inflammatory markers, mainly derived from activated microglia, are widely present in neurodegenerative diseases. Microglial inflammatory dysfunction, also linked to microglial senescence, has been extensively demonstrated and associated with cognitive impairment in neuropathological conditions related to aging. In fact, microglia polarization is known to influence cognitive function and has therefore become a main player in neurodegenerative diseases leading to dementia. As the life span of human beings increases, so does the prevalence of cognitive dysfunction. Thus, therapeutic strategies aimed to modify microglia polarization are currently being developed. Pharmacological approaches able to shift microglia from M1 pro-inflammatory to M2 neuroprotective phenotype are actually being studied, by acting on many different molecular targets, such as glycogen synthase kinase-3 (GSK3) β, AMP-activated protein kinase (AMPK), histone deacetylases (HDACs), etc. Furthermore, nutritional approaches can also modify microglia polarization and, consequently, impact cognitive function. Several bioactive compounds normally present in foods, such as polyphenols, can have anti-inflammatory effects on microglia. Both pharmacological and nutritional approaches seem to be promising, but still need further development. Here we review recent data on these approaches and propose that their combination could have a synergistic effect to counteract cognitive aging impairment and Alzheimer's disease (AD) through immunomodulation of microglia polarization, i.e., by driving the shift of activated microglia from the pro-inflammatory M1 to the neuroprotective M2 phenotype.

Keywords: immunomodulation, microglia, cognitive impairment, aging, Alzheimer's disease, drug therapy, bioactive compounds, nutrition

MICROGLIA AND THEIR POLARIZATION

Microglia are the resident mononuclear phagocytes of the central nervous system and constitute about 5%–20% of total brain cells displaying regional differences in density (Lawson et al., 1990). These cells are known for their plastic capability and the functional characteristic depending on their activation state; indeed, it is not difficult to find morphological changes these cells undergo depending on their function (Szabo and Gulya, 2013). Under physiological conditions, microglial cells are in a "resting" state of non-activation, and cell morphology is characterized by numerous processes that originate from the soma with distal arborization (Hailer et al., 1996). On the other hand, under conditions of stress, inflammation, injury or upon the effect of certain signals, microglia change their morphology and activation state, from a non-activated to an activated state (Stence et al., 2001). Microglial cells enlarge their cell body and their ramifications become shorter and less arborized. This morphological mutation can induce phagocytic functions and amoeboid ability that allows cells to move toward sites of injury (Tzeng and Wu, 1999). A typical feature of this state is the activation of microglia and subsequent release of inflammatory mediators that lead to an increased oxidative and nitrosative stress. This condition promotes the inflammatory process, and persisting microglial activation in this condition shows to be harmful to the nervous tissue (Csuka et al., 2000; Polazzi and Monti, 2010). Activated microglia have two different phenotypes: M1 and M2. Classically activated M1 microglia, activated by LPS or IFN-γ, have pro-inflammatory, neurotoxic properties, inhibiting the proliferation of lymphocytes; M1 activated macrophages secrete proinflammatory cytokines, such as interleukin IL-1α, IL-1β, tumor necrosis factors (TNF) and nitric oxide (NO). Alternatively activated M2 microglia are able to repair small damage, have an anti-inflammatory phenotype, contributing to trophic support of neurons, possess the ability to degrade toxic aggregates and increase the neuroprotective functions thanks to anti-inflammatory interleukin production (Michelucci et al., 2009; Choi et al., 2017). The M2 phenotype is further divided in three subtypes; M2a, M2b, M2c. They may have comparable biochemical functions, but are different in the mechanisms of action. The shift to the M2a subtype is driven by IL-3 and IL-4 and is involved in collagen formation, tissue repair and immunity against parasites whereas the transition to the M2b subtype is driven by the activation of Toll-like receptor (TLRs) agonists and is able to recruit regulatory T-cells. On the other hand, the M2c phenotype, induced by IL-10, TGFβ1 and glucocorticoids, is involved in the repair of damage and injury (Chhor et al., 2013; Mecha et al., 2015).

Regarding the beneficial or detrimental role of activated microglia on neuronal survival, the most accredited hypothesis today is that microglia may have a dual role, both neuroprotective and neurotoxic, depending on their activation state, which in turn depends on the nature, length and extension of the insult (Ransohoff and Perry, 2009). *In vitro* studies in cell cultures have shown the ambivalent role of microglial cells on neurons; neuroprotective, but also neurotoxic, while *in vivo* studies mainly support the neuroprotective potential of activated microglia (Streit, 2002).

COGNITIVE DEFICITS IN AGING AND AD

Aging is defined as "the gradual change in an organism that leads to increased risk of weakness, disease and death" (Merriam-Webster thesaurus). It takes place all throughout an organism and the brain is no exception. Aging leads to reduced brain size, neurotransmitter receptor alterations, dendrite loss/regression and electrophysiological changes such as cortical spreading depression alterations, possibly connected also to cortical microglial reactivity, as shown by Iba-1 immunolabeling (Landfield et al., 1978; Earnest et al., 1979; Jacobs et al., 1997; Hof et al., 2002; Duan et al., 2003; Luebke et al., 2004; Batista-de-Oliveira et al., 2012; Lima et al., 2014). These alterations lead to what is normally called "age related cognitive decline". Human cognitive function can be classified in basic cognitive functions: attention, working memory, long-term memory, perception; and higher-level cognitive functions: speech and language, decision making, executive control (Glisky, 2007). However, much research on cognitive function has mainly focused on memory, and this could account for variability between aged individuals. The term "mild cognitive impairment" (MCI) was first introduced with the Global Deterioration Scale (Reisberg et al., 1982) for those individuals whose cognitive performance is below normal according to age-matched healthy individuals, especially regarding memory-based performance. The term was further refined in 2004 by the International Working Group on MCI (Winblad et al., 2004), in which affected individuals are considered those that show evidence of cognitive decline after appropriate testing, but maintain normal everyday life activities and functions. MCI appears to be a risk factor for developing dementia as shown by a Chinese study in which about 30% of patients with MCI developed dementia within 2 years and high plasma C-reactive protein levels were associated with accelerated cognitive decline and increased risk of dementia (Xu et al., 2009). Moreover, in another recent study, about 20% of patients with MCI developed Alzheimer's disease (AD) within 2 years after diagnosis, as assessed through biochemical and magnetic resonance imaging (MRI) performed for brain volumetric assessment, among which hippocampal volume (Nesteruk et al., 2016). AD is a neurodegenerative disease characterized by progressive cognitive decline, present both as familial and sporadic cases. Aβ production and processing alterations are thought to be one of the causes that trigger the disease. Post-mortem brain studies have shown that AD pathology hallmarks are the deposition of extracellular Aβ plaques as well as intracellular neurofibrillary tangles (Lantos et al., 1992). Familial AD which accounts for 2% of all cases and may have a disease onset as early as 40–50 years, is caused by mutations in the amyloid precursor protein (APP) gene and presenilin 1–2 genes prevalently (Karlinsky et al., 1992; Levy-Lahad et al., 1995; Sherrington et al., 1995). However, also rare TREM2 receptor mutations increase the risk of developing

AD (Guerreiro et al., 2013; Jonsson et al., 2013). TREM2 is an innate immune receptor expressed by macrophages and dendritic cells, among other cell types, while in the central nervous system it is expressed mainly by microglia (Hickman and El Khoury, 2014) and is involved in inflammation and phagocytosis. Mutations in TREM2 may impair phagocytosis (Kleinberger et al., 2014), supporting microglial involvement in AD pathology. On the other hand, sporadic AD shows late disease onset around 60–70 years for which the apoliprotein E type 4 (APOE-ε-4) allele has been identified as a major risk factor (Corder et al., 1993). Currently, there is no cure available for AD, yet AD is responsible for 60%–80% of all dementia cases (Alzheimer's international statistics). Nearly 46.8 million people worldwide were affected by dementia in 2015 and this number is expected to reach 131.5 million cases by 2050 (Alzheimer's international statistics). Thus, dementia represents a burden to society and to healthcare systems.

IMMUNOMODULATION AS A PROMISING THERAPEUTIC STRATEGY TO COUNTERACT COGNITIVE IMPAIRMENT

Under physiological conditions, immune responses exert positive effects on the brain by regulating neuroplasticity, learning and memory, while injury or chronic stress lead to the increased production of inflammatory molecules such as IL-1, IL-6 and TNF-α which may disrupt neurotrophic factor production/signaling and impair learning and memory (Schneider et al., 1998; Parish et al., 2002; Avital et al., 2003; Balschun et al., 2004; Golan et al., 2004; Soiampornkul et al., 2008). Interestingly, increased pro-inflammatory IL-6 and reduced anti-inflammatory IL-10 levels have been detected in brains from aged mice (Ye and Johnson, 1999, 2001). Moreover, immune status can also influence brain function in humans as the Hoorn Study evidenced that increased levels of inflammatory plasma markers (TNF-α, IL-6, IL-8, C-reactive protein) were associated with cognitive decline (Heringa et al., 2014). Because M1 activated microglia produce inflammatory cytokines, and these seem to induce cognitive impairment, immunomodulation strategies aiming to attenuate M1 microglial activation or induce an M1 to M2 microglial shift may contribute to counteract, at least partially, cognitive impairment in aging and in neurodegenerative diseases such as AD. Thus pharmacological and nutritional approaches targeting immunomodulation are currently being developed, and a remarkable amount of data has been produced recently (**Figure 1**).

PHARMACOLOGICAL APPROACHES TOWARDS IMMUNOMODULATION AND THEIR POTENTIAL APPLICATION IN AGING/AD

Therapeutic strategies aimed to modify microglia polarization, and therefore leading to immunomodulation, are currently being developed. Pharmacological approaches able to shift microglia from the M1 pro-inflammatory to the M2 neuroprotective phenotype could become new therapeutic tools in neurodegenerative diseases such as AD and also in normal brain aging. In the following sections we discuss on potentially interesting and successful immunomodulatory targets including glycogen synthase kinase-3 (GSK3) β, b-site APP-cleaving enzymes (BACEs), Janus kinase (JNK), phosphodiesterases (PDEs), AMP-activated protein kinase (AMPK), histone deacetylases (HDACs) and peroxisome proliferator-activated receptor gamma (PPAR-γ) according to currently available evidence.

GSK-3 β

GSK-3 β is a serine/threonine kinase, involved in several signaling pathways such as cell proliferation and inflammation (Cui et al., 1998; Park et al., 2006). Notably, GSK-3β appears to be responsible for tau hyperphosphorylation (Sperber et al., 1995), detaching tau from microtubules and inducing tau precipitation as intracellular neurofibrillary tangles (NFTs; Ferrer et al., 2002), a hallmark of AD. Moreover, GSK-3β has been shown to mediate the release of inflammatory cytokines in LPS-activated microglia *in vitro* (Green and Nolan, 2012), thus GSK-3 could be a promising target. Tideglusib (NP031112), a thiadiazolidinine derivative, prevents inflammation and neurodegeneration in a kainic-acid inflammation rat model (Luna-Medina et al., 2007) and has reached phase II clinical trials on AD patients (Clincaltrials.gov identifier NCT00948259), appearing safe though not effective enough (del Ser et al., 2013; Lovestone et al., 2015). In another study, two triazolopyridine derivative GSK-3 inhibitors (C-7a and C-7b) reduced Aβ neurotoxicity and tau hyperphosphorylation *in vitro* and improved cognitive deficits in a transgenic AD mouse model (Noh et al., 2013), though no anti-inflammatory effects were investigated. More recently, triazinones displayed *in vitro* anti-GSK-3 and anti-BACE-1 activity plus neuroprotective and neurogenic effects besides good brain permeability *in vivo* (Prati et al., 2015), however no anti-inflammatory data are currently available. Lastly, L807mts, a highly selective GSK-3 peptide derivative inhibitor, reduced Aβ levels, reduced inflammation and enhanced autophagy in a transgenic AD mouse model (Licht-Murava et al., 2016).

BACEs

Aβ aggregates are generated by the cleavage of the membrane-associated APP by α, β and γ-secretases. Through two successive proteolytic cleavages by α-secretase and γ-secretase, a harmless peptide, p3, is produced. On the other hand, β-secretase operates a different cleavage leading to the production of two neurotoxic peptides of 40 and 42 amino acids each, called Aβ40 and Aβ42, respectively. The first β–secretase identified was BACE-1, a type I transmembrane aspartic protease (Vassar et al., 1999). Because Aβ can induce neuroinflammation, BACE-1 inhibitors can contribute indirectly to inhibiting microglial M1 activation and research on their potential application is ongoing. *In vivo* treatment with the aminoisoindole AZ-4217, a BACE-1 inhibitor, resulted in long term reduced Aβ deposition

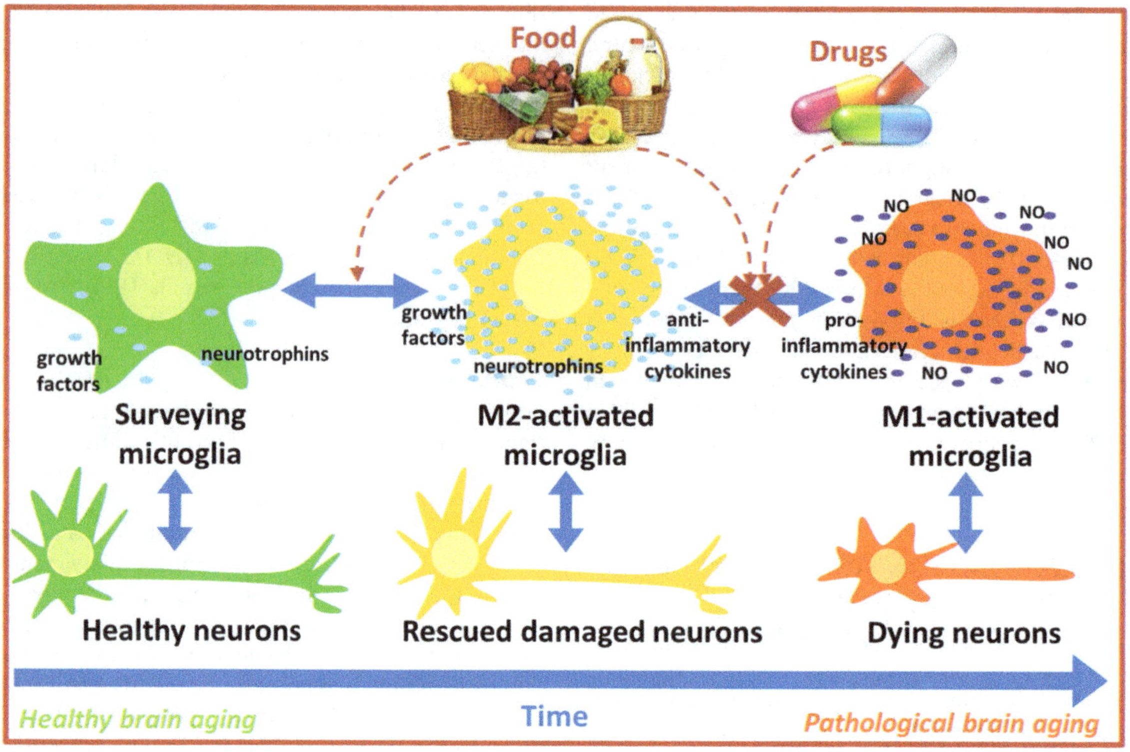

FIGURE 1 | Possible pharmacological and nutritional approaches towards immunomodulation to counteract pathological brain aging. Food bioactive compounds and/or synthetic compounds may influence microglial activation state contributing to neuronal survival and thus improve cognitive function during aging.

in an APP transgenic cerebral amyloidosis mouse model (Eketjäll et al., 2013). In another study, treatment with the BACE inhibitor RO5508887 reduced amyloid plaque load and formation in an AD transgenic mouse model and combined treatment with an anti-Aβ antibody (gantenerumab) further enhanced these effects (Jacobsen et al., 2014), however the impact on cognition was not investigated. Also, as previously stated, triazinones displayed anti-GSK-3 and anti-BACE-1 activity (Prati et al., 2015) while NB-360, another BACE-1 inhibitor was able to block Aβ deposition and the accumulation of inflammatory cells in a transgenic AD mouse model (Neumann et al., 2015). Noteworthy, a clinical trial to study the effect of the BACE-1 inhibitor LY3202626 on patients with mild AD dementia, as of February 2017 was recruiting patients (Clinicaltrials.gov identifier NCT02791191).

JNK

Mitogen-activated protein kinases (MAPKs) are serine–threonine kinases that mediate intracellular signaling. JNK is a major cellular stress response protein induced by oxidative stress and its activation is believed to be an early event in AD (Zhu et al., 2001). Among the MAPKs, JNK is one of the essential mediators of microglial proinflammatory functions (Waetzig et al., 2005), it is a component of signaling pathways that lead to inflammation, and it can control the synthesis and release of proinflammatory molecules by LPS-activated microglia (Hidding et al., 2002). Moreover, the JNK-AP1 signaling pathway mediates the increased expression of inflammatory genes induced by Aβ peptides in human brain endothelial cells and in AD brain (Vukic et al., 2009). Thus JNK is an attractive target for AD prevention/therapy. In one study, treatment of LPS-activated primary rat microglia with conserved dopamine neurotrophic factor (CDNF) resulted in reduced production of inflammatory cytokines by suppressing the phosphorylation of JNK and thus inhibiting JNK signaling (Zhao et al., 2014). Therefore, CDNF use *in vivo* seems promising. Another recent *in vivo* study showed that administration of the JNK inhibitor SP600125 resulted in cognitive deficit improvement in a transgenic AD mouse model by reducing Aβ production, inflammatory responses and synaptic loss (Zhou et al., 2015). Interestingly, *in vivo* administration of the small molecule LX2343 improved cognitive deficits in a transgenic AD mouse model by inhibiting both JNK and BACE-1 activity, reducing Aβ production and promoting autophagy (Guo et al., 2016), though no direct anti-inflammatory mechanisms were investigated.

PDEs

PDEs act as regulators of intracellular signaling cascades through the control of 2 second messengers, cyclic adenosine monophosphate and cyclic guanosine monophosphate. Recent findings point to PDE inhibitors as compounds able to affect different mechanisms underlying AD, as shown by active ongoing research with these molecules. Administration of sildenafil, a PDE-5 inhibitor, improved cognitive deficits, reduced Aβ levels and neuroinflammation in a transgenic AD mouse model (Zhang et al., 2013). Moreover, administration of another PDE-5 inhibitor, yonkenafil, resulted in improved cognitive function, increased neurogenesis in the dentate gyrus and reduced activation of microglia and astrocytes in a transgenic AD mouse model (Zhu et al., 2015), therefore showing also anti-inflammatory effects. In another study, the PDE-7 inhibitor S14 improved cognitive impairment, reduced Aβ deposition and tau phosphorylation in a transgenic AD mouse model (Perez-Gonzalez et al., 2013). Also in an *in vitro* study, the PDE-3 inhibitor cilostazol reduced Aβ production by increasing ADAM10 expression (Lee et al., 2014), though no anti-inflammatory effects were investigated. Noteworthy, a phase IV clinical trial to examine the additive effects of cilostazol on donepezil-treated mild to moderate AD patients has been completed (Clinicaltrials.gov identifier NCT01409564) and in a very recent small clinical trial, cilostazol administration as an add-on therapy reduced cognitive decline in AD patients (Tai et al., 2017). In another study, administration of GEBR-7b, a PDE-4D inhibitor, improved cognitive deficits in a transgenic AD mouse model (Sierksma et al., 2014) though the underlying mechanisms of action remain to be discovered. Lastly, in a very recent *in vivo* study, administration of the PDE-4 inhibitor FFM reversed cognitive deficits in a transgenic AD mouse model by increasing CREB phosphorylation and BDNF levels and reducing inducible NO synthase (iNOS), TNF-α and IL-1β levels (Guo et al., 2017).

AMPK

AMPK is a highly conserved energy sensor involved in mitochondrial biogenesis, cellular stress responses and regulation of inflammation (Corton et al., 1994; Zong et al., 2002; Giri et al., 2004). Because overactivated AMPK has been reported to accumulate in neurons containing tangles in AD brains (Vingtdeux et al., 2011) and AMPK can phosphorylate tau protein (Domise et al., 2016), AMPK may represent an interesting target, though its role in AD is not fully understood. While inhibition of AMPK with the compound C (CC) improved hippocampal synaptic plasticity impairment induced by Aβ in a transgenic AD mouse model (Ma et al., 2014) AMPK activators have also shown beneficial effects in AD models. An example are the anti-epileptic drugs topiramate and levetiracetam which improved cognitive deficits, reduced Aβ production, increased the activation of AMPK and inhibited HDAC activity in a transgenic AD mouse model (Shi et al., 2013). Moreover, a phase II levetiracetam clinical trial on MCI patients was completed in 2012, though no results were posted (Clinicaltrials.gov identifier NCT01044758). Also, while not tested in AD, telmisartan, an angiotensin II type 1 receptor blocker, increased brain AMPK activation and microglial M2 gene expression in an LPS-induced neuroinflammation mouse model (Xu et al., 2015) thus its application in AD may deserve attention. In another study, administration of the AMPK activator AICAR, improved cognitive deficits in a streptozotocin-induced AD rat model (Du et al., 2015) by restoring mitochondrial functions, though no anti-inflammatory effects were investigated. Lastly, treatment with the small molecule THSG exerted anti-inflammatory effects on LPS-activated microglia by reducing iNOS, COX-2, TNF-α and IL-6 levels and increased AMPK phosphorylation levels, thus confirming AMPK activation (Park et al., 2016).

HDACs

The effects of histone acetylation on the activation of gene expression were unknown until the 1960s (Allfrey et al., 1964). Acetylation reduces the positive charge of basic histone proteins thus decreasing their interaction with DNA and allowing gene expression. More in detail, this process is finely regulated by several Histone Acetyl Transferases (HATs) and HDACs. Recently, the effects of HDAC inhibitors on immunomodulation have increasingly generated interest due to a potential role in immunotherapy. In fact, class I HDAC inhibitors have been reported to increase transcription of neuronal genes, provide neuroprotective effects, and enhance cognitive abilities. Moreover, class I HDAC inhibitors such as valproic acid (VPA), trichostatin A (TSA), suberoylanilide hydroxamic acid (SAHA), sodium phenylbutyrate (SB) and MS-275 have been shown to enhance neurite outgrowth, synaptic plasticity, neurogenesis, neuronal differentiation and axon regeneration in cultured neurons and *in vivo* (Laeng et al., 2004; Siebzehnrubl et al., 2007; Koriyama et al., 2014). In one *in vivo* study, administration of the HDAC inhibitor SB, prevented cognitive deficits and reduced Aβ and GFAP levels, suggesting an anti-inflammatory effect in a transgenic AD mouse model (Ricobaraza et al., 2011). Another *in vivo* study showed that treatment with the benzamide HDAC inhibitor MS-275 improved cognitive deficits and reduced microglial activation and Aβ accumulation in a transgenic AD mouse model (Zhang and Schluesener, 2013). Lastly, in another *in vivo* study, SAHA treatment restored H3 acetylation and BDNF levels (Sharma and Taliyan, 2016) in mice fed a fat-enriched diet which developed insulin resistance-induced cognitive decline. While not being an AD study, insulin resistance is considered a risk factor for AD (Fava et al., 2017) and thus SAHA may deserve attention in AD research.

PPAR-γ

PPAR-γ is a nuclear receptor that, after binding peroxisome proliferators, binds to specific DNA PPAR response elements regulating the expression of genes involved in fatty acid peroxisomal beta-oxidation (Dreyer et al., 1993). Current evidence shows that PPAR-γ activation may prove useful in AD therapy. In one *in vitro* study pioglitazone, a PPAR-γ agonist, inhibited iNOS and the production of IL-1β, TNF-α and IL-6 in LPS-activated HAPI microglia (Ji et al., 2010). Unfortunately, a phase II pioglitazone clinical trial performed in mild to moderate AD patients completed in 2009 produced no results (Clinicaltrials.gov identifier

NCT00982202). In another *in vitro* study, the small molecule SNU-BP inhibited inflammatory cytokine production and iNOS in LPS-stimulated microglia by activating PPAR-γ. SNU-BP also increased IL-4 and arginase-1 expression, considered as M2 microglial phenotype markers (Song et al., 2016), thus SNU-BP may deserve *in vivo* testing as well. Interestingly, PPAR-γ agonists able to act on other targets are also being studied in AD therapy. Such is the case for T3D-959, a PPAR-γ and PPAR-δ agonist that reversed neurodegeneration in a streptozotocin-induced AD mouse model though no anti-inflammatory mechanisms were investigated (Tong et al., 2016). Noteworthy, a phase II clinical trial focused on TD3D-959 in mild to moderate AD patients as of June 2016 was being performed (Clinicaltrials.gov identifier NCT02560753). Lastly, MH84 a PPAR-γ agonist/γ-secretase modulator, reduced Aβ42 in HEK293APPwt cells, characterized by elevated Aβ42 levels, and improved mitochondrial dysfunction (Pohland et al., 2016), thus performing *in vivo* MH84 studies applied to AD therapy may be worth.

NUTRITIONAL APPROACHES TOWARDS IMMUNOMODULATION AND THEIR POTENTIAL APPLICATION IN AGING/AD

Interest in the role of diet in health developed after several epidemiological studies found an association between the Mediterranean diet and a lower risk of developing cardiovascular diseases and death (Menotti et al., 1996; Knoops et al., 2004). Nutritional approaches to target immunomodulation could become interesting strategies given that foods we consume on a daily basis, especially plant-based foods (widely present in the Mediterranean diet), besides providing nutrients contain also non-essential molecules, termed bioactive food compounds, able to exert multiple effects throughout the body by acting on different targets. Science has started understanding the effect of these molecules, and they could join the list of key players in immunomodulation strategies.

Bioactive compounds comprise a heterogeneous group of thousands of molecules. They can be classified into four/five major groups depending on authors: carotenoids (including carotenes and xantohpylls); phytosterols (including sterols and stanols); phenolic compounds (including chlorogenic acid); polyphenols (including flavonoids, stilbenes, lignans and curcuminoids) and sulfur compounds (including glucosinolates; Lozano et al., 2016).

Being a heterogeneous group of molecules with distinct chemical structures, bioactive compounds exert therefore different effects such as anti-inflammatory, antioxidant, hypoglycemic, cholesterol-lowering, estrogen mimicking, immunostimulant, neurogenic and neuroprotective effects.

Nutritional strategies based on the use of bioactive compounds can include dietary enrichment, by increasing the intake of foods containing naturally high amounts of bioactive compounds; intake of bioactive compound-enriched supplements, such as concentrated extracts or purified single molecules; intake of foods fortified with bioactive compounds. On the other hand, dietary supplements containing high amounts of bioactive compounds are already commercially available.

Given their multifaceted properties, many studies have focused on the effect of bioactive compounds which we summarize in the following sections and discuss on their potential use in aging/AD.

Carotenoids

Well-known carotenoids such as β-carotene, lycopene and lutein can be found in carrots, tomatoes, peaches and peppers among other foods (Lozano et al., 2016). Lycopene, highly concentrated in tomatoes, was able to reduce BV-2 microglial cell activation after LPS treatment *in vitro* by reducing COX-2 expression (Lin et al., 2014). Moreover, lycopene exerted anti-inflammatory effects and enhanced cognitive performance in a Aβ42-induced AD rat model by downregulating inflammatory cytokines such as TNF-α and IL1-B (Sachdeva and Chopra, 2015). Also lutein, highly present in parsley, was able to reduce LPS-induced neuroinflammation in BV-2 microglial cells, by significantly inhibiting iNOS and cyclooxygenase-2 activity, as well as by reducing TNF-α and IL-1β production (Wu et al., 2015). However, no *in vivo* data on the anti-inflammatory effect of lutein are currently available. Interestingly, a human study involving nearly 7000 participants aged 50 or older found an association between high levels of serum lycopene and lutein and a lower risk of mortality by AD (Min and Min, 2014). Current research on AD and bioactive compounds has also focused on less-known carotenoinds. For example, fucoxanthin, a carotenoid abundant in brown seaweeds, exerted anti-inflammatory effects and reduced reactive oxygen species levels in Aβ42 treated BV2 microglial cells (Pangestuti et al., 2013). Moreover, in another *in vitro* inflammation-induced microglial cell culture study, fucoxanthin was able to inhibit the secretion of inflammatory cytokines after LPS treatment (Zhao et al., 2017). However, no *in vivo* data on the anti-inflammatory effect of fucoxanthin are currently available.

On the other hand, carotenoids contained in saffron, such as crocin and crocetin, exerted *in vitro* anti-inflammatory effects on LPS-treated rat brain microglial cells by inhibiting NO synthesis from iNOS and the production of inflammatory cytokines (Nam et al., 2010). Also, in another study, trans-crocetin was able to improve Aβ degradation in monocytes derived from AD patients (Tiribuzi et al., 2017) thus it would be interesting to determine whether trans-crocetin may induce the same effect in microglia. Remarkably, crocin intraperitoneal administration showed neuroprotective effects *in vivo*, by blocking Aβ-induced apoptosis in an AD animal model (Asadi et al., 2015) which means crocin is able to cross the blood brain barrier, despite its hydrophilic nature.

Phytosterols

Phytosterols such as β-sitosterol, stigmasterol and campesterol can be found in vegetable oils, such as olive oil, cereals, legumes and nuts (Lozano et al., 2016). While a direct anti-inflammatory activity in AD has not been reported for most phytosterols, their anti-inflammatory effects may not have been thoroughly investigated. Stigmasterol, one of the most prevalent phytosterols in foods, exhibited beneficial effects *in vivo* in an AD animal model, mainly by reducing Aβ generation (Burg et al., 2013). In another *in vivo* study, a plant sterol-enriched diet was able to prevent cognitive impairment in SAMP8 mice, a non-transgenic AD animal model. This beneficial effect could derive from the fact that plant sterols may substitute lost cholesterol in SAMP8 mice brains (Pérez-Cañamás et al., 2016). AD studies have also focused on less common phytosterols. For example, spinasterol, isolated from *Aster scaber*, widely used in Korean cuisine, exerted anti-inflammatory effects on LPS-activated BV-2 microglial cells by upregulating heme-oxygenase-1 and reducing the production of TNF-α, IL-1β and PGE2 (Jeong et al., 2010). However, no anti-inflammatory effects for spinasterol in aging/AD models have been reported. Moreover, fucosterol, a phytosterol contained in brown seaweed, exerted anti-inflammatory effects on RAW264.7 macrophages by inhibiting the production of NO and the expression of iNOS and cyclooxygenase-2 (Jung et al., 2013). This suggests that fucosterol may exert the same anti-inflammatory effects on microglial cells. Interestingly, a recent *in vitro* study additionally shows that fucosterol may also exert BACE-1 inhibitory effects (Jung et al., 2016).

Phenolic Compounds/Polyphenols

Phenolic compounds such as tyrosol, capsaicin, coumaric, caffeic and chlorogenic acid can be found in citrus, olives, oats and soybeans wheras polyphenols, the most heterogeneous group of bioactive compounds, which includes quercetin, rutin, flavan-3-ols, catechins, anthocyanins, flavones (luteolin), isoflavones (phytoestrogens such as genistein, daidzein), curcumin and lignans can be found in onions, blueberries, red wine and tea (Lozano et al., 2016). Chemically speaking, phenolic acids belong to the supercategory of polyphenols, and thus we describe several examples together. In one *in vitro* study, caffeic acid, naturally present in honeybee propolis, exerted anti-inflammatory effects on BV-2 microglia by inhibiting the expression of iNOS and cyclooxygenase-2 (Tsai et al., 2015). Moreover, caffeic acid oral administration improved cognitive deficits in an Aβ25–35-induced AD animal model, possibly by inhibiting lipid peroxidation and NO production (Kim et al., 2015).

In another study, artoindonesianin O, a phenolic compound found in mulberries, blocked Aβ-42 toxicity in an *in vitro* model of AD (Qiao et al., 2015). While no *in vivo* anti-inflammatory properties for artoindonesianin O have been reported, a recent report showed that artoindonesianin O is a potent lipooxygenase inhibitor, thus it could also play an anti-inflammatory role *in vivo* (Lang et al., 2016).

On the other hand, carnosic acid found in rosemary and sage, was able to inhibit LPS-induced activation of MG6 microglial cells *in vitro*, by reducing iNOS levels (Yanagitai et al., 2012). Moreover, carnosic acid was able to improve cognitive deficits in an Aβ40-induced AD rat model (Rasoolijazi et al., 2013). In another study, oral administration of ferulic acid, found in seeds and cereals, particularly flaxseed (Beejmohun et al., 2007), inhibited microglial activation in an Aβ42-induced AD mouse model by decreasing IFN-gamma levels in the hippocampus (Kim et al., 2004). Moreover, ferulic acid administration was able to improve cognitive deficits in a transgenic AD mouse model (Mori et al., 2013).

Interest in the application of other polyphenols normally present in foods for AD research has constantly increased. In fact, oral administration of oleuropein aglycone, found in olive leaves, significantly attenuated astrocyte and microglial activation in an Aβ42-induced AD rat model (Luccarini et al., 2014). Moreover, oleuropein aglycone oral administration also improved cognitive deficits and reduced Aβ42 plaque area and number in a transgenic AD mouse model (Pantano et al., 2017). Also resveratrol, a polyphenol found in red grapes and wine, was able to inhibit Aβ-induced activation of BV-2 microglial cells by reducing the production of inflammatory factors such as TNF-α, IL-1β and NO (Yao et al., 2015). Moreover, resveratrol administration showed anti-inflammatory and anti-apoptotic effects *in vivo* in an Aβ42-induced AD mouse model by inhibiting PDE-4 signaling (Wang et al., 2016). Interestingly, dietary resveratrol also extended life span of SAMP8 mice, a non-transgenic AD mouse model through sirtuin activation (Porquet et al., 2013). However, a resveratrol phase II clinical trial on patients with mild to moderate AD, resulted in no benefit to patients (Turner et al., 2015; Clinicaltrials.gov identifier NCT01504854).

In another study, curcumin, mainly found in turmeric, inhibited Aβ induced microglial activation *in vitro* (Shi et al., 2015). Moreover, curcumin administration improved cognitive deficits in an AD transgenic rat model, possibly through an anti-inflammatory effect by activating PPAR-gamma (Liu et al., 2016) and a phase II curcumin clinical trial on mild to moderate AD patients was concluded in 2009 though no results were posted (Clinicaltrials.gov identifier NCT00099710).

Regarding phytoestrogens, genistein, the main isoflavone found in soy, exerted anti-inflammatory effects on LPS-activated BV-2 microglia by blocking TLR4 signaling (Jeong et al., 2014). Moreover, genistein improved cognitive deficits in an AD mouse model (Bonet-Costa et al., 2016). However, oral administration of soy isoflavones (100 mg/day) to AD patients for 6 months resulted in no cognitive deficit improvement (Gleason et al., 2015; Clinicaltrials.org identifier NCT00205179). This could be due to the fact that genistein is metabolized by the gut microbiome to its most active metabolite, equol, only in presence of specific bacteria in the gut microbiome such as Slackia isoflavoniconvertens (Matthies et al., 2009).

In another study, anthocyanin *in vitro* treatment inhibited LPS-induced BV-2 microglial activation by reducing IL-1β levels (Meireles et al., 2016). Moreover, a diet supplemented with 1% anthocyanin extracts was able to prevent cognitive deficits in a transgenic AD mouse model (Yamakawa et al., 2016) whereas pomegranate polyphenol administration exerted anti-inflammatory effects on a transgenic AD mouse model by reducing TNF-α brain levels and microgliosis (Rojanathammanee et al., 2013).

Even the polyphenol epigallocatechin from green tea, attenuated Aβ EOC 13.31 microglial activation *in vitro* (Cheng-Chung Wei et al., 2016). While no *in vivo* anti-inflammatory effects for green tea catechins in AD have been reported, green tea epicatechin administration combined with treadmill exercise improved cognitive deficits in an AD transgenic mouse model (Zhang et al., 2016). Also, a phase II epigallocatechin clinical trial on early stage AD patients was completed on 2016 though no results have been published yet (Clinicaltrials.gov identifier NCT00951834).

Lastly, rutin, a citrus flavonoid, exerted anti-inflammatory and antioxidant effects in an AD transgenic mouse model, improving spatial memory (Xu et al., 2014).

Interestingly, one *in vivo* study showed that dietary polyphenols may exert in part their beneficial effects after being converted into phenolic acids by intestinal microbiota (Wang et al., 2015).

Sulfur Compounds

Sulfur compounds such as glucosinolates (isothiocyanate, sulphoraphane) and Allium genus compounds (allin, allicin and ajoene) can be found in cabbage, broccoli, onions and garlic (Lozano et al., 2016). Sulforaphane, an isothiocyanate derived from glucoraphanin hydrolysis in broccoli, exerted anti-inflammatory effects *in vitro* on LPS-activated microglia by decreasing IL-1β, IL-6 and TNF-α expression (Brandenburg et al., 2010). Moreover, sulforaphane was able to extert anti-inflammatory effects against Aβ42-induced microglial activation in THP-1 macrophages through STAT-1 dephosphorylation and the activation of heme-oxygenase 1 (An et al., 2016). While no *in vivo* anti-inflammatory effects in AD disease have been reported for sulforaphane, sulforaphane administration exerted neuroprotective effects in an AD aluminum-induced mouse model (Zhang et al., 2015). Moreover, a very recent study showed that treatment with moringin, an isothiocyanate derived from the edible plant *Moringa oleifera*, exerted potent *in vitro* ant-inflammatory effects on LPS-activated RAW 264.7 macrophages (Giacoppo et al., 2017). Also, moringin showed *in vivo* anti-inflammatory effects in a Parkinson's disease mouse model (Giacoppo et al., 2017) and thus it would be worth testing moringin also on aging and AD models.

IN VITRO AND *IN VIVO* CONSIDERATIONS

Microglial cells are able to exert neuroprotective effects towards neurons challenged with toxic insults. Evidence shows that this mechanism can be exerted either through direct contact or through factors secreted by microglia, as shown by *in vitro* studies (Polazzi et al., 2001, 2009, 2013). On the other hand, nanomolar concentrations of Aβ induced neuronal death in mixed neuron-glial cerebellum cultures, possibly through a microglia mediated mechanism (Neniskyte et al., 2011), thus outlining a multifaceted role of microglial activation. Of remarkable importance are the limitations of the *in vitro* and *in vivo* studies here discussed. Regarding both pharmacological and nutritional *in vitro* studies, the abovementioned molecules may actually be metabolized by the liver cytochrome P450 systems and thus their properties may change, thus further research in *in vivo* models to understand the effect of liver metabolism will be required. Moreover, regarding nutritional *in vitro* studies, the bioactive compounds here cited may not all cross the blood brain barrier and thus may not reach the identified targets. Also, dietary bioactive compounds may be transformed by the gut microbiome, as is the case for genistein which is converted into equol, its most active derivative (Matthies et al., 2009). This means further research needs to be performed in order to understand whether food bioactive compounds used in *in vitro* studies are actually the same identical molecules crossing the blood brain barrier after being absorbed in the gastrointestinal tract. Also, most nutritional based studies have focused on the administration of a single bioactive compound. Bioactive compound mixtures, as present in foods, could modify/enhance their activity mutually. For example, as stated in the previous sections, brown seaweeds contain both the carotenoid fucoxanthin and the phytosterol fucosterol and thus may exert a synergistic effect on AD when brown seaweeds are consumed with the diet. However, one caveat of the above described nutritional approaches is that single compounds may have been used at concentrations much higher than those present in foods and thus the observed effects may not be attainable through food intake. In fact, in the previously described *in* vivo lycopene AD study (Sachdeva and Chopra, 2015), lycopene was used at concentrations reaching 4 mg/kg of body weight. In order to reach such dietary intake in humans, more than 2 kg of fresh tomatoes would need to be consumed (Kamiloglu et al., 2014). However, dietary bioactive compound supplementation may overcome this problem. Also, regarding nutritional approaches, intestinal absorption should not be underestimated as is the case for some carotenoids, which are partially absorbed at the intestinal level, as is the case for lycopene, which shows about 20% absorption levels (Moran et al., 2015) and thus, circulating blood carotenoid levels may be too low compared to those used in the previously described studies. Moreover, carotenoid polarity influences greatly their absorption, though dietary fat intake and food matrix also influence carotenoid intestinal absorption, as shown in an *in vitro* Caco-2 intestinal barrier model (Mashurabad et al., 2017). However, carotenoid absorption problems may also be overcome by avoiding oral carotenoid administration, for example, through intraperitoneal administration, as previously stated for crocin *in vivo* studies (Asadi et al., 2015). On the other hand, AD animal studies pose several limitations when compared to human studies, being species-specific differences the most important ones. While extremely useful, currently available transgenic AD models are based on the overexpression of one or more proteins, as suggested from familial AD genetic causes, involved in AD pathology in order for animals to develop AD. However, protein overexpression at much higher than physiological levels, such as APP transgenic mice which develop cerebral amyloidosis (Jacobsen et al., 2014; Neumann et al., 2015) may lead to negative results after compound administration perhaps not necessarily due to compound inefficacy but rather to forced protein expression levels much higher than in AD patients. At such high transgene expression levels, the studied molecules may not be able to exert detectable beneficial effects, while they could do so at physiological protein expression levels. Another issue regards compound metabolism since pharmacological and food bioactive compounds may be differently metabolized by rodents, the most widely used animal model for AD research. Moreover, gut microbiome differences present in humans which can influence bioactive compound metabolism, may not be as sharp in rodents and rodent intestinal permeability may differ from human intestinal permeability for the above mentioned pharmacological and food bioactive compounds. Noteworthy, the amount of pharmacological or food bioactive compounds used in animal studies, when extrapolated to human studies may be quite high. This suggests further consideration is needed when designing human studies. Despite these limitations, animal models continue to be an invaluable resource in AD research. Furthermore, regarding pharmacological approaches in human studies, compound delivery conditions may not be optimal: orally administered compounds may need to be increasingly stable and/or rendered more permeable to brain parenchyma in order to reach their targets in affected areas. Accordingly, pharmacological compound delivery methodologies should be further developed. One last consideration regarding human studies is that gut microbiome differences between different world populations may account for different outcomes in clinical trials when dealing with food bioactive compounds, in case these are metabolized by gut microbiota. Such is the case for genistein conversion into equol, its most active derivative, given that only about 30%–50% of the world population contains gut bacteria able to perform this specific chemical reaction (Atkinson et al., 2005).

CONCLUSION

Pharmacological and nutritional strategies aimed at modulating microglial activation (**Figure 2**) offer much potential for future

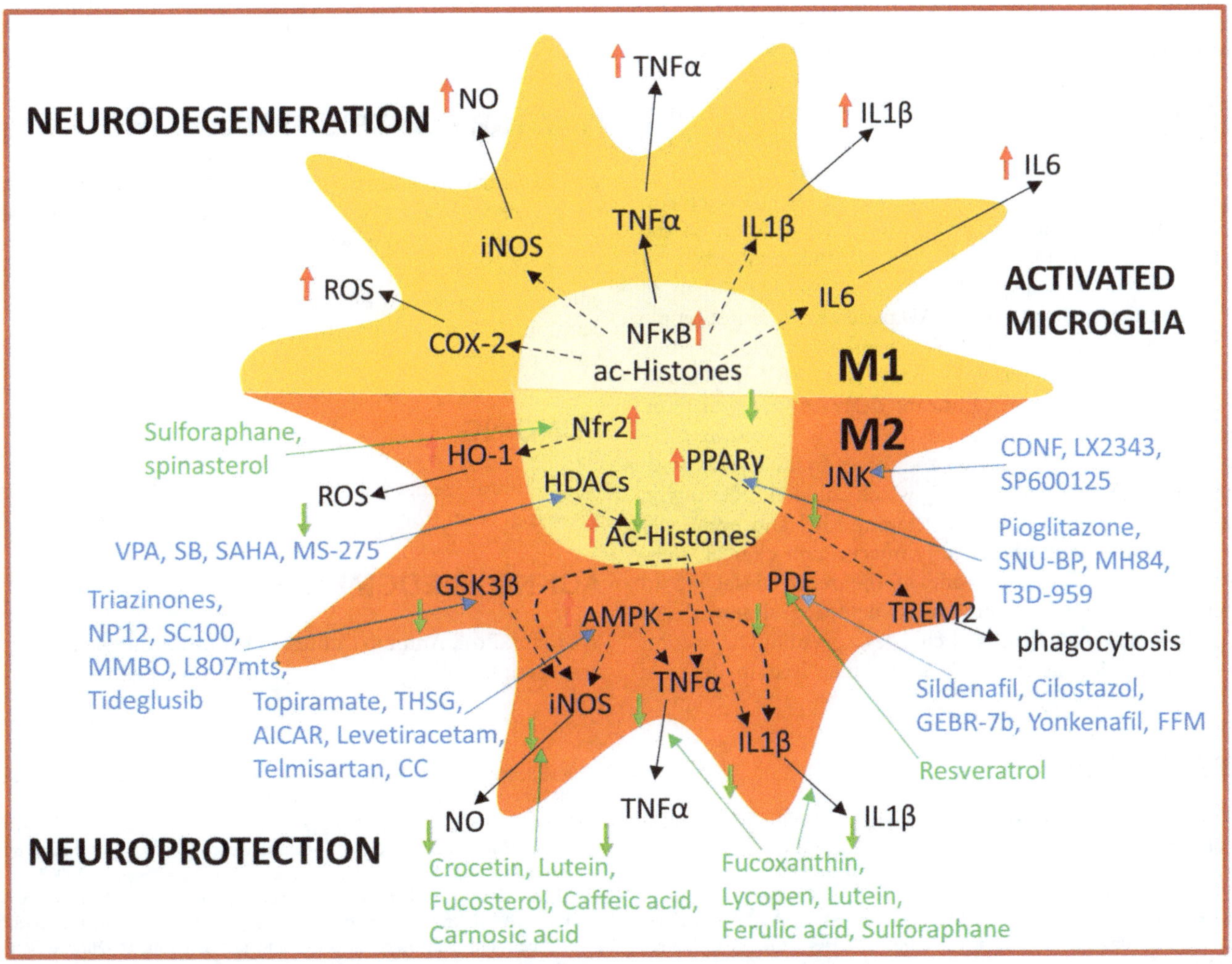

FIGURE 2 | Summary of immunomodulatory bioactive and synthetic compounds. Bioactive (green) and synthetic (blue) compounds are able to modulate microglial activation by shifting from the M1 neurotoxic to the M2 neuroprotective phenotype acting on several intracellular targets.

brain aging and AD therapy. However, they also represent a big challenge and further research is needed to understand their potential application in humans. Clinical trials focused on immunomodulation targets performed so far, have not resulted in AD patient improvement, however it has to be considered that immunomodulatory strategies may have preventive rather than protective effects. This could derive from the fact that initial AD pathology hallmarks such as Aβ accumulation may start years before symptoms manifest. In fact, protein tangles may already be present in early life and even in healthy aged people (Braak and Del Tredici, 2011), thus perhaps only when a combination of biochemical (Aβ deposition) and cellular factors (Aβ clearance dysfunction) are present, may AD pathology progress. A considerable amount of Aβ turnover is handled by the glymphatic system in the brain and perivascular circulation and dysfunction in these systems may contribute to Aβ accumulation as well (Tarasoff-Conway et al., 2015). Microglial activation thus may be initially beneficial in AD pathology as show by positron emission tomography imaging studies in AD patients and only after becoming chronic it may exacerbate disease (Hamelin et al., 2016; Fan et al., 2017). For example, Aβ direct interaction with the receptor for advance glycation end products (RAGE) increases oxidative stress in neurons, however it also enhances inflammatory response in microglia (Deane et al., 2012). By the time symptoms manifest, microglial dysfunction has already been established and it may be too late to apply current immunomodulation strategies for disease management. However, if compound administration starts as soon as the first biochemical alterations are detected, this may prove an effective preventive strategy. Therefore, a different design of clinical trials directed not towards AD patients, but rather people with MCI should be considered. This approach would hopefully allow to evaluate efficacy from a reduction of MCI individuals undergoing AD and/or a significant delay of this transition. Recent technological advances in MRI allow to discriminate healthy individuals with higher and lower brain levels of Aβ accumulation (Yasuno et al., 2016) which could aid identifying patients with a higher risk of developing MCI and eventually AD in order to better design early intervention clinical trials. If high brain Aβ levels are one of the required factors to trigger AD, yet not the only cause, detecting abnormal Aβ and perhaps tau conformational changes, spreading, deposition and mislocalization at early AD stages may lead to define a time frame in which initial beneficial microglial inflammatory responses are ongoing and immunomodulation strategies thus may prove more effective. Pharmacological therapies are currently experiencing a renaissance, thanks to multitarget drug design, in which already approved or discontinued drugs are fused with other drugs or food bioactive compounds. Thus the obtained hybrid molecule exerts multitarget directed activities derived from the original forming molecules, which may also act on different brain cell populations (Jeřábek et al., 2017). Regarding nutritional approaches, a first step could be adopting, the earlier the better, a healthy eating lifestyle, as close as possible to the Mediterranean diet, in order to increase the intake of bioactive compounds and contribute to healthy aging. Considering the multifactorial nature of cognitive impairment in aging, especially in AD, it is evident that a multitarget-based approach is essential to address this complex condition (Bolognesi, 2013). Interestingly, this multitarget approach can be obtained through either pharmacological or nutritional strategies, however the combined use of both approaches in order to obtain a synergistic effect could be even more effective most probably as a preventive AD/cognitive aging strategy and perhaps also as a therapeutic approach.

AUTHOR CONTRIBUTIONS

EP-A contributed to literature search, manuscript writing, editing, revision and final approval. SP contributed to literature search and manuscript writing. FM contributed to literature search and manuscript writing. MV contributed to manuscript editing and revision. MLB contributed to manuscript editing and revision. BM contributed to manuscript editing, revision and figure preparation.

FUNDING

All authors are supported by the University of Bologna as well as a research grant from Fondazione Umberto Veronesi to EP-A.

ACKNOWLEDGMENTS

We thank Prof. Antonio Contestabile for thoroughly reading the manuscript.

REFERENCES

Allfrey, V. G., Faulkner, R., and Mirsky, A. E. (1964). Acetylation and methylation of histones and their possible role in the regulation of RNA synthesis. *Proc. Natl. Acad. Sci. U S A* 51, 786–794. doi: 10.1073/pnas.51.5.786

An, Y. W., Jhang, K. A., Woo, S. Y., Kang, J. L., and Chong, Y. H. (2016). Sulforaphane exerts its anti-inflammatory effect against amyloid-β peptide via STAT-1 dephosphorylation and activation of Nrf2/HO-1 cascade in human THP-1 macrophages. *Neurobiol. Aging* 38, 1–10. doi: 10.1016/j.neurobiolaging.2015.10.016

Asadi, F., Jamshidi, A. H., Khodagholi, F., Yans, A., Azimi, L., Faizi, M., et al. (2015). Reversal effects of crocin on amyloid β-induced memory deficit: modification of autophagy or apoptosis markers. *Pharmacol. Biochem. Behav.* 139, 47–58. doi: 10.1016/j.pbb.2015.10.011

Atkinson, C., Frankenfeld, C. L., and Lampe, J. W. (2005). Gut bacterial metabolism of the soy isoflavone daidzein: exploring the relevance to human health. *Exp. Biol. Med.* 230, 155–170. doi: 10.1177/153537020523000302

Avital, A., Goshen, I., Kamsler, A., Segal, M., Iverfeldt, K., Richter-Levin, G., et al. (2003). Impaired interleukin-1 signaling is associated with deficits in hippocampal memory processes and neural plasticity. *Hippocampus* 13, 826–834. doi: 10.1002/hipo.10135

Balschun, D., Wetzel, W., Del Rey, A., Pitossi, F., Schneider, H., Zuschratter, W., et al. (2004). Interleukin-6: a cytokine to forget. *FASEB J.* 18, 1788–1790. doi: 10.1096/fj.04-1625fje

Batista-de-Oliveira, M., Lopes, A. A., Mendes-da-Silva, R. F., and Guedes, R. C. (2012). Aging-dependent brain electrophysiological effects in rats after distinct lactation conditions, and treadmill exercise: a spreading depression analysis. *Exp. Gerontol.* 47, 452–457. doi: 10.1016/j.exger.2012.03.016

Beejmohun, V., Fliniaux, O., Grand, E., Lamblin, F., Bensaddek, L., Christen, P., et al. (2007). Microwave-assisted extraction of the main phenolic compounds in flaxseed. *Phytochem. Anal.* 18, 275–282. doi: 10.1002/pca.973

Bolognesi, M. L. (2013). Polypharmacology in a single drug: multitarget drugs. *Curr. Med. Chem.* 20, 1639–1645. doi: 10.2174/0929867311320130004

Bonet-Costa, V., Herranz-Pérez, V., Blanco-Gandía, M., Mas-Bargues, C., Inglés, M., Garcia-Tarraga, P., et al. (2016). Clearing amyloid-β through PPARγ/ApoE activation by genistein is a treatment of experimental Alzheimer's disease. *J. Alzheimers Dis.* 51, 701–711. doi: 10.3233/JAD-151020

Braak, H., and Del Tredici, K. (2011). The pathological process underlying Alzheimer's disease in individuals under thirty. *Acta Neuropathol.* 121, 171–181. doi: 10.1007/s00401-010-0789-4

Brandenburg, L. O., Kipp, M., Lucius, R., Pufe, T., and Wruck, C. J. (2010). Sulforaphane suppresses LPS-induced inflammation in primary rat microglia. *Inflamm. Res.* 59, 443–450. doi: 10.1007/s00011-009-0116-5

Burg, V. K., Grimm, H. S., Rothhaar, T. L., Grösgen, S., Hundsdörfer, B., Haupenthal, V. J., et al. (2013). Plant sterols the better cholesterol in Alzheimer's disease? A mechanistical study. *J. Neurosci.* 33, 16072–16087. doi: 10.1523/JNEUROSCI.1506-13.2013

Cheng-Chung Wei, J., Huang, H. C., Chen, W. J., Huang, C. N., Peng, C. H., and Lin, C. L. (2016). Epigallocatechin gallate attenuates amyloid β-induced inflammation and neurotoxicity in EOC 13.31 microglia. *Eur. J. Pharmacol.* 770, 16–24. doi: 10.1016/j.ejphar.2015.11.048

Chhor, V., Le Charpentier, T., Lebon, S., Oré, M. V., Celador, I. L., Josserand, J., et al. (2013). Characterization of phenotype markers and neuronotoxic potential of polarised primary microglia *in vitro*. *Brain Behav. Immun.* 32, 70–85. doi: 10.1016/j.bbi.2013.02.005

Choi, J. Y., Kim, J. Y., Kim, J. Y., Park, J., Lee, W. T., and Lee, J. E. (2017). M2 phenotype microglia-derived cytokine stimulates proliferation and neuronal differentiation of endogenous stem cells in ischemic brain. *Exp. Neurobiol.* 26, 33–41. doi: 10.5607/en.2017.26.1.33

Corder, E. H., Saunders, A. M., Strittmatter, W. J., Schmechel, D. E., Gaskell, P. C., Small, G. W., et al. (1993). Gene dose of apolipoprotein E type 4 allele and the risk of Alzheimer's disease in late onset families. *Science* 261, 921–923. doi: 10.1126/science.8346443

Corton, J. M., Gillespie, J. G., and Hardie, D. G. (1994). Role of the AMP-activated protein kinase in the cellular stress response. *Curr. Biol.* 4, 315–324. doi: 10.1016/s0960-9822(00)00070-1

Csuka, E., Hans, V. H., Ammann, E., Trentz, O., Kossmann, T., and Morganti-Kossmann, M. C. (2000). Cell activation and inflammatory response following traumatic axonal injury in the rat. *Neuroreport* 11, 2587–2590. doi: 10.1097/00001756-200008030-00047

Cui, H., Meng, Y., and Bulleit, R. F. (1998). Inhibition of glycogen synthase kinase 3β activity regulates proliferation of cultured cerebellar granule cells. *Brain Res. Dev. Brain Res.* 111, 177–188. doi: 10.1016/s0165-3806(98)00136-9

Deane, R., Singh, I., Sagare, A. P., Bell, R. D., Ross, N. T., LaRue, B., et al. (2012). A multimodal RAGE-specific inhibitor reduces amyloid β-mediated brain disorder in a mouse model of Alzheimer disease. *J. Clin. Invest.* 122, 1377–1392. doi: 10.1172/JCI58642

del Ser, T., Steinwachs, K. C., Gertz, H. J., Andrés, M. V., Gómez-Carrillo, B., Medina, M., et al. (2013). Treatment of Alzheimer's disease with the GSK-3 inhibitor tideglusib: a pilot study. *J. Alzheimers Dis.* 33, 205–215. doi: 10.3233/JAD-2012-120805

Domise, M., Didier, S., Marinangeli, C., Zhao, H., Chandakkar, P., Buée, L., et al. (2016). AMP-activated protein kinase modulates tau phosphorylation and tau pathology *in vivo*. *Sci. Rep.* 6:26758. doi: 10.1038/srep26758

Dreyer, C., Keller, H., Mahfoudi, A., Laudet, V., Krey, G., and Wahli, W. (1993). Positive regulation of the peroxisomal β-oxidation pathway by fatty acids through activation of peroxisome proliferator-activated receptors (PPAR). *Biol. Cell* 77, 67–74. doi: 10.1016/s0248-4900(05)80176-5

Du, L. L., Chai, D. M., Zhao, L. N., Li, X. H., Zhang, F. C., Zhang, H. B., et al. (2015). AMPK activation ameliorates Alzheimer's disease-like pathology and spatial memory impairment in a streptozotocin-induced Alzheimer's disease model in rats. *J. Alzheimers Dis.* 43, 775–784. doi: 10.3233/JAD-140564

Duan, H., Wearne, S. L., Rocher, A. B., Macedo, A., Morrison, J. H., and Hof, P. R. (2003). Age-related dendritic and spine changes in corticocortically projecting neurons in macaque monkeys. *Cereb. Cortex* 13, 950–961. doi: 10.1093/cercor/13.9.950

Earnest, M. P., Heaton, R. K., Wilkinson, W. E., and Manke, W. F. (1979). Cortical atrophy, ventricular enlargement and intellectual impairment in the aged. *Neurology* 29, 1138–1143. doi: 10.1212/wnl.29.8.1138

Eketjäll, S., Janson, J., Jeppsson, F., Svanhagen, A., Kolmodin, K., Gustavsson, S., et al. (2013). AZ-4217: a high potency BACE inhibitor displaying acute central efficacy in different *in vivo* models and reduced amyloid deposition in Tg2576 mice. *J. Neurosci.* 33, 10075–10084. doi: 10.1523/jneurosci.1165-13.2013

Fan, Z., Brooks, D. J., Okello, A., and Edison, P. (2017). An early and late peak in microglial activation in Alzheimer's disease trajectory. *Brain* 140, 792–803. doi: 10.1093/brain/aww349

Fava, A., Colica, C., Plastino, M., Messina, D., Cristiano, D., Opipari, C., et al. (2017). Cognitive impairment is correlated with insulin resistance degree: the "PA-NICO-study". *Metab. Brain Dis.* 32, 799–810. doi: 10.1007/s11011-017-9977-4

Ferrer, I., Barrachina, M., and Puig, B. (2002). Glycogen synthase kinase-3 is associated with neuronal and glial hyperphosphorylated tau deposits in Alzheimer's disease, Pick's disease, progressive supranuclear palsy and corticobasal degeneration. *Acta Neuropathol.* 104, 583–591. doi: 10.1007/s00401-002-0587-8

Giacoppo, S., Rajan, T. S., De Nicola, G. R., Iori, R., Rollin, P., Bramanti, P., et al. (2017). The isothiocyanate isolated from moringa oleifera shows potent anti-inflammatory activity in the treatment of murine subacute Parkinson's disease. *Rejuvenation Res.* 20, 50–63. doi: 10.1089/rej.2016.1828

Giri, S., Nath, N., Smith, B., Viollet, B., Singh, A. K., and Singh, I. (2004). 5-aminoimidazole-4-carboxamide-1-β-4-ribofuranoside inhibits proinflammatory response in glial cells: a possible role of AMP-activated protein kinase. *J. Neurosci.* 24, 479–487. doi: 10.1523/jneurosci.4288-03.2004

Gleason, C. E., Fischer, B. L., Dowling, N. M., Setchell, K. D., Atwood, C. S., Carlsson, C. M., et al. (2015). Cognitive effects of soy isoflavones in patients with Alzheimer's disease. *J. Alzheimers Dis.* 47, 1009–1019. doi: 10.3233/jad-142958

Glisky, E. L. (2007). "Changes in cognitive function in human aging," in *Brain Aging: Models, Methods, and Mechanisms*, ed. D. R. Riddle (Boca Raton, FL: CRC Press/Taylor and Francis), Chapter 1, 3–20.

Golan, H., Levav, T., Mendelsohn, A., and Huleihel, M. (2004). Involvement of tumor necrosis factor alpha in hippocampal development and function. *Cereb. Cortex* 14, 97–105.

Green, H. F., and Nolan, Y. M. (2012). GSK-3 mediates the release of IL-1β, TNF-α and IL-10 from cortical glia. *Neurochem. Int.* 61, 666–671. doi: 10.1016/j.neuint.2012.07.003

Guerreiro, R., Wojtas, A., Bras, J., Carrasquillo, M., Rogaeva, E., Majounie, E., et al. (2013). TREM2 variants in Alzheimer's disease. *N. Engl. J. Med.* 368, 117–127. doi: 10.1056/NEJMoa1211851

Guo, H., Cheng, Y., Wang, C., Wu, J., Zou, Z., Niu, B., et al. (2017). FFPM, a PDE4 inhibitor, reverses learning and memory deficits in APP/PS1 transgenic mice via cAMP/PKA/CREB signaling and anti-inflammatory effects. *Neuropharmacology* 116, 260–269. doi: 10.1016/j.neuropharm.2017.01.004

Guo, X. D., Sun, G. L., Zhou, T. T., Xu, X., Zhu, Z. Y., Rukachaisirikul, V., et al. (2016). Small molecule LX2343 ameliorates cognitive deficits in AD model mice by targeting both amyloid β production and clearance. *Acta Pharmacol. Sin.* 37, 1281–1297. doi: 10.1038/aps.2016.80

Hailer, N. P., Jarhult, J. D., and Nitsch, R. (1996). Resting microglial cells *in vitro*: analysis of morphology and adhesion molecule expression in organotypic hippocampal slice cultures. *Glia* 18, 319–331. doi: 10.1002/(SICI)1098-1136(199612)18:4<319::AID-GLIA6>3.0.CO;2-S

Hamelin, L., Lagarde, J., Dorothée, G., Leroy, C., Labit, M., Comley, R. A., et al. (2016). Early and protective microglial activation in Alzheimer's disease: a prospective study using 18F-DPA-714 PET imaging. *Brain* 139, 1252–1264. doi: 10.1093/brain/aww017

Heringa, S. M., van den Berg, E., Reijmer, Y. D., Nijpels, G., Stehouwer, C. D., Schalkwijk, C. G., et al. (2014). Markers of low-grade inflammation and endothelial dysfunction are related to reduced information processing speed and executive functioning in an older population—the Hoorn Study. *Psychoneuroendocrinology* 40, 108–118. doi: 10.1016/j.psyneuen.2013.11.011

Hickman, S. E., and El Khoury, J. (2014). TREM2 and the neuroimmunology of Alzheimer's disease. *Biochem. Pharmacol.* 88, 495–498. doi: 10.1016/j.bcp.2013.11.021

Hidding, U., Mielke, K., Waetzig, V., Brecht, S., Hanisch, U., Behrens, A., et al. (2002). The c-Jun N-terminal kinases in cerebral microglia: immunological functions in the brain. *Biochem. Pharmacol.* 64, 781–788. doi: 10.1016/s0006-2952(02)01139-5

Hof, P. R., Duan, H., Page, T. L., Einstein, M., Wicinski, B., He, Y., et al. (2002). Age-related changes in GluR2 and NMDAR1 glutamate receptor subunit protein immunoreactivity in corticocortically projecting neurons in macaque and patas monkeys. *Brain Res.* 928, 175–186. doi: 10.1016/s0006-8993(01)03345-5

Jacobs, B., Driscoll, L., and Schall, M. (1997). Life-span dendritic and spine changes in areas 10 and 18 of human cortex: a quantitative Golgi study. *J. Comp. Neurol.* 386, 661–680. doi: 10.1002/(SICI)1096-9861(19971006)386:4<661::AID-CNE11>3.0.CO;2-N

Jacobsen, H., Ozmen, L., Caruso, A., Narquizian, R., Hilpert, H., Jacobsen, B., et al. (2014). Combined treatment with a BACE inhibitor and anti-Aβ antibody gantenerumab enhances amyloid reduction in APPLondon mice. *J. Neurosci.* 34, 11621–11630. doi: 10.1523/jneurosci.1405-14.2014

Jeong, J. W., Lee, H. H., Han, M. H., Kim, G. Y., Kim, W. J., and Choi, Y. H. (2014). Anti-inflammatory effects of genistein via suppression of the toll-like receptor 4-mediated signaling pathway in lipopolysaccharide-stimulated BV2 microglia. *Chem. Biol. Interact.* 212, 30–39. doi: 10.1016/j.cbi.2014.01.012

Jeong, G. S., Li, B., Lee, D. S., Kim, K. H., Lee, I. K., Lee, K. R., et al. (2010). Cytoprotective and anti-inflammatory effects of spinasterol via the induction of heme oxygenase-1 in murine hippocampal and microglial cell lines. *Int. Immunopharmacol.* 10, 1587–1594. doi: 10.1016/j.intimp.2010.09.013

Jeřábek, J., Uliassi, E., Guidotti, L., Korábecný, J., Soukup, O., Sepsova, V., et al. (2017). Tacrine-resveratrol fused hybrids as multi-target-directed ligands against Alzheimer's disease. *Eur. J. Med. Chem.* 127, 250–262. doi: 10.1016/j.ejmech.2016.12.048

Ji, H., Wang, H., Zhang, F., Li, X., Xiang, L., and Aiguo, S. (2010). PPARγ agonist pioglitazone inhibits microglia inflammation by blocking p38 mitogen-activated protein kinase signaling pathways. *Inflamm. Res.* 59, 921–929. doi: 10.1007/s00011-010-0203-7

Jonsson, T., Stefansson, H., Steinberg, S., Jonsdottir, I., Jonsson, P. V., Snaedal, J., et al. (2013). Variant of TREM2 associated with the risk of Alzheimer's disease. *N. Engl. J. Med.* 368, 107–116. doi: 10.1056/NEJMoa1211103

Jung, H. A., Ali, M. Y., Choi, R. J., Jeong, H. O., Chung, H. Y., and Choi, J. S. (2016). Kinetics and molecular docking studies of fucosterol and fucoxanthin, BACE1 inhibitors from brown algae Undaria pinnatifida and Ecklonia stolonifera. *Food Chem. Toxicol.* 89, 104–111. doi: 10.1016/j.fct.2016.01.014

Jung, H. A., Jin, S. E., Ahn, B. R., Lee, C. M., and Choi, J. S. (2013). Anti-inflammatory activity of edible brown alga Eisenia bicyclis and its constituents fucosterol and phlorotannins in LPS-stimulated RAW264.7 macrophages. *Food Chem. Toxicol.* 59, 199–206. doi: 10.1016/j.fct.2013.05.061

Kamiloglu, S., Demirci, M., Selen, S., Toydemir, G., Boyacioglu, D., and Capanoglu, E. (2014). Home processing of tomatoes (Solanum lycopersicum): effects on *in vitro* bioaccessibility of total lycopene, phenolics, flavonoids, and antioxidant capacity. *J. Sci. Food Agric.* 94, 2225–2233. doi: 10.1002/jsfa.6546

Karlinsky, H., Vaula, G., Haines, J. L., Ridgley, J., Bergeron, C., Mortilla, M., et al. (1992). Molecular and prospective phenotypic characterization of a pedigree with familial Alzheimer's disease and a missense mutation in codon 717 of the β-amyloid precursor protein gene. *Neurology* 42, 1445–1453. doi: 10.1212/WNL.42.8.1445

Kim, H. S., Cho, J. Y., Kim, D. H., Yan, J. J., Lee, H. K., Suh, H. W., et al. (2004). Inhibitory effects of long-term administration of ferulic acid on microglial activation induced by intracerebroventricular injection of β-amyloid peptide (1–42) in mice. *Biol. Pharm. Bull.* 27, 120–121. doi: 10.1248/bpb.27.120

Kim, J. H., Wang, Q., Choi, J. M., Lee, S., and Cho, E. J. (2015). Protective role of caffeic acid in an Aβ25–35-induced Alzheimer's disease model. *Nutr. Res. Pract.* 9, 480–488. doi: 10.4162/nrp.2015.9.5.480

Kleinberger, G., Yamanishi, Y., Suárez-Calvet, M., Czirr, E., Lohmann, E., Cuyvers, E., et al. (2014). TREM2 mutations implicated in neurodegeneration impair cell surface transport and phagocytosis. *Sci. Transl Med.* 6:243ra86. doi: 10.1126/scitranslmed.3009093

Knoops, K. T., de Groot, L. C., Kromhout, D., Perrin, A. E., Moreiras-Varela, O., Menotti, A., et al. (2004). Mediterranean diet, lifestyle factors, and 10-year mortality in elderly European men and women: the HALE project. *JAMA* 292, 1433–1439. doi: 10.1097/01.ieb.0000150381.96671.6b

Koriyama, Y., Sugitani, K., Ogai, K., and Kato, S. (2014). Neuritogenic activity of trichostatin A in adult rat retinal ganglion cells through acetylation of histone H3 lysine 9 and RARβ induction. *J. Pharmacol. Sci.* 124, 112–116. doi: 10.1254/jphs.13171sc

Laeng, P., Pitts, R. L., Lemire, A. L., Drabik, C. E., Weiner, A., Tang, H., et al. (2004). The mood stabilizer valproic acid stimulates GABA neurogenesis from rat forebrain stem cells. *J. Neurochem.* 91, 238–251. doi: 10.1111/j.1471-4159.2004.02725.x

Landfield, P. W., McGaugh, J. L., and Lynch, G. (1978). Impaired synaptic potentiation processes in the hippocampus of aged, memory-deficient rats. *Brain Res.* 150, 85–101. doi: 10.1016/0006-8993(78)90655-8

Lang, L., Dong, N., Wu, D., Yao, X., Lu, W., Zhang, C., et al. (2016). 2-Arylbenzo[*b*]furan derivatives as potent human lipoxygenase inhibitors. *J. Enzyme Inhib. Med. Chem.* 31, 98–105. doi: 10.1080/14756366.2016.1220376

Lantos, P. L., Luthert, P. J., Hanger, D., Anderton, B. H., Mullan, M., and Rossor, M. (1992). Familial Alzheimer's disease with the amyloid precursor protein position 717 mutation and sporadic Alzheimer's disease have the same cytoskeletal pathology. *Neurosci. Lett.* 137, 221–224. doi: 10.1016/0304-3940(92)90408-y

Lawson, L. J., Perry, V. H., Dri, P., and Gordon, S. (1990). Heterogeneity in the distribution and morphology of microglia in the normal adult mouse brain. *Neuroscience* 39, 151–170. doi: 10.1016/0306-4522(90)90229-w

Lee, H. R., Shin, H. K., Park, S. Y., Kim, H. Y., Lee, W. S., Rhim, B. Y., et al. (2014). Cilostazol suppresses β-amyloid production by activating a disintegrin and metalloproteinase 10 via the upregulation of SIRT1-coupled retinoic acid receptor-β. *J. Neurosci. Res.* 92, 1581–1590. doi: 10.1002/jnr.23421

Levy-Lahad, E., Wijsman, E. M., Nemens, E., Anderson, L., Goddard, K. A., Weber, J. L., et al. (1995). A familial Alzheimer's disease locus on chromosome 1. *Science* 269, 970–973. doi: 10.1126/science.7638621

Licht-Murava, A., Paz, R., Vaks, L., Avrahami, L., Plotkin, B., Eisenstein, M., et al. (2016). A unique type of GSK-3 inhibitor brings new opportunities to the clinic. *Sci. Signal.* 9:ra110. doi: 10.1126/scisignal.aah7102

Lima, C. B., Soares Gde, S., Vitor, S. M., Andrade-da-Costa, B. L., Castellano, B., and Guedes, R. C. (2014). Spreading depression features and Iba1 immunoreactivity in the cerebral cortex of developing rats submitted to treadmill exercise after treatment with monosodium glutamate. *Int. J. Dev. Neurosci.* 33, 98–105. doi: 10.1016/j.ijdevneu.2013.12.008

Lin, H. Y., Huang, B. R., Yeh, W. L., Lee, C. H., Huang, S. S., Lai, C. H., et al. (2014). Antineuroinflammatory effects of lycopene via activation of adenosine monophosphate-activated protein kinase-α1/heme oxygenase-1 pathways. *Neurobiol. Aging* 35, 191–202. doi: 10.1016/j.neurobiolaging.2013.06.020

Liu, Z. J., Li, Z. H., Liu, L., Tang, W. X., Wang, Y., Dong, M. R., et al. (2016). Curcumin attenuates β-amyloid-induced neuroinflammation via activation of peroxisome proliferator-activated receptor-γ function in a rat model of Alzheimer's disease. *Front. Pharmacol.* 7:261. doi: 10.3389/fphar.2016.00261

Lovestone, S., Boada, M., Dubois, B., Hüll, M., Rinne, J. O., Huppertz, H. J., et al. (2015). A phase II trial of tideglusib in Alzheimer's disease. *J. Alzheimers Dis.* 45, 75–88. doi: 10.3233/JAD-141959

Lozano, J., Matatagui, D., Santos, J. P., and Horrillo, C. (2016). "Electronic sensory systems for characterization of bioactive compounds," in *Frontiers in Bioactive Compounds* (Vol. 1), ed. C. Apetrei (Sharjah: Bentham Science Publishers), 190–217.

Luccarini, I., Ed Dami, T., Grossi, C., Rigacci, S., Stefani, M., and Casamenti, F. (2014). Oleuropein aglycone counteracts Aβ42 toxicity in the rat brain. *Neurosci. Lett.* 558, 67–72. doi: 10.1016/j.neulet.2013.10.062

Luebke, J. I., Chang, Y. M., Moore, T. L., and Rosene, D. L. (2004). Normal aging results in decreased synaptic excitation and increased synaptic inhibition of layer 2/3 pyramidal cells in the monkey prefrontal cortex. *Neuroscience* 125, 277–288. doi: 10.1016/j.neuroscience.2004.01.035

Luna-Medina, R., Cortes-Canteli, M., Sanchez-Galiano, S., Morales-Garcia, J. A., Martinez, A., Santos, A., et al. (2007). NP031112, a thiadiazolidinone compound, prevents inflammation and neurodegeneration under excitotoxic conditions: potential therapeutic role in brain disorders. *J. Neurosci.* 27, 5766–5776. doi: 10.1523/JNEUROSCI.1004-07.2007

Ma, T., Chen, Y., Vingtdeux, V., Zhao, H., Viollet, B., Marambaud, P., et al. (2014). Inhibition of AMP-activated protein kinase signaling alleviates impairments in hippocampal synaptic plasticity induced by amyloid β. *J. Neurosci.* 34, 12230–12238. doi: 10.1523/JNEUROSCI.1694-14.2014

Mashurabad, P. C., Palika, R., Jyrwa, Y. W., Bhaskarachary, K., and Pullakhandam, R. (2017). Dietary fat composition, food matrix and relative polarity modulate the micellarization and intestinal uptake of carotenoids from vegetables and fruits. *J. Food Sci. Technol.* 54, 333–341. doi: 10.1007/s13197-016-2466-7

Matthies, A., Blaut, M., and Braune, A. (2009). Isolation of a human intestinal bacterium capable of daidzein and genistein conversion. *Appl. Environ. Microbiol.* 75, 1740–1744. doi: 10.1128/AEM.01795-08

Mecha, M., Feliú, A., Carrillo-Salinas, F. J., Rueda-Zubiaurre, A., Ortega-Gutiérrez, S., de Sola, R. G., et al. (2015). Endocannabinoids drive the acquisition of an alternative phenotype in microglia. *Brain Behav. Immun.* 49, 233–245. doi: 10.1016/j.bbi.2015.06.002

Meireles, M., Marques, C., Norberto, S., Santos, P., Fernandes, I., Mateus, N., et al. (2016). Anthocyanin effects on microglia M1/M2 phenotype: consequence on neuronal fractalkine expression. *Behav. Brain Res.* 305, 223–228. doi: 10.1016/j.bbr.2016.03.010

Menotti, A., Kromhout, D., Nissinen, A., Giampaoli, S., Seccareccia, F., Feskens, E., et al. (1996). Short-term all-cause mortality and its determinants in elderly male populations in Finland, The Netherlands, and Italy: the FINE Study. Finland, Italy, Netherlands Elderly Study. *Prev Med.* 25, 319–326. doi: 10.1006/pmed.1996.0062

Michelucci, A., Heurtaux, T., Grandbarbe, L., Morga, E., and Heuschling, P. (2009). Characterization of the microglial phenotype under specific pro-inflammatory and anti-inflammatory conditions: effects of oligomeric and fibrillar amyloid-β. *J. Neuroimmunol.* 210, 3–12. doi: 10.1016/j.jneuroim.2009.02.003

Min, J. Y., and Min, K. B. (2014). Serum lycopene, lutein and zeaxanthin, and the risk of Alzheimer's disease mortality in older adults. *Dement. Geriatr Cogn. Disord.* 37, 246–256. doi: 10.1159/000356486

Moran, N. E., Cichon, M. J., Riedl, K. M., Grainger, E. M., Schwartz, S. J., Novotny, J. A., et al. (2015). Compartmental and noncompartmental modeling of ^{13}C-lycopene absorption, isomerization, and distribution kinetics in healthy adults. *Am. J. Clin. Nutr.* 102, 1436–1449. doi: 10.3945/ajcn.114.103143

Mori, T., Koyama, N., Guillot-Sestier, M. V., Tan, J., and Town, T. (2013). Ferulic acid is a nutraceutical β-secretase modulator that improves behavioral impairment and alzheimer-like pathology in transgenic mice. *PLoS One.* 8:e55774. doi: 10.1371/journal.pone.0055774

Nam, K. N., Park, Y. M., Jung, H. J., Lee, J. Y., Min, B. D., Park, S. U., et al. (2010). Anti-inflammatory effects of crocin and crocetin in rat brain microglial cells. *Eur. J. Pharmacol.* 648, 110–116. doi: 10.1016/j.ejphar.2010.09.003

Neniskyte, U., Neher, J. J., and Brown, G. C. (2011). Neuronal death induced by nanomolar amyloid β is mediated by primary phagocytosis of neurons by microglia. *J. Biol. Chem.* 286, 39904–39913. doi: 10.1074/jbc.M111.267583

Nesteruk, M., Nesteruk, T., Styczyńska, M., Mandecka, M., Barczak, A., and Barcikowska, M. (2016). Combined use of biochemical and volumetric biomarkers to assess the risk of conversion of mild cognitive impairment to Alzheimer's disease. *Folia Neuropathol.* 54, 369–374. doi: 10.5114/fn.2016.64815

Neumann, U., Rueeger, H., Machauer, R., Veenstra, S. J., Lueoend, R. M., Tintelnot-Blomley, M., et al. (2015). A novel BACE inhibitor NB-360 shows a superior pharmacological profile and robust reduction of amyloid-β and neuroinflammation in APP transgenic mice. *Mol. Neurodegener.* 10:44. doi: 10.1186/s13024-015-0033-8

Noh, M. Y., Chun, K., Kang, B. Y., Kim, H., Park, J. S., Lee, H. C., et al. (2013). Newly developed glycogen synthase kinase-3 (GSK-3) inhibitors protect neuronal cells death in amyloid-β induced cell model and in a transgenic mouse model of Alzheimer's disease. *Biochem. Biophys. Res. Commun.* 435, 274–281. doi: 10.1016/j.bbrc.2013.04.065

Pangestuti, R., Vo, T. S., Ngo, D. H., and Kim, S. K. (2013). Fucoxanthin ameliorates inflammation and oxidative reponses in microglia. *J. Agric. Food Chem.* 61, 3876–3883. doi: 10.1021/jf400015k

Pantano, D., Luccarini, I., Nardiello, P., Servili, M., Stefani, M., and Casamenti, F. (2017). Oleuropein aglycone and polyphenols from olive mill waste water ameliorate cognitive deficits and neuropathology. *Br. J. Clin. Pharmacol.* 83, 54–62. doi: 10.1111/bcp.12993

Parish, C. L., Finkelstein, D. I., Tripanichkul, W., Satoskar, A. R., Drago, J., and Horne, M. K. (2002). The role of interleukin-1, interleukin-6, and glia in inducing growth of neuronal terminal arbors in mice. *J. Neurosci.* 22, 8034–8041.

Park, C., Lee, S., Cho, I. H., Lee, H. K., Kim, D., Choi, S. Y., et al. (2006). TLR3-mediated signal induces proinflammatory cytokine and chemokine gene expression in astrocytes: differential signaling mechanisms of TLR3-induced IP-10 and IL-8 gene expression. *Glia* 53, 248–256. doi: 10.1002/glia.20278

Park, S. Y., Jin, M. L., Wang, Z., Park, G., and Choi, Y. W. (2016). 2,3,4',5-tetrahydroxystilbene-2-O-β-d-glucoside exerts anti-inflammatory effects on lipopolysaccharide-stimulated microglia by inhibiting NF-κB and activating AMPK/Nrf2 pathways. *Food Chem. Toxicol.* 97, 159–167. doi: 10.1016/j.fct.2016.09.010

Pérez-Cañamás, A., Sarroca, S., Melero-Jerez, C., Porquet, D., Sansa, J., Knafo, S., et al. (2016). A diet enriched with plant sterols prevents the memory impairment induced by cholesterol loss in senescence-accelerated mice. *Neurobiol. Aging* 48, 1–12. doi: 10.1016/j.neurobiolaging.2016.08.009

Perez-Gonzalez, R., Pascual, C., Antequera, D., Bolos, M., Redondo, M., Perez, D. I., et al. (2013). Phosphodiesterase 7 inhibitor reduced cognitive impairment and pathological hallmarks in a mouse model of Alzheimer's disease. *Neurobiol. Aging* 34, 2133–2145. doi: 10.1016/j.neurobiolaging.2013.03.011

Pohland, M., Hagl, S., Pellowska, M., Wurglics, M., Schubert-Zsilavecz, M., and Eckert, G. P. (2016). MH84: a novel γ-secretase modulator/PPARγ agonist—improves mitochondrial dysfunction in a cellular model of Alzheimer's disease. *Neurochem. Res.* 41, 231–242. doi: 10.1007/s11064-015-1765-0

Polazzi, E., Altamira, L. E., Eleuteri, S., Barbaro, R., Casadio, C., Contestabile, A., et al. (2009). Neuroprotection of microglial conditioned medium on 6-hydroxydopamine-induced neuronal death: role of transforming growth factor β-2. *J. Neurochem.* 110, 545–556. doi: 10.1111/j.1471-4159.2009.06117.x

Polazzi, E., Gianni, T., and Contestabile, A. (2001). Microglial cells protect cerebellar granule neurons from apoptosis: evidence for reciprocal signaling. *Glia* 36, 271–280. doi: 10.1002/glia.1115

Polazzi, E., Mengoni, I., Caprini, M., Peña-Altamira, E., Kurtys, E., and Monti, B. (2013). Copper-zinc superoxide dismutase (SOD1) is released by microglial cells and confers neuroprotection against 6-OHDA neurotoxicity. *Neurosignals* 21, 112–128. doi: 10.1159/000337115

Polazzi, E., and Monti, B. (2010). Microglia and neuroprotection: from *in vitro* studies to therapeutic applications. *Prog. Neurobiol.* 92, 293–315. doi: 10.1016/j.pneurobio.2010.06.009

Porquet, D., Casadesús, G., Bayod, S., Vicente, A., Canudas, A. M., Vilaplana, J., et al. (2013). Dietary resveratrol prevents Alzheimer's markers and increases life span in SAMP8. *Age* 35, 1851–1865. doi: 10.1007/s11357-012-9489-4

Prati, F., De Simone, A., Bisignano, P., Armirotti, A., Summa, M., Pizzirani, D., et al. (2015). Multitarget drug discovery for Alzheimer's disease: triazinones as BACE-1 and GSK-3β inhibitors. *Angew. Chem. Int. Ed Engl.* 54, 1578–1582. doi: 10.1002/anie.201410456

Qiao, A., Wang, Y., Zhang, W., and He, X. (2015). Neuroprotection of brain-targeted bioactive dietary artoindonesianin O (AIO) from mulberry on rat neurons as a novel intervention for Alzheimer's disease. *J. Agric. Food Chem.* 63, 3687–3693. doi: 10.1021/acs.jafc.5b00396

Ransohoff, R. M., and Perry, V. H. (2009). Microglial physiology: unique stimuli, specialized responses. *Annu. Rev. Immunol.* 27, 119–145. doi: 10.1146/annurev.immunol.021908.132528

Rasoolijazi, H., Azad, N., Joghataei, M. T., Kerdari, M., Nikbakht, F., and Soleimani, M. (2013). The protective role of carnosic acid against β-amyloid toxicity in rats. *ScientificWorldJournal* 2013:917082. doi: 10.1155/2013/917082

Reisberg, B., Ferris, S. H., de Leon, M. J., and Crook, T. (1982). The Global Deterioration Scale for assessment of primary degenerative dementia. *Am. J. Psychiatry* 139, 1136–1139. doi: 10.1176/ajp.139.9.1136

Ricobaraza, A., Cuadrado-Tejedor, M., and Garcia-Osta, A. (2011). Long-term phenylbutyrate administration prevents memory deficits in Tg2576 mice by decreasing Aβ. *Front. Biosci.* 3, 1375–1384. doi: 10.2741/340

Rojanathammanee, L., Puig, K. L., and Combs, C. K. (2013). Pomegranate polyphenols and extract inhibit nuclear factor of activated T-cell activity and microglial activation *in vitro* and in a transgenic mouse model of Alzheimer disease. *J. Nutr.* 143, 597–605. doi: 10.3945/jn.112.169516

Sachdeva, A. K., and Chopra, K. (2015). Lycopene abrogates Aβ(1–42)-mediated neuroinflammatory cascade in an experimental model of Alzheimer's disease. *J. Nutr. Biochem.* 26, 736–744. doi: 10.1016/j.jnutbio.2015.01.012

Schneider, H., Pitossi, F., Balschun, D., Wagner, A., del Rey, A., and Besedovsky, H. O. (1998). A neuromodulatory role of interleukin-1β in the hippocampus. *Proc. Natl. Acad. Sci. U S A* 95, 7778–7783. doi: 10.1073/pnas.95.13.7778

Sharma, S., and Taliyan, R. (2016). Epigenetic modifications by inhibiting histone deacetylases reverse memory impairment in insulin resistance induced cognitive deficit in mice. *Neuropharmacology* 105, 285–297. doi: 10.1016/j.neuropharm.2016.01.025

Sherrington, R., Rogaev, E. I., Liang, Y., Rogaeva, E. A., Levesque, G., Ikeda, M., et al. (1995). Cloning of a gene bearing missense mutations in early-onset familial Alzheimer's disease. *Nature* 375, 754–760. doi: 10.1038/375754a0

Shi, J. Q., Wang, B. R., Tian, Y. Y., Xu, J., Gao, L., Zhao, S. L., et al. (2013). Antiepileptics topiramate and levetiracetam alleviate behavioral deficits and reduce neuropathology in APPswe/PS1dE9 transgenic mice. *CNS Neurosci. Ther.* 19, 871–881. doi: 10.1111/cns.12144

Shi, X., Zheng, Z., Li, J., Xiao, Z., Qi, W., Zhang, A., et al. (2015). Curcumin inhibits Aβ-induced microglial inflammatory responses *in vitro*: involvement of ERK1/2 and p38 signaling pathways. *Neurosci. Lett.* 594, 105–110. doi: 10.1016/j.neulet.2015.03.045

Siebzehnrubl, F. A., Buslei, R., Eyupoglu, I. Y., Seufert, S., Hahnen, E., and Blumcke, I. (2007). Histone deacetylase inhibitors increase neuronal differentiation in adult forebrain precursor cells. *Exp. Brain Res.* 176, 672–678. doi: 10.1007/s00221-006-0831-x

Sierksma, A. S., van den Hove, D. L., Pfau, F., Philippens, M., Bruno, O., Fedele, E., et al. (2014). Improvement of spatial memory function in APPswe/PS1dE9 mice after chronic inhibition of phosphodiesterase type 4D. *Neuropharmacology* 77, 120–130. doi: 10.1016/j.neuropharm.2013.09.015

Soiampornkul, R., Tong, L., Thangnipon, W., Balazs, R., and Cotman, C. W. (2008). Interleukin-1β interferes with signal transduction induced by neurotrophin-3 in cortical neurons. *Brain Res.* 1188, 189–197. doi: 10.1016/j.brainres.2007.10.051

Song, G. J., Nam, Y., Jo, M., Jung, M., Koo, J. Y., Cho, W., et al. (2016). A novel small-molecule agonist of PPAR-γ potentiates an anti-inflammatory M2 glial phenotype. *Neuropharmacology* 109, 159–169. doi: 10.1016/j.neuropharm.2016.06.009

Sperber, B. R., Leight, S., Goedert, M., and Lee, V. M. (1995). Glycogen synthase kinase-3 β phosphorylates tau protein at multiple sites in intact cells. *Neurosci. Lett.* 197, 149–153. doi: 10.1016/0304-3940(95)11902-9

Stence, N., Waite, M., and Dailey, M. E. (2001). Dynamics of microglial activation: a confocal time-lapse analysis in hippocampal slices. *Glia* 33, 256–266. doi: 10.1002/1098-1136(200103)33:3<256::aid-glia1024>3.0.co;2-j

Streit, W. J. (2002). Microglia as neuroprotective, immunocompetent cells of the CNS. *Glia* 40, 133–139. doi: 10.1002/glia.10154

Szabo, M., and Gulya, K. (2013). Development of the microglial phenotype in culture. *Neuroscience* 241, 280–295. doi: 10.1016/j.neuroscience.2013.03.033

Tai, S. Y., Chen, C. H., Chien, C. Y., and Yang, Y. H. (2017). Cilostazol as an add-on therapy for patients with Alzheimer's disease in Taiwan: a case control study. *BMC Neurol.* 17:40. doi: 10.1186/s12883-017-0800-y

Tarasoff-Conway, J. M., Carare, R. O., Osorio, R. S., Glodzik, L., Butler, T., Fieremans, E., et al. (2015). Clearance systems in the brain-implications for Alzheimer disease. *Nat. Rev. Neurol.* 11, 457–470. doi: 10.1038/nrneurol.2015.119

Tiribuzi, R., Crispoltoni, L., Chiurchiù, V., Casella, A., Montecchiani, C., Del Pino, A. M., et al. (2017). Trans-crocetin improves amyloid-β degradation in monocytes from Alzheimer's disease patients. *J. Neurol. Sci.* 372, 408–412. doi: 10.1016/j.jns.2016.11.004

Tong, M., Dominguez, C., Didsbury, J., and de la Monte, S. M. (2016). Targeting Alzheimer's disease neuro-metabolic dysfunction with a small molecule nuclear receptor agonist (T3D-959) reverses disease pathologies. *J. Alzheimers Dis. Parkinsonism* 6:238. doi: 10.4172/2161-0460.1000238

Tsai, C. F., Kuo, Y. H., Yeh, W. L., Wu, C. Y., Lin, H. Y., Lai, S. W., et al. (2015). Regulatory effects of caffeic acid phenethyl ester on neuroinflammation in microglial cells. *Int. J. Mol. Sci.* 16, 5572–5589. doi: 10.3390/ijms16035572

Turner, R. S., Thomas, R. G., Craft, S., van Dyck, C. H., Mintzer, J., Reynolds, B. A., et al. (2015). A randomized, double-blind, placebo-controlled trial of resveratrol for Alzheimer disease. *Neurology* 85, 1383–1391. doi: 10.1212/WNL.0000000000002206

Tzeng, S. -F., and Wu, J. -P. (1999). Responses of microglia and neural progenitors to mechanical brain injury. *Neuroreport* 10, 2287–2292. doi: 10.1097/00001756-199908020-00012

Vassar, R., Bennett, B. D., Babu-Khan, S., Kahn, S., Mendiaz, E. A., Denis, P., et al. (1999). β-secretase cleavage of Alzheimer's amyloid precursor protein by the transmembrane aspartic protease BACE. *Science* 286, 735–741. doi: 10.1126/science.286.5440.735

Vingtdeux, V., Davies, P., Dickson, D. W., and Marambaud, P. (2011). AMPK is abnormally activated in tangle- and pre-tangle-bearing neurons in Alzheimer's disease and other tauopathies. *Acta Neuropathol.* 121, 337–349. doi: 10.1007/s00401-010-0759-x

Vukic, V., Callaghan, D., Walker, D., Lue, L. F., Liu, Q. Y., Couraud, P. O., et al. (2009). Expression of inflammatory genes induced by β-amyloid peptides in human brain endothelial cells and in Alzheimer's brain is mediated by the JNK-AP1 signaling pathway. *Neurobiol. Dis.* 34, 95–106. doi: 10.1016/j.nbd.2008.12.007

Waetzig, V., Czeloth, K., Hidding, U., Mielke, K., Kanzow, M., Brecht, S., et al. (2005). c-Jun N-terminal kinases (JNKs) mediate pro-inflammatory actions of microglia. *Glia* 50, 235–246. doi: 10.1002/glia.20173

Wang, G., Chen, L., Pan, X., Chen, J., Wang, L., Wang, W., et al. (2016). The effect of resveratrol on β amyloid-induced memory impairment involves inhibition of phosphodiesterase-4 related signaling. *Oncotarget* 7, 17380–17392. doi: 10.18632/oncotarget.8041

Wang, D., Ho, L., Faith, J., Ono, K., Janle, E. M., Lachcik, P. J., et al. (2015). Role of intestinal microbiota in the generation of polyphenol-derived phenolic acid mediated attenuation of Alzheimer's disease β-amyloid oligomerization. *Mol. Nutr. Food Res.* 59, 1025–1040. doi: 10.1002/mnfr.201400544

Winblad, B., Palmer, K., Kivipelto, M., Jelic, V., Fratiglioni, L., Wahlund, L. O., et al. (2004). Mild cognitive impairment—beyond controversies, towards a consensus: report of the international working group on mild cognitive impairment. *J. Intern. Med.* 256, 240–246. doi: 10.1111/j.1365-2796.2004.01380.x

Wu, W., Li, Y., Wu, Y., Zhang, Y., Wang, Z., and Liu, X. (2015). Lutein suppresses inflammatory responses through Nrf2 activation and NF-κB inactivation in lipopolysaccharide-stimulated BV-2 microglia. *Mol. Nutr. Food Res.* 59, 1663–1673. doi: 10.1002/mnfr.201500109

Xu, P. X., Wang, S. W., Yu, X. L., Su, Y. J., Wang, T., Zhou, W. W., et al. (2014). Rutin improves spatial memory in Alzheimer's disease transgenic mice by reducing Aβ oligomer level and attenuating oxidative stress and neuroinflammation. *Behav. Brain Res.* 264, 173–180. doi: 10.1016/j.bbr.2014.02.002

Xu, Y., Xu, Y., Wang, Y., Wang, Y., He, L., Jiang, Z., et al. (2015). Telmisartan prevention of LPS-induced microglia activation involves M2 microglia polarization via CaMKKβ-dependent AMPK activation. *Brain Behav. Immun.* 50, 298–313. doi: 10.1016/j.bbi.2015.07.015

Xu, G., Zhou, Z., Zhu, W., Fan, X., and Liu, X. (2009). Plasma C-reactive protein is related to cognitive deterioration and dementia in patients with mild cognitive impairment. *J. Neurol. Sci.* 284, 77–80. doi: 10.1016/j.jns.2009.04.018

Yamakawa, M. Y., Uchino, K., Watanabe, Y., Adachi, T., Nakanishi, M., Ichino, H., et al. (2016). Anthocyanin suppresses the toxicity of Aβ deposits through diversion of molecular forms in *in vitro* and *in vivo* models of Alzheimer's disease. *Nutr. Neurosci.* 19, 32–42. doi: 10.1179/1476830515Y.0000000042

Yanagitai, M., Itoh, S., Kitagawa, T., Takenouchi, T., Kitani, H., and Satoh, T. (2012). Carnosic acid, a pro-electrophilic compound, inhibits LPS-induced activation of microglia. *Biochem. Biophys. Res. Commun.* 418, 22–26. doi: 10.1016/j.bbrc.2011.12.087

Yao, Y., Li, J., Niu, Y., Yu, J. Q., Yan, L., Miao, Z. H., et al. (2015). Resveratrol inhibits oligomeric Aβ-nduced microglial activation via NADPH oxidase. *Mol. Med. Rep.* 12, 6133–6139. doi: 10.3892/mmr.2015.4199

Yasuno, F., Kazui, H., Morita, N., Kajimoto, K., Ihara, M., and Taguchi, A. (2016). Use of T1-weighted/T2-weighted magnetic resonance ratio to elucidate changes due to amyloid β accumulation in cognitively normal subjects. *Neuroimage Clin.* 13, 209–214. doi: 10.1016/j.nicl.2016.11.029

Ye, S. M., and Johnson, R. W. (1999). Increased interleukin-6 expression by microglia from brain of aged mice. *J. Neuroimmunol.* 93, 139–148. doi: 10.1016/s0165-5728(98)00217-3

Ye, S. M., and Johnson, R. W. (2001). An age-related decline in interleukin-10 may contribute to the increased expression of interleukin-6 in brain of aged mice. *Neuroimmunomodulation* 9, 183–192. doi: 10.1159/000049025

Zhang, J., Guo, J., Zhao, X., Chen, Z., Wang, G., Liu, A., et al. (2013). Phosphodiesterase-5 inhibitor sildenafil prevents neuroinflammation, lowers β-amyloid levels and improves cognitive performance in APP/PS1 transgenic mice. *Behav. Brain Res.* 250, 230–237. doi: 10.1016/j.bbr.2013.05.017

Zhang, R., Miao, Q. W., Zhu, C. X., Zhao, Y., Liu, L., Yang, J., et al. (2015). Sulforaphane ameliorates neurobehavioral deficits and protects the brain from amyloid β deposits and peroxidation in mice with Alzheimer-like lesions. *Am. J. Alzheimers Dis. Other Demen.* 30, 183–191. doi: 10.1177/1533317514542645

Zhang, Z. Y., and Schluesener, H. J. (2013). Oral administration of histone deacetylase inhibitor MS-275 ameliorates neuroinflammation and cerebral amyloidosis and improves behavior in a mouse model. *J. Neuropathol. Exp. Neurol.* 72, 178–185. doi: 10.1097/NEN.0b013e318283114a

Zhang, Z., Wu, H., and Huang, H. (2016). Epicatechin plus treadmill exercise are neuroprotective against moderate-stage amyloid precursor protein/presenilin 1 mice. *Pharmacogn. Mag.* 12, S139–S146. doi: 10.4103/0973-1296.182174

Zhao, H., Cheng, L., Liu, Y., Zhang, W., Maharjan, S., Cui, Z., et al. (2014). Mechanisms of anti-inflammatory property of conserved dopamine neurotrophic factor: inhibition of JNK signaling in lipopolysaccharide-induced microglia. *J. Mol. Neurosci.* 52, 186–192. doi: 10.1007/s12031-013-0120-7

Zhao, D., Kwon, S. H., Chun, Y. S., Gu, M. Y., and Yang, H. O. (2017). Anti-neuroinflammatory effects of fucoxanthin via inhibition of Akt/NF-κB and MAPKs/AP-1 pathways and activation of PKA/CREB pathway in lipopolysaccharide-activated BV-2 microglial cells. *Neurochem. Res.* 42, 667–677. doi: 10.1007/s11064-016-2123-6

Zhou, Q., Wang, M., Du, Y., Zhang, W., Bai, M., Zhang, Z., et al. (2015). Inhibition of c-Jun N-terminal kinase activation reverses Alzheimer disease phenotypes in APPswe/PS1dE9 mice. *Ann. Neurol.* 77, 637–654. doi: 10.1002/ana.24361

Zhu, X., Raina, A. K., Rottkamp, C. A., Aliev, G., Perry, G., Boux, H., et al. (2001). Activation and redistribution of c-jun N-terminal kinase/stress activated protein kinase in degenerating neurons in Alzheimer's disease. *J. Neurochem.* 76, 435–441. doi: 10.1046/j.1471-4159.2001.00046.x

Zhu, L., Yang, J. Y., Xue, X., Dong, Y. X., Liu, Y., Miao, F. R., et al. (2015). A novel phosphodiesterase-5 Inhibitor: yonkenafil modulates neurogenesis, gliosis to improve cognitive function and ameliorates amyloid burden in an APP/PS1 transgenic mice model. *Mech. Ageing Dev.* 150, 34–45. doi: 10.1016/j.mad.2015.07.002

Zong, H., Ren, J. M., Young, L. H., Pypaert, M., Mu, J., Birnbaum, M. J., et al. (2002). AMP kinase is required for mitochondrial biogenesis in skeletal muscle in response to chronic energy deprivation. *Proc. Natl. Acad. Sci. U S A* 99, 15983–15987. doi: 10.1073/pnas.252625599

8

The Role of Microglia in Prion Diseases: A Paradigm of Functional Diversity

*Juliane Obst†, Emilie Simon†, Renzo Mancuso† and Diego Gomez-Nicola**

Biological Sciences, University of Southampton, Southampton General Hospital, Southampton, United Kingdom

***Correspondence:**
Diego Gomez-Nicola
d.gomez-nicola@soton.ac.uk

†These authors have contributed equally to this work.

Inflammation is a major component of neurodegenerative diseases. Microglia are the innate immune cells in the central nervous system (CNS). In the healthy brain, microglia contribute to tissue homeostasis and regulation of synaptic plasticity. Under disease conditions, they play a key role in the development and maintenance of the neuroinflammatory response, by showing enhanced proliferation and activation. Prion diseases are progressive chronic neurodegenerative disorders associated with the accumulation of the scrapie prion protein PrP^{Sc}, a misfolded conformer of the cellular prion protein PrP^{C}. This review article provides the current knowledge on the role of microglia in the pathogenesis of prion disease. A large body of evidence shows that microglia can trigger neurotoxic pathways contributing to progressive degeneration. Yet, microglia are also crucial for controlling inflammatory, repair and regenerative processes. This dual role of microglia is regulated by multiple pathways and evidences the ability of these cells to polarize into distinct phenotypes with characteristic functions. The awareness that the neuroinflammatory response is inextricably involved in producing tissue damage as well as repair in neurodegenerative disorders, opens new perspectives for the modulation of the immune system. A better understanding of this complex process will be essential for developing effective therapies for neurodegenerative diseases, in order to improve the quality of life of patients and mitigating the personal, economic and social consequences derived from these diseases.

Keywords: microglia, Csf1r, proliferation, neuroinflammation, neurodegnerative diseases

---

Abbreviations: Aβ, amyloid-β; AD, Alzheimer's disease; ALS, amyotrophic lateral sclerosis; APP/PS1, APPswe/PSEN1dE9; Ara-C, cytosine arabinoside; ASC, apoptosis-associated speck-like protein containing a caspase recruitment domain; BBB, blood-brain barrier; CCL2, C-C motif chemokine ligand 2; CCR2, C-C chemokine receptor type 2; CD, Cluster of differentiation; C/EBPα, CCAAT/enhancer-binding protein alpha; COX, cyclooxygenase; CVO, circumventricular organs; CJD, Creutzfeldt-Jakob disease; CNS, Central nervous system; CR3, complement receptor 3; CSF, cerebrospinal fluid; CSF1, Colony stimulating factor; CSF1R, Colony stimulating factor 1 receptor; CTL/CTLD, C-type lectin/C-type lectin-like domain; CX3CL1, C-X3-C motif chemokine ligand 1; CX3CR1, C-X3-C motif chemokine receptor 1; DAP12, DNAX-activating protein of 12-kDa; EAE, Experimental autoimmune encephalomyelitis; EMP, Erythroid-myeloid progenitors; Iba1, Ionized calcium-binding adaptor molecule 1; IL-1β, Interleukin 1β; IL-34, Interleukin 34; IRF8, Interferon regulatory factor 8; LPS, lipopolysaccharide; MFGE8, Milk fβt globule-EGF factor 8 protein; MHC, Major histocompatibility complex; miR, microRNA; NFκB, Nuclear factor kappa-light-chain-enhancer of activated B cells; NLRP3, Nod-like receptor family pyrin domain containing 3; NSAID, Nonsteroidal anti-inflammatory drug; NO, nitric oxide; NOX2, Nicotinamide adenine dinucleotide phosphate-oxidase (NADPH) oxidase 2; PD, Parkinson's disease; PGE2, prostaglandin E2; pMac, pre-macrophage; poly I:C, Polyinosinic-polycytidylic acid; MM1, *PRNP* codon 129 Met/Met type 1; PrP^{C}, cellular prion protein; PrP^{Sc}, misfolded prion protein (scrapie); ROS, Reactive oxygen species; Runtl, Runt-related transcription factor 1; Sall1/3, Sal-like 1/3; SIRPα, Signal regulatory protein α; SOD1, superoxide dismutase 1; STAT1/3, Signal transducer and activator of transcription 1/3; Tie2, TEK receptor tyrosine kinase; TGFβ, Transforming growth factor β; TK, thymidine kinase; TIMD4, T-cell immunoglobulin and mucin domain containing 4; TNFα, Tumor nerosis factor α; TREM2, triggering receptor expressed on myeloid cells 2; VV2, *PRNP* codon 129 Val/Val type 2; YS, yolk sac.

MICROGLIA IN THE HEALTHY BRAIN

Origin and Turnover of Microglia

Since the initial description of microglial cells by Pio Del Rio Hortega (del Río-Hortega, 1920, 1932; del Río-Hortega and Penfield, 1927), their origin has been a source of debate. However, it has been recently established that tissue resident macrophages as microglia originate from erythroid-myeloid progenitors (EMPs) emerging from the yolk sac (YS) during primitive hemeatopoiesis at embryonic stages 7.0 (E7.0) to E9.5 (Cuadros et al., 1993; Alliot et al., 1999; Schulz et al., 2012; Gomez Perdiguero et al., 2015; Sheng et al., 2015; Wang et al., 2015). A pioneering study by Ginhoux et al. (2010) allowed finding the earliest microglial progenitors in the YS during mouse development, thanks to fate-mapping experiments that allowed tagging early YS blood-island cells and then follow the emergence of microglial cells into the central nervous system (CNS). Fate mapping of YS progenitors from E6.5 to E7.0 produced tagging of less than 4% of adult microglia, whereas mapping from E7.0 to E7.25 produced 29% microglia being labeled, allowing the definition that primitive EMPs that arise before E7.5 are the main contributors to the adult microglial population (Ginhoux et al., 2010). Then, several studies using tamoxifen-inducible Cre lines in which the Cre-ER-T2/Mer-Cre-Mer protein was expressed under the control of different genes such as Colony stimulating factor receptor 1 (*Csf1r*; Schulz et al., 2012), *C-kit* (Sheng et al., 2015), TEK Receptor Tyrosine Kinase (*Tie2*; Gomez Perdiguero et al., 2015) corroborated that microglial progenitors have a YS origin. A recent study by Mass et al. (2016) has allowed a more precise definition of the sequence of differentiation steps leading to the adult microglial population. In the YS, uncommitted EMPs (Kit^{+} CD45^{lo} Csf1r^{+} AA4.1^{+}) differentiate into pre-macrophage (pMac; kit^{-} CD45^{hi} F4/80^{-}) that do not yet have a microglial phenotype. From E9.5, as they initiate a core macrophage transcriptional program, those pMacs colonize the whole embryo in a C-X3-C motif chemokine receptor 1 (CX3CR1)-dependent manner. Indeed, at E9.5 and E10.5, CX3CR1-deficient embryos exhibit a delay in the colonization of progenitors and a decrease of pMacs and macrophages population in the head while they display an accumulation of pMacs in the YS and fetal liver (Mass et al., 2016). Immediately following colonization of the embryonic brain, a tissue specific transcriptional program is triggered and leads to the production of postnatal microglia, including a downregulation of T-cell immunoglobulin and mucin domain containing 4 (*Timd4*) and mannose receptor (*Cd206*) and an upregulation of Sal-like (*Sall*)*1* and *Sall3* (Lavin et al., 2014; Mass et al., 2016). As the embryo develops, microglia progenitors mature in a Interferon regulatory factor 8 (IRF8) and PU.1-dependant manner by expressing a set of different markers including CSF1R, Runt-related transcription factor (Runx1), ionized calcium-binding adaptor molecule 1 (Iba1), C-X3-C Motif Chemokine Receptor (CX3CR1), Tie2, the cluster of differentiation 45 (CD45) or C-kit (Kierdorf et al., 2013; Mass et al., 2016).

In humans, microglial cells are identified in the extracerebral mesenchyme around 4.5 gestational weeks. At 5 gestational weeks, they invade the parenchyma by entering the brain primordium via the developing meninges, ventricular zone and choroid plexus (Monier et al., 2006; Verney et al., 2010) and they only exhibit a ramified morphology around the 35th week (Hutchins et al., 1990; Esiri et al., 1991; Rezaie and Male, 1999).

In the adult, the microglial population is maintained by a self-renewal process (Lawson et al., 1992; Askew et al., 2017; **Figure 1**). A foundational study by Lawson et al. (1992) defined a remarkably slow turnover rate of adult murine microglia, by means of analyzing short-term ^{3}H tymidine incorporation. However, more recent insight arising from repopulation paradigms suggested that microglia could have a higher turnover capacity in the steady state. The pharmacological depletion of microglia, by using a potent CSF1R inhibitor, is followed by the rapid reconstitution of the microglia population by proliferation of resident microglia, without the contribution of circulating monocytes (Elmore et al., 2014). A transgenic paradigm, allowing the depletion of microglia by diphtheria toxin injection, validated this repopulating capacity, independent of circulating monocytes (Bruttger et al., 2015). Although these repopulation paradigms are distal from modeling a homeostatic system, they suggested a latent potential for microglial cells to proliferate more rapidly than thought before, allowing the colonization of an empty niche. In this line, a recent study from our group showed that in mice and humans the turnover of microglia in the steady state is remarkably fast, allowing the whole population to be renewed several times during a lifetime (Askew et al., 2017). Indeed, whereas the previous study in the healthy brain, using ^{3}H thymidine and immunohistochemistry for F4/80, had shown that, at a given time, only 0.05% of the microglia were proliferating (Lawson et al., 1992), Askew et al. (2017) recently demonstrated that 0.69% of the microglial population is proliferating by using more sensitive techniques (BrdU incorporation detected in Iba1^{+} cells and 2-photon live imaging). Microglial proliferation is balanced by microglial apoptosis, with these two mechanisms being synchronized in time and space, allowing for a rapid remodeling of the microglial landscape during a lifetime, without the contribution of circulating monocytes (Askew et al., 2017).

Distribution and Function of Microglia in the Adult Brain

The density and morphology of microglia varies considerably across the healthy adult brain. In the mouse brain, there are an estimated total number of 3.5×10^{6} microglial cells, however their distribution varies from 5% in the cortex and corpus callosum, to 12% in the substantia nigra (Lawson et al., 1990). In mice, microglia are more numerous in gray matter than white matter and areas as the hippocampus, basal ganglia and substantia nigra are particularly densely populated in microglia (Lawson et al., 1990). In comparison, the less densely populated areas include fiber tracts, cerebellum and much of the brainstem whereas the cerebral cortex, thalamus and hypothalamus have average cell densities (Lawson et al., 1990). This cell density remains constant from early postnatal development to aging, thanks to the constant turnover of the population (Askew et al., 2017). In the human brain, microglia has been estimated to make

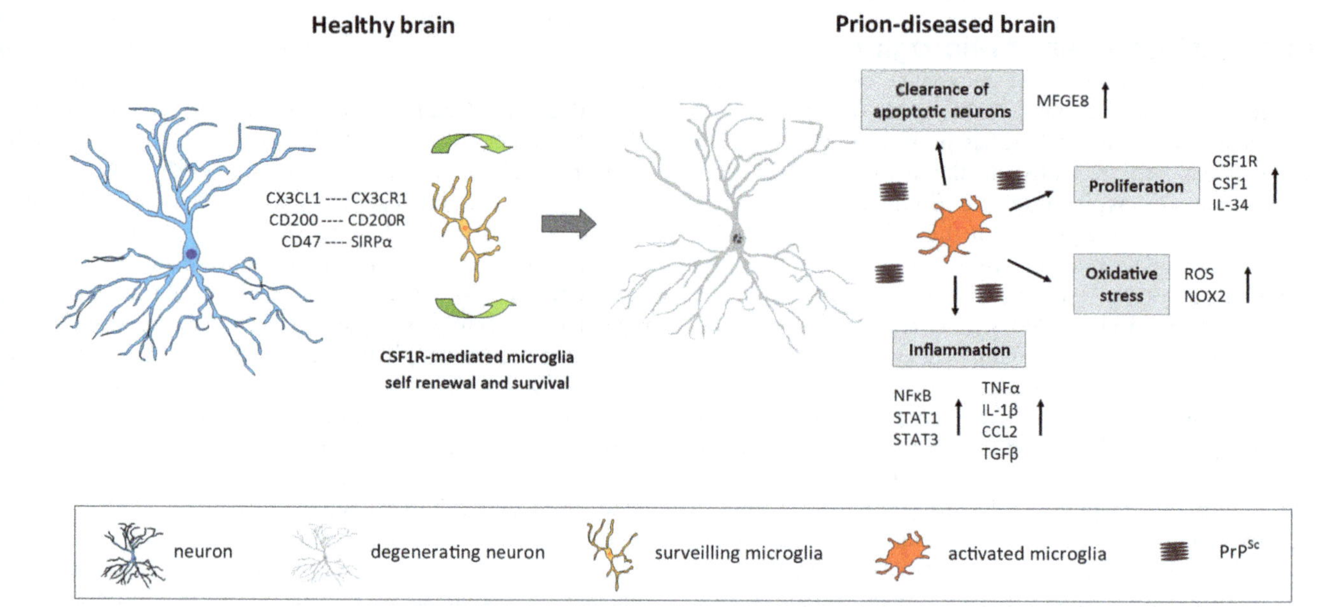

FIGURE 1 | Microglia in the prion-diseased brain. In the healthy brain, microglia constantly surveil their microenvironment for any disturbance of brain homeostasis and are kept in this surveiling state by signals mainly originating from healthy neurons. The microglial population is maintained by local self-renewal mediated via CSF1R and its ligands CSF1 and IL-34. In the context of neurodegeneration and protein accumulation present in the prion-diseased brain, the microglial response is characterized by functional changes involving increased proliferation, an inflammatory activation and the removal of apoptotic neurons. CX3CL1, C-X3-C motif chemokine ligand 1; CX3CR1, C-X3-C motif chemokine receptor 1; CD200, Cluster of differentiation 200; CD47, Cluster of differentiation 47; SIRPα, Signal regulatory protein α; CSF1R, Colony stimulating factor 1 receptor; CSF1, Colony stimulating factor; IL-34, Interleukin 34; MFGE8, Milk fat globule-EGF factor 8 protein; ROS, Reactive oxygen species; NOX2, Nicotinamide adenine dinucleotide phosphate-oxidase (NADPH) oxidase 2; NFκB, Nuclear factor kappa-light-chain-enhancer of activated B cells; STAT1/3, Signal transducer and activator of transcription 1/3; TNFα, Tumor nerosis factor α; IL-1β, Interleukin 1β; CCL2, C-C motif chemokine ligand 2; TGFβ, Transforming growth factor β; PrP^{Sc} misfolded prion protein (scrapie).

up 6%–18% of neocortical cells (Mittelbronn et al., 2001; Pelvig et al., 2008; Lyck et al., 2009). Similarly, microglial morphology varies considerably depending on specific regional properties. Whereas they are usually more ramified in gray matter, in white matter they display elongated somata and less ramified processes preferentially oriented along fiber tracts (Lawson et al., 1990; Mittelbronn et al., 2001; Torres-Platas et al., 2014). The molecular determinants of those anatomical differences in diversity and morphology are not clearly defined, however recent studies showed that microglia have a distinct region-dependent and age-dependent transcriptomic signature corroborating the existence of the regional heterogeneity of microglial phenotypes (Hickman et al., 2013; Grabert et al., 2016; Soreq et al., 2017).

In the healthy brain, microglia display a "surveilling" phenotype characterized by a small cell body and long branching processes serving to continuously sense the microenvironment to detect any alteration of CNS homeostasis (Kettenmann et al., 2013; **Figure 1**). Microglia show invariant soma positions but continually and rapidly moving processes (average velocity around 2.5 μm/min; Davalos et al., 2005; Nimmerjahn et al., 2005; Wake et al., 2009). Microglias rapidly change their surveilling phenotype into a diversity of "activated" phenotypes after the alteration of the CNS homeostasis or presence of a threat to neuronal integrity. They adopt a more amoeboid and less ramified phenotype with a large soma and rapidly trigger appropriate responses, which could range from upregulation or *de novo* synthesis of cell-surface molecules such as CD68 and major histocompatibility complex (MHC) class II to phagocytosis or the release of molecular mediators, including immune and non-immune factors (Kettenmann et al., 2011; **Figure 1**). Consequently, this activated phenotype is a generalized term that fails to take into account that microglia can adopt numerous functionally different phenotypes, depending on the exact nature of the stimulus (Perry et al., 2010).

In the healthy brain, microglia is involved in several mechanisms regulating CNS physiology. Microglia are in direct contact with dendritic spines, axons and synapses, suggesting that they participate in the regulation of synaptic structure and function (Wake et al., 2009; Paolicelli et al., 2011; Squarzoni et al., 2014). One of these mechanisms is synaptic pruning, a process by which excess synapses formed in the developing brain are eliminated to thereby increase the efficiency of the neural network. In this process, microglia has been shown in direct contact with the synapses and removing unwanted elements by phagocytosis (Paolicelli et al., 2011). Electron microscopy and high resolution *in vivo* engulfment assays have showed also the presence of presynaptic and postsynaptic elements inside microglial lysosomes (Berbel and Innocenti, 1988; Tremblay et al., 2010; Schafer et al., 2012). Some proteins as complement receptor 3 (CR3/CD11b), CX3CR1 or the adaptor protein DNAX-activating protein of 12-kDa (DAP12), highly expressed by microglia, are involved in the process of synaptic pruning. Indeed it has been shown that disruption of one of those proteins resulted in synaptic abnormalities in both prenatal and postnatal brain development (Stevens et al., 2007; Paolicelli et al., 2011; Squarzoni et al., 2014).

As mentioned above, the interactions between microglia and their surrounding cells have a major role in the determination of the microglial phenotype. Healthy neurons maintain microglia in their surveilling state via secreted and membrane bound signals. The interaction of neuronal CD200 with microglial CD200R leads to inactivation of microglia and plays a critical role in neuroprotection (Lyons et al., 2007). In CD200-deficient mice, microglia are more numerous, form more aggregate-like structures, display less ramifications with shorter processes and show an upregulation of CD45 and CD11b, which are markers of activation (Hoek et al., 2000). The bidirectional signaling between SIRPα and CD47 that can be co-expressed by both neurons and microglia maintains microglia in their surveilling state by inhibiting phagocytosis and inducing the synthesis of the anti-inflammatory cytokines (Zhang et al., 2015). The interaction of neuronal CX3CL1 with microglial CX3CR1 constrains microglial activation (Lyons et al., 2009). In models for Parkinson's disease (PD) under a CX3CR1-deficient background, microglia exhibit an over-activated phenotype and neuronal cell death is enhanced (Bhaskar et al., 2010; Cho et al., 2011). The neurotoxicity induced by activated microglia in neurodegenerative diseases seems to be worsened in CX3CR1-deficient mice, suggesting that the signaling through CX3CL1/CX3CR1 regulates the phenotype of microglia (Cardona et al., 2006). Another receptor involved in the maintenance of the microglial surveilling state is the triggering receptor expressed on myeloid cells 2 (TREM2) associated with the adaptor protein DAP12. TREM2 is essential for phagocytosis process by microglia (Takahashi et al., 2007) and has recently been shown to interact with specific lipids to promote microglial survival (Wang et al., 2015). Mutations leading to a loss of function in TREM2 or DAP12 underlie the Nasu–Hakola disease, in which patients display progressive presenile dementia (Paloneva et al., 2000, 2002).

Microglia also express receptors that trigger essential cellular survival and developmental signals. CSF1R plays a major role in microglial development and survival. Expressed by microglia (Akiyama et al., 1994; Raivich et al., 1998), CSF1R is activated by two homodimeric glycoprotein ligands, CSF1 (Stanley and Heard, 1977) and Interleukin 34 (IL-34; Lin et al., 2008). In the brain, IL-34 is primarily expressed by neurons (Mizuno et al., 2011; Wang et al., 2012) whereas CSF1 is mainly expressed by microglia (Chitu et al., 2016). These two ligands present different patterns of regional expression in the prenatal and postnatal brain. CSF1 is highly expressed in the neocortex, corpus callosum, cerebellum and spinal cord, whereas IL-34 is highly expressed in the forebrain (neocortex, olfactory bulb and striatum; Wei et al., 2010; Nandi et al., 2012). The binding of CSF1 or IL-34 to CSF1R leads to the oligomerization and transphosphorylation of CSF1R followed by the phosphorylation and activation of downstream cytoplasmic mediators that promote microglia development, survival and proliferation (Ségaliny et al., 2015). As described previously, the development of tissue-resident macrophages including microglia is dependent on *Csf1r* expression from the first stages of development (Mass et al., 2016). Moreover, IL-34-deficient and CSF1-deficient mice display fewer microglia in various regions of the brain while Csf1r-deficient mice are completely devoid of them (Dai et al., 2002; Ginhoux et al., 2010).

In addition to their manifold functions in maintaining homeostasis in the healthy brain, microglia have been shown to play a major role in driving innate inflammatory responses in many neurodegenerative diseases. Prion disease is characterized by progressive neurodegeneration, which is accompanied by a pronounced microglia-mediated immune response, therefore being an extraordinary model to study the role of microglia in chronic neurodegenerative diseases. In this review, we will explore the molecular determinants of the contribution of microglia to the pathogenic cascade in prion disease, aiming to address some of the most relevant remaining unknowns of the role of microglia in prion disease: is microglial activation merely a bystander effect of prion pathology, or what aspects of microglia-mediated immune response are contributing to disease outcome in a beneficial or detrimental manner? Can the microglia-derived inflammatory response directly harm neurons and lead to neuronal degeneration, or is neuronal loss a consequence of misfolded prion protein (scrapie) (PrP^{sc}) accumulation, or a combination of both? In the following sections, we will provide a comprehensive picture defining many aspects of microglial biology in prion disease.

PRION PATHOLOGY

Transmissible spongiform encephalopathies or prion diseases, such as Creutzfeldt-Jakob disease (CJD), are fatal neurodegenerative disorders that affect humans and many other mammals (Aguzzi and Calella, 2009). The infectious agent consists of PrP^{Sc}. PrP^{Sc} can aggregate, recruit and convert benign cellular prion protein (PrP^{C}) into abnormal pathological isoforms (Aguzzi and Calella, 2009). Thereby, prions act as "seeds" that trigger a chain reaction of PrP misfolding and aggregation (Jarrett and Lansbury, 1993). Prion diseases have a heterogeneous etiology, as they can be genetic, infectious or sporadic. Infectivity requires the transfer of prion seeds from affected individuals into healthy hosts, whereas in genetic and idiopathic cases prion protein undergoes a spontaneous misfolding of PrP molecules into self-propagating seeds. In humans, sporadic CJD (sCJD) is the most common prion disease, followed by genetic CJD (gCJD) and transmitted CJD (iatrogenic CJD and variant CJD; Aguzzi and Calella, 2009). CJD has been also shown to be transmitted through blood or blood derivatives (Llewelyn et al., 2004; Bishop et al., 2013).

The prion neuropathology is characterized by spongiform degeneration, synaptic and neuronal loss, gliosis and the accumulation of aggregated PrP^{SC} (DeArmond and Prusiner, 1995; Cunningham et al., 2003; Wadsworth and Collinge, 2011; Hilton et al., 2013). Prion disease typically has long incubation times and a rapid disease progression, and can be manifested in different ways, with behavioral and pathological differences within and across species (Prusiner, 1998; Tanaka et al., 2006; Collinge and Clarke, 2007; Colby and Prusiner, 2011). Interestingly, different strains of prion (e.g., ME7, 79A, 22L, 22A) preferentially affect specific regions of the brain in mice (Cunningham et al., 2005a). The simplest explanation for such regional selectivity would be a differential tropism of prion strains and thereby a regional aggregation and toxicity. However, recent experiments assessing prion misfolding using highly sensitive techniques showed that prion protein seeds accumulate in all brain regions irrespective of neurodegeneration (Alibhai et al., 2016).

Prions disease also provides an interesting experimental approach to model many aspects of neurodegenerative diseases associated with protein misfolding. In mouse models of prion disease, microglia become activated early in the disease process thereby representing a valuable tool for elucidating the impact of neuroinflammation in chronic neurodegenerative disorders.

MICROGLIAL PROLIFERATION AND ACTIVATION IN PRION DISEASE

Prion disease is characterized by an increase in the number of microglia, associated with an activated and phagocytic phenotype (Perry et al., 2002; Perry and O'Connor, 2010; **Figure 1**). The relative contribution of local proliferation of microglia vs. the infiltration of bone-marrow derived progenitors to this increase has been a source of debate during recent years (Gomez-Nicola and Perry, 2015). However, a recent study demonstrated that, in a murine model of prion disease, local proliferation of resident microglial cells is a major component in the evolution of chronic neurodegeneration (Gómez-Nicola et al., 2013). The increase in microglial density and proliferative activity varies across different regions such as the hippocampus (CA1) and the thalamus, the later showing the biggest increase in cell numbers (Gómez-Nicola et al., 2013). This increase in microglial numbers is independent of the recruitment of circulating monocytes, evidenced by comparing microglial density in prion diseased mice with a C-C chemokine receptor type 2 $(CCR2)^{-/-}$ background with WT mice (Gómez-Nicola et al., 2014).

The proliferation of microglia in prion disease is regulated by the activation of CSF1R and the transcription factors PU.1 and CCAAT/enhancer-binding protein alpha (C/EBPα, being this system also active in human variant CJD and Alzheimer's disease (AD; Gómez-Nicola et al., 2013; Olmos-Alonso et al., 2016). The inhibition of CSF1R blocks the proliferation of microglia, leading to a decrease in neuronal death in the hippocampus (Gómez-Nicola et al., 2013). A recent study showed that prolonged inhibition of CSF1R in APPswe/PSEN1dE9 (APP/PS1) mice, a model of AD-like pathology, blocks microglial proliferation and leads to the prevention of synaptic degeneration and to an improvement of performance in memory and exploratory tasks (Olmos-Alonso et al., 2016). CSF1R blockade also showed positive effect in mutant superoxide dismutase 1 (SOD1) models of Amyotrophic Lateral Sclerosis (ALS) by reducing microglial proliferation in the spinal cord and macrophage infiltration into peripheral nerves (Martínez-Muriana et al., 2016). The studies focused to targeting CSF1R suggest that microglial proliferation in prion disease, AD and ALS has a net detrimental contribution to the disease progression.

Targeting microglial proliferation by the specific inhibition of CSF1R renders a different experimental outcome than the unspecific removal of microglia. Some studies have aimed at eliminating microglial cells in prion disease, either by the transgenic expression of thymidine kinase (TK) and "suicide" of proliferating CD11b+ cells (Zhu et al., 2016), or by the non-specific blocker of mitosis cytosine arabinoside (Ara-C; Gómez-Nicola et al., 2013). These approaches indicated a neutral or beneficial role of microglia, as their elimination did not change the trajectory of the disease. However, the technical limitations of these targeting approaches difficult the interpretation. For example, the use of CD11b-TK mice leads to a prominent and uncontrolled death of microglia in the context of on-going neurodegeneration, not providing a physiologically silent way to address the contribution of the cells. Also, the TK transgene in CD11b-TK mice is activated by the administration of ganciclovir, an agent recently identified to have a potent anti-proliferative impact on microglia during brain pathology (Ding et al., 2014). Similarly, the use of Ara-C causes a shift in the microglial phenotype towards a detrimental pro-inflammatory profile, independent from its effects on cell proliferation, accelerating neuronal death (Gómez-Nicola et al., 2013). Together, these findings suggest that the specific and selective targeting of microglial proliferation, instead to their elimination, is an optimal approach to understand the contribution of these cells to the pathology.

Activation of microglia is detectable from early stages of prion disease pathogenesis (Betmouni et al., 1996) and becomes more widespread as the disease progresses, closely associated with the spread of neurodegeneration (Perry, 2016). Microglial activation appears simultaneously with first behavioral deficits (Guenther et al., 2001), at a time point when synapses start to degenerate in the stratum radiatum of the hippocampus, but no neuronal loss occurs yet (Cunningham et al., 2003; Gray et al., 2009). Whether microglia activation is directly caused by accumulating misfolded PrP^{sc} or as a response to synaptic damage cannot be reliably concluded. While studies *in vitro* have demonstrated that microglia can be activated directly by PrP and subsequently damage neurons (Brown et al., 1996; Giese et al., 1998), there is limited evidence of a direct response to PrP^{Sc} aggregates *in vivo*. In contrast, the mere presence of misfolded prion protein, as detected in various brain regions using high sensitivity techniques, might not be sufficient to induce a microglia-mediated immune response in all brain regions (Alibhai et al., 2016). However, it is widely accepted that microglia activation precedes neuronal degeneration and the onset of clinical disease (Williams et al., 1997; Giese et al., 1998).

The cytokine profile in the prion-diseased brain is associated with the expression of both pro- and anti-inflammatory molecules (Perry, 2016; **Figure 1**). While a number of studies demonstrated a profile shifted to the anti-inflammatory spectrum, dominated by the expression of transforming growth factor β (TGFβ, C-C Motif Chemokine Ligand 2 (CCL2) and prostaglandin E2 (PGE2) with a limited pro-inflammatory response characterized by IL-1β and tumor necrosis factor α (TNFa; Minghetti et al., 2000; Walsh et al., 2001; Cunningham et al., 2002, 2005b; Perry et al., 2002), other studies have reported that also pro-inflammatory factors are up-regulated in the prion brain (Campbell et al., 1994; Williams et al., 1994; Kordek et al., 1996), suggestive of a mixed inflammatory profile. The lack of consensus regarding the inflammatory profile in the prion brain may arise from the fact that different prion strains, stages of disease and techniques of detection were used. Recent studies using a broader panel of markers support the hypothesis that both pro-and anti-inflammatory factors contribute to the immune response in prion disease. Vincenti et al. (2015) re-analyzed a large transcriptomic database of brains from multiple mouse strains exposed to various prion strains and collected at different stages of disease progression (Hwang et al., 2009) and proposed that most of the differentially expressed genes in the prion brain were of microglial origin and associated with the inflammatory response. Microglia isolated from 79A-infected mice showed increased expression of IL-1β, TNFα and CSF1, but not IL-6, IL-10 or TGFβ, which correlates with disease progression and indicates a classical activation phenotype of microglia in this prion model (Vincenti et al., 2015). A recent longitudinal study reported new inflammatory genes upregulated early in the prion brain, including genes involved in inflammation, monocyte recruitment and growth regulation (Carroll et al., 2015). Concerning signal transduction pathways, an early activation predominantly of the Signal transducer and activator of transcription (STAT)- and Nuclear factor kappa-light-chain-enhancer of activated B cells (NFkB) pathways has been observed in prion disease models, determined by the up-regulation of STAT- and NFkB-responsive genes, including many cytokines and chemokines, as well as by the detection of increased phosphorylation of STAT1 and STAT3 specifically (Llorens et al., 2014; Carroll et al., 2015). The inflammatory response seems to be quite consistent between different murine prion strains. Although prion strains 22L, RML and ME7 revealed cellular and regional differences in PrP^{Sc} accumulation, they showed a similar up-regulation mainly of pro-inflammatory genes and chemokines which correlated with the deposition of PrP^{Sc} and the onset of glial activation (Carroll et al., 2016).

Targeting individual immune pathways which are dysregulated in prion disease have shown differential effects in modifying pathology. The absence of CCL2 does not drastically affect the disease course (Felton et al., 2005; O'Shea et al., 2008) and similarly, reducing PGE2 levels using dapsone or Nonsteroidal anti-inflammatory drugs (NSAIDs) did not impact disease progression (Guenther et al., 2001; Perry, 2010). On the contrary, inhibition of TGFβ enhanced neurodegeneration, indicating that this immune mediator is critically involved in regulation of the innate immune response in prion disease (Boche et al., 2006). TNFα as well as TNF receptor 1 knockout mice show normal prion disease progression after intracerebral injection of the prion protein (Klein et al., 1997; Mabbott et al., 2000), whereas deficiency of IL-1 receptor type 1 prolongs prion incubation time (Tamgüney et al., 2008) and delays disease onset and protein aggregation and increases survival of diseased mice (Schultz et al., 2004). PrP fibrils have been found to induce IL-1β secretion by microglia *in vitro*, dependent on components of the Nod-like receptor family pyrin domain containing 3 (NLRP3) inflammasome, is sufficient to induce neuronal toxicity (Hafner-Bratkovič et al., 2012; Shi et al., 2012). However, an *in vivo* study using mice deficient in NLRP3 or the adaptor protein apoptosis-associated speck-like protein containing a caspase recruitment domain (ASC) and thereby lacking functional NLRP3 inflammasome, failed to demonstrate a significant impact on prion pathogenesis, indicating that inflammasomes do not contribute to prion progression (Nuvolone et al., 2015).

Numerous studies have reported signs of oxidative stress in brains of CJD patients as well as in murine models of prion disease (Guentchev et al., 2002; Van Everbroeck et al., 2004; Yun et al., 2006), which might play a role in disease progression by contributing to neurotoxicity and neurodegeneration. Stimulation of microglia with PrP fragments *in vitro* has been shown to induce growth arrest and the release of nitric oxide (NO) and PGE2 (Villa et al., 2016). Furthermore, in patients with CJD as well as in a mouse model of prion, production of NADPH oxidase 2 (NOX2) was up-regulated specifically by microglia in the affected brain regions (Sorce et al., 2014). Prion-induced mice deficient in NOX2 demonstrated decreased production of reactive oxygen species (ROS), a delayed onset of motor deficits and an increased survival time, indicating that microglia-specific NOX2 production leads to the release of ROS and affects prion pathology (Sorce et al., 2014).

It has been shown that microglia are able to engulf and clear apoptotic neurons (Hughes et al., 2010; Kranich et al., 2010). The phagocytic function of microglia is increased in the prion-diseased brain and associated with enhanced expression of scavenger receptors, cathepsins, and proteins of the respiratory burst, while phagocytic microglia were characterized by a lack of IL-1β expression (Hughes et al., 2010). While microglia were efficient in the uptake of injected latex beads and apoptotic cells, they were unable to remove prion protein aggregates, even upon additional stimulation with lipopolysaccharide (LPS; Hughes et al., 2010). Phagocytosis of apoptotic neurons by microglia has been shown to be dependent on milk fat globule epidermal growth factor 8 (MFGE8). Ablation of mfge8 resulted in accelerated prion pathology, with reduced clearance of apoptotic bodies and increased prion protein accumulation, indicating that microglia phagocytosis via MFGE8 is a protective mechanism in prion disease (Kranich et al., 2010). While *in vitro* studies using microglia cells or organotypic brain slices proposed that microglia can clear PrP and thereby decrease prion titers (McHattie et al., 1999; Falsig et al., 2009; Kranich et al., 2010; Zhu et al., 2016), evidence that they do so *in vivo* is still missing. It is possible that the removal of misfolded prion protein is simply inefficient or that PrP^{sc} is not a sufficient trigger to induce phagocytosis, a similar concept to that proposed for phagocytosis of amyloid β (Aβ in AD (Guillot-Sestier and Town, 2013; Prokop et al., 2013). Furthermore, while the phagocytic function of microglia in prion disease is mostly considered to be beneficial and protective, it is also conceivable that microglia, by taking up cell debris from prion infected cells or possibly PrP aggregates, might even contribute to the spreading of the pathogenic protein (Baker et al., 2002).

TREM2 has been implicated in several neurodegenerative diseases such as AD (Jonsson et al., 2012; Guerreiro R. J. et al., 2013), frontotemporal dementia (Guerreiro R. et al., 2013) and ALS (Cady et al., 2014). TREM2 is an innate immune cell receptor expressed on microglia and other myeloid cells is thought to be involved in phagocytosis of apoptotic neurons and promoting an anti-inflammatory phenotype (Takahashi et al., 2005, 2007; Hsieh et al., 2009). In the context of prion disease, TREM2 has been demonstrated to be up-regulated after prion infection, but the depletion of TREM2 did neither change incubation time and survival, nor microglia immune phenotype during prion disease (Zhu et al., 2015).

Recently, there has been evidence of the involvement of non-coding microRNAs (miR) in regulating the microglia inflammatory response in prion disease. A number of miRs implicated in the regulation of gliosis, glial cell proliferation, the innate-immune response, inflammatory signaling, deficits in neurotrophic signaling and synaptogenesis have been found to be upregulated in human prion disease cases (Zhao et al., 2016). Among them, miR-146a was observed to influence immune response and activation state of microglia (Saba et al., 2012).

While increasing evidence indicates that microglia activation seems to contribute to prion pathogenesis, not much is known about the mechanistic underpinnings. We have shown recently that microglial expansion negatively affects prion disease pathology (Gómez-Nicola et al., 2013), pointing towards a net detrimental role of microglia during chronic neurodegeneration. Another recent study emphasized a protective role of microglia in prion disease, demonstrating accelerated disease pathology upon microglia ablation in the brain (Zhu et al., 2016). This dual role of microglia during prion disease provides further proof that microglia function is highly dynamic and versatile, by promoting neurotoxic effects through facilitating a potentially aberrant and harmful inflammation in prion disease, but also by provoking a protective response through tissue maintenance and repair.

SYSTEMIC INFLAMMATION AND MICROGLIAL PRIMING

The study of immune to brain communication is gaining interest, with the immune system as a transducer of both endogenous and exogenous challenges to the host. It is known that systemic infection and inflammation are able to produce behavioral changes, known as "sickness behaviors", that include fever, malaise, anorexia, lethargy and depression (Dantzer et al., 1998), demonstrating an important influence of the immune system on CNS processes. LPS challenge in healthy humans has been shown to produce sickness behavior with fever and neuropsychological symptoms, including reduced declarative memory performance (Krabbe et al., 2005) and increased symptoms of depression (DellaGioia et al., 2012). Systemic inflammation communicates with the brain by several neural and humoral pathways. Receptors for inflammatory mediators present on vagus nerve fibers can respond to inflammatory signals and inform the nucleus of the solitary tract and other regions of the brain (Wang et al., 2003). Macrophages in the circumventricular organs (CVOs), which are regions of the CNS without a tight blood-brain barrier (BBB), are also able to communicate with systemic inflammatory mediators. Signals generated in the CVOs subsequently travel to other regions of the brain (Lacroix et al., 1998). A third route of communication involves cerebral endothelial cells of the BBB, which can transduce signals from blood to the CNS (Laflamme and Rivest, 1999). The molecular pathways by which systemic inflammation alters brain function leading to sickness behavior are not completely elucidated. It has been suggested that the link between the systemic immune system and the CNS is located at the level of the hypothalamus, the main brain region controlling the neuroendocrine system. Systemic inflammation or ageing can modify the hypothalamic function though NFkB activation and microglial-neuronal crosstalk (Li et al., 2012; Zhang et al., 2013). Further studies are needed to elucidate the exact mechanism underpinning the alteration of neuronal function by systemic inflammation.

It is known that microglia play an important role in immune-to-brain communication (Perry and Teeling, 2013). Within this context, the concept of microglial priming has been proposed. Microglial priming occurs as a result of damage associated with chronic neurodegenerative conditions (e.g., misfolded protein, neuronal debris or vascular changes), or several other stressors affecting the nervous system, such as maternal separation, acute injury or aging. It consists of an exaggerated or heightened microglial response—much stronger than that observed in stimulus-naïve microglia—to a second inflammatory stimulus. Most of the evidence supporting the hypothesis of microglial priming in chronic neurodegenerative conditions arises from the study of prion models. In fact, microglial priming was first described in prion brains subjected to a systemic challenge mimicking systemic infection (Combrinck et al., 2002). Cunningham et al. (2005b) showed how intracerebral LPS injection in prion mice results in exacerbated IL-1β expression, neutrophil infiltration and NO expression, accompanied with increased cell death. Systemic injection of LPS (Cunningham et al., 2009), Polyinosinic-polycytidylic acid (poly I:C; Cunningham et al., 2002, 2005b, 2007; Field et al., 2010) or TNFα (Hennessy et al., 2017) in prion mice also leads to exacerbated in the brain, with increased expression of pro-inflammatory cytokines and chemokines including IL-1β TNFα and CCL2. Interestingly, the increased inflammation triggered by LPS in ME7 prion brain is independent on circulating IL-1β and IL-6 (Murray et al., 2011; Hennessy et al., 2017). Although the exact mechanism by which microglia is primed is still unknown, it has been suggested that cyclooxygenase 1 (COX-1) expression in microglia mediates the systemic effects of LPS in the prion brain (Griffin et al., 2013). More recently, Hennessy et al.

(2017) reported that astrocytes could be also primed in the prion brain, and generate exaggerated levels of cytokines and chemokines after systemic LPS challenge. Although these findings suggest that microglia in the prion diseased brain are primed by the ongoing pathology and that a secondary stimulus switches these cells to an aggressive phenotype, there is still no defining criteria to classify this state, and it remains unclear whether different patterns of priming result from different forms of neurodegeneration or different systemic inflammatory stimuli.

Interestingly, priming observations and the impact of the immune system on the CNS are not restricted to prion disease (Perry, 2010; Cunningham, 2013). Systemic LPS injection can induce degeneration of cells in the substantia nigra (Gao et al., 2002; Qin et al., 2007) and systemic challenge with IL-1β in an animal model of PD leads to enhanced degeneration of substantia nigra neurons and pro-inflammatory cytokine production (Pott-Godoy et al., 2008). Systemic challenge with LPS or other bacterial toxins in an experimental model of multiple sclerosis, Experimental autoimmune encephalomyelitis (EAE), can also exacerbate neurological symptoms (Schiffenbauer et al., 1993). Systemic LPS challenge caused increased synthesis of pro-inflammatory cytokines in the CNS of transgenic mouse models of AD-like pathology (Sly et al., 2001), and tau phosphorylation (Roe et al., 2011). Chronic systemic inflammation in the form of osteoarthritis results in accelerated neuroinflammation and Aβ pathology in APP/PS1/Col1-IL1βXAT mice (Kyrkanides et al., 2011). There is also evidence about the impact of the immune system upon human neurodegenerative diseases. Systemic infection and increased systemic inflammation have been associated to an enhanced cognitive decline in AD patients (Holmes et al., 2003, 2009, 2011), and systemic infections are associated with relapses in multiple sclerosis in patients (Buljevac et al., 2002).

Overall, evidence suggests that systemic inflammation contributes to the pathology during chronic neurodegenerative conditions, with microglia acting as a hub of communication between the systemic and CNS compartments. According to this view, it is likely that a correct treatment and management of systemic inflammation could potentially delay the progression of neurodegenerative disorders.

ROLE OF MICROGLIA IN HUMAN PRION DISEASES

Evidence from the literature supports a role of microglia-mediated inflammation in human prion diseases. Activated microglia are found in the brains of CJD patients (Sasaki et al., 1993; Szpak et al., 2006) where they appear to be closely associated with PrP^{Sc} deposits (Miyazono et al., 1991; Guiroy et al., 1994; Muhleisen et al., 1995). However the degree of microglial reactivity seems to depend on the subtype of prion disease and the type of biochemical PrP^{Sc} (Puoti et al., 2005; Shi et al., 2013). Increased levels of inflammatory cytokines such as IL-8, CCL2, TGFβ, TNFα and IL-1β have been found in the cerebrospinal fluid (CSF) of sporadic CJD cases (Sharief et al., 1999; Stoeck et al., 2006, 2014) and the inflammatory response seems to correlate with the severity of lesions (Van Everbroeck et al., 2002). A recent study demonstrated subtype-specific and region-specific changes in glia activation and the expression of inflammatory mediators in CJD, with inflammation being pre-dominant in the cerebral cortex in the CJD subtype *PRNP* codon 129 Met/Met type 1 (MM1) and in the cerebellum in *PRNP* codon 129 Val/Val type 2 (VV2) cases (Llorens et al., 2014). Microglia markers such as CD11b, Iba-1 and CD68 were found to be up-regulated in a region- and subtype-specific manner which correlated with the up-regulation of pro- and anti-inflammatory cytokines, members of the complement system, the integrin family and C-type lectin/C-type lectin-like domain (CTL/CTLD) superfamily, toll-like receptors, colony-stimulating factors and cathepsins (Llorens et al., 2014). Additionally, regulatory proteins IL-34, PU.1 and C/EBPα involved in microglial proliferation are increased in variant CJD (Gómez-Nicola et al., 2013). The increased inflammatory response observed in the two subtypes of CJD was further associated with an activation of NFkB and STAT1, 3 signaling pathways (Llorens et al., 2014). The finding that key regulators of inflammationCOX-1/2 and PGE2, are elevated in brains of CJD (Minghetti et al., 2000; Deininger et al., 2003; Llorens et al., 2014) further speaks for a crucial role of inflammatory processes in human prion disease, however the exact role of microglia-mediated inflammation during the course of the fatal disease remains to be elucidated.

CONCLUSION

Increasing evidence highlights the major contribution of the expansion and activation of microglia to the pathogenesis of prion disease. Activated microglia adopts a variety of functionally diverse phenotypes depending on the disease stage and systemic influences. While their response is manifold during prion disease, targeting the microglia-mediated immune response appears to be a useful approach to modify the disease course. Determining the exact mechanistic underpinnings of the neuroinflammatory processes in prion disease is an informative step in order to develop novel treatment strategies targeting neurodegenerative disease.

AUTHOR CONTRIBUTIONS

JO, ES and RM jointly wrote the manuscript and contributed to the drafting. DG-N designed the contents of the revision and drafted the manuscript.

FUNDING

We would like to acknowledge the Medical Research Council, Wellcome Trust and Alzheimer's Research UK for funding the experimental work of the lab.

REFERENCES

Aguzzi, A., and Calella, A. M. (2009). Prions: protein aggregation and infectious diseases. *Physiol. Rev.* 89, 1105–1152. doi: 10.1152/physrev.00006.2009

Akiyama, H., Nishimura, T., Kondo, H., Ikeda, K., Hayashi, Y., and McGeer, P. L. (1994). Expression of the receptor for macrophage colony stimulating factor by brain microglia and its upregulation in brains of patients with Alzheimer's disease and amyotrophic lateral sclerosis. *Brain Res.* 639, 171–174. doi: 10.1016/0006-8993(94)91779-5

Alibhai, J., Blanco, R. A., Barria, M. A., Piccardo, P., Caughey, B., Perry, V. H., et al. (2016). Distribution of misfolded prion protein seeding activity alone does not predict regions of neurodegeneration. *PLoS Biol.* 14:e1002579. doi: 10.1371/journal.pbio.1002579

Alliot, F., Godin, I., and Pessac, B. (1999). Microglia derive from progenitors, originating from the yolk sac and which proliferate in the brain. *Dev. Brain Res.* 117, 145–152. doi: 10.1016/s0165-3806(99)00113-3

Askew, K., Li, K., Olmos-Alonso, A., Garcia-Moreno, F., Liang, Y., Richardson, P., et al. (2017). Coupled proliferation and apoptosis maintain the rapid turnover of microglia in the adult brain. *Cell Rep.* 18, 391–405. doi: 10.1016/j.celrep.2016.12.041

Baker, C. A., Martin, D., and Manuelidis, L. (2002). Microglia from Creutzfeldt-Jakob disease-infected brains are infectious and show specific mRNA activation profiles. *J. Virol.* 76, 10905–10913. doi: 10.1128/jvi.76.21.10905-10913.2002

Berbel, P., and Innocenti, G. M. (1988). The development of the corpus callosum in cats: a light- and electron-microscopic study. *J. Comp. Neurol.* 276, 132–156. doi: 10.1002/cne.902760109

Betmouni, S., Perry, V. H., and Gordon, J. L. (1996). Evidence for an early inflammatory response in the central nervous system of mice with scrapie. *Neuroscience* 74, 1–5. doi: 10.1016/0306-4522(96)00212-6

Bhaskar, K., Konerth, M., Kokiko-Cochran, O. N., Cardona, A., Ransohoff, R. M., and Lamb, B. T. (2010). Regulation of tau pathology by the microglial fractalkine receptor. *Neuron* 68, 19–31. doi: 10.1016/j.neuron.2010.08.023

Bishop, M. T., Bishop, M. T., Diack, A. B., Ritchie, D. L., Ironside, J. W., Will, R. G., et al. (2013). Prion infectivity in the spleen of aPRNP heterozygous individual with subclinical variant Creutzfeldt-Jakob disease. *Brain* 136, 1139–1145. doi: 10.1093/brain/awt032

Boche, D., Cunningham, C., Docagne, F., Scott, H., and Perry, V. H. (2006). TGFβ1 regulates the inflammatory response during chronic neurodegeneration. *Neurobiol. Dis.* 22, 638–650. doi: 10.1016/j.nbd.2006.01.004

Brown, D. R., Schmidt, B., and Kretzschmar, H. A. (1996). Role of microglia and host prion protein in neurotoxicity of a prion protein fragment. *Nature* 380, 345–347. doi: 10.1038/380345a0

Bruttger, J., Karram, K., Wortge, S., Regen, T., Marini, F., Hoppmann, N., et al. (2015). Genetic cell ablation reveals clusters of local self-renewing microglia in the mammalian central nervous system. *Immunity* 43, 92–106. doi: 10.1016/j.immuni.2015.06.012

Buljevac, D., Flach, H. Z., Hop, W. C., Hijdra, D., Laman, J. D., Savelkoul, H. F., et al. (2002). Prospective study on the relationship between infections and multiple sclerosis exacerbations. *Brain* 125, 952–960. doi: 10.1093/brain/awf098

Cady, J., Koval, E. D., Benitez, B. A., Zaidman, C., Jockel-Balsarotti, J., Allred, P., et al. (2014). *TREM2* variant p.R47H as a risk factor for sporadic amyotrophic lateral sclerosis. *JAMA Neurol.* 71, 449–453. doi: 10.1001/jamaneurol.2013.6237

Campbell, I. L., Eddleston, M., Kemper, P., Oldstone, M. B., and Hobbs, M. V. (1994). Activation of cerebral cytokine gene expression and its correlation with onset of reactive astrocyte and acute-phase response gene expression in scrapie. *J. Virol.* 68, 2383–2387.

Cardona, A. E., Pioro, E. P., Sasse, M. E., Kostenko, V., Cardona, S. M., Dijkstra, I. M., et al. (2006). Control of microglial neurotoxicity by the fractalkine receptor. *Nat. Neurosci.* 9, 917–924. doi: 10.1038/nn1715

Carroll, J. A., Striebel, J. F., Race, B., Phillips, K., and Chesebro, B. (2015). Prion infection of mouse brain reveals multiple new upregulated genes involved in neuroinflammation or signal transduction. *J. Virol.* 89, 2388–2404. doi: 10.1128/jvi.02952-14

Carroll, J. A., Striebel, J. F., Rangel, A., Woods, T., Phillips, K., Peterson, K. E., et al. (2016). Prion strain differences in accumulation of PrPSc on neurons and glia are associated with similar expression profiles of neuroinflammatory genes: comparison of three prion strains. *PLoS Pathog.* 12:e1005551. doi: 10.1371/journal.ppat.1005551

Chitu, V., Gokhan, S., Nandi, S., Mehler, M. F., and Stanley, E. R. (2016). Emerging roles for CSF-1 receptor and its ligands in the nervous system. *Trends Neurosci.* 39, 378–393. doi: 10.1016/j.tins.2016.03.005

Cho, S.-H., Sun, B., Zhou, Y., Kauppinen, T. M., Halabisky, B., Wes, P., et al. (2011). CX3CR1 protein signaling modulates microglial activation and protects against plaque-independent cognitive deficits in a mouse model of Alzheimer disease. *J. Biol. Chem.* 286, 32713–32722. doi: 10.1074/jbc.m111.254268

Colby, D. W., and Prusiner, S. B. (2011). Prions. *Cold Spring Harb. Perspect. Biol.* 3:a006833. doi: 10.1101/cshperspect.a006833

Collinge, J., and Clarke, A. R. (2007). A general model of prion strains and their pathogenicity. *Science* 318, 930–936. doi: 10.1126/science.1138718

Combrinck, M. I., Perry, V. H., and Cunningham, C. (2002). Peripheral infection evokes exaggerated sickness behaviour in pre-clinical murine prion disease. *Neuroscience* 112, 7–11. doi: 10.1016/s0306-4522(02)00030-1

Cuadros, M. A., Martin, C., Coltey, P., Almendros, A., and Navascués, J. (1993). First appearance, distribution and origin of macrophages in the early development of the avian central nervous system. *J. Comp. Neurol.* 330, 113–129. doi: 10.1002/cne.903300110

Cunningham, C. (2013). Microglia and neurodegeneration: the role of systemic inflammation. *Glia* 61, 71–90. doi: 10.1002/glia.22350

Cunningham, C., Boche, D., and Perry, V. H. (2002). Transforming growth factor β1, the dominant cytokine in murine prion disease: influence on inflammatory cytokine synthesis and alteration of vascular extracellular matrix. *Neuropathol. Appl. Neurobiol.* 28, 107–119. doi: 10.1046/j.1365-2990.2002.00383.x

Cunningham, C., Campion, S., Lunnon, K., Murray, C. L., Woods, J. F., Deacon, R. M., et al. (2009). Systemic inflammation induces acute behavioral and cognitive changes and accelerates neurodegenerative disease. *Biol. Psychiatry* 65, 304–312. doi: 10.1016/j.biopsych.2008.07.024

Cunningham, C., Campion, S., Teeling, J., Felton, L., and Perry, V. H. (2007). The sickness behaviour and CNS inflammatory mediator profile induced by systemic challenge of mice with synthetic double-stranded RNA (poly I:C). *Brain Behav. Immun.* 24, 590–602. doi: 10.1016/j.bbi.2006.12.007

Cunningham, C., Deacon, R. M., Chan, K., Boche, D., Rawlins, J. N., and Perry, V. H. (2005a). Neuropathologically disctint prion strains give rise to similar temporal profiles of behavioral deficits. *Neurobiol. Dis.* 18, 258–269. doi: 10.1016/j.nbd.2004.08.015

Cunningham, C., Wilcockson, D. C., Campion, S., Lunnon, K., and Perry, V. H. (2005b). Central and systemic endotoxin challenges exacerbate the local inflammatory response and increase neuronal death during chronic neurodegeneration. *J. Neurosci.* 25, 9275–9284. doi: 10.1523/jneurosci.2614-05.2005

Cunningham, C., Deacon, R., Wells, H., Boche, D., Waters, S., Diniz, C. P., et al. (2003). Synaptic changes characterize early behavioural signs in the ME7 model of murine prion disease. *Eur. J. Neurosci.* 17, 2147–2155. doi: 10.1046/j.1460-9568.2003.02662.x

Dai, X. M., Ryan, G. R., Hapel, A. J., Dominguez, M. G., Russell, R. G., Kapp, S., et al. (2002). Targeted disruption of the mouse colony-stimulating factor 1 receptor gene results in osteopetrosis, mononuclear phagocyte deficiency, increased primitive progenitor cell frequencies and reproductive defects. *Blood* 99, 111–120. doi: 10.1182/blood.v99.1.111

Dantzer, R., Bluthé, R. M., Layé, S., Bret-Dibat, J. L., Parnet, P., and Kelley, K. W. (1998). Cytokines and sickness behavior. *Ann. N Y Acad. Sci.* 840, 586–590. doi: 10.1111/j.1749-6632.1998.tb09597.x

Davalos, D., Grutzendler, J., Yang, G., Kim, J. V., Zuo, Y., Jung, S., et al. (2005). ATP mediates rapid microglial response to local brain injury *in vivo*. *Nat. Neurosci.* 8, 752–758. doi: 10.1038/nn1472

DeArmond, S. J., and Prusiner, S. B. (1995). Etiology and pathogenesis of prion diseases. *Am. J. Pathol.* 146, 785–811.

Deininger, M. H., Bekure-Nemariam, K., Trautmann, K., Morgalla, M., Meyermann, R., and Schluesener, H. J. (2003). Cyclooxygenase-1 and -2 in brains of patients who died with sporadic Creutzfeldt-Jakob disease. *J. Mol. Neurosci.* 20, 25–30. doi: 10.1385/jmn:20:1:25

del Río-Hortega, P. (1920). Estudios sobre la neuroglía. La microglia y su transformación en células en bastoncito y cuerpos gránulo-adiposos. *Trab. Lab Inv. Biol.* 18, 37–82.

del Río-Hortega, P. (1932). "Microglia," in *Cytology and Cellular Pathology of the Nervous System* (Vol. 2), ed. W. Penfield (New York, NY: P.B. Hoeber, Inc.), 483–534.

del Río-Hortega, P., and Penfield, W. G. (1927). Cerebral cicatrix: the reaction of neuroglia and microglia to brain wounds. *Bull. John Hopkins. Hosp.* 41, 278–303.

DellaGioia, N., Devine, L., Pittman, B., and Hannestad, J. (2012). Bupropion pre-treatment of endotoxin-induced depressive symptoms. *Brain Behav. Immun.* 31, 197–204. doi: 10.1016/j.bbi.2012.10.008

Ding, Z., Mathur, V., Ho, P. P., James, M. L., Lucin, K. M., Hoehne, A., et al. (2014). Antiviral drug ganciclovir is a potent inhibitor of microglial proliferation and neuroinflammation. *J. Exp. Med.* 211, 189–198. doi: 10.1084/jem.201 20696

Elmore, M. R., Najafi, A. R., Koike, M. A., Dagher, N. N., Spangenberg, E. E., Rice, R. A., et al. (2014). Colony-stimulating factor 1 receptor signaling is necessary for microglia viability, unmasking a microglia progenitor cell in the adult brain. *Neuron* 82, 380–397. doi: 10.1016/j.neuron.2014.02.040

Esiri, M. M., al Izzi, M. S., and Reading, M. C. (1991). Macrophages, microglial cells and HLA-DR antigens in fetal and infant brain. *J. Clin. Pathol.* 44, 102–106. doi: 10.1136/jcp.44.2.102

Falsig, J., Julius, C., Margalith, I., Schwarz, P., Heppner, F. L., and Aguzzi, A. (2009). A versatile prion replication assay in organotypic brain slices. *Nat. Neurosci.* 11, 109–117. doi: 10.1038/nn2028

Felton, L. M., Cunningham, C., Rankine, E. L., Waters, S., Boche, D., and Perry, V. H. (2005). MCP-1 and murine prion disease: Separation of early behavioural dysfunction from overt clinical disease. *Neurobiol. Dis.* 20, 283–295. doi: 10.1016/j.nbd.2005.03.008

Field, R., Campion, S., Warren, C., Murray, C., and Cunningham, C. (2010). Systemic challenge with the TLR3 agonist poly I:C induces amplified IFNα/β and IL-1β responses in the diseased brain and exacerbates chronic neurodegeneration. *Brain Behav. Immun.* 24, 996–1007. doi: 10.1016/j.bbi. 2010.04.004

Gao, H. M., Jiang, J., Wilson, B., Zhang, W., Hong, J. S., and Liu, B. (2002). Microglial activation-mediated delayed and progressive degeneration of rat nigral dopaminergic neurons: relevance to Parkinson's disease. *J. Neurochem.* 81, 1285–1297. doi: 10.1046/j.1471-4159.2002.00928.x

Giese, A., Brown, D. R., Groschup, M. H., Feldmann, C., Haist, I., and Kretzschmar, H. A. (1998). Role of microglia in neuronal cell death in prion disease. *Brain Pathol.* 8, 449–457. doi: 10.1111/j.1750-3639.1998.tb00167.x

Ginhoux, F., Greter, M., Leboeuf, M., Nandi, S., See, P., Gokhan, S., et al. (2010). Fate mapping analysis reveals that adult microglia derive from primitive macrophages. *Science* 330, 841–845. doi: 10.1126/science.1194637

Gomez Perdiguero, E., Klapproth, K., Schulz, C., Busch, K., Azzoni, E., Crozet, L., et al. (2015). Tissue-resident macrophages originate from yolk-sac-derived erythro-myeloid progenitors. *Nature* 518, 547–551. doi: 10.1038/nature13989

Gómez-Nicola, D., Fransen, N. L., Suzzi, S., and Perry, V. H. (2013). Regulation of microglial proliferation during chronic neurodegeneration. *J. Neurosci.* 33, 2481–2493. doi: 10.1523/JNEUROSCI.4440-12.2013

Gomez-Nicola, D., and Perry, V. H. (2015). Microglial dynamics and role in the healthy and diseased brain: a paradigm of functional plasticity. *Neuroscientist* 21, 169–184. doi: 10.1177/1073858414530512

Gómez-Nicola, D., Schetters, S. T., and Perry, V. H. (2014). Differential role of CCR2 in the dynamics of microglia and perivascular macrophages during prion disease. *Glia* 62, 1041–1052. doi: 10.1002/glia.22660

Grabert, K., Michoel, T., Karavolos, M. H., Clohisey, S., Baillie, J. K., Stevens, M. P., et al. (2016). Microglial brain region-dependent diversity and selective regional sensitivities to aging. *Nat. Neurosci.* 19, 504–516. doi: 10.1038/nn.4222

Gray, B. C., Siskova, Z., Perry, V. H., and O'Connor, V. (2009). Selective presynaptic degeneration in the synaptopathy associated with ME7-induced hippocampal pathology. *Neurobiol. Dis.* 35, 63–74. doi: 10.1016/j.nbd. 2009.04.001

Griffin, É. W., Skelly, D. T., Murray, C. L., and Cunningham, C. (2013). Cyclooxygenase-1-dependent prostaglandins mediate susceptibility to systemic inflammation-induced acute cognitive dysfunction. *J. Neurosci.* 38, 15248–15258. doi: 10.1523/JNEUROSCI.6361-11.2013

Guentchev, M., Siedlak, S. L., Jarius, C., Tagliavini, F., Castellani, R. J., Perry, G., et al. (2002). Oxidative damage to nucleic acids in human prion disease. *Neurobiol. Dis.* 9, 275–281. doi: 10.1006/nbdi.2002.0477

Guenther, K., Deacon, R. M., Perry, V. H., and Rawlins, J. N. (2001). Early behavioural changes in scrapie-affected mice and the influence of dapsone. *Eur. J. Neurosci.* 14, 401–409. doi: 10.1046/j.0953-816x.2001.01645.x

Guerreiro, R. J., Lohmann, E., Brás, J. M., Gibbs, J. R., Rohrer, J. D., Gurunlian, N., et al. (2013). Using exome sequencing to reveal mutations in *TREM2* presenting as a frontotemporal dementia-like syndrome without bone involvement. *JAMA Neurol.* 70, 78–84. doi: 10.1001/jamaneurol.2013.579

Guerreiro, R., Wojtas, A., Bras, J., Carrasquillo, M., Rogaeva, E., Majounie, E., et al. (2013). *TREM2* variants in Alzheimer's disease. *N. Engl. J. Med.* 368, 117–127. doi: 10.1056/NEJMoa1211851

Guillot-Sestier, M.-V., and Town, T. (2013). Innate immunity in Alzheimer's disease: a complex affair. *CNS Neurol. Disord. Drug Targets* 12, 593–607. doi: 10.2174/1871527311312050008

Guiroy, D. C., Wakayama, I., Liberski, P. P., and Gajdusek, D. C. (1994). Relationship of microglia and scrapie amyloid-immunoreactive plaques in kuru, Creutzfeldt-Jakob disease and Gerstmann-Sträussler syndrome. *Acta Neuropathol.* 87, 526–530. doi: 10.1007/s004010050119

Hafner-Bratkovič, I., Benčina, M., Fitzgerald, K. A., Golenbock, D., and Jerala, R. (2012). NLRP3 inflammasome activation in macrophage cell lines by prion protein fibrils as the source of IL-1β and neuronal toxicity. *Cell. Mol. Life Sci.* 69, 4215–4228. doi: 10.1007/s00018-012-1140-0

Hennessy, E., Gormley, S., Lopez-Rodriguez, A. B., Murray, C., Murray, C., and Cunningham, C. (2017). Systemic TNF-α produces acute cognitive dysfunction and exaggerated sickness behavior when superimposed upon progressive neurodegeneration. *Brain. Behav. Immun.* 59, 233–244. doi: 10.1016/j.bbi.2016. 09.011

Hickman, S. E., Kingery, N. D., Ohsumi, T. K., Borowsky, M. L., Wang, L. C., Means, T. K., et al. (2013). The microglial sensome revealed by direct RNA sequencing. *Nat. Neurosci.* 16, 1896–1905. doi: 10.1038/nn.3554

Hilton, K. J., Cunningham, C., Reynolds, R. A., and Perry, V. H. (2013). Early hippocampal synaptic loss precedes neuronal loss and associates with early behavioral deficits in three distinct strains of prion disease. *PLoS One* 8:e68062. doi: 10.1371/journal.pone.0068062

Hoek, R. M., Ruuls, S. R., Murphy, C. A., Wright, G. J., Goddard, R., Zurawski, S. M., et al. (2000). Down-regulation of the macrophage lineage through interaction with OX2 (CD200). *Science* 290, 1768–1771. doi: 10.1126/science.290.5497.1768

Holmes, C., Arranz, M., Collier, D., Powell, J., and Lovestone, S. (2003). Depression in Alzheimer's disease: the effect of serotonin receptor gene variation. *Am. J. Med. Genet. B Neuropsychiatr. Genet.* 119B, 40–43. doi: 10.1002/ajmg.b.10068

Holmes, C., Cunningham, C., Zotova, E., Culliford, D., and Perry, V. H. (2011). Proinflammatory cytokines, sickness behavior, and Alzheimer disease. *Neurology* 77, 212–218. doi: 10.1212/WNL.0b013e318225ae07

Holmes, C., Cunningham, C., Zotova, E., Woolford, J., Dean, C., Kerr, S., et al. (2009). Systemic inflammation and disease progression in Alzheimer disease. *Neurology* 73, 768–774. doi: 10.1212/WNL.0b013e3181b6bb95

Hsieh, C. L., Koike, M., Spusta, S. C., Niemi, E. C., Yenari, M., Nakamura, M. C., et al. (2009). A role for TREM2 ligands in the phagocytosis of apoptotic neuronal cells by microglia. *J. Neurochem.* 109, 1144–1156. doi: 10.1111/j.1471-4159.2009.06042.x

Hughes, M. M., Field, R. H., Perry, V. H., Murray, C. L., and Cunningham, C. (2010). Microglia in the degenerating brain are capable of phagocytosis of beads asncd of apoptotic cells, but do not efficiently remove PrPSc, even upon LPS stimulation. *Glia* 58, 2017–2030. doi: 10.1002/glia.21070

Hutchins, K. D., Dickson, D. W., Rashbaum, W. K., and Lyman, W. D. (1990). Localization of morphologically distinct microglial populations in the developing human fetal brain: implications for ontogeny. *Dev. Brain Res.* 55, 95–102. doi: 10.1016/0165-3806(90)90109-c

Hwang, D., Lee, I. Y., Yoo, H., Gehlenborg, N., Cho, J.-H., Petritis, B., et al. (2009). A systems approach to prion disease. *Mol. Syst. Biol.* 5:252. doi: 10.1038/msb. 2009.10

Jarrett, J. T., and Lansbury, P. T. Jr. (1993). Seeding "one-dimensional crystallization" of amyloid: a pathogenic mechanism in Alzheimer's disease and scrapie? *Cell* 73, 1055–1058. doi: 10.1016/0092-8674(93)90635-4

Jonsson, T., Atwal, J. K., Steinberg, S., Snaedal, J., Jonsson, P. V., Bjornsson, S., et al. (2012). A mutation in *APP* protects against Alzheimer's disease and age-related cognitive decline. *Nature* 488, 96–99. doi: 10.1038/nature11283

Kettenmann, H., Hanisch, U. K., Noda, M., and Verkhratsky, A. (2011). Physiology of microglia. *Physiol. Rev.* 91, 461–553. doi: 10.1152/physrev.00011.2010

Kettenmann, H., Kirchhoff, F., and Verkhratsky, A. (2013). Microglia: new roles for the synaptic stripper. *Neuron* 77, 10–18. doi: 10.1016/j.neuron.2012.12.023

Kierdorf, K., Erny, D., Goldmann, T., Sander, V., Schulz, C., Perdiguero, E. G., et al. (2013). Microglia emerge from erythromyeloid precursors via Pu.1- and Irf8-dependent pathways. *Nat. Neurosci.* 16, 273–280. doi: 10.1038/nn.3318

Klein, M. A., Frigg, R., Flechsig, E., Raeber, A. J., Kalinke, U., Bluethmann, H., et al. (1997). A crucial role for B cells in neuroinvasive scrapie. *Nature* 390, 687–690.

Kordek, R., Nerurkar, V. R., Liberski, P. P., Isaacson, S., Yanagihara, R., and Gajdusek, D. C. (1996). Heightened expression of tumor necrosis factor α, interleukin 1 α and glial fibrillary acidic protein in experimental Creutzfeldt-Jakob disease in mice. *Proc. Natl. Acad. Sci. U S A* 93, 9754–9758. doi: 10.1073/pnas.93.18.9754

Krabbe, K. S., Reichenberg, A., Yirmiya, R., Smed, A., Pedersen, B. K., and Bruunsgaard, H. (2005). Low-dose endotoxemia and human neuropsychological functions. *Brain Behav. Immun.* 19, 454–460. doi: 10.1016/j.bbi.2005.04.010

Kranich, J., Krautler, N. J., Falsig, J., Ballmer, B., Li, S., Hutter, G., et al. (2010). Engulfment of cerebral apoptotic bodies controls the course of prion disease in a mouse strain-dependent manner. *J. Exp. Med.* 207, 2271–2281. doi: 10.1084/jem.20092401

Kyrkanides, S., Tallents, R. H., Miller, J.-N., Olschowka, M. E., Johnson, R., Yang, M., et al. (2011). Osteoarthritis accelerates and exacerbates Alzheimer's disease pathology in mice. *J. Neuroinflammation* 8:112. doi: 10.1186/1742-2094-8-112

Lacroix, S., Feinstein, D., and Rivest, S. (1998). The bacterial endotoxin lipopolysaccharide has the ability to target the brain in upregulating its membrane CD14 receptor within specific cellular populations. *Brain Pathol.* 8, 625–640. doi: 10.1111/j.1750-3639.1998.tb00189.x

Laflamme, N., and Rivest, S. (1999). Effects of systemic immunogenic insults and circulating proinflammatory cytokines on the transcription of the inhibitory factor κBα within specific cellular populations of the rat brain. *J. Neurochem.* 73, 309–321. doi: 10.1046/j.1471-4159.1999.0730309.x

Lavin, Y., Winter, D., Blecher-Gonen, R., David, E., Keren-Shaul, H., Merad, M., et al. (2014). Tissue-resident macrophage enhancer landscapes are shaped by the local microenvironment. *Cell* 159, 1312–1326. doi: 10.1016/j.cell.2014.11.018

Lawson, L. J., Perry, V. H., and Gordon, S. (1992). Turnover of resident microglia in the normal adult mouse brain. *Neuroscience* 48, 405–415. doi: 10.1016/0306-4522(92)90500-2

Lawson, L. J., Perry, V. H., Dri, P., and Gordon, S. (1990). Heterogeneity in the distribution and morphology of microglia in the normal adult mouse brain. *Neuroscience* 39, 151–170. doi: 10.1016/0306-4522(90)90229-w

Li, J., Tang, Y., and Cai, D. (2012). IKKβ/NF-κB disrupts adult hypothalamic neural stem cells to mediate a neurodegenerative mechanism of dietary obesity and pre-diabetes. *Nat. Cell Biol.* 14, 999–1012. doi: 10.1038/ncb2562

Lin, H., Lee, E., Hestir, K., Leo, C., Huang, M., Bosch, E., et al. (2008). Discovery of a cytokine and its receptor by functional screening of the extracellular proteome. *Science* 320, 807–811. doi: 10.1126/science.1154370

Llewelyn, C. A., Hewitt, P. E., Knight, R. S., Amar, K., Cousens, S., Mackenzie, J., et al. (2004). Possible transmission of variant Creutzfeldt-Jakob disease by blood transfusion. *Lancet* 363, 417–421. doi: 10.1016/s0140-6736(04)15486-x

Llorens, F., López-González, I., Thüne, K., Carmona, M., Zafar, S., Andéoletti, O., et al. (2014). Subtype and regional-specific neuroinflammation in sporadic creutzfeldt-jakob disease. *Front. Aging Neurosci.* 6:198. doi: 10.3389/fnagi.2014.00198

Lyck, L., Santamaria, I. D., Pakkenberg, B., Chemnitz, J., Schrøder, H. D., Finsen, B., et al. (2009). An empirical analysis of the precision of estimating the numbers of neurons and glia in human neocortex using a fractionator-design with sub-sampling. *J. Neurosci. Methods* 182, 143–156. doi: 10.1016/j.jneumeth.2009.06.003

Lyons, A., Downer, E. J., Crotty, S., Nolan, Y. M., Mills, K. H., and Lynch, M. A. (2007). CD200 ligand receptor interaction modulates microglial activation *in vivo* and *in vitro*: a role for IL-4. *J. Neurosci.* 27, 8309–8313. doi: 10.1523/JNEUROSCI.1781-07.2007

Lyons, A., Lynch, A. M., Downer, E. J., Hanley, R., O'Sullivan, J. B., Smith, A., et al. (2009). Fractalkine-induced activation of the phosphatidylinositol-3 kinase pathway attentuates microglial activation *in vivo* and *in vitro*. *J. Neurochem.* 110, 1547–1556. doi: 10.1111/j.1471-4159.2009.06253.x

Mabbott, N. A., Williams, A., Farquhar, C. F., Pasparakis, M., Kollias, G., and Bruce, M. E. (2000). Tumor necrosis factor α-deficient, but not interleukin-6-deficient, mice resist peripheral infection with scrapie. *J. Virol.* 74, 3338–3344. doi: 10.1128/jvi.74.7.3338-3344.2000

Martínez-Muriana, A., Mancuso, R., Francos-Quijorna, I., Olmos-Alonso, A., Osta, R., Perry, V. H., et al. (2016). CSF1R blockade slows the progression of amyotrophic lateral sclerosis by reducing microgliosis and invasion of macrophages into peripheral nerves. *Sci. Rep.* 6:25663. doi: 10.1038/srep25663

Mass, E., Ballesteros, I., Farlik, M., Halbritter, F., Günther, P., Crozet, L., et al. (2016). Specification of tissue-resident macrophages during organogenesis. *Science* 353:aaf4238. doi: 10.1126/science.aaf4238

McHattie, S. J., Brown, D. R., and Bird, M. M. (1999). Cellular uptake of the prion protein fragment PrP106–126 *in vitro*. *J. Neurocytol.* 28, 149–159. doi: 10.1023/A:1007028323666

Minghetti, L., Greco, A., Cardone, F., Puopolo, M., Ladogana, A., Almonti, S., et al. (2000). Increased brain synthesis of prostaglandin E2 and F2-isoprostane in human and experimental transmissible spongiform encephalopathies. *J. Neuropathol. Exp. Neurol.* 59, 866–871. doi: 10.1093/jnen/59.10.866

Mittelbronn, M., Dietz, K., Schluesener, H. J., and Meyermann, R. (2001). Local distribution of microglia in the normal adult human central nervous system differs by up to one order of magnitude. *Acta Neuropathol.* 101, 249–255. doi: 10.1007/s004010000284

Miyazono, M., Iwaki, T., Kitamoto, T., Kaneko, Y., Doh-ura, K., and Tateishi, J. (1991). A comparative immunohistochemical study of Kuru and senile plaques with a special reference to glial reactions at various stages of amyloid plaque formation. *Am. J. Pathol.* 139, 589–598.

Mizuno, T., Doi, Y., Mizoguchi, H., Jin, S., Noda, M., Sonobe, Y., et al. (2011). Interleukin-34 selectively enhances the neuroprotective effects of microglia to attenuate oligomeric amyloid-β neurotoxicity. *Am. J. Pathol.* 179, 2016–2027. doi: 10.1016/j.ajpath.2011.06.011

Monier, A., Evrard, P., Gressens, P., and Verney, C. (2006). Distribution and differentiation of microglia in the human encephalon during the first two trimesters of gestation. *J. Comp. Neurol.* 499, 565–582. doi: 10.1002/cne.21123

Muhleisen, H., Gehrmann, J., and Meyermann, R. (1995). Reactive microglia in Creutzfeldt-Jakob disease. *Neuropathol. Appl. Neurobiol.* 21, 505–517. doi: 10.1111/j.1365-2990.1995.tb01097.x

Murray, C. L., Skelly, D. T., and Cunningham, C. (2011). Exacerbation of CNS inflammation and neurodegeneration by systemic LPS treatment is independent of circulating IL-1β and IL-6. *J. Neuroinflammation* 8:50. doi: 10.1186/1742-2094-8-50

Nandi, S., Gokhan, S., Dai, X. M., Wei, S., Enikolopov, G., Lin, H., et al. (2012). The CSF-1 receptor ligands IL-34 and CSF-1 exhibit distinct developmental brain expression patterns and regulate neural progenitor cell maintenance and maturation. *Dev. Biol.* 367, 100–113. doi: 10.1016/j.ydbio.2012.03.026

Nimmerjahn, A., Kirchhoff, F., and Helmchen, F. (2005). Resting microglial cells are highly dynamic surveillants of brain parenchyma *in vivo*. *Science* 308, 1314–1318. doi: 10.1126/science.1110647

Nuvolone, M., Sorce, S., Schwarz, P., and Aguzzi, A. (2015). Prion pathogenesis in the absence of NLRP3/ASC inflammasomes. *PLoS One* 10:e0117208. doi: 10.1371/journal.pone.0117208

O'Shea, M., Maytham, E. G., Linehan, J. M., Brandner, S., Collinge, J., and Lloyd, S. E. (2008). Investigation of mcp1 as a quantitative trait gene for prion disease incubation time in mouse. *Genetics* 180, 559–566. doi: 10.1534/genetics.108.090894

Olmos-Alonso, A., Schetters, S. T., Sri, S., Askew, K., Mancuso, R., Vargas-Caballero, M., et al. (2016). Pharmacological targeting of CSF1R inhibits microglial proliferation and prevents the progression of Alzheimer's-like pathology. *Brain* 139, 891–907. doi: 10.1093/brain/awv379

Paloneva, J., Kestilä, M., Wu, J., Salminen, A., Böhling, T., Ruotsalainen, V., et al. (2000). Loss-of-function mutations in TYROBP (DAP12) result in a presenile dementia with bone cysts. *Nat. Genet.* 25, 357–361. doi: 10.1038/77153

Paloneva, J., Manninen, T., Christman, G., Hovanes, K., Mandelin, J., Adolfsson, R., et al. (2002). Mutations in two genes encoding different subunits of a receptor signaling complex result in an identical disease phenotype. *Am. J. Hum. Genet.* 71, 656–662. doi: 10.1086/342259

Paolicelli, R. C., Bolasco, G., Pagani, F., Maggi, L., Scianni, M., Panzanelli, P., et al. (2011). Synaptic pruning by microglia is necessary for normal brain development. *Science* 333, 1456–1458. doi: 10.1126/science.1202529

Pelvig, D. P., Pakkenberg, H., Stark, A. K., and Pakkenberg, B. (2008). Neocortical glial cell numbers in human brains. *Neurobiol Aging* 29, 1754–1762. doi: 10.1016/j.neurobiolaging.2007.04.013

Perry, V. H. (2010). Contribution of systemic inflammation to chronic neurodegeneration. *Acta Neuropathol.* 120, 277–286. doi: 10.1007/s00401-010-0722-x

Perry, V. H. (2016). Microglia. *Microbiol. Spectr.* 4:3. doi: 10.1128/microbiolspec.MCHD-0003-2015

Perry, V. H., Cunningham, C., and Boche, D. (2002). Atypical inflammation in the central nervous system in prion disease. *Curr. Opin. Neurol.* 15, 349–354. doi: 10.1097/00019052-200206000-00020

Perry, V. H., Nicoll, J. A., and Holmes, C. (2010). Microglia in neurodegenerative disease. *Nat. Rev. Neurol.* 6, 193–201. doi: 10.1038/nrneurol.2010.17

Perry, V. H., and O'Connor, V. (2010). The role of microglia in synaptic stripping and synaptic degeneration: a revised perspective. *ASN Neuro* 2:e00047. doi: 10.1042/AN20100024

Perry, V. H., and Teeling, J. (2013). Microglia and macrophages of the central nervous system: the contribution of microglia priming and systemic inflammation to chronic neurodegeneration. *Semin. Immunopathol.* 35, 601–612. doi: 10.1007/s00281-013-0382-8

Pott-Godoy, M. C., Tarelli, R., Ferrari, C. C., Sarchi, M. I., and Pitossi, F. J. (2008). Central and systemic IL-1 exacerbates neurodegeneration and motor symptoms in a model of Parkinson's disease. *Brain* 131, 1880–1894. doi: 10.1093/brain/awn101

Prokop, S., Miller, K. R., and Heppner, F. L. (2013). Microglia actions in Alzheimer's disease. *Acta Neuropathol.* 126, 461–477. doi: 10.1007/s00401-013-1182-x

Prusiner, S. B. (1998). Prions. *Proc. Natl. Acad. Sci. U S A* 95, 13363–13383. doi: 10.1073/pnas.95.23.13363

Puoti, G., Giaccone, G., Mangieri, M., Limido, L., Fociani, P., Zerbi, P., et al. (2005). Sporadic Creutzfeldt-Jakob disease: the extent of microglia activation is dependent on the biochemical type of PrPSc. *J. Neuropathol. Exp. Neurol.* 64, 902–909. doi: 10.1097/01.jnen.0000183346.19447.55

Qin, L., Wu, X., Block, M. L., Liu, Y., Breese, G. R., Hong, J. S., et al. (2007). Systemic LPS causes chronic neuroinflammation and progressive neurodegeneration. *Glia* 55, 453–462. doi: 10.1002/glia.20467

Raivich, G., Haas, S., Werner, A., Klein, M. A., Kloss, C., and Kreutzberg, G. W. (1998). Regulation of MCSF receptors on microglia in the normal and injured mouse central nervous system: a quantitative immunofluorescence study using confocal laser microscopy. *J. Comp. Neurol.* 395, 342–358. doi: 10.1002/(SICI)1096-9861(19980808)395:3<342::aid-cne6>3.0.co;2-2

Rezaie, P., and Male, D. (1999). Colonisation of the developing human brain and spinal cord by microglia: a review. *Microsc. Res. Tech.* 45, 359–382. doi: 10.1002/(sici)1097-0029(19990615)45:6<359::aid-jemt4>3.3.co;2-4

Roe, A. D., Staup, M. A., Serrats, J., Sawchenko, P. E., and Rissman, R. A. (2011). Lipopolysaccharide-induced tau phosphorylation and kinase activity—modulation, but not mediation, by corticotropin-releasing factor receptors. *Eur. J. Neurosci.* 34, 448–456. doi: 10.1111/j.1460-9568.2011.07764.x

Saba, R., Gushue, S., Huzarewich, R. L., Manguiat, K., Medina, S., Robertson, C., et al. (2012). MicroRNA 146a (miR-146a) is over-expressed during prion disease and modulates the innate immune response and the microglial activation state. *PLoS One* 7:e30832. doi: 10.1371/journal.pone.0030832

Sasaki, A., Hirato, J., and Nakazato, Y. (1993). Immunohistochemical study of microglia in the Creutzfeldt-Jakob diseased brain. *Acta Neuropathol.* 86, 337–344. doi: 10.1007/bf00369445

Schafer, D. P., Lehrman, E. K., Kautzman, A. G., Koyama, R., Mardinly, A. R., Yamasaki, R., et al. (2012). Microglia sculpt postnatal neural circuits in an activity and complement-dependent manner. *Neuron* 74, 691–705. doi: 10.1016/j.neuron.2012.03.026

Schiffenbauer, J., Johnson, H. M., Butfiloski, E. J., Wegrzyn, L., and Soos, J. M. (1993). Staphylococcal enterotoxins can reactivate experimental allergic encephalomyelitis. *Proc. Natl. Acad. Sci. U S A* 90, 8543–8854. doi: 10.1073/pnas.90.18.8543

Schultz, J., Schwarz, A., Neidhold, S., Burwinkel, M., Riemer, C., Simon, D., et al. (2004). Role of interleukin-1 in prion disease-associated astrocyte activation. *Am. J. Pathol.* 165, 671–678. doi: 10.1016/s0002-9440(10)63331-7

Schulz, C., Gomez Perdiguero, E., Chorro, L., Szabo-Rogers, H., Cagnard, N., Kierdorf, K., et al. (2012). A lineage of myeloid cells independent of Myb and hematopoietic stem cells. *Science* 336, 86–90. doi: 10.1126/science.1219179

Ségaliny, A. I., Brion, R., Brulin, B., Maillasson, M., Charrier, C., Téletchéa, S., et al. (2015). IL-34 and M-CSF form a novel heteromeric cytokine and regulate the M-CSF receptor activation and localization. *Cytokine* 76, 170–181. doi: 10.1016/j.cyto.2015.05.029

Sharief, M. K., Green, A., Dick, J. P., Gawler, J., and Thompson, E. J. (1999). Heightened intrathecal release of proinflammatory cytokines in Creutzfeldt-Jakob disease. *Neurology* 52, 1289–1291. doi: 10.1212/wnl.52.6.1289

Sheng, J., Ruedl, C., and Karjalainen, K. (2015). Most tissue-resident macrophages except microglia are derived from fetal hematopoietic stem cells. *Immunity* 43, 382–393. doi: 10.1016/j.immuni.2015.07.016

Shi, Q., Xie, W.-L., Zhang, B., Chen, L.-N., Xu, Y., Wang, K., et al. (2013). Brain microglia were activated in sporadic CJD but almost unchanged in fatal familial insomnia and G114V genetic CJD. *Virol. J.* 10:216. doi: 10.1186/1743-422x-10-216

Shi, F., Yang, L., Kouadir, M., Yang, Y., Wang, J., Zhou, X., et al. (2012). The NALP3 inflammasome is involved in neurotoxic prion peptide-induced microglial activation. *J. Neuroinflammation* 9:73. doi: 10.1186/1742-2094-9-73

Sly, L. M., Krzesicki, R. F., Brashler, J. R., Buhl, A. E., McKinley, D. D., Carter, D. B., et al. (2001). Endogenous brain cytokine mRNA and inflammatory responses to lipopolysaccharide are elevated in the Tg2576 transgenic mouse model of Alzheimer's disease. *Brain Res. Bull.* 56, 581–588. doi: 10.1016/s0361-9230(01)00730-4

Sorce, S., Nuvolone, M., Keller, A., Falsig, J., Varol, A., Schwarz, P., et al. (2014). The role of the NADPH oxidase NOX2 in prion pathogenesis. *PLoS Pathog.* 10:e1004531. doi: 10.1371/journal.ppat.1004531

Soreq, L., UK Brain Expression Consortium, North American Brain Expression Consortium, Rose, J., Soreq, E., Hardy, J., et al. (2017). Major shifts in glial regional identity are a transcriptional hallmark of human brain aging. *Cell Rep.* 18, 557–570. doi: 10.1016/j.celrep.2016.12.011

Squarzoni, P., Oller, G., Hoeffel, G., Pont-Lezica, L., Rostaing, P., Low, D., et al. (2014). Microglia modulate wiring of the embryonic forebrain. *Cell Rep.* 8, 1271–1279. doi: 10.1016/j.celrep.2014.07.042

Stanley, E. R., and Heard, P. M. (1977). Factors regulating macrophage production and growth. Purification and some properties of the colony stimulating factor from medium conditioned by mouse L cells. *J. Biol. Chem.* 252, 4305–4312.

Stevens, B., Allen, N. J., Vazquez, L. E., Howell, G. R., Christopherson, K. S., Nouri, N., et al. (2007). The classical complement cascade mediates CNS synapse elimination. *Cell* 131, 1164–1178. doi: 10.1016/j.cell.2007.10.036

Stoeck, K., Bodemer, M., and Zerr, I. (2006). Pro- and anti-inflammatory cytokines in the CSF of patients with Creutzfeldt-Jakob disease. *J. Neuroimmunol.* 172, 175–181. doi: 10.1016/j.jneuroim.2005.10.008

Stoeck, K., Schmitz, M., Ebert, E., Schmidt, C., and Zerr, I. (2014). Immune responses in rapidly progressive dementia: a comparative study of neuroinflammatory markers in Creutzfeldt-Jakob disease, Alzheimer's disease and multiple sclerosis. *J. Neuroinflammation* 11:170. doi: 10.1186/s12974-014-0170-y

Szpak, G. M., Lewandowska, E., Lechowicz, W., Wierzba-Bobrowicz, T., Kulczycki, J., Bertrand, E., et al. (2006). The brain immune response in human prion diseases. Microglial activation and microglial disease. I. Sporadic Creutzfeldt-Jakob disease. *Folia Neuropathol.* 44, 202–213.

Takahashi, K., Prinz, M., Stagi, M., Chechneva, O., and Neumann, H. (2007). TREM2-transduced myeloid precursors mediate nervous tissue debris clearance and facilitate recovery in an animal model of multiple sclerosis. *PLoS Med.* 4:e124. doi: 10.1371/journal.pmed.0040124

Takahashi, K., Rochford, C. D. P., and Neumann, H. (2005). Clearance of apoptotic neurons without inflammation by microglial triggering receptor expressed on myeloid cells-2. *J. Exp. Med.* 201, 647–657. doi: 10.1084/jem.200 41611

Tamgüney, G., Giles, K., Glidden, D. V., Lessard, P., Wille, H., Tremblay, P., et al. (2008). Genes contributing to prion pathogenesis. *J. Gen. Virol.* 89, 1777–1788. doi: 10.1099/vir.0.2008/001255-0

Tanaka, M., Collins, S. R., Toyama, B. H., and Weissman, J. S. (2006). The physical basis of how prion conformations determine strain phenotypes. *Nature* 442, 585–589. doi: 10.1038/nature04922

Torres-Platas, S. G., Comeau, S., Rachalski, A., Bo, G. D., Cruceanu, C., Turecki, G., et al. (2014). Morphometric characterization of microglial phenotypes in human cerebral cortex. *J. Neuroinflammation* 11:12. doi: 10.1186/1742-2094-11-12

Tremblay, M. E., Lowery, R. L., and Majewska, A. K. (2010). Microglial interactions with synapses are modulated by visual experience. *PLoS Biol.* 8:e1000527. doi: 10.1371/journal.pbio.1000527

Van Everbroeck, B., Dewulf, E., Pals, P., Lübke, U., Martin, J.-J., and Cras, P. (2002). The role of cytokines, astrocytes, microglia and apoptosis in Creutzfeldt-Jakob disease. *Neurobiol. Aging* 23, 59–64. doi: 10.1016/s0197-4580(01)00236-6

Van Everbroeck, B., Dobbeleir, I., De Waele, M., De Leenheir, E., Lübke, U., Martin, J.-J., et al. (2004). Extracellular protein deposition correlates with glial activation and oxidative stress in Creutzfeldt-Jakob and Alzheimer's disease. *Acta Neuropathol.* 108, 194–200. doi: 10.1007/s00401-004-0879-2

Verney, C., Monier, A., Fallet-Bianco, C., and Gressens, P. (2010). Early microglial colonization of the human forebrain and possible involvement in periventricular white-matter injury of preterm infants. *J. Anat.* 217, 436–448. doi: 10.1111/j.1469-7580.2010.01245.x

Villa, V., Thellung, S., Corsaro, A., Novelli, F., Tasso, B., Colucci-D'Amato, L., et al. (2016). Celecoxib inhibits prion protein 90-231-mediated pro-inflammatory responses in microglial cells. *Mol. Neurobiol.* 53, 57–72. doi: 10.1007/s12035-014-8982-4

Vincenti, J. E., Murphy, L., Grabert, K., McColl, B. W., Cancellotti, E., Freeman, T. C., et al. (2015). Defining the microglia response during the time course of chronic neurodegeneration. *J. Virol.* 90, 3003–3017. doi: 10.1128/jvi.02613-15

Wadsworth, J. D., and Collinge, J. (2011). Molecular pathology of human prion disease. *Acta Neuropathol.* 121, 69–77. doi: 10.1007/s00401-010-0735-5

Wake, H., Moorhouse, A. J., Jinno, S., Kohsaka, S., and Nabekura, J. (2009). Resting microglia directly monitor the functional state of synapses *in vivo* and determine the fate of ischemic terminals. *J. Neurosci.* 29, 3974–3980. doi: 10.1523/JNEUROSCI.4363-08.2009

Walsh, D. T., Betmouni, S., and Perry, V. H. (2001). Absence of detectable IL-1β production in murine prion disease: a model of chronic neurodegeneration. *J. Neuropathol. Exp. Neurol.* 60, 173–182. doi: 10.1093/jnen/60.2.173

Wang, Y., Cella, M., Mallinson, K., Ulrich, J. D., Young, K. L., Robinette, M. L., et al. (2015). TREM2 lipid sensing sustains the microglial response in an Alzheimer's disease model. *Cell* 160, 1061–1071. doi: 10.1016/j.cell.2015.01.049

Wang, Y., Szretter, K. J., Vermi, W., Gilfillan, S., Rossini, C., Cella, M., et al. (2012). IL-34 is a tissue-restricted ligand of CSF1R required for the development of Langerhans cells and microglia. *Nat. Immunol.* 13, 753–760. doi: 10.1038/ni.2360

Wang, H., Yu, M., Ochani, M., Amella, C. A., Tanovic, M., Susarla, S., et al. (2003). Nicotinic acetylcholine receptor α7 subunit is an essential regulator of inflammation. *Nature* 421, 384–388. doi: 10.1038/nature01339

Wei, S., Nandi, S., Chitu, V., Yeung, Y.-G., Yu, W., Huang, M., et al. (2010). Functional overlap but differential expression of CSF-1 and IL-34 in their CSF-1 receptor-mediated regulation of myeloid cells. *J. Leukoc. Biol.* 88, 495–505. doi: 10.1189/jlb.1209822

Williams, A., Lucassen, P. J., Ritchie, D., and Bruce, M. (1997). PrP deposition, microglial activation, and neuronal apoptosis in murine scrapie. *Exp. Neurol.* 144, 433–438. doi: 10.1006/exnr.1997.6424

Williams, A. E., van Dam, A. M., Man-A-Hing, W. K., Berkenbosch, F., Eikelenboom, P., and Fraser, H. (1994). Cytokines, prostaglandins and lipocortin-1 are present in the brains of scrapie-infected mice. *Brain Res.* 654, 200–206. doi: 10.1016/0197-4580(94)92818-5

Yun, S.-W., Gerlach, M., Riederer, P., and Klein, M. A. (2006). Oxidative stress in the brain at early preclinical stages of mouse scrapie. *Exp. Neurol.* 201, 90–98. doi: 10.1016/j.expneurol.2006.03.025

Zhang, G., Li, J., Purkayastha, S., Tang, Y., Zhang, H., Yin, Y., et al. (2013). Hypothalamic programming of systemic ageing involving IKK-β, NF-κB and GnRH. *Nature* 497, 211–216. doi: 10.1038/nature12143

Zhang, H., Li, F., Yang, Y., Chen, J., and Hu, X. (2015). SIRP/CD47 signaling in neurological disorders. *Brain Res.* 1623, 74–80. doi: 10.1016/j.brainres.2015.03.012

Zhao, Y., Jaber, V., and Lukiw, W. J. (2016). Over-expressed pathogenic miRNAs in Alzheimer's disease (AD) and prion disease (PrD) drive deficits in TREM2-mediated Aβ42 peptide clearance. *Front. Aging Neurosci.* 8:140. doi: 10.3389/fnagi.2016.00140

Zhu, C., Herrmann, U. S., Falsig, J., Abakumova, I., Nuvolone, M., Schwarz, P., et al. (2016). A neuroprotective role for microglia in prion diseases. *J. Exp. Med.* 213, 1047–1059. doi: 10.1084/jem.20151000

Zhu, C., Herrmann, U. S., Li, B., Abakumova, I., Moos, R., Schwarz, P., et al. (2015). Triggering receptor expressed on myeloid cells-2 is involved in prion-induced microglial activation but does not contribute to prion pathogenesis in mouse brains. *Neurobiol. Aging* 36, 1994–2003. doi: 10.1016/j.neurobiolaging.2015.02.019

9

Acute Hypoxia Induced an Imbalanced M1/M2 Activation of Microglia through NF-κB Signaling in Alzheimer's Disease Mice and Wild-Type Littermates

Feng Zhang [1,2†], *Rujia Zhong* [1,2†], *Song Li* [1,2], *Zhenfa Fu* [1,2], *Cheng Cheng* [1,2], *Huaibin Cai* [3] *and Weidong Le* [1,2,4*]

[1]Liaoning Provincial Center for Clinical Research on Neurological Diseases, The First Affiliated Hospital, Dalian Medical University, Dalian, China, [2]Liaoning Provincial Key Laboratory for Research on the Pathogenic Mechanisms of Neurological Diseases, The First Affiliated Hospital, Dalian Medical University, Dalian, China, [3]Laboratory of Neurogenetics, National Institute on Aging, National Institutes of Health, Bethesda, MD, United States, [4]Collaborative Innovation Center for Brain Science, The First Affiliated Hospital, Dalian Medical University, Dalian, China

***Correspondence:**
Weidong Le
wdle@sibs.ac.cn

† These authors have contributed equally to this work.

Alzheimer's disease (AD) is the most common neurodegenerative disease mainly caused by abnormal tau phosphorylation, amyloid β (Aβ) deposition and neuroinflammation. As an important environmental factor, hypoxia has been reported to aggravate AD via exacerbating Aβ and tau pathologies. However, the link between hypoxia and neuroinflammation, especially the changes of pro-inflammatory M1 or anti-inflammation M2 microglia phenotypes in AD, is still far from being clearly investigated. Here, we evaluated the activation of microglia in the brains of $APP^{swe}/PS1^{dE9}$ transgenic (Tg) mice and their wild type (Wt) littermates, after a single episode of acute hypoxia (24 h) exposure. We found that acute hypoxia activated M1 microglia in both Tg and Wt mice as evidenced by the elevated M1 markers including cluster of differentiation 86 (CD86), tumor necrosis factor-α (TNF-α), interleukin-6 (IL-6), C-C motif chemokine ligand 2 (CCL2) and CCL3. In addition, the markers of M2 microglia phenotype (arginase-1 (Arg-1), CD206, IL-4 and IL-10) were decreased after acute hypoxia exposure, suggesting an attenuated M2 phenotype of microglia. Moreover, the activation of microglia and the release of cytokines and chemokines were associated with Nuclear factor-κB (NF-κB) induction through toll-like receptor 4 (TLR4). In summary, our findings revealed that acute hypoxia modulated microglia M1/M2 subgroup profile, indicating the pathological role of hypoxia in the neuroinflammation of AD.

Keywords: hypoxia, Alzheimer's disease, neuroinflammation, microglia, M1/M2 phenotypes

INTRODUCTION

Neuroinflammation plays pivotal roles in various neurodegenerative diseases, including Alzheimer's disease (AD). However, whether it is protective or harmful is still under debate. Although immune response is intended to be protective, excessive inflammatory response may cause tissue damage (Calsolaro and Edison, 2016). Senile plaques composed of amyloid-β (Aβ) polypeptides and neurofibrillary tangles (NFTs) made by abnormally phosphorylated tau proteins are pathological hallmarks of AD. In AD brain, Aβ and NFTs can directly cause neuronal damage and cell death. Indirectly, Aβ and NFTs can also activate immune response and lead to the release of inflammatory cytokines, chemokines, and neurotoxins including reactive oxygen species (ROS), nitric oxide (NO), and excitatory amino acids, which may contribute to the neuronal degeneration. Besides their neurotoxic effects, pro-inflammatory cytokines, such as interleukin-1β (IL-1β), tumor necrosis factor-α (TNF-α), and activated glial cells are believed to promote Aβ production (Azizi et al., 2014; Calsolaro and Edison, 2016). Senile plaques deposition is a result of imbalanced Aβ production and removal. Clearance of Aβ is a complex process mediated by various cellular machinery, including engulfment and degradation by resident microglia and infiltrating innate immune cells. In AD brain, aging and toxic conditions favor the chronic activation of microglia and reduce their phagocytic capacity and prolong neuroinflammation (Zuroff et al., 2017).

Microglia and astrocytes are the main immune cells in the central nervous system (CNS). As the resident macrophages of CNS, microglial cells act as the first and main form of active immune defense (Filiano et al., 2015). Activated microglia could execute many functions such as phagocytosis of toxic products, releasing of cytokines, promotion of repair and antigen-presenting (Morales et al., 2014). It is generally considered that microglia have two different phenotypes of activation: pro-inflammatory M1 and immunosuppressive M2. M1 phenotype, a classical activation, is associated with massive inflammatory response releasing IL-1β, TNF-α and expressing inducible nitric oxide synthase (iNOS). M2 includes the states of both alternative activation and acquired deactivation with an anti-inflammatory profile. Alternative activation responds to IL-4 or IL-13 and promotes resolution of inflammation and tissue repair. Acquired deactivation results from uptake of apoptotic cells or exposure to anti-inflammatory cytokines such as IL-10 and transforming growth factor-β (TGF-β) and alleviates acute inflammation (Orihuela et al., 2016; Tang and Le, 2016). In AD, microglia surrounding and infiltrating the Aβ plaques are generally activated as YM-1 positive M2 phenotype (Jimenez et al., 2008). Pro-inflammatory cytokines, such as interferon-γ (IFN-γ), IL-1β and TNF-α, which shift microglia to M1 activation, attenuate the phagocytosis of Aβ (Koenigsknecht-Talboo and Landreth, 2005). For misfolded tau protein, pro-inflammation cytokines can affect the tau pathological metamorphosis, increasing tau phosphorylation and accelerating tangle formation (Zilka et al., 2012).

Hypoxia, as one of the environmental risk factors, was reported to contribute to the pathogenesis of AD (Zhang and Le, 2010). Previous studies have indicated that hypoxia may increase Aβ production (Li et al., 2009), decrease Aβ degradation (Wang et al., 2011) and enhance tau phosphorylation (Gao et al., 2013; Yagishita et al., 2017), thereafter may further aggravate the pathological changes of AD. Hypoxia is also reported to be associated with neuroinflammation. The results of chronic hypoxia studies showed that intermittent hypoxia increased pro-inflammatory cytokines in microglia and in dorsal hippocampus of mice (Smith et al., 2013; Sapin et al., 2015). These results imply that neuroinflammation may be one of the mechanisms of hypoxia-induced cognitive impairment. Here, we determined the activation status of microglia and the secretion of cytokines after acute hypoxia exposure, and investigated the possible transition of M1/M2 phenotypes in AD mouse model.

MATERIALS AND METHODS

Animals and Hypoxic Treatment

Adult male $APP^{swe}/PS1^{dE9}$ transgenic (Tg) mice at the age of 6 months and their age-matched wild-type (Wt) littermates were included. Tg mice were purchased from the Jackson Laboratory (No. 004462, Bar Harbor, MA, USA). All the mice were housed under the condition of controlled light (12 h/12 h light/dark cycle), constant room temperature 22 ± 1°C and relative humidity 50 ± 10%. The mice were randomized into four groups: Tg with acute hypoxia (H-Tg), Tg with normoxia (N-Tg), Wt with acute hypoxia (H-Wt), Wt with normoxia (N-Wt), with 10 mice in each group. The hypoxia groups were exposed to a continued hypoxic condition (oxygen 7%) in a hypoxic chamber for 24 h. The normoxia groups were kept in a similar chamber with normoxic condition. After hypoxic exposure, the mice were immediately sacrificed for pathological and biochemical tests. Animal care and procedures were carried out in accordance with the Laboratory Animal Care Guidelines approved by the Institutional Animal Care Committee at Dalian Medical University. The protocol was approved by the Institutional Animal Care Committee at Dalian Medical University.

Gene Expression

Protocols for total RNA extraction, cDNA synthesis and quantitative real-time polymerase chain reaction (PCR) were described previously (Tang et al., 2014). Mice were sacrificed immediately after the 24-h hypoxia episode. Bilateral hippocampus (n = 4 in each group) were dissected and extracted for total RNA with RNAiso Plus (Total RNA extraction reagent; Takara, Shiga, Japan). According to Revertra Ace qPCR RT kit (Takara, Shiga, Japan) instructions, total RNA was synthesized to cDNA. Real-time PCR was performed with TransStart Top Green qPCR SuperMix (TransGen Biotech, Beijing, China) and monitored by the Real-time PCR System (Applied Biosystems 7500 Real-Time PCR Systems). The primer sequences were provided upon request as summarized in **Table 1**. The relative expression levels of each primer sequences mRNA were analyzed by the $2^{-\Delta\Delta Ct}$ algorithm normalizing to GAPDH and relative to the control groups.

Western Blotting

Western blotting was performed according to our previous protocols (Liu et al., 2015, 2016; Qiu et al., 2016). Bilateral hippocampus (n = 3 in each group) were dissected and sonicated in ice cold lysis buffer (P10013B, Beyotime Institute of

TABLE 1 | Primer sequences for real-time polymerase chain reaction (PCR).

	Forward (5′ to 3′)	Reverse (5′ to 3′)
GAPDH	TGTGTCCGTCGTGGATCTGA	TTGCTGTTGAAGTCG CAGGAG
IL-1β	AAGGGGACATTAGGCAGCAC	ATGAAAGACCTCAG TGCGGG
TNF-α	CCAGTGTGGGAAGCTGTCTT	AAGCAAAAGAGGAG GCAACA
TGF-β	CACTCCCGTGGCTTCTAGTG	CTTCGATGCGCTTC CGTTTC
CCL2	GCATCCACGTGTTGGCTCA	CTCCAGCCTACTCATTG GGATCA
CCR2	ACAGCTCAGGATTAACAGGGACTTG	ACCACTTGCATGCACA CATGAC
CCL3	GCTCAACATCATGAAGGTCTCC	TGCCGGTTTCTCTTA GTCAGG
CD86	ACGATGGACCCCAGATGCACCA	GCGTCTCCACGGAA ACAGCA
CD206	TCAGCTATTGGACGCGAGGCA	TCCGGGTTGCAAGT TGCCGT
Arg-1	CTTGCGAGACGTAGACCCTG	TCCATCACCTTGCC AATCCC
TLR4	AGGCAGCAGGTGGAATTGTATC	TCGAGGCTTTTCCATC CAATAG

Biotechnology, China). The lysate was centrifuged at 12,000× *g* for 10 min at 4°C. Then the supernatant fraction was collected for Western blotting analysis. Nucleoprotein and cytoplasmic protein were extracted with Nucleoprotein and Cytoplasmic Protein Extraction Kit (KeyGEN BioTECH, China). BCA Protein Assay Kit (T9300A, Takara, Shiga, Japan) was used to detect the protein concentration. The primary antibodies used in Western blotting analysis were as follows: Rabbit Anti-Nuclear factor-κB (NFκB; P105/P50; 13586S, 1:1000; Cell Signaling, Chicago, IL, USA), Mouse Anti-NFκB (P65; 6956S, 1:1000; Cell Signaling, Chicago, IL, USA), Rabbit Anti-inhibitor of NF-κB α (IκBα; 4814S, 1:1000; Cell Signaling, Chicago, IL, USA), Rabbit Anti-P-IκBα (9246S, 1:1000; Cell Signaling, Chicago, IL, USA), Rabbit Anti-GAPDH (14C10; 2118S, 1:1000; Cell Signaling, Chicago, IL, USA). The secondary antibodies were Anti-Rabbit/Mouse IgG, HRP-linked antibody (7076/7074, 1:2000, Cell Signaling, Chicago, IL, USA). The target protein bands were quantified by using FluorChem Q system (ProteinSimple, San Jose, CA, USA).

Immunostaining

For histological analysis, mice were anesthetized and perfused transcardially with cold phosphate buffer solution (PBS) and 4% paraformaldehyde (PFA). The whole brains were post-fixed with 4% PFA overnight and then dehydrated in 15% and 30% sucrose solutions. The brain tissues were then coated with Tissue-Tek optimal cutting temperature compound (OCT, Tissue-Tek, 4583, SAKURA, Torrance, CA, USA). All brain tissues were cut coronally into 10 μm coronal sections with Leica cryostat (CM-1950S, Leica, Germany). The slices were used for immunofluorescent staining with Ionized Calcium Binding Adapter Molecule 1 (Iba1) antibody (019-19741, 1:1000; Wako, Japan) to detect microglia. As for M1 or M2 staining, Anti-Mouse Cluster of Differentiation 86 (CD86) antibody (553689, 1:1000; BD Biosciences, San Jose, CA, USA) was used to detect M1 microglia, Mouse Macrophage Mannose Receptor (MMR)/CD206 antibody (AF2535, 1:40; R&D Systems, Minneapolis, MN, USA) was used to detect M2 microglia. For astrocytes, Glial Fibrillary Acidic Protein (GFAP) antibody (Z0334, 1:2000; Dako, Denmark) was used. The secondary antibodies were Anti-Rabbit IgG (H + L), F(ab')$_2$ Fragment (Alexa Fluor® 594/488 Conjugate; 8889S/4412S, 1:2000; Cell Signaling, Chicago, IL, USA); Cy3 Goat Anti-Rat IgG (H + L; A0507, 1:2000; Beyotime, China); Alexa Fluor® 555 Donkey Anti-Rabbit TgG (H + L; A0453, 1:2000; Beyotime, China) and IFKine Green, AffiniPure, Donkey Anti-Goat IgG (H + L; A24221, 1:2000; Abbkine Scientific, California, CA, USA). Pictures were visualized and photographed by a fluorescent microscope equipped with a DP80 CCD digital camera (Olympus, Tokyo, Japan). Three microscopic fields, 0.1 mm^2 per slice were captured with the same reference position of hippocampus. The integrated density of positive staining was measured and recorded by ImageJ software on 10 slices per animal ($n = 3$ in each group).

Statistical Analysis

All data were presented as mean ± standard error of the mean (SEM) values. Statistical significance was determined using one-way analysis of variance (ANOVA) by GraphPad Prism 7 (GraphPad Software Inc., La Jolla, CA, USA). The results were considered significant when p-value was less than 0.05. The n values in each figure legend represent the number of animals referred to the statistical analysis.

RESULTS

Acute Hypoxia Induced Microglial Activation in Mouse Hippocampus

To investigate whether acute hypoxia affected microglia activation status in AD mice, immunofluorescence staining was performed to detect microglia using anti-Iba1 antibody in hippocampus of each group. As shown in **Figure 1**, Iba1 positive staining increased in both H-Tg and H-Wt groups, compared with N-Tg and N-Wt groups, respectively. Quantitative analysis results showed that the integrated density in hypoxia groups increased significantly when compared to normoxia groups. Interestingly, the GFAP immunostaining revealed no alterations in hippocampal astrocytes after acute hypoxia exposure (**Figure 2**). All these data suggested that acute hypoxia induced microglial activation in hippocampus of both Tg and Wt mice.

Acute Hypoxia Altered M1/M2 Phenotype in Mouse Hippocampus

In order to further investigate the possible impacts of acute hypoxia on hippocampal M1/M2 phenotypes transition, double staining of CD86 (M1 marker) or CD206 (M2 marker) with Iba1 was performed. The fluorescent immunostaining together with quantitative analysis clearly showed an enhanced M1 but a declined M2 phenotype of microglia, as evidenced

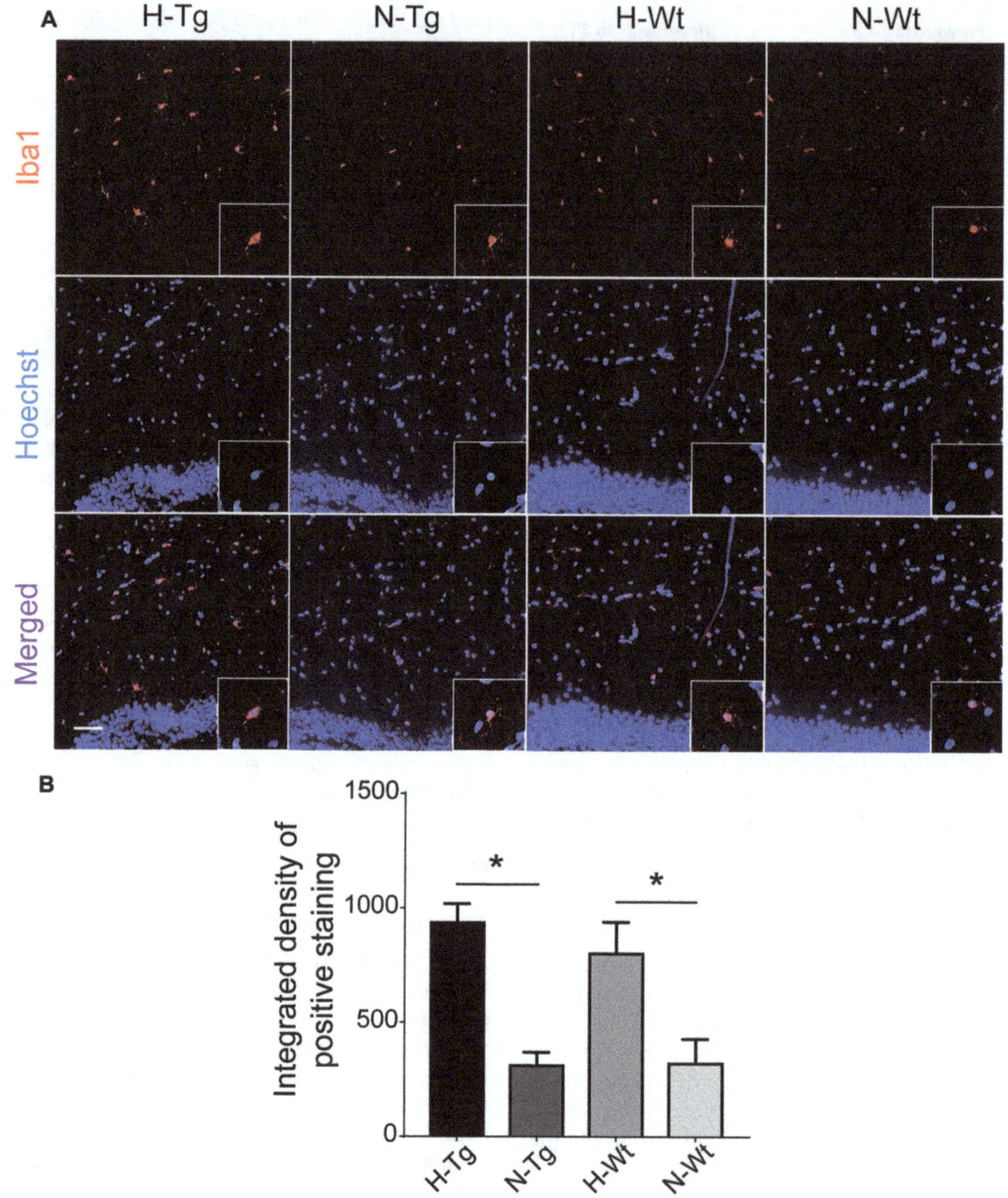

FIGURE 1 | Immunoflourescence staining of microglia cells in mouse hippocampus after acute hypoxia. Microglia were detected by ionized calcium binding adapter molecule 1 (Iba1) antibody **(A)**. Iba1 positive staining was increased in H-Tg and H-Wt groups vs. N-Tg and N-Wt groups, respectively **(B)**. Scale bar: 50 μm, $n = 3$ in each group. Data were the mean ± standard error of the mean (SEM) values. $^*p < 0.05$ by one-way analysis of variance (ANOVA).

by the increased CD86$^+$/Iba1$^+$ (**Figure 3**) and the decreased CD206$^+$/Iba1$^+$ (**Figure 4**) microglia cells, respectively.

The mRNA levels of M1/M2 markers were further evaluated by real-time PCR. Consistent with fluorescent immunostaining, our results showed that M1 marker CD86 was increased in H-Tg group, whereas mRNA levels of M2 markers CD206 and arginase-1 (Arg-1) were decreased in H-Tg and H-Wt groups (**Figure 5**). Consequently, the CD86/CD206 and CD86/Arg-1 ratios increased significantly in H-Tg group (**Figure 5**). These data indicated that acute hypoxia enhanced M1 activation and attenuated M2 activation in hippocampus.

Acute Hypoxia Changed the Cytokines and Chemokines Levels in Mouse Hippocampus

We next tested the mRNA levels of cytokines and chemokines in hypoxia-treated mice to confirm the above mentioned

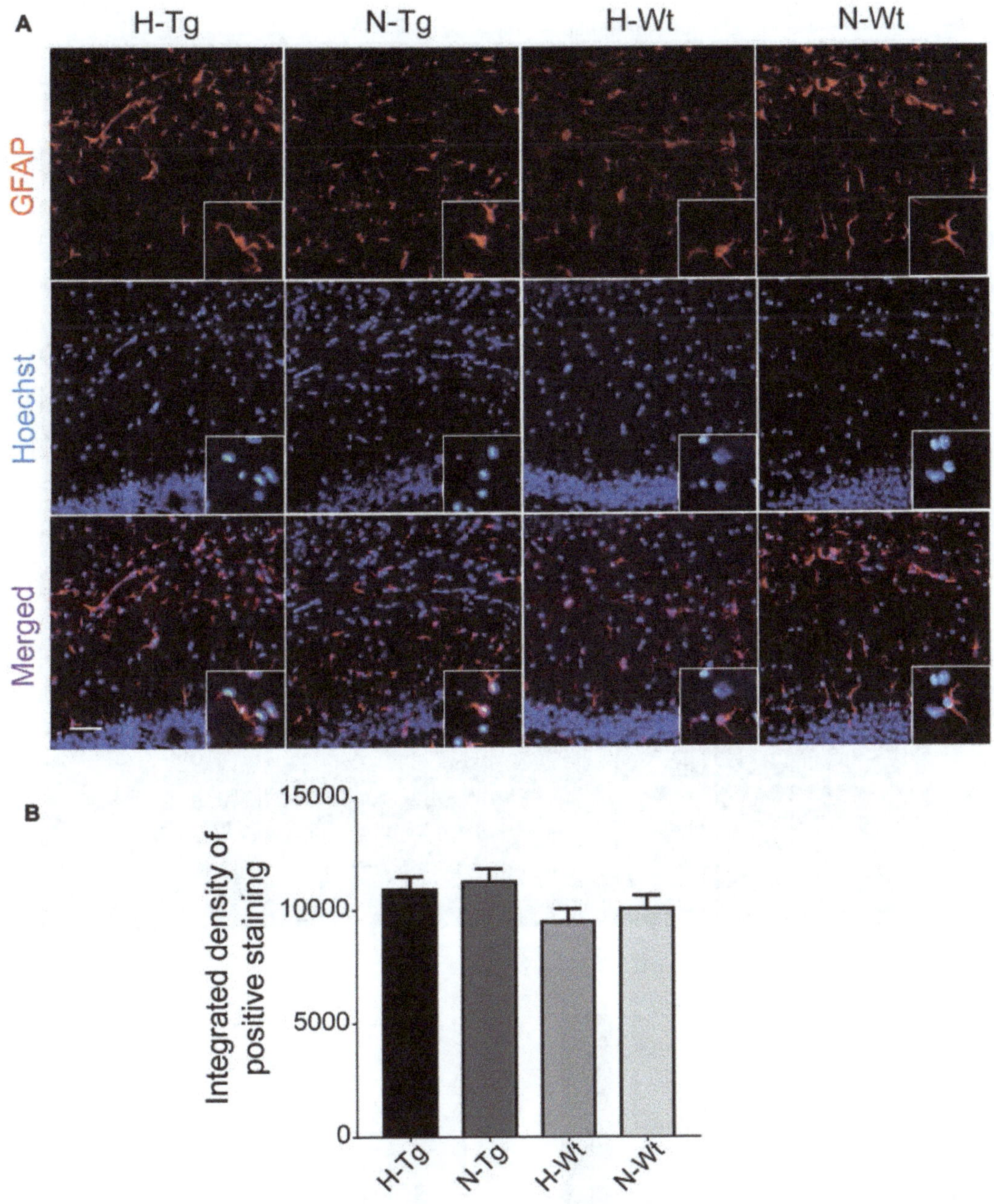

FIGURE 2 | Immunoflourescence staining of astrocytes in mouse hippocampus after acute hypoxia. Astrocytes were detected by glial fibrillary acidic protein (GFAP) antibody **(A)**. The GFAP immunostaining revealed no alteration in hippocampal astrocytes after acute hypoxia exposure **(B)**. Scale bar: 50 μm, *n* = 3 in each group. Data were the mean ± SEM values.

M1/M2 phenotype change. As shown in **Figure 6**, the relative mRNA levels of pro-inflammatory cytokines IL-6 and TNF-α were increased in H-Tg group. In contrast, the levels of two anti-inflammatory cytokines, IL-4 and IL-10, were decreased in hypoxia groups, compared to normoxia groups. These data implied that acute hypoxia induced an imbalanced M1/M2 phenotype which resulted in increased level of pro-inflammatory cytokines and decreased level of anti-inflammatory cytokines. Consistently, chemokine C-C motif ligand 2 (CCL2) and CCL3 were also increased in the mouse hippocampus of hypoxia groups. These chemokines were critical for the accumulation of activated glial cells, monocytes and lymphocytes, which might play important roles in neuroinflammation (Azizi et al., 2014).

Acute Hypoxia Activated NF-κB Signaling in Mouse Hippocampus

NF-κB family of transcription factors plays a crucial role in inflammation (Cao et al., 2006). Here, protein levels

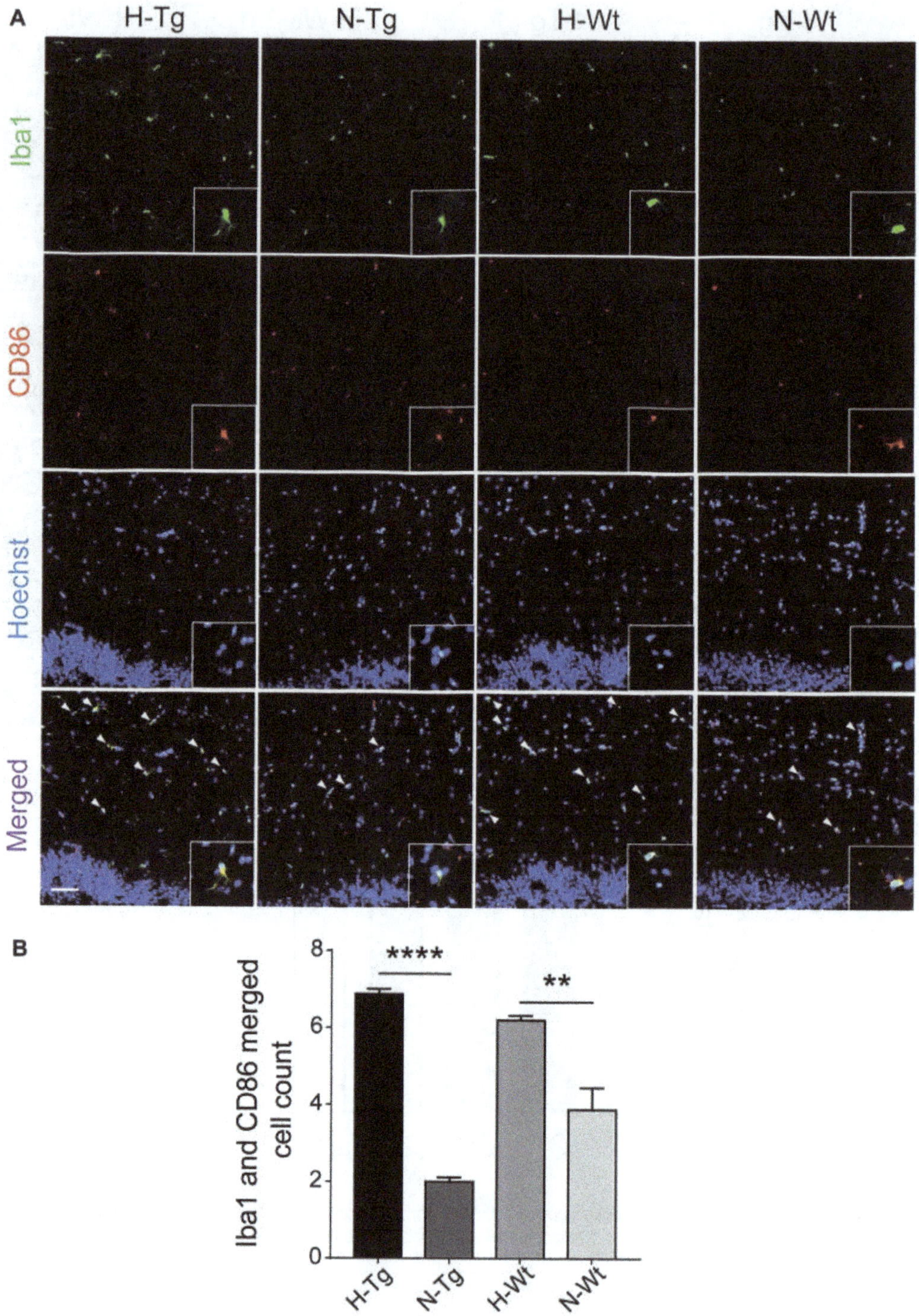

FIGURE 3 | Double immunostaining of cluster of differentiation 86 (CD86; M1 marker) and Iba1 positive microglial cells in hippocampus. CD86 (red) and Iba (green) co-stained microglial cells (yellow, arrow head) were increased significantly in H-Tg and H-Wt groups vs. N-Tg and N-Wt groups, respectively **(A,B)**. Scale bar: 50 μm, $n = 3$ in each group. Data were the mean ± SEM values. $^{**}p < 0.01$, $^{****}p < 0.0001$ by one-way ANOVA.

of NF-κB p50, p65 and IκBα were detected by western blotting. Our data showed that both NF-κB p50 and p65 levels were increased in H-Tg and H-Wt groups. In addition, the phosphorylation of the inhibitor of NF-κB, IκBα, increased significantly as evidenced by the increased ratio of phosphorylated IκBα (p-IκBα)/IκBα in H-Tg group, suggesting an activated NF-κB signaling pathway after acute hypoxia (**Figure 7**). Moreover, the nuclear NF-κB p65 was increased significantly in H-Tg group, which implied a translocation of NF-κB p65 into nucleus.

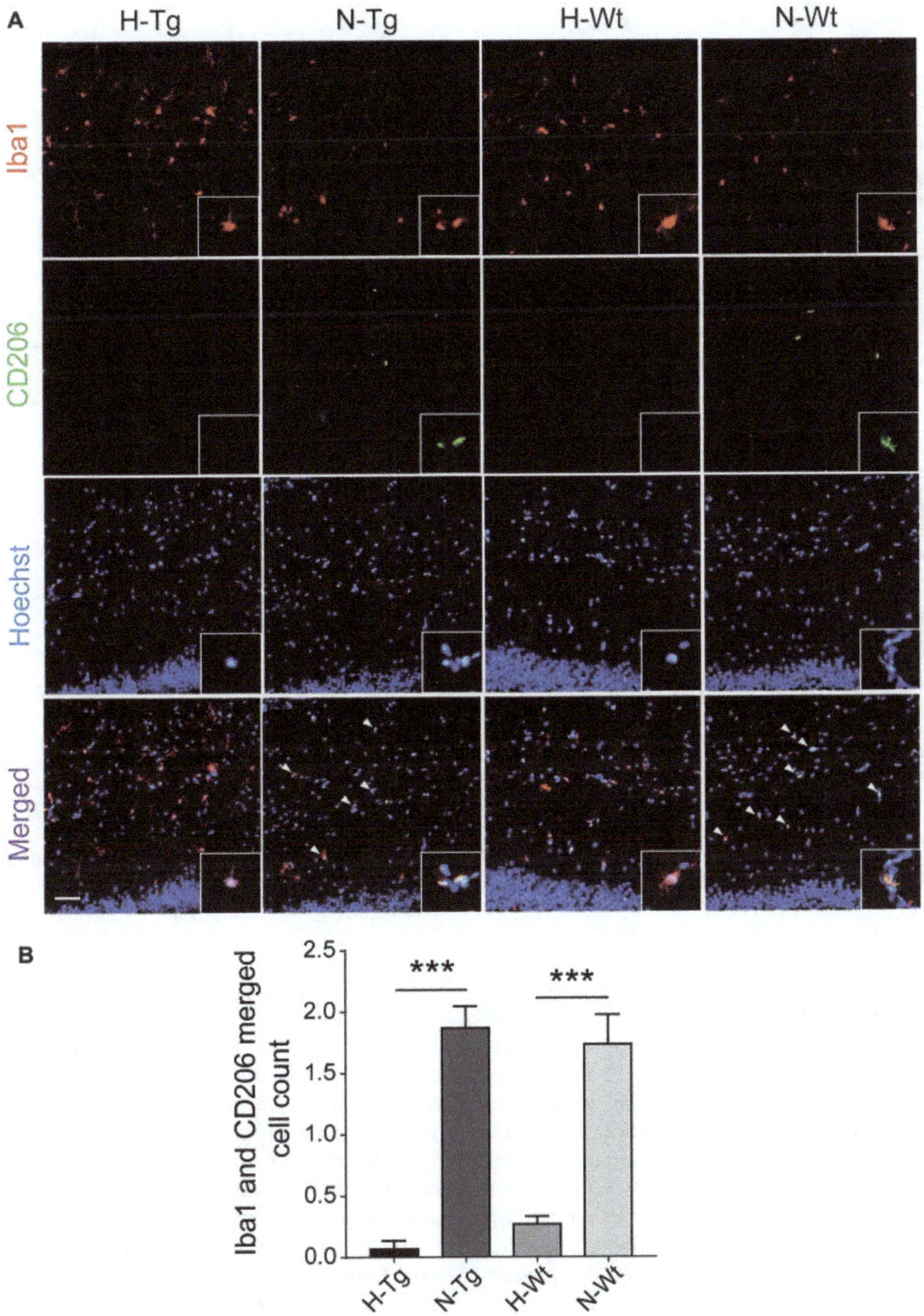

FIGURE 4 | Double immunostaining of CD206 (M2 marker) and Iba1 positive microglial cells in hippocampus. CD206 (green) and Iba (red) co-stained microglial cells (yellow, arrow head) were decreased significantly in H-Tg and H-Wt groups vs. N-Tg and N-Wt groups, respectively **(A,B)**. Scale bar: 50 μm, $n = 3$ in each group. Data were the mean ± SEM values. ***$p < 0.001$ by one-way ANOVA.

Since NF-κB could be activated by toll-like receptor 4 (TLR4; Ha et al., 2011), we then investigated the relative mRNA level of TLR4 with real-time PCR. As expected, both H-Tg and H-Wt group showed a significant increase of TLR4 mRNA level.

DISCUSSION

Hypoxia is believed to be an important risk factor for AD, contributing to the pathological changes of Aβ and tau in AD. We have previously reported that chronic hypoxia aggravated

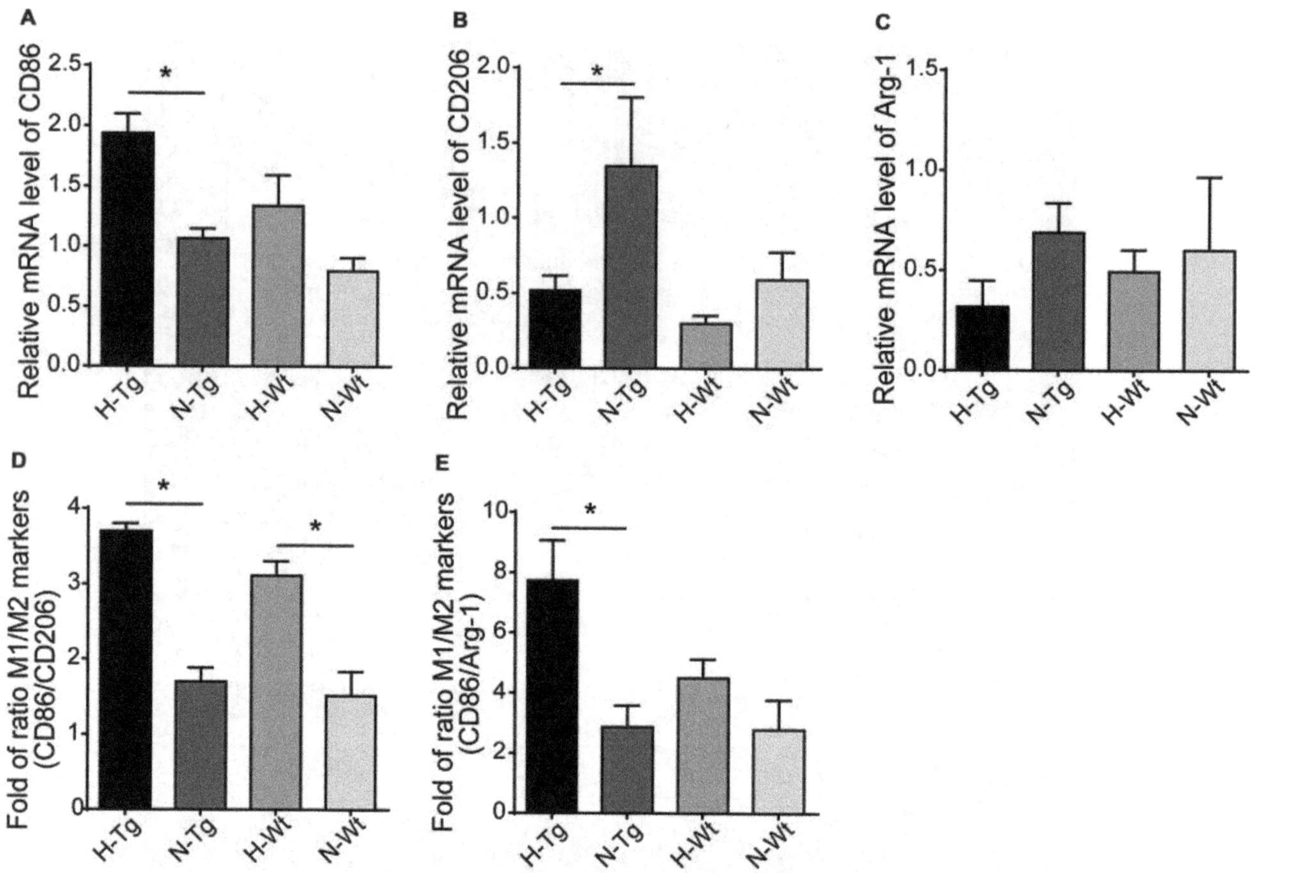

FIGURE 5 | mRNA levels of M1 and M2 markers were evaluated by real-time polymerase chain reaction (PCR). M1 marker, CD86, increased in H-Tg group **(A)** and M2 markers, CD206 and arginase-1 (Arg-1), decreased in hypoxia groups **(B,C)**. The ratio of CD86/CD206 **(D)** and CD86/Arg-1 **(E)** increased significantly in hypoxia groups, $n = 4$ in each group. Data were the mean ± SEM values. $^*p < 0.05$ by one-way ANOVA.

Aβ production though epigenetic modifications of γ-secretase (Liu et al., 2016) and induced autophagy in AD mouse model (Liu et al., 2015). Other studies have confirmed that hypoxia could increase tau phosphorylation (Zhang et al., 2014; Yagishita et al., 2017). Furthermore, our group and others have demonstrated that hypoxia can significantly activate microglia which is believed to play an important role in the pathogenesis of AD (Zhang et al., 2013; Sapin et al., 2015). It is known that pro-inflammatory cytokines released by microglia can increase Aβ production and decrease its clearance (Cai et al., 2014). Persistent increase of pro-inflammatory cytokines and chronic activation of microglia may cause chronic inflammatory status leading to neuronal damage and neurodegeneration (Calsolaro and Edison, 2016). With more knowledge of the interplay among hypoxia, neuroinflammation and AD pathogenesis, anti-inflammatory treatment is likely to be successful in AD. And more therapeutic targets could be found in studies of mechanisms of hypoxia-induced neuroinflammation.

Microglia can be activated as M1 and M2 phenotypes. The pro-inflammatory M1 phenotype predominates at the site of neuroinflammation and is associated with the release of pro-inflammatory cytokines and chemokines which may cause cell death and tissue damage. In contrast, M2 microglial phenotype appears later and is related to repair processes with anti-inflammatory property (Bolós et al., 2017). Previous study has reported that short-term hypoxia could increase the expression of pro-inflammatory cytokines and favored M1 activation of microglia *in vitro*. An increased iNOS and decreased Trem2 and Arg-1 have been reported in cultured primary rat microglia after 3-h hypoxia (Habib et al., 2014). Another study of neonatal hypoxic-ischemic brain injury in mice showed that CD86 positive cells were increased and relative proportion of CD206 positive cells were reduced after injury, indicating that hypoxia might facilitate M1 polarization and attenuate M2 activation (Hellström Erkenstam et al., 2016). Consistently, in current study, we found that acute hypoxia increased M1 marker CD86 and reduced M2 markers, CD206 and Arg-1, along with the increased levels of pro-inflammatory cytokines and the reduced levels of anti-inflammatory cytokines in hippocampus of AD mouse model.

Moreover, the levels of chemokines, CCL2 and CCL3, increased significantly in hypoxia groups. CCL2, also known as

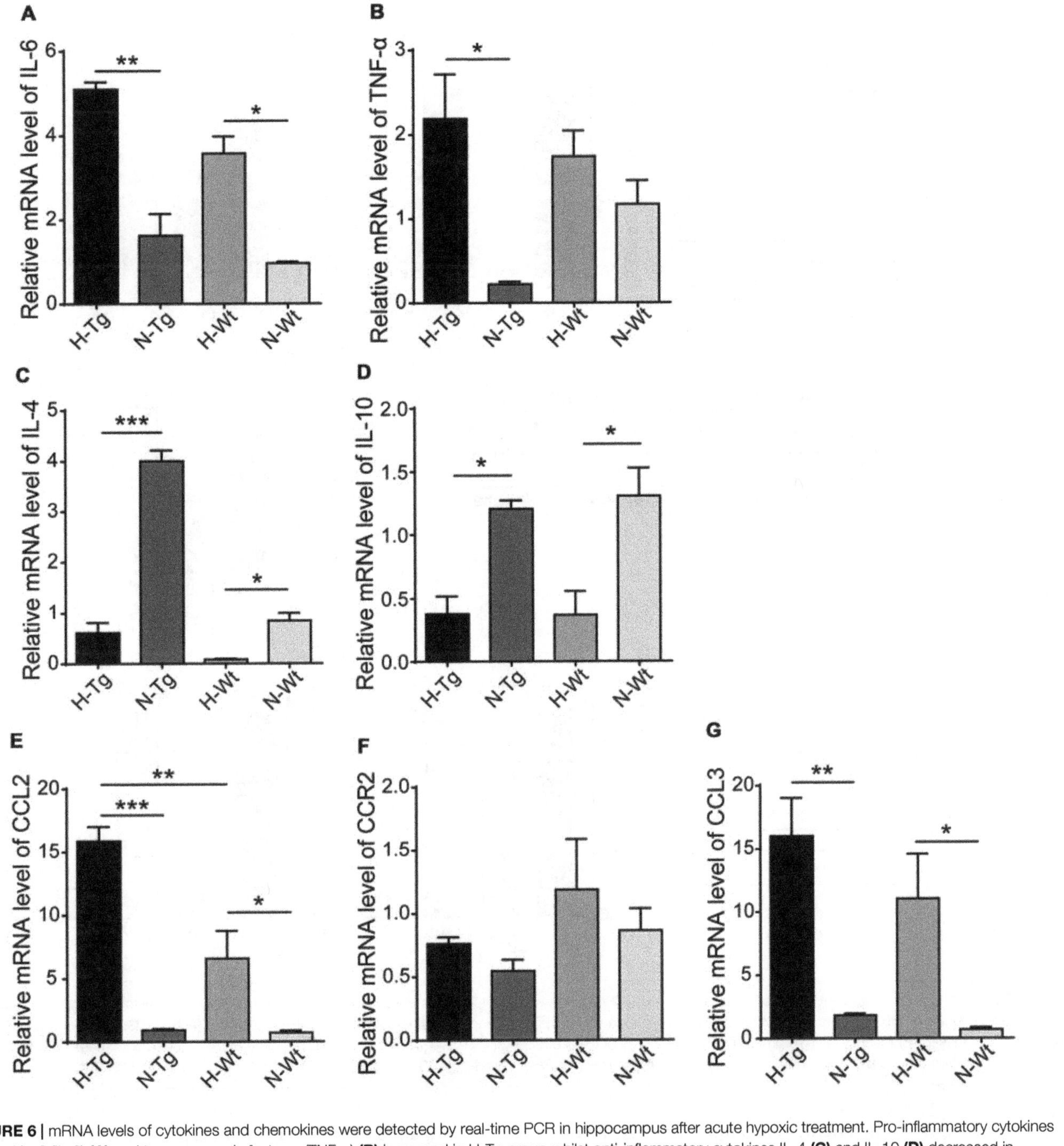

FIGURE 6 | mRNA levels of cytokines and chemokines were detected by real-time PCR in hippocampus after acute hypoxic treatment. Pro-inflammatory cytokines interleukin-6 (IL-6) **(A)** and tumor necrosis factor-α (TNF-α) **(B)** increased in H-Tg group whilst anti-inflammatory cytokines IL-4 **(C)** and IL-10 **(D)** decreased in hypoxia groups. Chemokines C-C motif ligand 2 (CCL2) **(E)** and CCL3 **(G)** increased in hypoxia groups, whereas the change of C-C motif chemokine receptor 2 (CCR2) remained modest **(F)**. $n = 4$ in each group. Data were the mean ± SEM values. *$p < 0.05$, **$p < 0.01$, ***$p < 0.001$ by one-way ANOVA.

monocyte chemoattractant protein 1 (MCP1), is a chemokine produced by neurons and glial cells and induces chemotaxis of monocytes and microglia, which contributes to the pathological microgliosis (Westin et al., 2012). Activated monocytes recruited into the brain are further differentiated into macrophages producing neurotoxic molecules (Azizi et al., 2014). Previous study reported that CCL2 overexpression induced microglial accumulation and facilitated Aβ oligomer formation, resulted in an enhanced plaque formation and accelerated memory deficits in APP/CCL2 bigenic mice (Kiyota et al., 2009). CCL2 overexpression was also reported to elevate the expression of apolipoprotein E and thus increase Aβ deposition by reducing the clearance (Yamamoto et al., 2005). CCL3 or human macrophage inflammatory protein 1α (MIP-1α)

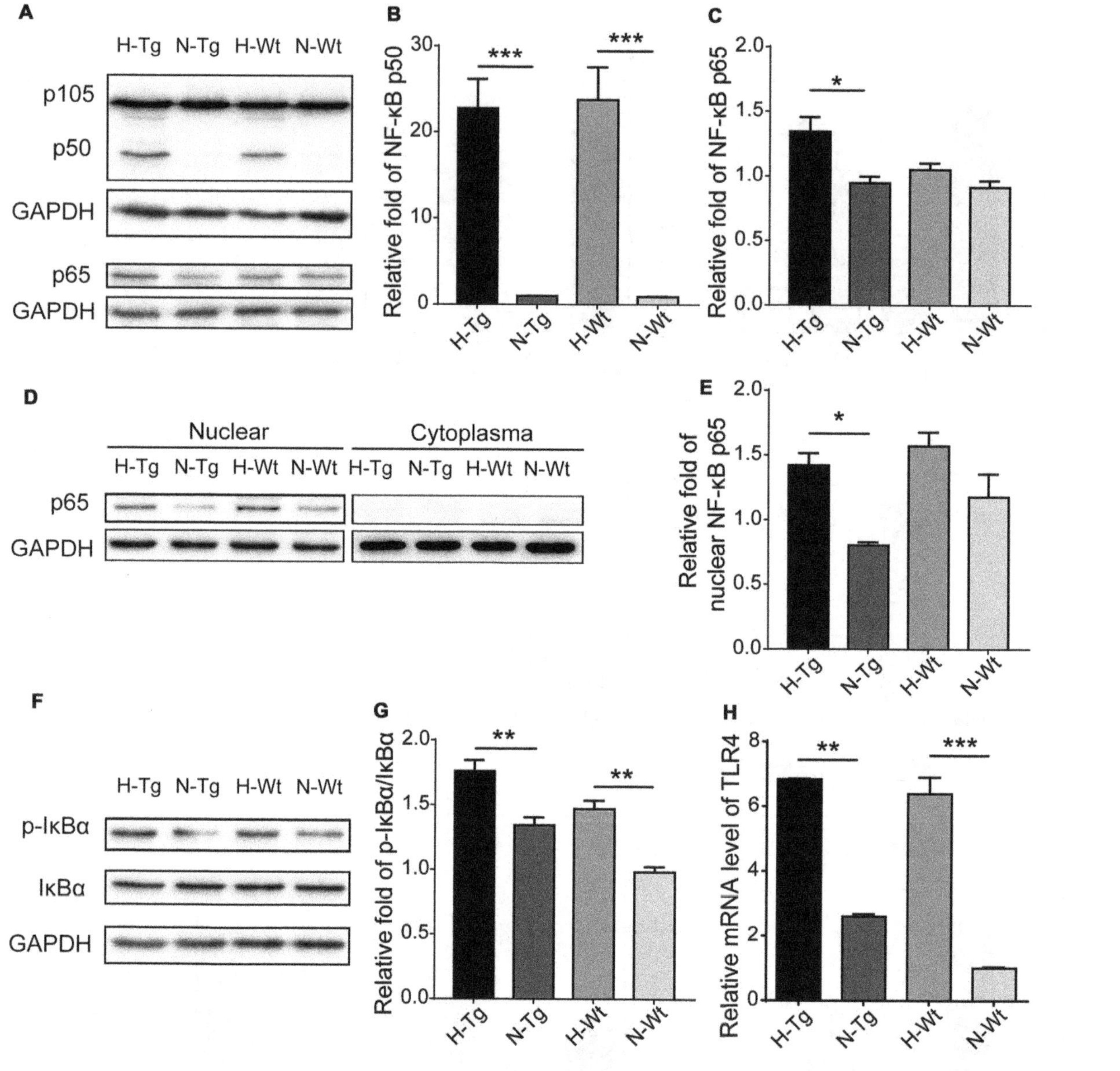

FIGURE 7 | Acute hypoxic treatment activated Nuclear factor-κB (NF-κB) pathway. Protein levels of key players in NF-κB pathway were tested with western blotting. Protein levels of NF-κB p65, p50 and p-IκBα/IκBα increased significantly in hypoxia group indicating activation of NF-κB pathway **(A,B,C,F,G)**. Nucleoprotein level of NF-κB p65 increased significantly in H-Tg group **(D,E)**. mRNA level of toll-like receptor 4 (TLR4) was evaluated by real-time PCR. Significant increase of TLR4 was observed in hypoxia groups **(H)**. $n = 3$ in each group. Data were the mean ± SEM values. *$p < 0.05$, **$p < 0.01$, ***$p < 0.001$, by one-way ANOVA.

is a member of β-chemokine subfamily and is involved in the recruitment and activation of polymorphonuclear leukocytes. Previous study found that AD patients had a higher level of CCL3 in peripheral T lymphocytes compared to age-matched healthy controls (Man et al., 2007). CCL3 induced the expression of CCR5, a potential receptor of CCL3, on brain microvascular endothelial cells constituting the blood-brain barrier and resulted in an increased T cells transendothelial migration from blood to the brain (Man et al., 2007). Then, the accumulated T cells might lead to the increased levels of pro-inflammatory cytokines and cause chronic inflammation, which enhanced neurotoxicity and impaired functions of microglia (Mietelska-Porowska and Wojda, 2017). T cell infiltrating the brain might also contribute to the cognitive impairment of tau pathology. One recent study found that hippocampal T cells might modulate microglial and/or astrocytic activation status and lead to detrimental impact on synaptic plasticity (Laurent et al., 2017).

NF-κB family of transcription factors plays a crucial role in inflammation, immunity and cell proliferation (Viatour et al., 2005). Activation of NF-κB pathway is triggered by a variety of extracellular stimuli and recruited IκB-kinase (IKK) complex. Once activated, the IKK complex phosphorylates IκB proteins, which leads to the proteasome-mediated degradation of IκB proteins and allows the NF-κB to translocate to the nucleus to execute transcription of target genes (Viatour et al., 2005; Kawai and Akira, 2007). In the present study, we further investigated protein levels of key players in NF-κB pathway and found that both NF-κB p50 and p65 subunit and nucleoprotein level of NF-κB p65 increased in hypoxia groups with a higher ratio of p-IκBα/IκBα, indicating that the increased pro-inflammatory cytokines and chemokines might be associated with activated NF-κB pathway. TLR4 is a type-I transmembrane receptor expressed in neurons, astrocytes and microglia. Its activation is involved in microglia-mediated inflammation responding to many insults and leads to the production and release of cytokines including IL-1β, IL-6, TNF-α and iNOS (Smith et al., 2013). NF-κB is one of the most important downstream transcription factors in TLR signaling pathways. TLR4 signaling induces the phosphorylation of IκB and the subsequent degradation, which promotes the nuclear translocation of NF-κB, stimulating the transcription of various target genes (Ha et al., 2011). Previous studies showed that chronic intermittent hypoxia activated NF-κB pathway through TLR4 signaling and might contribute to hippocampal neuronal damage (Smith et al., 2013; Deng et al., 2015). In our study, we found an increased mRNA level of TLR4 in acute hypoxia groups which might indicate that acute hypoxia could activate NF-κB pathway through TLR4 signaling.

In summary, here we investigated microglia activation and cytokines levels in hippocampus of APP/PS1 mouse model after acute hypoxic treatment. We found that acute hypoxia favored M1 activation and attenuated M2 activation, which resulted in the release of pro-inflammatory cytokines and chemokines, such as IL-6, TNF-α, CCL2 and CCL3, and contributed to the pathogenesis of AD. Acute hypoxia induced activation of microglia might be associated with the activation of NF-κB pathway through TLR4 signaling.

AUTHOR CONTRIBUTIONS

WL designed the project of this manuscript; FZ, RZ and ZF carried out all the experiments. FZ, RZ, SL and CC contributed to statistical analyses and results interpretation. FZ, RZ, ZF and SL contributed to drafting of the manuscript. RZ, SL, HC and WL revised the manuscript. WL contributed to research concept, research administration. All authors edited and approved the final version of the manuscript.

ACKNOWLEDGMENTS

This work was supported in part by funding from the National Natural Sciences Foundation of China (NSFC 81430021 and 81370470), the Program for Liaoning Innovative Research Team in University (LT2015009), Liaoning Science and Technology Project (2015225008), and the intramural program of National Institute on Aging, National Institutes of Health, USA (1-ZIA-AG000959).

REFERENCES

Azizi, G., Khannazer, N., and Mirshafiey, A. (2014). The potential role of chemokines in Alzheimer's disease pathogenesis. *Am. J. Alzheimers Dis. Other Demen.* 29, 415–425. doi: 10.1177/1533317513518651

Bolós, M., Perea, J. R., and Avila, J. (2017). Alzheimer's disease as an inflammatory disease. *Biomol. Concepts* 8, 37–43. doi: 10.1515/bmc-2016-0029

Cai, Z., Hussain, M. D., and Yan, L. J. (2014). Microglia, neuroinflammation, and beta-amyloid protein in Alzheimer's disease. *Int. J. Neurosci.* 124, 307–321. doi: 10.3109/00207454.2013.833510

Calsolaro, V., and Edison, P. (2016). Neuroinflammation in Alzheimer's disease: current evidence and future directions. *Alzheimers Dement.* 12, 719–732. doi: 10.1016/j.jalz.2016.02.010

Cao, S., Zhang, X., Edwards, J. P., and Mosser, D. M. (2006). NF-kappaB1 (p50) homodimers differentially regulate pro- and anti-inflammatory cytokines in macrophages. *J. Biol. Chem.* 281, 26041–26050. doi: 10.1074/jbc.m602222200

Deng, Y., Yuan, X., Guo, X. L., Zhu, D., Pan, Y. Y., and Liu, H. G. (2015). Efficacy of atorvastatin on hippocampal neuronal damage caused by chronic intermittent hypoxia: involving TLR4 and its downstream signaling pathway. *Respir. Physiol. Neurobiol.* 218, 57–63. doi: 10.1016/j.resp.2015.07.006

Filiano, A. J., Gadani, S. P., and Kipnis, J. (2015). Interactions of innate and adaptive immunity in brain development and function. *Brain Res.* 1617, 18–27. doi: 10.1016/j.brainres.2014.07.050

Gao, L., Tian, S., Gao, H., and Xu, Y. (2013). Hypoxia increases Aβ-induced tau phosphorylation by calpain and promotes behavioral consequences in AD transgenic mice. *J. Mol. Neurosci.* 51, 138–147. doi: 10.1007/s12031-013-9966-y

Ha, T., Liu, L., Kelley, J., Kao, R., Williams, D., and Li, C. (2011). Toll-like receptors: new players in myocardial ischemia/reperfusion injury. *Antioxid. Redox Signal.* 15, 1875–1893. doi: 10.1089/ars.2010.3723

Habib, P., Slowik, A., Zendedel, A., Johann, S., Dang, J., and Beyer, C. (2014). Regulation of hypoxia-induced inflammatory responses and M1-M2 phenotype switch of primary rat microglia by sex steroids. *J. Mol. Neurosci.* 52, 277–285. doi: 10.1007/s12031-013-0137-y

Hellström Erkenstam, N., Smith, P. L., Fleiss, B., Nair, S., Svedin, P., Wang, W., et al. (2016). Temporal characterization of microglia/macrophage phenotypes in a mouse model of neonatal hypoxic-ischemic brain injury. *Front. Cell. Neurosci.* 10:286. doi: 10.3389/fncel.2016.00286

Jimenez, S., Baglietto-Vargas, D., Caballero, C., Moreno-Gonzalez, I., Torres, M., Sanchez-Varo, R., et al. (2008). Inflammatory response in the hippocampus of PS1M146L/APP751SL mouse model of Alzheimer's disease: age-dependent switch in the microglial phenotype from alternative to classic. *J. Neurosci.* 28, 11650–11661. doi: 10.1523/jneurosci.3024-08.2008

Kawai, T., and Akira, S. (2007). Signaling to NF-κB by Toll-like receptors. *Trends Mol. Med.* 13, 460–469. doi: 10.1016/j.molmed.2007.09.002

Kiyota, T., Yamamoto, M., Xiong, H., Lambert, M. P., Klein, W. L., Gendelman, H. E., et al. (2009). CCL2 accelerates microglia-mediated Aβ oligomer formation and progression of neurocognitive dysfunction. *PLoS One* 4:e6197. doi: 10.1371/journal.pone.0006197

Koenigsknecht-Talboo, J., and Landreth, G. E. (2005). Microglial phagocytosis induced by fibrillar β-amyloid and IgGs are differentially regulated by proinflammatory cytokines. *J. Neurosci.* 25, 8240–8249. doi: 10.1523/jneurosci.1808-05.2005

Laurent, C., Dorothée, G., Hunot, S., Martin, E., Monnet, Y., Duchamp, M., et al. (2017). Hippocampal T cell infiltration promotes neuroinflammation and cognitive decline in a mouse model of tauopathy. *Brain* 140, 184–200. doi: 10.1093/brain/aww270

Li, L., Zhang, X., Yang, D., Luo, G., Chen, S., and Le, W. (2009). Hypoxia increases Aβ generation by altering β- and γ-cleavage of APP. *Neurobiol. Aging* 30, 1091–1098. doi: 10.1016/j.neurobiolaging.2007.10.011

Liu, H., Qiu, H., Xiao, Q., and Le, W. (2015). Chronic hypoxia-induced autophagy aggravates the neuropathology of Alzheimer's disease through AMPK-mTOR signaling in the APPSwe/PS1dE9 mouse model. *J. Alzheimers Dis.* 48, 1019–1032. doi: 10.3233/jad-150303

Liu, H., Qiu, H., Yang, J., Ni, J., and Le, W. (2016). Chronic hypoxia facilitates Alzheimer's disease through demethylation of γ-secretase by downregulating DNA methyltransferase 3b. *Alzheimers Dement.* 12, 130–143. doi: 10.1016/j.jalz.2015.05.019

Man, S.-M., Ma, Y.-R., Shang, D.-S., Zhao, W.-D., Li, B., Guo, D.-W., et al. (2007). Peripheral T cells overexpress MIP-1α to enhance its transendothelial migration in Alzheimer's disease. *Neurobiol. Aging* 28, 485–496. doi: 10.1016/j.neurobiolaging.2006.02.013

Mietelska-Porowska, A., and Wojda, U. (2017). T lymphocytes and inflammatory mediators in the interplay between brain and blood in Alzheimer's disease: potential pools of new biomarkers. *J. Immunol. Res.* 2017:4626540. doi: 10.1155/2017/4626540

Morales, I., Guzmán-Martínez, L., Cerda-Troncoso, C., Farías, G. A., and Maccioni, R. B. (2014). Neuroinflammation in the pathogenesis of Alzheimer's disease. A rational framework for the search of novel therapeutic approaches. *Front. Cell. Neurosci.* 8:112. doi: 10.3389/fncel.2014.00112

Orihuela, R., McPherson, C. A., and Harry, G. J. (2016). Microglial M1/M2 polarization and metabolic states. *Br. J. Pharmacol.* 173, 649–665. doi: 10.1111/bph.13139

Qiu, H., Zhong, R., Liu, H., Zhang, F., Li, S., and Le, W. (2016). Chronic sleep deprivation exacerbates learning-memory disability and Alzheimer's disease-like pathologies in $A\beta PP^{swe}/PS1^{\Delta E9}$ mice. *J. Alzheimers Dis.* 50, 669–685. doi: 10.3233/jad-150774

Sapin, E., Peyron, C., Roche, F., Gay, N., Carcenac, C., Savasta, M., et al. (2015). Chronic intermittent hypoxia induces chronic low-grade neuroinflammation in the dorsal hippocampus of mice. *Sleep* 38, 1537–1546. doi: 10.5665/sleep.5042

Smith, S. M., Friedle, S. A., and Watters, J. J. (2013). Chronic intermittent hypoxia exerts CNS region-specific effects on rat microglial inflammatory and TLR4 gene expression. *PLoS One* 8:e81584. doi: 10.1371/journal.pone.0081584

Tang, Y., and Le, W. (2016). Differential roles of M1 and M2 microglia in neurodegenerative diseases. *Mol. Neurobiol.* 53, 1181–1194. doi: 10.1007/s12035-014-9070-5

Tang, Y., Li, T., Li, J., Yang, J., Liu, H., Zhang, X. J., et al. (2014). Jmjd3 is essential for the epigenetic modulation of microglia phenotypes in the immune pathogenesis of Parkinson's disease. *Cell Death Differ.* 21, 369–380. doi: 10.1038/cdd.2013.159

Viatour, P., Merville, M. P., Bours, V., and Chariot, A. (2005). Phosphorylation of NF-κB and IκB proteins: implications in cancer and inflammation. *Trends Biochem. Sci.* 30, 43–52. doi: 10.1016/j.tibs.2004.11.009

Wang, Z., Yang, D., Zhang, X., Li, T., Li, J., Tang, Y., et al. (2011). Hypoxia-induced down-regulation of neprilysin by histone modification in mouse primary cortical and hippocampal neurons. *PLoS One* 6:e19229. doi: 10.1371/journal.pone.0019229

Westin, K., Buchhave, P., Nielsen, H., Minthon, L., Janciauskiene, S., and Hansson, O. (2012). CCL2 is associated with a faster rate of cognitive decline during early stages of Alzheimer's disease. *PLoS One* 7:e30525. doi: 10.1371/journal.pone.0030525

Yagishita, S., Suzuki, S., Yoshikawa, K., Iida, K., Hirata, A., Suzuki, M., et al. (2017). Treatment of intermittent hypoxia increases phosphorylated tau in the hippocampus via biological processes common to aging. *Mol. Brain* 10:2. doi: 10.1186/s13041-016-0282-7

Yamamoto, M., Horiba, M., Buescher, J. L., Huang, D., Gendelman, H. E., Ransohoff, R. M., et al. (2005). Overexpression of monocyte chemotactic protein-1/CCL2 in β-amyloid precursor protein transgenic mice show accelerated diffuse β-amyloid deposition. *Am. J. Pathol.* 166, 1475–1485. doi: 10.1016/s0002-9440(10)62364-4

Zhang, C. E., Yang, X., Li, L., Sui, X., Tian, Q., Wei, W., et al. (2014). Hypoxia-induced tau phosphorylation and memory deficit in rats. *Neurodegener. Dis.* 14, 107–116. doi: 10.1159/000362239

Zhang, X., and Le, W. (2010). Pathological role of hypoxia in Alzheimer's disease. *Exp. Neurol.* 223, 299–303. doi: 10.1016/j.expneurol.2009.07.033

Zhang, X., Li, L., Zhang, X., Xie, W., Li, L., Yang, D., et al. (2013). Prenatal hypoxia may aggravate the cognitive impairment and Alzheimer's disease neuropathology in $APP^{Swe}/PS1^{A246E}$ transgenic mice. *Neurobiol. Aging* 34, 663–678. doi: 10.1016/j.neurobiolaging.2012.06.012

Zilka, N., Kazmerova, Z., Jadhav, S., Neradil, P., Madari, A., Obetkova, D., et al. (2012). Who fans the flames of Alzheimer's disease brains? Misfolded tau on the crossroad of neurodegenerative and inflammatory pathways. *J. Neuroinflammation* 9:47. doi: 10.1186/1742-2094-9-47

Zuroff, L., Daley, D., Black, K. L., and Koronyo-Hamaoui, M. (2017). Clearance of cerebral Aβ in Alzheimer's disease: reassessing the role of microglia and monocytes. *Cell. Mol. Life Sci.* 74, 2167–2201. doi: 10.1007/s00018-017-2463-7

10

Microglial Activation in Traumatic Brain Injury

*Cornelius K. Donat, Gregory Scott, Steve M. Gentleman and Magdalena Sastre **

Division of Brain Sciences, Department of Medicine, Imperial College London, London, United Kingdom

***Correspondence:**
Magdalena Sastre
m.sastre@imperial.ac.uk

Microglia have a variety of functions in the brain, including synaptic pruning, CNS repair and mediating the immune response against peripheral infection. Microglia rapidly become activated in response to CNS damage. Depending on the nature of the stimulus, microglia can take a number of activation states, which correspond to altered microglia morphology, gene expression and function. It has been reported that early microglia activation following traumatic brain injury (TBI) may contribute to the restoration of homeostasis in the brain. On the other hand, if they remain chronically activated, such cells display a classically activated phenotype, releasing pro-inflammatory molecules, resulting in further tissue damage and contributing potentially to neurodegeneration. However, new evidence suggests that this classification is over-simplistic and the balance of activation states can vary at different points. In this article, we review the role of microglia in TBI, analyzing their distribution, morphology and functional phenotype over time in animal models and in humans. Animal studies have allowed genetic and pharmacological manipulations of microglia activation, in order to define their role. In addition, we describe investigations on the *in vivo* imaging of microglia using translocator protein (TSPO) PET and autoradiography, showing that microglial activation can occur in regions far remote from sites of focal injuries, in humans and animal models of TBI. Finally, we outline some novel potential therapeutic approaches that prime microglia/macrophages toward the beneficial restorative microglial phenotype after TBI.

Keywords: traumatic brain injury, CCI, microglia, neuroinflammation, TSPO, polarization states

INTRODUCTION

Traumatic brain injury (TBI) is the biggest cause of death and disability in the under 40s in the developed world (Langlois et al., 2006; Hyder et al., 2007), both in the civilian and military context. The overall majority of TBIs is a single event; however, repeated injuries among soldiers and athletes are associated with the development of Chronic Traumatic Encephalopathy (CTE) although the pathology of CTE can also be seen after single TBI and its causation remains uncertain (Omalu et al., 2011; Goldstein et al., 2012). Survivors often suffer from debilitating cognitive, emotional and physical impairments. This is further aggravated by the constant failure of clinical trials (reviewed in Loane and Faden, 2010; Gruenbaum et al., 2016), leaving patients without any treatment.

Brain injury can trigger neurodegeneration, which is a major determinant of long-term outcome. Head injury is a major risk factor for the development of dementia, suggested by the presence of amyloid-β (Aβ) plaques in around 30% of post-mortem brain tissue from TBI patients (Roberts et al., 1994). Additionally, amyloid plaques have been observed in surgically removed tissue surrounding contusions in brains of survivors of TBI (Ikonomovic et al., 2004; DeKosky et al., 2007). Recently, it has been shown by Positron Emission Tomography (PET) imaging that the distribution of amyloid plaque in TBI survivors overlaps with that in patients with Alzheimer's disease (AD) but also involves the cerebellum, an area of the brain not typically involved in AD (Scott et al., 2016). Other pathological features of AD are also present in TBI, including increased phosphorylated tau and acetylcholine deficiency (Jordan, 2000; Tran et al., 2011; Goldstein et al., 2012; McKee and Daneshvar, 2015; Shin and Dixon, 2015). In particular, repetitive mild TBI leading to CTE is characterized by perivascular tau pathology, which is also irregularly distributed in the depths of cortical sulci. Another AD susceptibility factor is the Apolipoprotein E isoform 4 (ApoE4), which has been linked with exiguous neurological outcome after TBI (Verghese et al., 2011). This has been associated with alterations in the integrity of the blood brain barrier (BBB) in individuals with ApoE4 genotype (Methia et al., 2001; Nishitsuji et al., 2011).

Additionally, TBI has been linked with Parkinson's disease (Jafari et al., 2013), various psychiatric disorders leading to increased risk of suicide, an overall increase in mortality (McMillan et al., 2011) and peripheral immune suppression (Hazeldine et al., 2015). There are currently no neuroprotective drug treatments available and a major challenge is to understand how brain trauma causes neurodegeneration and other long-term impairments.

A common feature of the neurological pathologies developing as a consequence of TBI is that they initiate and are potentiated by an inflammatory response. Microglial activation occurs early after experimental (Chiu et al., 2016) and human TBI (Ramlackhansingh et al., 2011; Johnson et al., 2013) and can persist for years, detectable both *in vivo* and post-mortem. Sites of activation often coincide with neuronal degeneration and axonal abnormality (Maxwell et al., 2010; Giunta et al., 2012). It was hypothesized that the inflammatory response to TBI therefore could be associated with the subsequent development of neurodegenerative disorders. However, new evidence indicates that glial activation may have also reparative/restorative effects. Thus, it is critical to investigate what causes this inflammatory response, what are the consequences for neuronal degeneration and survival and whether this can be modified with anti-inflammatory therapeutic approaches.

In this review, we analyse the role of microglia in TBI patients and animal models, from imaging studies used to visualize changes in microglia activation *in vivo* and *ex vivo* to studies in post-mortem brains of TBI patients and the prospects of therapies targeting microglia activation in TBI.

MICROGLIA ACTIVATION STATES IN TBI

TBI occurs when brain structure and physiology are disrupted due to an extrinsic biomechanical insult to the cranium, resulting in neuronal, axonal and vascular damage. In response to TBI, the brain orchestrates a complex immunological tissue reaction similar to ischemic reperfusion injury (Werner and Engelhard, 2007). It was suggested that, as macrophages, microglia can migrate to the site of the injury, in order to establish a protective environment mitigating deleterious consequences of the injury (Faden et al., 2016). The acute function of microglia in response to TBI is to eradicate cellular and molecular debris. Microglial removal of damaged cells is a very important step in the restoration of the normal brain environment. Damaged cells release Danger-associated molecular patterns (DAMPs), which can become potent inflammatory stimuli, resulting in further tissue damage (Solito and Sastre, 2012; Zhang et al., 2012). Moreover, activated microglia are also capable of releasing noxious substances such as pro-inflammatory cytokines, reactive oxygen species (ROS), nitrogen species and excitatory neurotransmitters i.e., glutamate, which exacerbate damage (Kreutzberg, 1996). While pro-inflammatory cytokines are directly deleterious, they also stimulate the release of glutamate from microglia in an autocrine/paracrine fashion. Therefore, depending on the released amount, this can lead to direct neurotoxic effects on neurons, synapses and dendrites, through ionotropic glutamate receptors and interfere with the glutamate buffering ability of astrocytes by inhibiting astrocytic glutamate transporters (Takaki et al., 2012).

It was initially hypothesized that there is a temporary transition in function of the inflammatory milieu, which in the latter phases favors a protracted inflammatory profile associated with chronic microglial activation, precipitating neurological manifestations, although this view has been found to be far too simplistic.

As in other CNS injuries, it seems that microglia activation in TBI results in different phenotypes, corresponding to neurotoxic or neuroprotective priming states. Depending on the stage of the disease and the chronicity, microglia are stimulated differentially and this leads to particular activation states, which correspond to altered microglia morphology, gene expression and function. Microglia are activated in-situ by pro-inflammatory cytokines such as IFN-γ, IL-1α, IL-6, and TNF-α (Ziebell and Morganti-Kossmann, 2010) and become primed. Microglia morphology can switch from a "normal," ramified shape to a hypertrophic, "bushy" morphology. In response to extensive tissue damage or pathogen invasion, microglia can change into an amoeboid morphology, primarily acting in a phagocytic/macrophage fashion and being difficult to differentiate from infiltrating macrophages (**Figure 1**). In general, these activation states are classified along a spectrum with M1 or "classically activated" at one end and M2 or "alternatively activated" and the opposite end, similar to macrophages. The proinflammatory M1 phenotype favors the production and release of cytokines that can exacerbate neural injury (Hu et al., 2015). In contrast, the M2 is associated with the release of neurotrophic factors that promote repair and a phagocytic role. However, in recent years, transcriptomic analysis has revealed that microglia and macrophages display a much broader transcriptional repertoire than M1 and M2, depending on the different environmental signals received (Hickman et al., 2013; Xue et al., 2014). Therefore, it is rare to find clear M1 or M2 microglial phenotypes in chronic diseases, since these states are transitory and eventually include mixed activation states. This seems particularly important in TBI as indicated by the many animal studies showing a mixed expression of different markers associated with both M1 and M2 phenotype (**Table 1**), also described as transitory state (Mtrans) by some authors (Kumar et al., 2016a). Additionally, the inevitable recruitment of bone

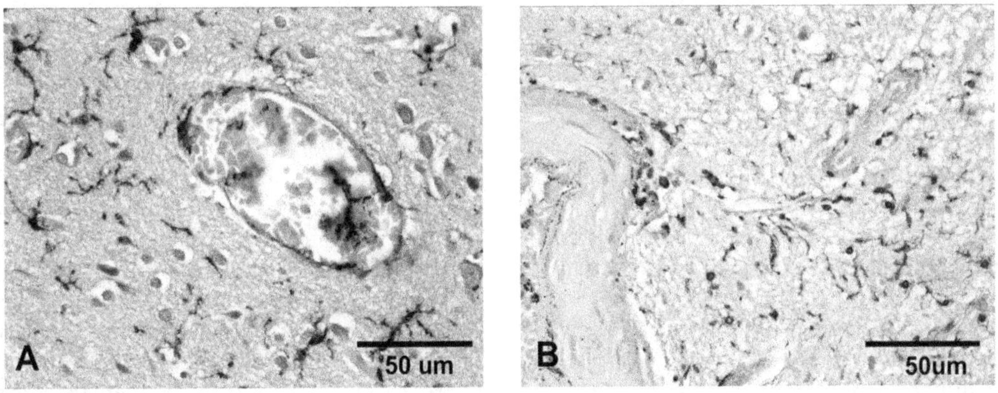

FIGURE 1 | Iba-1 staining illustrating the ramified microglial morphology associated with normal surveillance activity **(A)** compared to that seen in patients where there has been damage to the vasculature and the microglia take on a more rounded phagocytic appearance **(B)**. Scale bar corresponds to 50 μM.

marrow-derived monocytes into the injured brain parenchyma following experimental TBI and the subsequent differentiation into macrophages complicates the interpretation of the findings, especially with regard to the ability of these cells to change phenotype.

Additional complications arise from the clinical observation that outcome after TBI can be different between male and female adults and post-pubescent adolescents in some but not all studies (Coimbra et al., 2003), with females having lower mortality and less complications (Phelan et al., 2007; Berry et al., 2009; Ley et al., 2013). This can be attributed, at least partially, to astrocytes and microglia, as recently reviewed (Caplan et al., 2017). Gonadal steroid hormones such as progesterone and estradiol are directly involved in the glial response under injury conditions in and during development (Lenz and McCarthy, 2015). Moreover, as progesterone can shift macrophage polarization from M1 to M2 phenotype (Menzies et al., 2011), is seems possible that similar effects could occur in microglia as well, whether the concept of microglia polarization is accepted or not.

The polarization states of microglia could therefore be relevant in the progression of TBI into other neurological disorders such as AD and could interfere with the recovery of the patients and the effectiveness of particular anti-inflammatory treatment.

In addition, the role of infiltrating macrophages and other immune cells are also relevant in the context of microglia dynamics; injury type and parameters may play an important role, with focal models of TBI generally eliciting a more pronounced and localized inflammatory response due to significant tissue damage and pronounced infiltration of peripheral immune cells through the compromised BBB. In line with this, factors that have been implicated in BBB breakdown after injury, such as ApoE (mentioned above) and the extracellular enzymes matrix metalloproteinases (MMPs) have been found to contribute to contusion expansion and vasogenic edema after TBI (Guilfoyle et al., 2015).

MICROGLIAL ACTIVATION IN ANIMAL MODELS OF TBI

In the past five decades, several animal models have been developed to characterize the biomechanical and pathophysiological patterns of TBI and to provide reliably ways to test treatment strategies. These models almost exclusively employ a single-hit injury and only in the past decade repeated injury models emerged that try to mimic the effect of repetitive injuries. The different animal models address distinct pathophysiological aspects of TBI and have different etiological and construct validity (O'Connor et al., 2011). The most widely applied models of TBI are open-head models, that induce an injury via the intact dura mater upon the underlying cortical tissue (reviewed in Xiong et al., 2013), with focal, diffuse and/or mixed injury patterns, depending on the type of injury. In order to do so, rigid impactors (Controlled Cortical Impact, CCI; weight drop, WD), fluidic pressure (Fluid Percussion Injury, FPI) and blast waves are employed. Additionally, high-velocity probes or projectiles are used to model penetrating brain injury. The CCI, FPI and the various WD models have a long history and were extensively characterized in the past, including assessment of long-term outcome (Kochanek et al., 2002; Immonen et al., 2009).

With the recognition that multiple head injuries, even of sub-threshold severity, are connected to chronic sequel, such as CTE (McKee et al., 2016; Vile and Atkinson, 2017), new models were developed to account for those findings. A growing number of studies in repeated injury rodent models (Shitaka et al., 2011; Klemenhagen et al., 2013; Mannix et al., 2014; Semple et al., 2016; Robinson et al., 2017) indicate that the glial response, in particular increases in microglia numbers and changes in morphology, shares an overall similar pattern with the traditional single-injury models. Interestingly, a few studies showed that repeated injuries can exacerbate the glial response, e.g., microglia or astrocyte cell density, as compared to a single injury (Ojo et al., 2013; Petraglia et al., 2014; Xu et al., 2016; Gao et al., 2017; Tyburski et al., 2017). Recent findings in human post-mortem tissue support the overall notion that repeated injuries result in a stronger glial response by showing that repeated head injury was a predictor of CD68 cell density and phosphorylated tau (Cherry et al., 2016).

The involvement of microglia in the complex pathophysiological cascade following brain injury has long been recognized. Shortly after the description of microglia by Del Rio-Hortega, accumulation of "microglia-like" cells were reported in the tissue around autologous blood injections and a cortical stab wound (Carmichael, 1929; Dunning and Stevenson, 1934) in the rabbit. Similar to reactive astrocytes, microglia are versatile cells, which is exemplified by their heterogeneous morphology (Boche et al., 2013). Perivascular microglia respond to pressure on the thinned mouse skull (Roth et al., 2014) by changing into jellyfish morphology; CCI causes some microglia to align with axon initial segment, the site where action potentials are generated (Baalman et al., 2015) and midline FPI yields several rod-like microglia (Ziebell et al., 2012).

Depending on the employed markers and methods, significantly increasing microglia activation in animal models of TBI is usually apparent from day 1 to 3 post-injury (p.i.) (Bye et al., 2007; Elliott et al., 2011) and can persist chronically beyond 28 days p.i., a usual cut-off time-point for many animal studies. A few studies have elegantly emphasized the long-term nature of microglia activation after experimental TBI, primarily with immunohistochemical analysis showing that major histocompatibility complex (MHC)-II positive cells were still present in the ipsilateral hemisphere at 3 months after WD injury (Holmin and Mathiesen, 1999). Recently, a significant loss of ramified, but increase of hypertrophic microglia in the injured rodent cortex at 1 year after moderate CCI in mice was demonstrated (Loane et al., 2014a). This suggests that, although microglial activation occurs early after TBI, it can change the phenotype and function over time (see **Table 1**).

Manipulation of Microglial Activation in Animal Models of TBI

Several studies have investigated the effects of microglial elimination in brain injury models, in order to understand their function and the potential as therapeutic approach. The use of the transgenic CD11b-HSVTK mice in response to ganciclovir (GCV) treatment allowed the study of the depletion of proliferating microglia in models of brain or peripheral nerve injury. These transgenic mice express a mutant form of the gene herpes simplex virus 1 thymidine kinase (HSV-1 TKmt-30) driven by the myeloid specific promoter CD11b. HSV-1 TK is capable of phosphorylating specific nucleoside analogs such as GCV, which lead to inhibition of DNA synthesis and cell death during cell proliferation (Cheng et al., 1983; Faulds and Heel, 1990; Black et al., 1996).

Unexpectedly, eliminating proliferative CD11b positive cells and therefore microglia and potentially macrophages in a model of hypoglossal nerve axotomy did not result in pronounced changes in motor neuron loss (Gowing et al., 2006). In another study, employing a repeated closed-head injury in the CD11b-TK mice, low dose of GCV reduced the microglial population after TBI but did not alter the extent of axonal injury as visualized by silver staining. Additionally, higher doses were found to be toxic and aggravated the TBI induced damage (Bennett and Brody, 2014).

Rapid elimination of ~95% of all microglia can be achieved by administration of the colony stimulating factor 1 receptor (CSF1R) inhibitor PLX3397. This approach was used in a model of neuronal injury (Rice et al., 2015) consisting of a diphtheria toxin-induced neuronal lesion in transgenic mice carrying a transgene for the diphtheria toxin A-chain. The diphtheria toxin was activated in transgenic mice by feeding them food without doxycycline, triggering neurotoxicity. The treatment with PLX3397 had different outcomes depending on whether microglia elimination took place in the recovery period only or was administered during the lesion as well as the recovery period. Elimination of microglia after the lesion resulted in improved functional recovery, while microglia depletion during the insult led to greater neuronal loss (Rice et al., 2015). Therefore, in models of CNS damage, it seems that chronically activated microglia display a pro-inflammatory phenotype that may contribute to further synaptic loss. In addition, using the same approach of treatment with the CSF1R inhibitor, it was recently shown that microglia are involved in changes in neuronal network activity and spreading depolarization after excitotoxic lesions and ischemia. Depletion of microglia led to dysregulated neuronal calcium responses, calcium overload and increased neuronal death and infarct size (Szalay et al., 2016), with similar reports in a mouse model of transient focal cerebral ischemia and reperfusion (Jin et al., 2017).

From these findings, it seems obvious that general ablation of microglia is not a productive strategy and perhaps it would be more effective to suppress a specific phenotype at a particular time-point. One approach would be to characterize the different microglial functions based on morphology and phenotype markers in order to find the right time for a microglia-targeting therapeutic strategy.

Polarization of Microglia in TBI Models

The polarization of microglia is a relatively new concept, not seen without controversy (Ransohoff, 2016), which has been already investigated in a number of studies, primarily in the CCI model in mice. Only a few studies employed rats or other established TBI models, such as FPI and WD. Data from clinically relevant repeated and penetrating models is lacking even for rodents. To the knowledge of the authors, no study has investigated microglia polarization in gyrencephalic models such as ferrets, sheep or pigs, even though these species had previously been employed in CCI, FPI, penetrating, and blast models.

In the established rodent models (see **Table 1**), data indicates that microglia and infiltrating macrophages, responding to injury, do not lean toward an extreme end of the spectrum, as shown in several studies through the expression of both M1 and M2-like markers in the "acute" phase. However, it seems that in the subsequent "subacute" and "chronic" phase, the expression of M2-like markers is reduced, while M1-like markers are still expressed, indicating that the pro-inflammatory action of microglia/macrophages exacerbates the pathology. In

TABLE 1 | Microglia/macrophage polarization in experimental models of Traumatic Brain Injury.

References	Species, strain, sex	Model, severity and injury details	Time post injury	Key markers	Simplified key results of M1/M2-like marker analysis
Jin et al., 2012	Mouse C57B6/J ♂	CCI, moderate 3 mm	dpi: 1, 3, 7 14, and 28	**M1**: CD86 **M2**: CD206	**M1**: ▲ 7 + 28 dpi **M2**: ▲ 1 dpi, Sham levels 28 dpi
Bedi et al., 2013	Mouse C57B6 ♂	CCI, moderate ns	dpi: 1	**M1**: $F_C\gamma$RII/III (CD16a/b) **M2**: CD206	**M1/2 ratio**: ▲ at 24 hpi
Walker et al., 2012	Mouse C57B6 ♂	CCI, moderate ns	hpi: 24, 48, 72, 120	**M2/M1** ratio of CD206/CD86	**M1**: ▲ 24–72 hpi
Hsieh et al., 2013	Mouse C57BL/6 ♂, YARG/Yet40 knock-in	CCI, moderate 2 mm flat	dpi: 1, 4, 7, 14	**M1**: IL-12p40 **M2**: Arg-1	**M1**: ▲ macrophages 1–14 dpi **M2**: ▲ macrophages 1 dpi Mixed M1/M2 expression
Tchantchou and Zhang, 2013	Mouse C57B6 ♂	CCI, moderate 3 mm flat	dpi: 3,7, 21	**M1**: iNOS **M2**: Arg-1	**M1**: ▲ 3 + 7 dpi, **M2**: no Arg-1
Wang et al., 2013	Mouse C57B6 ♂	CCI, moderate 3 mm flat	dpi: 1, 3, 5, 7, 14	**M1**: CD16/32, iNOS, CD11b, CD86 **M2**: CD206, IL-10, Ym1/2, TGF-β, Arg-1, CCL22	**M1**: ▲ 5–14 dpi **M2**: ▲ 3–5 dpi
Wang et al., 2015	Mouse C57B6 ♂	CCI, moderate 3 mm flat	dpi: 7, 35	**M1**: CD16, iNOS **M2**: CD206, IL-10	**M1**: ▲ 7 dpi **M2**: ▲ 7 dpi
Kumar et al., 2013	Mouse C57B6 ♂,	CCI, severe 3.5 mm flat	dpi: 1, 7	**M1**: IL-1β, TNF-α, CD86, iNOS, CCL2, CCL3 **M2a**: Arg-1, Ym1, CD206/MRC, Fizz-1 **M2c**: IL-4Rα, SOCS3, TGF-β	Mixed M1/M2 expression **M1**: aged > young **M2a**: marker specific ▲▼ **M2c**: young > aged Aged animals ▲ Ym1 on highly activated microglia/macrophages Young animals ▲Ym1 on ramified cells
Loane et al., 2014a	Mouse C57Bl/6 ♂	CCI, severe 3.5 mm flat	wpi: 1, 5, 12, 52	**M1**: MHC II **M2**: Ym-1	M1/MHC II: ▲ 1–52 wpi **M2**: ▲ 1–5 wpi, absent 12–54 wpi
Loane et al., 2014b	Mouse C57Bl/6 ♂	CCI, severe 3.5 mm flat	dpi: 28	**M1**: iNOS **M2**: Arg-1	**M1**: ▲ iNOS/CD11b **M2**: ▼Arg-1/CD11b
Kumar et al., 2016a	Mouse C57Bl/6 ♂	CCI, severe 3.5 mm flat	hpi: 1, 6, 24 dpi: 7	mRNA: **M1**: IL-1β, IL-12, TNF-α, IL-6, iNOS **M2a**: Arg-1, Ym1, CD206, Fizz-1, IL-1rn **M2c**: IL-4Rα, SOCS3, TGF-β Flow cytometry: **M1**: iNOS, IL-12 **M2**: TGF-β, Ym1, CD206, Arg-1 Histology: **M1**: CD16/32, iNOS **Mtrans**: CD16/32+TGF-β, iNOS+, Arg-1 **M2**: TGF-β, Arg-1	Mixed expression of M1/M2 mRNA and protein M1/trans dominate contusion and peri-contusional tissue at 7 dpi

(Continued)

TABLE 1 | Continued

References	Species, strain, sex	Model, severity and injury details	Time post injury	Key markers	Simplified key results of M1/M2-like marker analysis
Kumar et al., 2016b	Mouse C57Bl/6 ♂ NOX2 −/−	CCI, severe 3.5 mm flat	dpi: 1, 3, 5, 7, 21, 28	**M1**: IL-1β, NOS2, TNF-α, IL-6, IL-12b **M2**: Arg-1, Ym1, SOCS3, Fizz-1, IL1rn, IL-4Rα **M2c**: IL-4Rα, SOCS3, TGF-β	Mixed expression of M1/2 up to 7 dpi
Morganti et al., 2015	Mouse Dbl-Het C57Bl/6 ♂/♀	CCI, moderate 3 mm convex	hpi: 3, 6, 12 dpi: 1, 2, 7, 14, 28	**M1**: CD68, CD45, MHC II, MARCO, NOS2, TNF-α, CCL2, IL-1β, IL-6, INF-γ **M2a**: Arg-1, Ym1, Fizz1, CD206, IL-4, IL-13 **M2c**: CD36, CD163, TGF-β, IL-10, IL-4Rα, IL-1Ra	Mixed expression of M1 and M2a/c marker mRNA in leucocytes **M1**: ▲ 3 hpi – 14 dpi **M2a**: ▲12 hpi – 7dpi **M2c**: ▲ 6 hpi – 7dpi
Morganti et al., 2016	Mouse C57Bl6/J ♂	CCI, moderate 3 mm convex	dpi: 1, 2, 7	**M1**: CCL2, CCL3, CCL4, CCL6, CCL7, CCL9, CCL12, CCL19, CCL25, CD14, CXCL1, CXCL2, CXCL3, CXCL9, CXCL10, CXCL16, DUSP1, IL-1β, IL-15, IL-16, PTX3, TLR2, TNF-α **M2**: Arg-1, CD36, CX3CL1, IL4R, IL25, TGF-βm TGM2, TLR1, TLR8	Mixed expression of M1 and M2 marker mRNA **M1**: ▲ 3–7 dpi **M2**: ▲ 3–7 dpi Lower fold changes in M2 expression compared to M1
Zanier et al., 2014	Mouse C57Bl/6 ♂	CCI, moderate 3 mm	dpi: 3, 7	**M1**: CD11b, TNF-α, CD68, CD86, IL-1β **M2a/c**: Ym1, Arg-1, CD206, SOCS3, IL-10	Mixed expression of M1 and M2 marker mRNA **M1**: ▲ at 3 + 7 dpi **M2**: ▲ Ym1, Arg-1, SOCS3 at 3 dpi
Febinger et al., 2015	Mouse CX3CR1−/− CX3CR1+/+ ♂	CCI, mild 3 mm	dpi: 7, 15, 30	**M1**: IL-1β, CD86, iNOS, MARCO **M2**: TGF-β, Arg-1, CD206	**M2a**: ▲ Ym1, CD206 in CX3CR1−/− only at 7 dpi ▲ TGF-β in CX3CR1−/− mRNA **M1**: ▼ iNOS, IL-1β 30 dpi: ▲ M1: Marco, CD68
Zanier et al., 2016	Mouse CX3CR1−/− CX3CR1+/+ ♂	CCI, Moderate 3 mm	dpi: 1, 2, 4, 7 wpi: 5	**M1**: CD11b, CD68, iNOS, IL-1β,TNF-α **M2**: Ym1	CX3CR1−/−, 4 dpi: ▲ sensorimotor performance ▼TUNEL positive cells ▼ M1, CD68, iNOS CX3CR1−/− 5 wpi: ▼ sensorimotor performance ▲TUNEL positive cells ▲ M1 iNOS
Desai et al., 2016	Mouse C57BL6/N ♂	CCI, moderate 3 mm flat	hpi: 4 dpi: 1, 4	**M1**: CD16, CD32 **M2**: CD-206, Arg-1, Ym1	**M1**: ▲ CD16, CD32 at 1–4 dpi **M2**: ▲ CD206, Arg-1, Ym1 at 1–4 dpi
Braun et al., 2017	Mouse C57BL/6 CD-1 C3H/OuJ C3H/HeJ CX3CR1 ♂	CCI, severe 3 mm convex	hpi: 24, 72 wpi: 3	**M1**: TNF-α, IL-12 **M2**: TGF-β, IL-10	**M1/M2 ratio**: ▲ 24 + 72 hpi, 3 wpi

(Continued)

TABLE 1 | Continued

References	Species, strain, sex	Model, severity and injury details	Time post injury	Key markers	Simplified key results of M1/M2-like marker analysis
Ansari, 2015	Rat Sprague-Dawley ♂	CCI, severe 5 mm flat	hpi: 2, 4, 6, 10, 24	**M1**: TNF-α, IL-1β, IL-6, IFN-γ **M2**: IL-4, IL-10, IL-13, Arg-1, Ym1, Fizz1, MRC-1	Mixed response **M1**: ▲ TNF-α, IL-1β, IL-6 mRNA/protein at 2-10 hpi **M2**: ▲ Arg-1: 6-24 hpi; Ym1: 6 hpi, Fizz1: 4-24 hpi
Turtzo et al., 2014	Rat Wistar ♀	CCI, severe 5 mm flat	dpi: 1, 3, 5, 7, 14, 30 wpi: 8	**M1**: CD40, CD68, TNF-α, CD86, CD80, NOS2 **M2**: CD163, CD206	Mixed expression of M1 and M2 protein expression and mRNA **M1**: ▲CD86 at 5, 7 dpi, TNF-α 1, 3 dpi **M2**: ▲ CD163 at 5, 7 dpi, CD206 at 7 dpi
Barrett et al., 2017	Mouse C57Bl/6 ♂ NOX2 −/−	CCI, severe 3.5 mm flat	dpi: 72	**M2**: IL-4Rα, SOCS3, TGF-β, SHIP1, Arg-1, Ym1, IL-10	NOX2 −/− mice show a robust increase in M2 markers ▲ IL-4Rα, SOCS3, TGF-β, SHIP1, Arg-1, Ym1, IL-10 at 72 hpi vs WT
Cao et al., 2012	Rat Sprague-Dawley ♂	mFPI, moderate 2 atm 4.8 mm craniotomy	dpi: 7, 28	**M1**: TNF-α, CD45 **M2a**: Arg-1 **M2c**: TGF-βI, TGF-βRII	M1 and M2c marker expression Cortex: M1 and M2c: ▲ nonsignificant CD45, TGF-βI, TGF-βRII at 7 dpi, no change in M2a (Arg-1) Thalamus: M1 and M2c: π CD45, TGF-βI, TGF-βRII at 7 and 28 dpi, no change in M2a (Arg-1)
Bachstetter et al., 2013	Mouse p38α MAPK −/− C57BL/6J ♂/♀	mFPI, moderate 1.2 atm 3 mm craniotomy	hpi: 3, 9, 24 dpi 7	**M1**: IL-1β, IL-6, TNF-α, CCL2, CCL5, CXCL1, CD45, CD68, MHC **M2**: Arg-1, Ym1	Mixed expression of M1 and M2 markers mRNA and cytokines/chemokines M1: ▲ IL-6, TNF-α, CCL3 3, 9 hpi, elevated at 7 dpi M2: ▲ Arg-1, Ym1 9 hpi, ▼ below sham levels at 7 dpi, Rod-like microglia p38α MAPK −/−: ▲ M1 and M2 response (mRNA/protein) at 6 hpi ▲ motor performance ▼ Synaptic loss, microglia activation
Fenn et al., 2014	Mouse BALB/c ♂	mFPI, moderate 1.2 -1.5 atm 3 mm craniotomy	hpi: 4, 72	**M1**: IL-1β, CD14, TNF-α, iNOS, IFN-γ, CCL2 **M2**: Arg-1, IL-4Rα, IGF-1, IL-10, IL4	Mixed mRNA expression in ipsilateral cortex and hippocampus, M2 markers less expressed at 72 hpi Cortex, 4 hpi: M1: ▲ IL-1β, CD14, TNF-α, CCL2; M2: ▲ Arg-1, IGF-1 72 hpi: M1: ▲ IFN-γ, CCL2, iNOS; M2: ▲ IL4 Hippocampus, 4 hpi: M1: ▲ IL-1β, CD14, TNF-α, CCL2; M2: ▲ IL-4, IL-10 72 hpi: M1: ▲ IL-1β, CD14, TNF-α, iNOS; M2 ▲ IL-10 ▲ Primed microglia
Fenn et al., 2015	Mouse BALB/c ♂	mFPI, moderate 1.2 -1.5 atm 3 mm craniotomy	dpi: 1	**M1**: IL-1β, CD14, TNF-α, iNOS **M2**: Arg-1, IL-10	Mixed expression at 1 dpi Hippocampus: **M1**: ▲ IL-1β, CD14, TNF-α, CCL2; **M2**: ▲ Arg-1

(Continued)

TABLE 1 | Continued

References	Species, strain, sex	Model, severity and injury details	Time post injury	Key markers	Simplified key results of M1/M2-like marker analysis
					Whole brain CD11b positive cells: **M1**: ▲ IL-1β, CD14, TNF-α, CCL2, iNOS; **M2**: ▲ Arg-1
Truettner et al., 2016	Rat Sprague-Dawley ♂	mFPI, moderate 1.8–2.2 atm 4.8 mm craniotomy	hpi: 4, 24	**M1**: iNOS, IL-1β, IL-1α, TNF-α, IL-6. IL-12, CCL2 **M2**: Arg-1, CD163, CD206, IL-10, Ym1, TGF- β **M1/M2**: iNOS/Arg-1 ratio	Mixed expression of M1 and M2 mRNA at 4 and 24 hpi, M1 more pronounced ▲ M1 ratio at 4 h, similar M1/M2 ratio at 24 h in microglia mRNA 4 h: **M1**: ▲ all; **M2**: ▲ (lower relative expression) mRNA 24 h: **M1**: ▲ TNF-α ▲ CD206, TGF-β
Chhor et al., 2016	Mouse OF-1 Postnatal day 7 ♂/♀	WD, closed 2 mm footplate 10 g weight dropped 10 cm	hpi: 2, 6, 14, 24 dpi: 5	**M1** (Cytotoxic): IL-1 α, IL-1β, IL-3, IL-6, IL-9, IL-12p40, IL-12p70, IL-17, INF-γ, TNF-α, CXCL1, CCL3, CCL4, CCL5, Cox-2, iNOS, CD32, CD86 **M2a** (Reparative/regenerative): IL4, IL-13, G-CSF, CCL2, Arg-1, CD206, IGF-1, Gal-3 **M2c** (Immunomodulatory): IL-5, IL-10, SphK1, IL-1rn, SOCS3, IL-4ra	Moderate mixed increase in M1 and M2a/c mRNA Ipsilateral hemisphere: **M1**: ▲ all markers except TNF-α and IL-12(p70) between 6, 14 and 24 hpi **M2a/c**: ▲ all markers except TNF-α and IL-12(p70) between 6, 14 and 24 hpi CD11b+ isolated microglia/macrophages: **M1**: ▲CD32/CD86 up to 1 dpi **M2a/c**: ▲Arg-1, CD206, SOCS3, IL-1rn, Gal3 up to 1 dpi, IGF-1 at 5 dpi Pronounced contralateral effects
Semple et al., 2010	Mouse CCL2 −/− C57Bl/6 ♂	WD, closed 333 g weight dropped 2 cm, silicone tip	hpi: 2, 4, 12, 24 dpi: 4, 7, 14, 28	**M1**: IL-1α, IL-1β, IL-6, IL-12p40, IL-12p70, CCL3, CXCL1, CXCL2, CCL5, TNF-α, INF-γ, **M2a**: G-CSF, IL-10	Primarily M1 driven response **M1**: ▲ IL-1α, IL-6, IL-12p40, CCL5 at 12 hpi **M2**: ▲ G-CSF1, IL-10 only at 12 hpi in CCL2 −/− CCL2 −/−: ▼lesion volume, macrophage accumulation and astrocyte activation at 14, 28 dpi

Levels of severity for CCI: Mild: 0.5 mm, Moderate: 0.95–1.5 mm; Severe: >2.0 mm.
CCI, Controlled Cortical Impact; mFPI, midline Fluid Percussion Injury, WD, Weight drop.
Dpi, Days post injury; hpi, hours post injury; wpi, weeks post injury.

contrast, studies in non-human primates suggest a trophic role for chronically activated microglia after TBI, indicating a restorative phenotype in the chronic phase (Nagamoto-Combs et al., 2007, 2010).

Another issue is the apparent differences in the expression of murine and human markers of potential microglia polarization, which have been found for macrophages (reviewed in Murray and Wynn, 2011). However, the employed cellular markers of M1-like and the different M2-like microglia/macrophages are not always clearly indicative of the presumed phenotype, which calls for new and more specific markers in murine models (Jablonski et al., 2015). Additionally, mRNA extraction of brain homogenates does not always yield reliable information on the M1/2-like spectrum. Ideally, microglia and macrophages are to be separated by flow cytometry and then assayed for their activation spectrum using transcriptomic analysis (Hickman et al., 2013; Xue et al., 2014).

The studies that employed different therapeutic strategies show that an increase in M2-like markers is often associated with a better cognitive and histopathological outcome (**Table 2**). It seems therefore imperative for future studies targeting microglia polarization as therapeutic strategies, to assess several markers in the target cells within a sufficient temporal window in order to show a long-term positive outcome.

IMAGING OF MICROGLIA ACTIVATION IN TBI

Measurement of microglial activation *in vivo* has become possible using PET and Single Photon Emission Computed

TABLE 2 | Treatments in experimental models of TBI targeting inflammation and microglia.

References	Species, Strain, sex	Treatment	Injury	Simplified treatment outcomes
Thal et al., 2011	Mouse C57BL6/CrIN ♂	Pioglitazone, rosiglitazone, PPARγ agonists	CCI	Pioglitazone: ▼ Lesion volume at 24 hpi **M1** ▼: iNOS, TNF-α, IL-1β mRNA at 24 hpi No beneficial effect of rosiglitazone
Besson et al., 2005	Rat Sprague-Dawley ♂	Fenofibrate, PPARα agonist	FPI	24 hpi: ▼ Neurologic deficits ▼ Oedema 7 dpi: ▼ Neurologic deficits
Bye et al., 2007	Mouse C57BL6 ♂	Minocycline	Closed-head WD	4 hpi: ▼ IL-1 β 1 dpi: ▼ Lesion volume ▼ Activated microglia accumulation (F4/80) ▲ Motor performance 4 dpi: Beneficial effects on lesion size and motor function loss No effect on apoptotic cell death, neutrophil infiltration
Homsi et al., 2010	Mouse Swiss ♂	Minocycline	Closed-head WD	1 dpi: ▼ Lesion volume ▼ Microglia/macrophages (CD11b) 2 dpi -12 wpi: ▼ Hyper-locomotor activity ▲ Body weight
Kovesdi et al., 2012	Rat Sprague-Dawley ♂	Minocycline	Blast injury, mild	▼ Serum biomarkers of inflammation, vascular and neuronal injury at 51 dpi ▼ Brain biomarkers in multiple brain regions at 51 dpi ▲ Locomotor activity, spatial memory ▼ Anxiety
Hanlon et al., 2016	Rat PD 11 Sprague-Dawley ♂/♀	Minocycline	Closed-head CCI, repeated	▼ Microglia/macrophages (ED1) accumulation at 3 dpi, Effect lost at 7 dpi, trend toward increase at 21 dpi ▼ Spatial memory vs vehicle No effect: Iba1 cells, axonal injury, white matter loss and neurodegeneration
Hanlon et al., 2017	Rat PD 11 Sprague-Dawley ♂/♀	Minocycline	Closed-head CCI	Short-term treatment (3 days): ▼ Microglia reactivity in cortex, hippocampus and white matter at 3 but not 7 dpi ▲ Neurodegeneration at 3 but not 7 dpi Long-term treatment (9 days): ▲ Microglial reactivity and neurodegeneration up to 15 dpi in cortex and hippocampus ▼ Spatial memory vs vehicle No effects of sex

(Continued)

TABLE 2 | Continued

References	Species, Strain, sex	Treatment	Injury	Simplified treatment outcomes
Chhor et al., 2016	Mouse OF-1 Postnatal day 7 ♂/♀	Minocycline	Closed-head WD	24 hpi: **M1**: ▼ IL-1β, IL-6 **M2a/c**: ▲ IGF-1, IL-1rn ▼ Ventricular volume ▼ Cleaved caspase 3 positive cells in cortex, hippocampus and striatum ▼ Iba1 positive cells in cortex but not hippocampus/striatum No beneficial effects at 5 dpi
Lloyd et al., 2008	Mouse CD-1 ♂	Minozac	Closed-head CCI	12 hpi: **M1** ▼: cytokines levels, IL-1β, IL-6, TNF-α, CCL2 in hippocampus and cortex 28 dpi: ▼ Astrogliosis ▼ Exploratory deficits
Tchantchou and Zhang, 2013	Mouse C57B6 ♂	WWL70, alpha/beta hydrolase domain 6 inhibitor	CCI	▼ iNOS ▲ ARG-1 staining ▼ BBB disruption, lesion size, neurodegeneration ▲ Motor/working memory performance
Loane et al., 2014b	Mouse C57Bl/6 ♂	VU0360172, mGlu5 positive allosteric modulator	CCI	**M1**: ▼iNOS/CD11b **M2**: ▲ Arg-1/CD11b ▲ motor performance ▼ lesion size, neurodegeneration
Wang et al., 2015	Mouse C57B6 ♂	Scriptaid, class I/II histone deacetylase inhibitor	CCI	**M1**: ▼ CD16 cells ▼CD16+iNOS mRNA **M2**: ▲ CD206 cells ▲ CD206 mRNA ▲ Sensorimotor performance ▲ White matter integrity
Morganti et al., 2015	Mouse Dbl-Het C57Bl/6 ♂/♀	CCX872, CCR2 selective antagonist	CCI	Acute phase: **M1** ▼: CD68, CD45, CCL2, IL-1β, IL-6 **M2a** ▼: Arg-1, Fizz1 **M2c** ▼: TGF-β and IL-10 Chronic phase: **M1** ▼: CD68, CD45, CCL2, IL-1β, TNF-α **M2a** ▼: Fizz1 ▲ Spatial learning/memory ▼ Macrophage invasion
Kumar et al., 2016a,b	Mouse C57Bl/6 NOX −/− ♂	gp91ds-tat, selective NOX2 inhibitor	CCI	**M1**: ▼CD16/32 **M2**: ▲ TGF-β **M1**: ▼ Nox2 **M2**: ▲ Ym1, Arg-1 ▼ lesion size, neurodegeneration ▲ motor/spatial memory performance
Menzel et al., 2017	Mouse Progranulin −/− and WT ♂	Recombinant progranulin, pre-injury	CCI	▼ **M1** cytokines mRNA at 5 dpi in progranulin −/− mice ▼ Neurological severity score ▼ Lesion size and white matter damage ▼ Astrogliosis

(Continued)

TABLE 2 | Continued

References	Species, Strain, sex	Treatment	Injury	Simplified treatment outcomes
Cao et al., 2012	Rat Sprague-Dawley ♂	Ibuprofen	FPI	▼ TGF-βI nonsignificant ▼ in TSPO, CD45 at 7 dpi in the thalamus
Chio et al., 2013; Cheong et al., 2013	Rat Sprague-Dawley ♂	Etanercept (TNF-α antagonist)	FPI	3/7 dpi: ▼ Neurological severity score ▼ Iba1/TNF-α positive cells in multiple brain regions ▼ TNF-α protein levels ▼ Oedema ▲ Neurogenesis

CCI, Controlled Cortical Impact; FPI, Fluid percussion injury, WD, Weight drop.
Dpi, Days post injury, hpi, hours post injury; wpi, weeks post injury;
Green color indicates beneficial, while red indicates detrimental actions of the treatment.

Tomography (SPECT) due to the development of radioligands that bind to the 18-kDa translocator protein (TSPO). TSPO is a five-transmembrane domain protein localized in the outer mitochondrial membrane (Jaremko et al., 2014). The best studied putative function of TSPO relates to its role in transporting cholesterol into the mitochondrial inner membrane space, the rate-limiting step of steroid and neurosteroid biosynthesis (Papadopoulos et al., 2006). However, this function has been lately questioned due to the findings from knockout mice that did not show abnormal steroidogenesis (Morohaku et al., 2014; Tu et al., 2014). Despite almost 40 years of study, the precise functional role of TSPO is far from clear (Selvaraj and Stocco, 2015).

Imaging of Activated Microglia after Experimental TBI

Autoradiographic studies and PET using TSPO ligands in experimental TBI have informed our understanding of the time-course and spatial distribution of microglial activation following brain trauma. The first TSPO ligand, PK11195, was synthesized in the 1980s. Autoradiographic studies localized binding of radiolabelled PK11195 to activated microglia (Banati et al., 1997) and, as a result, [^{11}C]PK11195 was adopted as a PET radioligand to image neuroinflammation *in vivo* (Liu et al., 2014). Increased TSPO-specific radioligand binding was detected as early as 6 h after CCI in rats, with significantly elevated radioligand binding in the ipsilateral and contralateral cortices at 24 h and delayed thalamic upregulation at 28 days p.i. (Donat et al., 2016). Additionally, we previously observed a small increase of [^{3}H]PK11195 binding in several brain regions of newborn piglets subjected to FPI at 6 h p.i. (Donat et al., 2014). Similarly, increased TSPO up-regulation indicative of microglia activation was reported in models including FPI (Yu et al., 2010; Cao et al., 2012), CCI (Venneti et al., 2007; Folkersma et al., 2011b; Wang et al., 2014), penetrating brain injury (Miyazawa et al., 1995; Grossman et al., 2012), closed-head injury (CHI) (Grossman et al., 2003) and dynamic cortical deformation (Soustiel et al., 2008).

In vivo studies employing [^{11}C]PK11195 PET in rats following CCI 1 day after injury showed no differences in whole brain uptake compared to baseline values or sham-treated controls, whereas scans at 10 days showed significantly increased uptake (Folkersma et al., 2011b). In another CCI rat model, uptake of [^{18}F]DPA-714 (a second-generation TSPO ligand) was observed on day 2 after injury, peaking on day 6, and remaining elevated to day 16 (Wang et al., 2014). Similar findings were seen in a weight-drop mouse model, no differences were observed in [^{18}F]DPA-714 binding at day 1, but increased uptake in focal brain lesions on repeated scans at days 7 and 16 (Israel et al., 2016).

Several experimental studies have also shown that TSPO expression increases not only in the vicinity of lesioned areas but also at locations remote from sites of focal damage. Following CCI in rats, the ipsilateral thalamus and hippocampus show increased [^{3}H]PK11195 binding between 3 and 14 days after injury (Raghavendra Rao et al., 2000). In the FPI model, increased uptake of [^{18}F]-fluoroethyl-DAA1106 (a second-generation TSPO ligand) appears in the ipsilateral striatum up to 4 weeks' post-injury (Yu et al., 2010). In our own study, using a CCI model in rats, we found increased binding of [^{123}I]CLINDE (a second-generation TSPO ligand) in contralateral motor cortex early after injury (24 h), whereas increased binding in the ipsilateral thalamus was observed first at 28 days post-injury (Donat et al., 2016).

However, TSPO up-regulation does not appear to relay any information on potential polarization pattern (Kim and Yu, 2015). In a mouse model of intracranial hemorrhage, microglia exclusively expressed TSPO and in these cells CD16/32 (M1-like) or CD206 (M2-like) were evenly distributed (Bonsack et al., 2016).

While TSPO seems a more general biomarker of glia activation, likely showing the mitochondrial changes due to the increased metabolic demand resulting from glia activation and cell proliferation (Liu et al., 2014), other targets expressed by microglia (e.g., cannabinoid type 2 receptor, P2X7 and P2Y12 receptors) could be more indicative of microglial polarization, although less tracers are available for these targets.

Imaging Microglia in Humans

In humans, [^{11}C]PK11195 PET has demonstrated increased TSPO expression in a variety of neuroinflammatory conditions (Owen and Matthews, 2011), including herpes encephalitis (Cagnin et al., 2001b), Alzheimer's disease (Cagnin et al., 2001a),

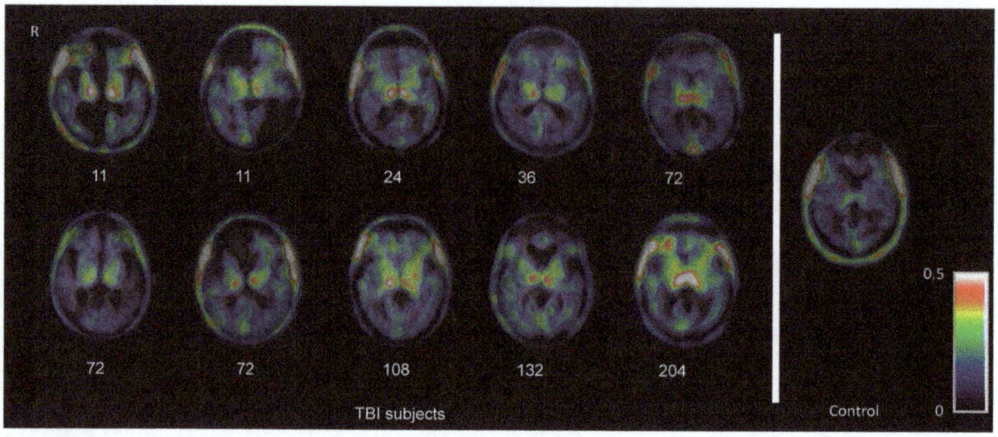

FIGURE 2 | Imaging of chronic microglial activation after TBI. Images of [11C]PK11195 PET images are shown superimposed on the T1 MRI scan at the level of the thalamus for 10 TBI patients, 11 months to 17 years after injury, and a representative control participant. Numbers indicate time since injury (months). *R* = right. The figure has been reproduced with permission of the copyright holder (Ramlackhansingh et al., 2011).

multiple sclerosis (Banati et al., 2000), and stroke (Gerhard et al., 2005). In the normal human brain, [^{11}C]PK11195 uptake is generally low, but with relatively high binding in subcortical structures, including midbrain, thalamus and putamen (Kumar et al., 2012; Kobayashi et al., 2017). The relatively increased TSPO ligand binding observed in midbrain, thalamus and basal ganglia (Kumar et al., 2012) is in keeping with the high density of microglia found in these regions in the mouse (Lawson et al., 1990) and human brain (Mittelbronn et al., 2001) in comparison to the cerebral cortex. However, increased TSPO ligand binding may reflect an increase in TSPO density rather than the number of cells expressing TSPO. These regions are highly connected through white matter to widespread brain regions. Owing to their dense connectivity, it is possible that even subtle neuronal injury, as may arise in normal aging, may result in the accumulation of secondary microglial activation in these regions, and therefore increased TSPO binding.

PET imaging with TSPO ligands provides a method to visualize microglial activity following TBI *in vivo*, although the specificity of TSPO for microglia still remains controversial. In an early study, we used [^{11}C]PK11195 PET to investigate a group of 10 patients in the chronic phase 11 months to 17 years after single moderate-severe TBI (**Figure 2**; Ramlackhansingh et al., 2011). [^{11}C]PK11195 binding potential was significantly increased in subcortical structures, particularly the thalami, putamen, and parts of the white matter. In keeping with animal work, this chronic microglial activation was seen in regions remote from focal damage and was also reduced around areas of focal injury. High [^{11}C]PK11195 binding in the thalamus was associated with more severe cognitive impairment, suggesting either that microglial activation might be directly contributing to cognitive impairment or that this was a response to underlying brain injury that caused the cognitive impairment.

These initial findings have been replicated and extended in further studies. A second study by another group also used [^{11}C]PK11195 PET following TBI (Folkersma et al., 2011a). They again showed increased binding in subcortical regions remote from the focal traumatic pathology, which included the thalamus, putamen, pons, and hippocampus. Increased microglial activation has also been observed in sportsmen exposed to repetitive TBI (Coughlin et al., 2015, 2017). A group of 14 active or recently retired National Football League players with a history of concussions were studied using the second generation TSPO ligand [^{11}C]DPA-713. Increased binding was seen predominantly in medial temporal lobe regions in sportsmen who also showed subtle evidence of white matter damage on diffusion MRI. In our follow-up study, we used the second generation TSPO ligand [^{11}C]PBR28 (Scott et al., 2015). A similar distribution of subcortical microglial activation was again seen years after single moderate/severe TBI. Prominent white matter microglial activation in areas of white matter damage was measured using magnetic resonance imaging (MRI). In addition, areas with high microglial activation showed high levels of brain atrophy over the next 6 months. This suggests that chronically activated microglia are seen in areas of persistent white matter damage, which are progressively degenerating even many years after injury.

These studies consistently show microglial activation in regions far removed from sites of focal injuries. Whilst at first glance surprising, the observation is in keeping with the evolution of microglial activation after experimental TBI (Donat et al., 2016) and is likely to reflect slowly progressive changes within damaged white matter, in particular Wallerian degeneration (**Figure 3**). In our initial study, the level of thalamic microglial activation after TBI showed a strong correlation with the level of traumatic axonal injury in thalamo-cortical projections. This suggests that traumatic axonal injury might be playing a causative role in increasing chronic microglial activation (Scott et al., 2015). The effect is not specific to TBI and a similar progression of microglial activity is seen following lacunar infarcts. This suggests that as the after effects of axonal injury develop and Wallerian degeneration progresses, microglial activation might be observed in cortical and subcortical regions remote from the initial injury.

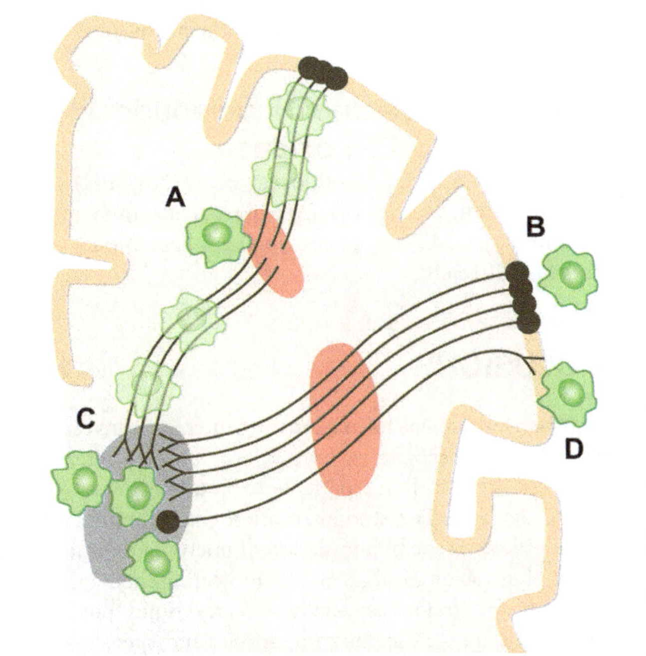

FIGURE 3 | How chronic microglial activation and axonal injury may be linked after TBI. Microglial activation (green cells) and traumatic axonal injury in thalamo-cortical white matter tracts (red areas) have been demonstrated after TBI. Sites of chronic microglial activation can co-localize with axonal abnormality **(A)** as well as along the entire axonal tract affected by injury. Remote from sites of primary axonal injury, microglia may be observed both in retrograde projection areas, toward the cell bodies of damaged neurons **(B)**, and in anterograde areas **(C,D)**. The thalamus is a highly-connected structure. Thalamic microglial activation may be observed after TBI because of the high density of connections to damaged axons. The number of cortico-thalamic projections far exceeds thalamo-cortical projections. If microglial activation preferentially favors anterograde involvement, then relatively increased activation would be expected in the thalamus **(C)** compared to corresponding cortical areas **(B)**.

A number of factors might explain the thalamic rather than cortical preponderance of microglial activation after TBI. Firstly, there is a high density of projection neurons converging in the thalamus, which might lead to a regional amplification of widespread, but sub-threshold cortical pathology (Cagnin et al., 2003). Secondly, as cortico-thalamic projections are 10 times more numerous that thalamo-cortical projections, a more intense microglial reaction to anterograde neurodegeneration might contribute to the persistent microglial reaction in the thalamus (**Figure 3**).

ANTI-INFLAMMATORY TREATMENTS TARGETING MICROGLIA ACTIVATION IN TBI

The relevance of microglia in the general pathophysiological response to TBI is recognized as a potential therapeutic avenue (reviewed in Chio et al., 2015) and has prompted several studies to investigate the effects of certain drugs on microglial polarization in brain injury models. Although studies in animal models indicate that microglia/macrophages respond to TBI with a transient M2 phenotype, followed by a shift to M1, and that the number of M1 cells is strongly correlated with the severity of white matter injury (Koh and DiPietro, 2011), this may differ in non-human and human primates. Therefore, therapies that prime microglia/macrophages toward the beneficial M2 phenotype after TBI may offer new anti-inflammatory strategies (**Table 2**). Several of these drugs, including minocycline, minozac, etanercept and the PPAR agonists fenofibrate and pioglitazone are FDA approved (Garrido-Mesa et al., 2013; Kim et al., 2014) confirming their safety and tolerability.

Progranulin

In response to TBI, microglia/macrophages and astrocytes release inflammatory mediators with dual effects on secondary brain damage progression. The neurotrophic and anti-inflammatory glycoprotein progranulin (PGRN) attenuates neuronal damage and microglia/macrophage activation in brain injury but mechanisms are still elusive. Intracerebroventricular administration of recombinant PGRN in mice immediately before trauma reduced brain damage and neurological deficits, and restored normal levels of cytokine transcription, axonal injury and astrogliosis 5 days after TBI in granulin knockout mice (Menzel et al., 2017).

Minocycline

Minocycline is a tetracycline derivative with anti-inflammatory and neuroprotective properties. Some of the proposed mechanisms for the anti-inflammatory properties for minocycline include the inhibitory effects on the activities of key enzymes, like iNOS, MMPs and PLA2 (Garrido-Mesa et al., 2013). In particular, it has been shown that it is able to inhibit M1 polarization state of microglia (Kobayashi et al., 2013), through the inhibition of NFκB and the interference with MAPK pathways. Minocycline significantly inhibited retinal neuroinflammation in an ischemia reperfusion (IR) model, characterized by inflammatory gene expression, leukocyte adhesion and invasion, and vascular permeability, however it failed to block neurodegeneration (Abcouwer et al., 2013). The effects of minocycline treatment in an animal model of TBI (closed head CCI in the neonate rat) revealed that the protective effects could be detected short term after injury (3 days after minocycline treatment) but not in chronic treatment (for 9 days after injury), in which microglial reactivity and neurodegeneration in all regions examined were exacerbated in minocycline-treated brain-injured animals (Hanlon et al., 2016, 2017). However, in other TBI models, such as blast injury, minocycline appears to prevent the development of neurobehavioral abnormalities (Kovesdi et al., 2012).

Minozac

Minozac (Mzc) is an anti-inflammatory molecule that selectively reduces excessive pro-inflammatory cytokine production by activated glia toward basal levels. There is evidence that administration of Mzc in a mouse closed-head, CCI at 3 and 9 h following TBI attenuates the acute increase in proinflammatory cytokine and chemokine levels and reduces the longer-term astrocyte activation, neurologic injury and neurobehavioral deficits observed over a 28-day recovery period (Lloyd et al., 2008)

Pharmacological Inhibition of TNF-α

Pharmacological inhibition of TNF-α using etanercept has been shown to reduce the expression of microglial TNF-α in rodents subjected to FPI (Cheong et al., 2013; Chio et al., 2013) and improve the neurological outcome after stroke and TBI in humans (Tobinick et al., 2012). Etanercept also seems to be able to stimulate neurogenesis in rats (Cheong et al., 2013).

Modulation of Glutamate Receptors

Although glutamate released by microglia may be related to a neurotoxic effect, it was shown that activation of metabotropic glutamate receptor 5 (mGluR5) on microglia is a novel mechanism to attenuate M1-like microglial activation and associated microglial-mediated neurotoxicity, suggesting a self-regulatory mechanism. Positive allosteric activation of mGluR5 has powerful neuroprotective effects in experimental models of CNS injury (Loane et al., 2014b).

PPAR Agonists

In traumatic brain injury, the PPARα agonist fenofibrate appears to represent a highly promising new anti-inflammatory compound. Besson et al. (2005) assessed the pharmacological role of fenofibrate in the FPI model in adult male Sprague-Dawley rats. The study revealed that the administration of fenofibrate during a clinically relevant therapeutic "time window of opportunity" at 1 h after trauma mediated a significant post-traumatic neuroprotection. This was demonstrated by improved neurological scores in the fenofibrate group at 24 h and 7 days after trauma, compared to vehicle-treated animals (Besson et al., 2005). In the case of PPARγ agonists, both pioglitazone and rosiglitazone seem to have protective effects, in particular pioglitazone reduced the histological damage and inflammation in the CCI model of TBI (Thal et al., 2011).

HDAC Inhibition

HDAC inhibitors have been found to have anti-inflammatory and neuroprotective effect in models of TBI. Scriptaid, a novel inhibitor of class I/II HDACs, was found to facilitate and enhance recovery of motor functions after CCI and protected white matter up to 35 day after TBI, as shown by reductions in abnormally dephosphorylated neurofilament protein, increases in myelin basic protein, anatomic preservation of myelinated axons, and improved nerve conduction (Wang et al., 2015). Furthermore, Scriptaid shifted microglia/macrophage polarization toward the protective M2 phenotype and mitigated inflammation. In primary co-cultures of microglia and oligodendrocytes, Scriptaid increased expression of microglial glycogen synthase kinase 3 beta (GSK3β), which phosphorylated and inactivated phosphatase and tensin homolog (PTEN), thereby enhancing phosphatidylinositide 3-kinases (PI3K)/Akt signaling and polarizing microglia toward M2. The increase in GSK3β in microglia and their phenotypic switch to M2 was associated with increased preservation of neighboring oligodendrocytes.

Nicotinamide Adenine Dinucleotide Phosphate (NADPH) oxidase

Nicotinamide adenine dinucleotide phosphate (NADPH) oxidase inhibitors were able to alter M1-/M2-like balance in favor of the anti-inflammatory M2-like phenotype in a CCI model of TBI (Kumar et al., 2016a,b).

CONCLUSIONS

In recent years, there has been a growing interest in investigating the activation of microglia in TBI, because of the potential role in the progression of those patients to neurodegenerative and psychiatric diseases. The studies of microglia in animal models of TBI have allowed the manipulation of microglial numbers (by genetic or pharmacological ablation), indicating their important role in neuroprotection especially at early times post-injury, although this sequence seems to be model and species-specific. In addition, this has provided insights into the time course of the different profile of microglial activation phenotypes in the injury site and the spreading of inflammation to other areas of the brain, such as the thalamus.

In vivo molecular imaging of TSPO potentially provides an extremely useful biomarker of microglial activation and the effect of immunomodulatory drugs. In TBI patients, it has allowed the observation of chronically activated microglia located in areas of persistent white matter damage, even long time post injury. However, it currently only provides a one-dimensional measure, i.e., the amount of microglial activation within a particular brain region. It is clearly too simplistic to describe microglial activation *in vivo* along a single dimension (i.e., from "low activity" to "high activity"). Crucially, on the basis of current evidence, TSPO molecular imaging cannot discriminate activation phenotype, but probably reflects the (potentially uneven) summation of activity from microglia across all functional states.

In addition, there has been some debate regarding the possibility that certain TSPO ligands also recognize astrocytes or other immune cells in the brains of TBI patients. Other limitations of the application of second-generation ligands include that the binding affinities are influenced by a common polymorphism (rs6971) in the TSPO gene which causes a single amino acid substitution (A147T) in the protein (Owen et al., 2012). Because 147T TSPO binds ligands with lower affinity than 147A, this produces three classes of binding affinity across a population, which studies must therefore control for. Even after accounting for TSPO genotype, however, many second-generation TSPO ligands show high between-subject variability in uptake when using analysis methods which rely on measurement of the ligand in arterial blood (Guo et al., 2012). As for $[^{11}C]$PK11195, high and variable plasma protein binding may be a factor (Lockhart et al., 2003). Methods of analysis such as the simplified reference tissue model (SRTM) have been developed that do not require arterial blood data, but rather use the PET imaging data from a reference region (or reference tissue) instead (Gunn et al., 1997).

To improve the interpretation of the TSPO signal, a detailed characterization is needed of how TSPO expression in humans varies with the diversity of microglial phenotypes seen *in vivo*. Future TBI work needs to provide a description of the time-course of microglial phenotype change after TBI and its relationship to TSPO expression. Novel PET ligands showing specificity for distinct functional subtypes of microglial activation would be of great utility, with cannabinoid type 2 and purinergic receptors, such as P2Y12 and P2X7, possibly providing suitable targets in the future. Another option is to combine TSPO PET imaging with different biomarkers that disambiguate the TSPO signal in a particular context, in particular neurofilament light (NFL). NFL levels in CSF have been proposed as a valid biomarker to accurately assess the level of trauma and predict the clinical outcome of the patient (Zhang et al., 2016).

Recent investigations have indicated that simple suppression of microglia activation can exert only limited beneficial effect and the inhibition of M1-like responses might be detrimental similar to a simple stimulation of M2-like phenotypes, as indicated by increased fibrosis which seems modulated by Arginase-1 in peripheral and central infection (Hesse et al., 2001; Aldrich and Kielian, 2011). In addition, pharmacological treatment with the anti-inflammatory drugs tested in several models may not have similar effects when administered in TBI patients, as seen in clinical trials for AD (Lleo et al., 2007), limiting the potential therapeutic impact. It seems therefore imperative for future studies that target microglia polarization as therapeutic strategies, to assess several markers in the target cells within a sufficient temporal window in order to show a long-term positive outcome.

AUTHOR CONTRIBUTIONS

MS wrote most of the introduction, the manipulation of microglia in animal models and the treatments section; CD wrote most of the section on animal models of TBI and preclinical TSPO imaging in animal models, made the tables, the references and wrote part of the conclusions; GS wrote most of the part of the imaging with TSPO, made two figures and part of the conclusions; SG contributed with the image of microglia (**Figure 1**) and edited the manuscript.

FUNDING

ISSF Networks of Excellence award 2015 (reference 105603/Z/14/Z, Wellcome Trust).

ACKNOWLEDGMENTS

We thank Prof. David J. Sharp (Imperial College London) for critical reading of the manuscript.

REFERENCES

Abcouwer, S. F., Lin, C. M., Shanmugam, S., Muthusamy, A., Barber, A. J., and Antonetti, D. A. (2013). Minocycline prevents retinal inflammation and vascular permeability following ischemia-reperfusion injury. *J. Neuroinflammat.* 10:149. doi: 10.1186/1742-2094-10-149

Aldrich, A., and Kielian, T. (2011). Central nervous system fibrosis is associated with fibrocyte-like infiltrates. *Am. J. Pathol.* 179, 2952–2962. doi: 10.1016/j.ajpath.2011.08.036

Ansari, M. A. (2015). Temporal profile of M1 and M2 responses in the hippocampus following early 24 h of neurotrauma. *J. Neurol. Sci.* 357, 41–49. doi: 10.1016/j.jns.2015.06.062

Baalman, K., Marin, M. A., Ho, T. S., Godoy, M., Cherian, L., Robertson, C., et al. (2015). Axon initial segment-associated microglia. *J. Neurosci.* 35, 2283–2292. doi: 10.1523/JNEUROSCI.3751-14.2015

Bachstetter, A. D., Rowe, R. K., Kaneko, M., Goulding, D., Lifshitz, J., and Van Eldik, L. J. (2013). The p38alpha MAPK regulates microglial responsiveness to diffuse traumatic brain injury. *J. Neurosci.* 33, 6143–6153. doi: 10.1523/JNEUROSCI.5399-12.2013

Banati, R. B., Myers, R., and Kreutzberg, G. W. (1997). PK ('peripheral benzodiazepine')--binding sites in the CNS indicate early and discrete brain lesions: microautoradiographic detection of [3H]PK11195 binding to activated microglia. *J. Neurocytol.* 26, 77–82. doi: 10.1023/A:1018567510105

Banati, R. B., Newcombe, J., Gunn, R. N., Cagnin, A., Turkheimer, F., Heppner, F., et al. (2000). The peripheral benzodiazepine binding site in the brain in multiple sclerosis: quantitative *in vivo* imaging of microglia as a measure of disease activity. *Brain* 123 (Pt 11), 2321–2337. doi: 10.1093/brain/123.11.2321

Barrett, J. P., Henry, R. J., Villapol, S., Stoica, B. A., Kumar, A., Burns, M. P., et al. (2017). NOX2 deficiency alters macrophage phenotype through an IL-10/STAT3 dependent mechanism: implications for traumatic brain injury. *J. Neuroinflammat.* 14, 65. doi: 10.1186/s12974-017-0843-4

Bedi, S. S., Smith, P., Hetz, R. A., Xue, H., and Cox, C. S. (2013). Immunomagnetic enrichment and flow cytometric characterization of mouse microglia. *J. Neurosci. Methods* 219, 176–182. doi: 10.1016/j.jneumeth.2013.07.017

Bennett, R. E., and Brody, D. L. (2014). Acute reduction of microglia does not alter axonal injury in a mouse model of repetitive concussive traumatic brain injury. *J. Neurotrauma.* 31, 1647–1663. doi: 10.1089/neu.2013.3320

Berry, C., Ley, E. J., Tillou, A., Cryer, G., Margulies, D. R., and Salim, A. (2009). The effect of gender on patients with moderate to severe head injuries. *J. Trauma* 67, 950–953. doi: 10.1097/TA.0b013e3181ba3354

Besson, V. C., Chen, X. R., Plotkine, M., and Marchand-Verrecchia, C. (2005). Fenofibrate, a peroxisome proliferator-activated receptor alpha agonist, exerts neuroprotective effects in traumatic brain injury. *Neurosci. Lett.* 388, 7–12. doi: 10.1016/j.neulet.2005.06.019

Black, M. E., Newcomb, T. G., Wilson, H. M., and Loeb, L. A. (1996). Creation of drug-specific herpes simplex virus type 1 thymidine kinase mutants for gene therapy. *Proc. Natl. Acad. Sci. U.S.A.* 93, 3525–3529. doi: 10.1073/pnas.93.8.3525

Boche, D., Perry, V. H., and Nicoll, J. A. (2013). Review: activation patterns of microglia and their identification in the human brain. *Neuropathol. Appl. Neurobiol.* 39, 3–18. doi: 10.1111/nan.12011

Bonsack, F. IV, Alleyne, C. H. Jr., and Sukumari-Ramesh, S. (2016). Augmented expression of TSPO after intracerebral hemorrhage: a role in inflammation? *J. Neuroinflammat.* 13:151. doi: 10.1186/s12974-016-0619-2

Braun, M., Vaibhav, K., Saad, N., Fatima, S., Brann, D. W., Vender, J. R., et al. (2017). Activation of Myeloid TLR4 Mediates T Lymphocyte polarization after Traumatic Brain Injury. *J. Immunol.* 198, 3615–3626. doi: 10.4049/jimmunol.1601948

Bye, N., Habgood, M. D., Callaway, J. K., Malakooti, N., Potter, A., Kossmann, T., et al. (2007). Transient neuroprotection by minocycline following traumatic brain injury is associated with attenuated microglial activation but no changes in cell apoptosis or neutrophil infiltration. *Exp. Neurol.* 204, 220–233. doi: 10.1016/j.expneurol.2006.10.013

Cagnin, A., Brooks, D. J., Kennedy, A. M., Gunn, R. N., Myers, R., Turkheimer, F. E., et al. (2001a). *In-vivo* measurement of activated microglia in dementia. *Lancet* 358, 461–467. doi: 10.1016/S0140-6736(01)05625-2

Cagnin, A., Gerhard, A., and Banati, R. B. (2003). *In vivo Imaging of Neuroinflammation in Neurodegenerative Diseases. (Neuroinflammation: Mechanisms and Management).* Totowa, NJ: Humana Press Inc.

Cagnin, A., Myers, R., Gunn, R. N., Lawrence, A. D., Stevens, T., Kreutzberg, G. W., et al. (2001b). *In vivo* visualization of activated glia by [11C] (R)-PK11195-PET following herpes encephalitis reveals projected neuronal damage beyond the primary focal lesion. *Brain* 124(Pt 10), 2014–2027. doi: 10.1093/brain/124.10.2014

Cao, T., Thomas, T. C., Ziebell, J. M., Pauly, J. R., and Lifshitz, J. (2012). Morphological and genetic activation of microglia after diffuse traumatic brain injury in the rat. *Neuroscience* 225, 65–75. doi: 10.1016/j.neuroscience.2012.08.058

Caplan, H. W., Cox, C. S., and Bedi, S. S. (2017). Do microglia play a role in sex differences in TBI? *J. Neurosci. Res.* 95, 509–517. doi: 10.1002/jnr.23854

Carmichael, E. A. (1929). Microglia: an experimental study in rabbits after intracerebral injection of blood. *J. Neurol. Psychopathol.* 9, 209–216. doi: 10.1136/jnnp.s1-9.35.209

Cheng, Y. C., Huang, E. S., Lin, J. C., Mar, E. C., Pagano, J. S., Dutschman, G. E., et al. (1983). Unique spectrum of activity of 9-[(1,3-dihydroxy-2-propoxy)methyl]-guanine against herpesviruses *in vitro* and its mode of action against herpes simplex virus type 1. *Proc. Natl. Acad. Sci. U.S.A.* 80, 2767–2770. doi: 10.1073/pnas.80.9.2767

Cheong, C. U., Chang, C. P., Chao, C. M., Cheng, B. C., Yang, C. Z., and Chio, C. C. (2013). Etanercept attenuates traumatic brain injury in rats by reducing brain TNF- alpha contents and by stimulating newly formed neurogenesis. *Mediat. Inflamm.* 2013:620837. doi: 10.1155/2013/620837

Cherry, J. D., Tripodis, Y., Alvarez, V. E., Huber, B., Kiernan, P. T., Daneshvar, D. H., et al. (2016). Microglial neuroinflammation contributes to tau accumulation in chronic traumatic encephalopathy. *Acta Neuropathol. Commun.* 4, 112. doi: 10.1186/s40478-016-0382-8

Chhor, V., Moretti, R., Le Charpentier, T., Sigaut, S., Lebon, S., Schwendimann, L., et al. (2016). Role of microglia in a mouse model of paediatric traumatic brain injury. *Brain Behav. Immun.* 63, 197–209. doi: 10.1016/j.bbi.2016.11.001

Chio, C. C., Chang, C. H., Wang, C. C., Cheong, C. U., Chao, C. M., Cheng, B. C., et al. (2013). Etanercept attenuates traumatic brain injury in rats by reducing early microglial expression of tumor necrosis factor-alpha. *BMC Neurosci.* 14:33. doi: 10.1186/1471-2202-14-33

Chio, C. C., Lin, M. T., and Chang, C. P. (2015). Microglial activation as a compelling target for treating acute traumatic brain injury. *Curr. Med. Chem.* 22, 759–770. doi: 10.2174/0929867321666141106124657

Chiu, C. C., Liao, Y. E., Yang, L. Y., Wang, J. Y., Tweedie, D., Karnati, H. K., et al. (2016). Neuroinflammation in animal models of traumatic brain injury. *J. Neurosci. Methods* 272, 38–49. doi: 10.1016/j.jneumeth.2016.06.018

Coimbra, R., Hoyt, D. B., Potenza, B. M., Fortlage, D., and Hollingsworth-Fridlund, P. (2003). Does sexual dimorphism influence outcome of traumatic brain injury patients? The answer is no! *J. Trauma.* 54, 689–700. doi: 10.1097/01.TA.0000058314.31655.5F

Coughlin, J. M., Wang, Y., Minn, I., Bienko, N., Ambinder, E. B., Xu, X., et al. (2017). Imaging of glial cell activation and white matter integrity in brains of active and recently retired national football league players. *JAMA Neurol.* 74, 67–74. doi: 10.1001/jamaneurol.2016.3764

Coughlin, J. M., Wang, Y., Munro, C. A., Ma, S., Yue, C., Chen, S., et al. (2015). Neuroinflammation and brain atrophy in former NFL players: an *in vivo* multimodal imaging pilot study. *Neurobiol. Dis.* 74, 58–65. doi: 10.1016/j.nbd.2014.10.019

DeKosky, S. T., Abrahamson, E. E., Ciallella, J. R., Paljug, W. R., Wisniewski, S. R., Clark, R. S., et al. (2007). Association of increased cortical soluble abeta42 levels with diffuse plaques after severe brain injury in humans. *Arch. Neurol.* 64, 541–544. doi: 10.1001/archneur.64.4.541

Desai, A., Park, T., Barnes, J., Kevala, K., Chen, H., and Kim, H. Y. (2016). Reduced acute neuroinflammation and improved functional recovery after traumatic brain injury by alpha-linolenic acid supplementation in mice. *J. Neuroinflammat.* 13:253. doi: 10.1186/s12974-016-0714-4

Donat, C. K., Fischer, F., Walter, B., Deuther-Conrad, W., Brodhun, M., Bauer, R., et al. (2014). Early increase of cannabinoid receptor density after experimental traumatic brain injury in the newborn piglet. *Acta Neurobiol. Exp. (Wars)* 74, 197–210.

Donat, C. K., Gaber, K., Meixensberger, J., Brust, P., Pinborg, L. H., Hansen, H. H., et al. (2016). Changes in binding of [(123)I]CLINDE, a high-affinity translocator protein 18 kDa (TSPO) selective radioligand in a rat model of traumatic brain injury. *Neuromol. Med.* 18, 158–169. doi: 10.1007/s12017-016-8385-y

Dunning, H. S., and Stevenson, L. (1934). Microglia-like cells and their reaction following injury to the liver, spleen and kidney. *Am. J. Pathol.* 10, 343–348.7

Elliott, M. B., Tuma, R. F., Amenta, P. S., Barbe, M. F., and Jallo, J. I. (2011). Acute effects of a selective cannabinoid-2 receptor agonist on neuroinflammation in a model of traumatic brain injury. *J. Neurotrauma* 28, 973–981. doi: 10.1089/neu.2010.1672

Faden, A. I., Wu, J., Stoica, B. A., and Loane, D. J. (2016). Progressive inflammation-mediated neurodegeneration after traumatic brain or spinal cord injury. *Br. J. Pharmacol.* 173, 681–691. doi: 10.1111/bph.13179

Faulds, D., and Heel, R. C. (1990). Ganciclovir. A review of its antiviral activity, pharmacokinetic properties and therapeutic efficacy in cytomegalovirus infections. *Drugs* 39, 597–638. doi: 10.2165/00003495-199039040-00008

Febinger, H. Y., Thomasy, H. E., Pavlova, M. N., Ringgold, K. M., Barf, P. R., George, A. M., et al. (2015). Time-dependent effects of CX3CR1 in a mouse model of mild traumatic brain injury. *J. Neuroinflammat.* 12:154. doi: 10.1186/s12974-015-0386-5

Fenn, A. M., Gensel, J. C., Huang, Y., Popovich, P. G., Lifshitz, J., and Godbout, J. P. (2014). Immune activation promotes depression 1 month after diffuse brain injury: a role for primed microglia. *Biol. Psychiatry* 76, 575–584. doi: 10.1016/j.biopsych.2013.10.014

Fenn, A. M., Skendelas, J. P., Moussa, D. N., Muccigrosso, M. M., Popovich, P. G., Lifshitz, J., et al. (2015). Methylene blue attenuates traumatic brain injury-associated neuroinflammation and acute depressive-like behavior in mice. *J. Neurotrauma.* 32, 127–138. doi: 10.1089/neu.2014.3514

Folkersma, H., Boellaard, R., Yaqub, M., Kloet, R. W., Windhorst, A. D., Lammertsma, A. A., et al. (2011a). Widespread and prolonged increase in (R)-11C-PK11195 binding after traumatic brain injury. *J. Nucl. Med.* 52, 1235–1239. doi: 10.2967/jnumed.110.084061

Folkersma, H., Foster Dingley, J. C., van Berckel, B. N., Rozemuller, A., Boellaard, R., Huisman, M. C., et al. (2011b). Increased cerebral (R)-[11C]-PK11195 uptake and glutamate release in a rat model of traumatic brain injury: a longitudinal pilot study. *J. Neuroinflammat.* 8:67. doi: 10.1186/1742-2094-8-67

Gao, H., Han, Z., Bai, R., Huang, S., Ge, X., Chen, F., et al. (2017). The accumulation of brain injury leads to severe neuropathological and neurobehavioral changes after repetitive mild traumatic brain injury. *Brain Res.* 1657, 1–8. doi: 10.1016/j.brainres.2016.11.028

Garrido-Mesa, N., Zarzuelo, A., and Galvez, J. (2013). Minocycline: far beyond an antibiotic. *Br. J. Pharmacol.*, 169, 337–352. doi: 10.1111/bph.12139

Gerhard, A., Schwarz, J., Myers, R., Wise, R., and Banati, R. B. (2005). Evolution of microglial activation in patients after ischemic stroke: a [11C](R)-PK11195 PET study. *Neuroimage* 24, 591–595. doi: 10.1016/j.neuroimage.2004.09.034

Giunta, B., Obregon, D., Velisetty, R., Sanberg, P. R., Borlongan, C. V., and Tan, J. (2012). The immunology of traumatic brain injury: a prime target for Alzheimer's disease prevention. *J. Neuroinflammat.* 9:185. doi: 10.1186/1742-2094-9-185

Goldstein, L. E., Fisher, A. M., Tagge, C. A., Zhang, X. L., Velisek, L., Sullivan, J. A., et al. (2012). Chronic traumatic encephalopathy in blast-exposed military veterans and a blast neurotrauma mouse model. *Sci. Transl. Med.* 4, 134ra160. doi: 10.1126/scitranslmed.3003716

Gowing, G., Vallieres, L., and Julien, J. P. (2006). Mouse model for ablation of proliferating microglia in acute CNS injuries. *Glia* 53, 331–337. doi: 10.1002/glia.20288

Grossman, R., Paden, C. M., Fry, P. A., Rhodes, R. S., and Biegon, A. (2012). Persistent region-dependent neuroinflammation, NMDA receptor loss and atrophy in an animal model of penetrating brain injury. *Fut. Neurol.* 7, 329–339. doi: 10.2217/fnl.12.25

Grossman, R., Shohami, E., Alexandrovich, A., Yatsiv, I., Kloog, Y., and Biegon, A. (2003). Increase in peripheral benzodiazepine receptors and loss of glutamate NMDA receptors in a mouse model of closed head injury: a quantitative autoradiographic study. *Neuroimage* 20, 1971–1981. doi: 10.1016/j.neuroimage.2003.06.003

Gruenbaum, S. E., Zlotnik, A., Gruenbaum, B. F., Hersey, D., and Bilotta, F. (2016). Pharmacologic neuroprotection for functional outcomes after traumatic Brain injury: a systematic review of the clinical literature. *CNS Drugs* 30, 791–806. doi: 10.1007/s40263-016-0355-2

Guilfoyle, M. R., Carpenter, K. L., Helmy, A., Pickard, J. D., Menon, D. K., and Hutchinson, P. J. (2015). Matrix metalloproteinase expression in contusional traumatic brain injury: a paired microdialysis study. *J. Neurotrauma* 32, 1553–1559. doi: 10.1089/neu.2014.3764

Gunn, R. N., Lammertsma, A. A., Hume, S. P., and Cunningham, V. J. (1997). Parametric imaging of ligand-receptor binding in PET using a simplified reference region model. *Neuroimage* 6, 279–287. doi: 10.1006/nimg.1997.0303

Guo, Q., Owen, D. R., Rabiner, E. A., Turkheimer, F. E., and Gunn, R. N. (2012). Identifying improved TSPO PET imaging probes through biomathematics: the impact of multiple TSPO binding sites *in vivo*. *Neuroimage* 60, 902–910. doi: 10.1016/j.neuroimage.2011.12.078

Hanlon, L. A., Huh, J. W., and Raghupathi, R. (2016). Minocycline transiently reduces microglia/macrophage activation but exacerbates cognitive deficits following repetitive traumatic brain injury in the neonatal rat. *J. Neuropathol. Exp. Neurol.* 75, 214–226. doi: 10.1093/jnen/nlv021

Hanlon, L. A., Raghupathi, R., and Huh, J. W. (2017). Differential effects of minocycline on microglial activation and neurodegeneration following closed head injury in the neonate rat. *Exp. Neurol.* 290, 1–14. doi: 10.1016/j.expneurol.2016.12.010

Hazeldine, J., Lord, J. M., and Belli, A. (2015). Traumatic brain injury and peripheral immune suppression: primer and prospectus. *Front. Neurol.* 6:235. doi: 10.3389/fneur.2015.00235

Hesse, M., Modolell, M., La Flamme, A. C., Schito, M., Fuentes, J. M., Cheever, A. W., et al. (2001). Differential regulation of nitric oxide synthase-2 and arginase-1 by type 1/type 2 cytokines *in vivo*: granulomatous pathology is shaped by the pattern of L-arginine metabolism. *J. Immunol.* 167, 6533–6544. doi: 10.4049/jimmunol.167.11.6533

Hickman, S. E., Kingery, N. D., Ohsumi, T. K., Borowsky, M. L., Wang, L. C., Means, T. K., et al. (2013). The microglial sensome revealed by direct RNA sequencing. *Nat. Neurosci.* 16, 1896–1905. doi: 10.1038/nn.3554

Holmin, S., and Mathiesen, T. (1999). Long-term intracerebral inflammatory response after experimental focal brain injury in rat. *Neuroreport* 10, 1889–1891. doi: 10.1097/00001756-199906230-00017

Homsi, S., Piaggio, T., Croci, N., Noble, F., Plotkine, M., Marchand-Leroux, C., et al. (2010). Blockade of acute microglial activation by minocycline promotes neuroprotection and reduces locomotor hyperactivity after closed head injury in mice: a twelve-week follow-up study. *J. Neurotrauma* 27, 911–921. doi: 10.1089/neu.2009.1223

Hsieh, C. L., Kim, C. C., Ryba, B. E., Niemi, E. C., Bando, J. K., Locksley, R. M., et al. (2013). Traumatic brain injury induces macrophage subsets in the brain. *Eur. J. Immunol.* 43, 2010–2022. doi: 10.1002/eji.201243084

Hu, X., Leak, R. K., Shi, Y., Suenaga, J., Gao, Y., Zheng, P., et al. (2015). Microglial and macrophage polarization-new prospects for brain repair. *Nat. Rev. Neurol.* 11, 56–64. doi: 10.1038/nrneurol.2014.207

Hyder, A. A., Wunderlich, C. A., Puvanachandra, P., Gururaj, G., and Kobusingye, O. C. (2007). The impact of traumatic brain injuries: a global perspective. *NeuroRehabilitation* 22, 341–353.

Ikonomovic, M. D., Uryu, K., Abrahamson, E. E., Ciallella, J. R., Trojanowski, J. Q., Lee, V. M., et al. (2004). Alzheimer's pathology in human temporal cortex surgically excised after severe brain injury. *Exp. Neurol.* 190, 192–203. doi: 10.1016/j.expneurol.2004.06.011

Immonen, R. J., Kharatishvili, I., Grohn, H., Pitkanen, A., and Grohn, O. H. (2009). Quantitative MRI predicts long-term structural and functional outcome after experimental traumatic brain injury. *Neuroimage* 45, 1–9. doi: 10.1016/j.neuroimage.2008.11.022

Israel, I., Ohsiek, A., Al-Momani, E., Albert-Weissenberger, C., Stetter, C., Mencl, S., et al. (2016). Combined [(18)F]DPA-714 micro-positron emission tomography and autoradiography imaging of microglia activation after closed head injury in mice. *J. Neuroinflammat.* 13:140. doi: 10.1186/s12974-016-0604-9

Jablonski, K. A., Amici, S. A., Webb, L. M., Ruiz-Rosado Jde, D., Popovich, P. G., Partida-Sanchez, S., et al. (2015). Novel Markers to Delineate Murine M1 and M2 Macrophages. *PLoS ONE* 10:e0145342. doi: 10.1371/journal.pone.0145342

Jafari, S., Etminan, M., Aminzadeh, F., and Samii, A. (2013). Head injury and risk of Parkinson disease: a systematic review and meta-analysis. *Mov. Disord.* 28, 1222–1229. doi: 10.1002/mds.25458

Jaremko, L., Jaremko, M., Giller, K., Becker, S., and Zweckstetter, M. (2014). Structure of the mitochondrial translocator protein in complex with a diagnostic ligand. *Science* 343, 1363–1366. doi: 10.1126/science.1248725

Jin, W. N., Shi, S. X., Li, Z., Li, M., Wood, K., Gonzales, R. J., et al. (2017). Depletion of microglia exacerbates postischemic inflammation and brain injury. *J. Cereb. Blood Flow Metab.* 37, 2224–2236. doi: 10.1177/0271678x17694185

Jin, X., Ishii, H., Bai, Z., Itokazu, T., and Yamashita, T. (2012). Temporal changes in cell marker expression and cellular infiltration in a controlled cortical impact model in adult male C57BL/6 mice. *PLoS ONE* 7:e41892. doi: 10.1371/journal.pone.0041892

Johnson, V. E., Stewart, J. E., Begbie, F. D., Trojanowski, J. Q., Smith, D. H., and Stewart, W. (2013). Inflammation and white matter degeneration persist for years after a single traumatic brain injury. *Brain* 136(Pt 1), 28–42. doi: 10.1093/brain/aws322

Jordan, B. D. (2000). Chronic traumatic brain injury associated with boxing. *Semin. Neurol.* 20, 179–185. doi: 10.1055/s-2000-9826

Kim, J. H., Jenrow, K. A., and Brown, S. L. (2014). Mechanisms of radiation-induced normal tissue toxicity and implications for future clinical trials. *Radiat. Oncol. J.* 32, 103–115. doi: 10.3857/roj.2014.32.3.103

Kim, E. J., and Yu, S. W. (2015). Translocator protein 18 kDa (TSPO): old dogma, new mice, new structure, and new questions for neuroprotection. *Neural Regen. Res.* 10, 878–880. doi: 10.4103/1673-5374.158338

Klemenhagen, K. C., O'Brien, S. P., and Brody, D. L. (2013). Repetitive concussive traumatic brain injury interacts with post-injury foot shock stress to worsen social and depression-like behavior in mice. *PLoS ONE* 8:e74510. doi: 10.1371/journal.pone.0074510

Kobayashi, K., Imagama, S., Ohgomori, T., Hirano, K., Uchimura, K., Sakamoto, K., et al. (2013). Minocycline selectively inhibits M1 polarization of microglia. *Cell Death Dis.* 4:e525. doi: 10.1038/cddis.2013.54

Kobayashi, M., Jiang, T., Telu, S., Zoghbi, S. S., Gunn, R. N., Rabiner, E. A., et al. (2017). 11C-DPA-713 has much greater specific binding to translocator protein 18 kDa (TSPO) in human brain than 11C-(R)-PK11195. *J. Cereb. Blood Flow Metab.* 271678x17699223. doi: 10.1177/0271678x17699223

Kochanek, P. M., Hendrich, K. S., Dixon, C. E., Schiding, J. K., Williams, D. S., and Ho, C. (2002). Cerebral blood flow at one year after controlled cortical impact in rats: assessment by magnetic resonance imaging. *J. Neurotrauma* 19, 1029–1037. doi: 10.1089/089771502760341947

Koh, T. J., and DiPietro, L. A. (2011). Inflammation and wound healing: the role of the macrophage. *Expert Rev. Mol. Med.* 13:e23. doi: 10.1017/s1462399411001943

Kovesdi, E., Kamnaksh, A., Wingo, D., Ahmed, F., Grunberg, N. E., Long, J. B., et al. (2012). Acute minocycline treatment mitigates the symptoms of mild blast-induced traumatic brain injury. *Front. Neurol.* 3:111. doi: 10.3389/fneur.2012.00111

Kreutzberg, G. W. (1996). Microglia: a sensor for pathological events in the CNS. *Trends Neurosci.* 19, 312–318. doi: 10.1016/0166-2236(96)10049-7

Kumar, A., Alvarez-Croda, D. M., Stoica, B. A., Faden, A. I., and Loane, D. J. (2016a). Microglial/Macrophage polarization dynamics following traumatic brain injury. *J. Neurotrauma* 33, 1732–1750. doi: 10.1089/neu.2015.4268

Kumar, A., Barrett, J. P., Alvarez-Croda, D. M., Stoica, B. A., Faden, A. I., and Loane, D. J. (2016b). NOX2 drives M1-like microglial/macrophage activation and neurodegeneration following experimental traumatic brain injury. *Brain Behav. Immun.* 58, 291–309. doi: 10.1016/j.bbi.2016.07.158

Kumar, A., Muzik, O., Shandal, V., Chugani, D., Chakraborty, P., and Chugani, H. T. (2012). Evaluation of age-related changes in translocator protein (TSPO) in human brain using (11)C-[R]-PK11195 PET. *J. Neuroinflammat.* 9:232. doi: 10.1186/1742-2094-9-232

Kumar, A., Stoica, B. A., Sabirzhanov, B., Burns, M. P., Faden, A. I., and Loane, D. J. (2013). Traumatic brain injury in aged animals increases lesion size and chronically alters microglial/macrophage classical and alternative activation states. *Neurobiol. Aging* 34, 1397–1411. doi: 10.1016/j.neurobiolaging.2012.11.013

Langlois, J. A., Rutland-Brown, W., and Wald, M. M. (2006). The epidemiology and impact of traumatic brain injury: a brief overview. *J. Head Trauma Rehabil*, 21, 375–378. doi: 10.1097/00001199-200609000-00001

Lawson, L. J., Perry, V. H., Dri, P., and Gordon, S. (1990). Heterogeneity in the distribution and morphology of microglia in the normal adult mouse brain. *Neuroscience* 39, 151–170. doi: 10.1016/0306-4522(90)90229-W

Lenz, K. M., and McCarthy, M. M. (2015). A starring role for microglia in brain sex differences. *Neuroscientist* 21, 306–321. doi: 10.1177/1073858414536468

Ley, E. J., Short, S. S., Liou, D. Z., Singer, M. B., Mirocha, J., Melo, N., et al. (2013). Gender impacts mortality after traumatic brain injury in teenagers. *J. Trauma Acute Care Surg.* 75, 682–686. doi: 10.1097/TA.0b013e31829d024f

Liu, G. J., Middleton, R. J., Hatty, C. R., Kam, W. W., Chan, R., Pham, T., et al. (2014). The 18 kDa translocator protein, microglia and neuroinflammation. *Brain Pathol.* 24, 631–653. doi: 10.1111/bpa.12196

Lleo, A., Galea, E., and Sastre, M. (2007). Molecular targets of non-steroidal anti-inflammatory drugs in neurodegenerative diseases. *Cell Mol. Life Sci.* 64, 1403–118. doi: 10.1007/s00018-007-6516-1

Lloyd, E., Somera-Molina, K., Van Eldik, L. J., Watterson, D. M., and Wainwright, M. S. (2008). Suppression of acute proinflammatory cytokine and chemokine upregulation by post-injury administration of a novel small molecule improves long-term neurologic outcome in a mouse model of traumatic brain injury. *J. Neuroinflammat.* 5:28. doi: 10.1186/1742-2094-5-28

Loane, D. J., and Faden, A. I. (2010). Neuroprotection for traumatic brain injury: translational challenges and emerging therapeutic strategies. *Trends Pharmacol. Sci.* 31, 596–604. doi: 10.1016/j.tips.2010.09.005

Loane, D. J., Kumar, A., Stoica, B. A., Cabatbat, R., and Faden, A. I. (2014a). Progressive neurodegeneration after experimental brain trauma: association with chronic microglial activation. *J. Neuropathol. Exp. Neurol.* 73, 14–29. doi: 10.1097/NEN.0000000000000021

Loane, D. J., Stoica, B. A., Tchantchou, F., Kumar, A., Barrett, J. P., Akintola, T., et al. (2014b). Novel mGluR5 positive allosteric modulator improves functional recovery, attenuates neurodegeneration, and alters microglial polarization after experimental traumatic brain injury. *Neurotherapeutics* 11, 857–869. doi: 10.1007/s13311-014-0298-6

Lockhart, A., Davis, B., Matthews, J. C., Rahmoune, H., Hong, G., Gee, A., et al. (2003). The peripheral benzodiazepine receptor ligand PK11195 binds with high affinity to the acute phase reactant alpha1-acid glycoprotein: implications for the use of the ligand as a CNS inflammatory marker. *Nucl. Med. Biol.* 30, 199–206. doi: 10.1016/S0969-8051(02)00410-9

Mannix, R., Berglass, J., Berkner, J., Moleus, P., Qiu, J., Andrews, N., et al. (2014). Chronic gliosis and behavioral deficits in mice following repetitive mild traumatic brain injury. *J. Neurosurg.* 121, 1342–1350. doi: 10.3171/2014.7.JNS14272

Maxwell, W. L., MacKinnon, M. A., Stewart, J. E., and Graham, D. I. (2010). Stereology of cerebral cortex after traumatic brain injury matched to the Glasgow outcome score. *Brain* 133(Pt 1), 139–160. doi: 10.1093/brain/awp264

McKee, A. C., Alosco, M. L., and Huber, B. R. (2016). Repetitive head impacts and chronic traumatic encephalopathy. *Neurosurg. Clin. N. Am.* 27, 529–535. doi: 10.1016/j.nec.2016.05.009

McKee, A. C., and Daneshvar, D. H. (2015). The neuropathology of traumatic brain injury. *Handb. Clin. Neurol.* 127, 45–66. doi: 10.1016/B978-0-444-52892-6.00004-0

McMillan, T. M., Teasdale, G. M., Weir, C. J., and Stewart, E. (2011). Death after head injury: the 13 year outcome of a case control study. *J. Neurol. Neurosurg. Psychiatr.* 82, 931–935. doi: 10.1136/jnnp.2010.222232

Menzel, L., Kleber, L., Friedrich, C., Hummel, R., Dangel, L., Winter, J., et al. (2017). Progranulin protects against exaggerated axonal injury and astrogliosis following traumatic brain injury. *Glia* 65, 278–292. doi: 10.1002/glia.23091

Menzies, F. M., Henriquez, F. L., Alexander, J., and Roberts, C. W. (2011). Selective inhibition and augmentation of alternative macrophage activation by progesterone. *Immunology* 134, 281–291. doi: 10.1111/j.1365-2567.2011.03488.x

Methia, N., Andre, P., Hafezi-Moghadam, A., Economopoulos, M., Thomas, K. L., and Wagner, D. D. (2001). ApoE deficiency compromises the blood brain barrier especially after injury. *Mol. Med.* 7, 810–815.

Mittelbronn, M., Dietz, K., Schluesener, H. J., and Meyermann, R. (2001). Local distribution of microglia in the normal adult human central nervous system differs by up to one order of magnitude. *Acta Neuropathol.* 101, 249–255.

Miyazawa, N., Diksic, M., and Yamamoto, Y. (1995). Chronological study of peripheral benzodiazepine binding sites in the rat brain stab wounds using [3H] PK-11195 as a marker for gliosis. *Acta Neurochir. (Wien).* 137, 207–216. doi: 10.1007/BF02187195

Morganti, J. M., Jopson, T. D., Liu, S., Riparip, L. K., Guandique, C. K., Gupta, N., et al. (2015). CCR2 antagonism alters brain macrophage polarization and ameliorates cognitive dysfunction induced by traumatic brain injury. *J. Neurosci.* 35, 748–760. doi: 10.1523/JNEUROSCI.2405-14.2015

Morganti, J. M., Riparip, L. K., and Rosi, S. (2016). Call Off the Dog(ma): M1/M2 polarization is concurrent following traumatic brain injury. *PLoS ONE* 11:e0148001. doi: 10.1371/journal.pone.0148001

Morohaku, K., Pelton, S. H., Daugherty, D. J., Butler, W. R., Deng, W., and Selvaraj, V. (2014). Translocator protein/peripheral benzodiazepine receptor is not required for steroid hormone biosynthesis. *Endocrinology* 155, 89–97. doi: 10.1210/en.2013-1556

Murray, P. J., and Wynn, T. A. (2011). Obstacles and opportunities for understanding macrophage polarization. *J. Leukoc. Biol.* 89, 557–563. doi: 10.1189/jlb.0710409

Nagamoto-Combs, K., McNeal, D. W., Morecraft, R. J., and Combs, C. K. (2007). Prolonged microgliosis in the rhesus monkey central nervous system after traumatic brain injury. *J. Neurotrauma* 24, 1719–1742. doi: 10.1089/neu.2007.0377

Nagamoto-Combs, K., Morecraft, R. J., Darling, W. G., and Combs, C. K. (2010). Long-term gliosis and molecular changes in the cervical spinal cord of the rhesus monkey after traumatic brain injury. *J. Neurotrauma* 27, 565–585. doi: 10.1089/neu.2009.0966

Nishitsuji, K., Hosono, T., Nakamura, T., Bu, G., and Michikawa, M. (2011). Apolipoprotein E regulates the integrity of tight junctions in an isoform-dependent manner in an *in vitro* blood-brain barrier model. *J. Biol. Chem.* 286, 17536–17542. doi: 10.1074/jbc.M111.225532

O'Connor, W. T., Smyth, A., and Gilchrist, M. D. (2011). Animal models of traumatic brain injury: a critical evaluation. *Pharmacol. Ther.* 130, 106–113. doi: 10.1016/j.pharmthera.2011.01.001

Ojo, J. O., Mouzon, B., Greenberg, M. B., Bachmeier, C., Mullan, M., and Crawford, F. (2013). Repetitive mild traumatic brain injury augments tau pathology and glial activation in aged hTau mice. *J. Neuropathol. Exp. Neurol.* 72, 137–151. doi: 10.1097/NEN.0b013e3182814cdf

Omalu, B., Bailes, J., Hamilton, R. L., Kamboh, M. I., Hammers, J., Case, M., et al. (2011). Emerging histomorphologic phenotypes of chronic traumatic encephalopathy in American athletes. *Neurosurgery* 69, 173–183; discussion 183. doi: 10.1227/neu.0b013e318212bc7b

Owen, D. R., and Matthews, P. M. (2011). Imaging brain microglial activation using positron emission tomography and translocator protein-specific radioligands. *Int. Rev. Neurobiol.* 101, 19–39. doi: 10.1016/B978-0-12-387718-5.00002-X

Owen, D. R., Yeo, A. J., Gunn, R. N., Song, K., Wadsworth, G., Lewis, A., et al. (2012). An 18-kDa translocator protein (TSPO) polymorphism explains differences in binding affinity of the PET radioligand PBR28. *J. Cereb. Blood Flow Metab.* 32, 1–5. doi: 10.1038/jcbfm.2011.147

Papadopoulos, V., Baraldi, M., Guilarte, T. R., Knudsen, T. B., Lacapere, J. J., Lindemann, P., et al. (2006). Translocator protein (18kDa): new nomenclature for the peripheral-type benzodiazepine receptor based on its structure and molecular function. *Trends Pharmacol. Sci.* 27, 402–409. doi: 10.1016/j.tips.2006.06.005

Petraglia, A. L., Plog, B. A., Dayawansa, S., Dashnaw, M. L., Czerniecka, K., Walker, C. T., et al. (2014). The pathophysiology underlying repetitive mild traumatic brain injury in a novel mouse model of chronic traumatic encephalopathy. *Surg. Neurol. Int.* 5:184. doi: 10.4103/2152-7806.147566

Phelan, H. A., Shafi, S., Parks, J., Maxson, R. T., Ahmad, N., Murphy, J. T., et al. (2007). Use of a pediatric cohort to examine gender and sex hormone influences on outcome after trauma. *J. Trauma* 63, 1127–1131. doi: 10.1097/TA.0b013e318154c1b8

Raghavendra Rao, V. L., Dogan, A., Bowen, K. K., and Dempsey, R. J. (2000). Traumatic brain injury leads to increased expression of peripheral-type benzodiazepine receptors, neuronal death, and activation of astrocytes and microglia in rat thalamus. *Exp. Neurol.* 161, 102–114. doi: 10.1006/exnr.1999.7269

Ramlackhansingh, A. F., Brooks, D. J., Greenwood, R. J., Bose, S. K., Turkheimer, F. E., Kinnunen, K. M., et al. (2011). Inflammation after trauma: microglial activation and traumatic brain injury. *Ann. Neurol.* 70, 374–383. doi: 10.1002/ana.22455

Ransohoff, R. M. (2016). A polarizing question: do M1 and M2 microglia exist? *Nat. Neurosci.* 19, 987–991. doi: 10.1038/nn.4338

Rice, R. A., Spangenberg, E. E., Yamate-Morgan, H., Lee, R. J., Arora, R. P., Hernandez, M. X., et al. (2015). Elimination of microglia improves functional outcomes following extensive neuronal loss in the hippocampus. *J. Neurosci.* 35, 9977–9989. doi: 10.1523/JNEUROSCI.0336-15.2015

Roberts, G. W., Gentleman, S. M., Lynch, A., Murray, L., Landon, M., and Graham, D. I. (1994). Beta amyloid protein deposition in the brain after severe head injury: implications for the pathogenesis of Alzheimer's disease. *J. Neurol. Neurosurg. Psychiatr.* 57, 419–425. doi: 10.1136/jnnp.57.4.419

Robinson, S., Berglass, J. B., Denson, J. L., Berkner, J., Anstine, C. V., Winer, J. L., et al. (2017). Microstructural and microglial changes after repetitive mild traumatic brain injury in mice. *J. Neurosci. Res.* 95, 1025–1035. doi: 10.1002/jnr.23848

Roth, T. L., Nayak, D., Atanasijevic, T., Koretsky, A. P., Latour, L. L., and McGavern, D. B. (2014). Transcranial amelioration of inflammation and cell death after brain injury. *Nature* 505, 223–228. doi: 10.1038/nature12808

Scott, G., Hellyer, P. J., Ramlackhansingh, A. F., Brooks, D. J., Matthews, P. M., and Sharp, D. J. (2015). Thalamic inflammation after brain trauma is associated with thalamo-cortical white matter damage. *J. Neuroinflammat.* 12:224. doi: 10.1186/s12974-015-0445-y

Scott, G., Ramlackhansingh, A. F., Edison, P., Hellyer, P., Cole, J., Veronese, M., et al. (2016). Amyloid pathology and axonal injury after brain trauma. *Neurology* 86, 821-828. doi: 10.1212/WNL.0000000000002413

Selvaraj, V., and Stocco, D. M. (2015). The changing landscape in translocator protein (TSPO) function. *Trends Endocrinol. Metab.* 26, 341–348. doi: 10.1016/j.tem.2015.02.007

Semple, B. D., Bye, N., Rancan, M., Ziebell, J. M., and Morganti-Kossmann, M. C. (2010). Role of CCL2 (MCP-1) in traumatic brain injury (TBI): evidence from severe TBI patients and CCL2−/− mice. *J. Cereb. Blood Flow Metab.* 30, 769–782. doi: 10.1038/jcbfm.2009.262

Semple, B. D., Sadjadi, R., Carlson, J., Chen, Y., Xu, D., Ferriero, D. M., et al. (2016). Long-term anesthetic-dependent hypoactivity after repetitive mild traumatic brain injuries in adolescent mice. *Dev. Neurosci.* 38, 220–238. doi: 10.1159/000448089

Shin, S. S., and Dixon, C. E. (2015). Alterations in cholinergic pathways and therapeutic strategies targeting cholinergic system after Traumatic Brain injury. *J. Neurotrauma* 32, 1429–1440. doi: 10.1089/neu.2014.3445

Shitaka, Y., Tran, H. T., Bennett, R. E., Sanchez, L., Levy, M. A., Dikranian, K., et al. (2011). Repetitive closed-skull traumatic brain injury in mice causes persistent multifocal axonal injury and microglial reactivity. *J. Neuropathol. Exp. Neurol.* 70, 551–567. doi: 10.1097/NEN.0b013e31821f891f

Solito, E., and Sastre, M. (2012). Microglia function in Alzheimer's disease. *Front. Pharmacol.* 3:14. doi: 10.3389/fphar.2012.00014

Soustiel, J. F., Palzur, E., Vlodavsky, E., Veenman, L., and Gavish, M. (2008). The effect of oxygenation level on cerebral post-traumatic apoptotsis is modulated by the 18-kDa translocator protein (also known as peripheral-type benzodiazepine receptor) in a rat model of cortical contusion. *Neuropathol. Appl. Neurobiol.* 34, 412–423. doi: 10.1111/j.1365-2990.2007.00906.x

Szalay, G., Martinecz, B., Lenart, N., Kornyei, Z., Orsolits, B., Judak, L., et al. (2016). Microglia protect against brain injury and their selective elimination dysregulates neuronal network activity after stroke. *Nat. Commun.* 7:11499. doi: 10.1038/ncomms11499

Takaki, J., Fujimori, K., Miura, M., Suzuki, T., Sekino, Y., and Sato, K. (2012). L-glutamate released from activated microglia downregulates astrocytic L-glutamate transporter expression in neuroinflammation: the 'collusion' hypothesis for increased extracellular L-glutamate concentration in neuroinflammation. *J. Neuroinflammat.* 9:275. doi: 10.1186/1742-2094-9-275

Tchantchou, F., and Zhang, Y. (2013). Selective inhibition of alpha/beta-hydrolase domain 6 attenuates neurodegeneration, alleviates blood brain barrier breakdown, and improves functional recovery in a mouse model of traumatic brain injury. *J. Neurotrauma* 30, 565–579. doi: 10.1089/neu.2012.2647

Thal, S. C., Heinemann, M., Luh, C., Pieter, D., Werner, C., and Engelhard, K. (2011). Pioglitazone reduces secondary brain damage after experimental brain trauma by PPAR-gamma-independent mechanisms. *J. Neurotrauma* 28, 983–993. doi: 10.1089/neu.2010.1685

Tobinick, E., Kim, N. M., Reyzin, G., Rodriguez-Romanacce, H., and DePuy, V. (2012). Selective TNF inhibition for chronic stroke and traumatic brain injury: an observational study involving 629 consecutive patients treated with perispinal etanercept. *CNS Drugs* 26, 1051–1070. doi: 10.1007/s40263-012-0013-2

Tran, H. T., LaFerla, F. M., Holtzman, D. M., and Brody, D. L. (2011). Controlled cortical impact traumatic brain injury in 3xTg-AD mice causes acute intra-axonal amyloid-beta accumulation and independently accelerates the development of tau abnormalities. *J. Neurosci.* 31, 9513–9525. doi: 10.1523/JNEUROSCI.0858-11.2011

Truettner, J. S., Bramlett, H. M., and Dietrich, W. D. (2016). Posttraumatic therapeutic hypothermia alters microglial and macrophage polarization toward a beneficial phenotype. *J. Cereb. Blood Flow Metab.* 271678X16680003. doi: 10.1177/0271678x16680003

Tu, L. N., Morohaku, K., Manna, P. R., Pelton, S. H., Butler, W. R., Stocco, D. M., et al. (2014). Peripheral benzodiazepine receptor/translocator protein global knock-out mice are viable with no effects on steroid hormone biosynthesis. *J. Biol. Chem.* 289, 27444–27454. doi: 10.1074/jbc.M114.578286

Turtzo, L. C., Lescher, J., Janes, L., Dean, D. D., Budde, M. D., and Frank, J. A. (2014). Macrophagic and microglial responses after focal traumatic brain injury in the female rat. *J. Neuroinflammation* 11:82. doi: 10.1186/1742-2094-11-82

Tyburski, A. L., Cheng, L., Assari, S., Darvish, K., and Elliott, M. B. (2017). Frequent mild head injury promotes trigeminal sensitivity concomitant with microglial proliferation, astrocytosis, and increased neuropeptide levels in the trigeminal pain system. *J. Headache Pain* 18:16. doi: 10.1186/s10194-017-0726-1

Venneti, S., Wagner, A. K., Wang, G., Slagel, S. L., Chen, X., Lopresti, B. J., et al. (2007). The high affinity peripheral benzodiazepine receptor ligand DAA1106 binds specifically to microglia in a rat model of traumatic brain injury: implications for PET imaging. *Exp. Neurol.* 207, 118–127. doi: 10.1016/j.expneurol.2007.06.003

Verghese, P. B., Castellano, J. M., and Holtzman, D. M. (2011). Apolipoprotein E in Alzheimer's disease and other neurological disorders. *Lancet Neurol.*, 10, 241–252. doi: 10.1016/S1474-4422(10)70325-2

Vile, A. R., and Atkinson, L. (2017). Chronic traumatic encephalopathy: the cellular sequela to repetitive brain injury. *J. Clin. Neurosci.* 41, 24–29. doi: 10.1016/j.jocn.2017.03.035

Walker, P. A., Bedi, S. S., Shah, S. K., Jimenez, F., Xue, H., Hamilton, J. A., et al. (2012). Intravenous multipotent adult progenitor cell therapy after traumatic brain injury: modulation of the resident microglia population. *J. Neuroinflammat.* 9:228. doi: 10.1186/1742-2094-9-228

Wang, G., Shi, Y., Jiang, X., Leak, R. K., Hu, X., Wu, Y., et al. (2015). HDAC inhibition prevents white matter injury by modulating microglia/macrophage polarization through the GSK3beta/PTEN/Akt axis. *Proc. Natl. Acad. Sci. U.S.A.* 112, 2853–2858. doi: 10.1073/pnas.1501441112

Wang, G., Zhang, J., Hu, X., Zhang, L., Mao, L., Jiang, X., et al. (2013). Microglia/macrophage polarization dynamics in white matter after traumatic brain injury. *J. Cereb. Blood Flow Metab.* 33, 1864–1874. doi: 10.1038/jcbfm.2013.146

Wang, Y., Yue, X., Kiesewetter, D. O., Niu, G., Teng, G., and Chen, X. (2014). PET imaging of neuroinflammation in a rat traumatic brain injury model with radiolabeled TSPO ligand DPA-714. *Eur. J. Nucl. Med. Mol. Imaging* 41, 1440–1449. doi: 10.1007/s00259-014-2727-5

Werner, C., and Engelhard, K. (2007). Pathophysiology of traumatic brain injury. *Br. J. Anaesth.* 99, 4–9. doi: 10.1093/bja/aem131

Xiong, Y., Mahmood, A., and Chopp, M. (2013). Animal models of traumatic brain injury. *Nat. Rev. Neurosci.* 14, 128–142. doi: 10.1038/nrn3407

Xu, L., Nguyen, J. V., Lehar, M., Menon, A., Rha, E., Arena, J., et al. (2016). Repetitive mild traumatic brain injury with impact acceleration in the mouse: multifocal axonopathy, neuroinflammation, and neurodegeneration in the visual system. *Exp Neurol* 275(Pt 3), 436–449. doi: 10.1016/j.expneurol.2014.11.004

Xue, J., Schmidt, S. V., Sander, J., Draffehn, A., Krebs, W., Quester, I., et al. (2014). Transcriptome-based network analysis reveals a spectrum model of human macrophage activation. *Immunity* 40, 274–288. doi: 10.1016/j.immuni.2014.01.006

Yu, I., Inaji, M., Maeda, J., Okauchi, T., Nariai, T., Ohno, K., et al. (2010). Glial cell-mediated deterioration and repair of the nervous system after traumatic brain injury in a rat model as assessed by positron emission tomography. *J. Neurotrauma* 27, 1463–1475. doi: 10.1089/neu.2009.1196

Zanier, E. R., Marchesi, F., Ortolano, F., Perego, C., Arabian, M., Zoerle, T., et al. (2016). Fractalkine receptor deficiency is associated with early protection but late worsening of outcome following Brain Trauma in mice. *J. Neurotrauma* 33, 1060–1072. doi: 10.1089/neu.2015.4041

Zanier, E. R., Pischiutta, F., Riganti, L., Marchesi, F., Turola, E., Fumagalli, S., et al. (2014). Bone marrow mesenchymal stromal cells drive protective M2 microglia polarization after brain trauma. *Neurotherapeutics* 11, 679–695. doi: 10.1007/s13311-014-0277-y

Zhang, J., Puvenna, V., and Janigro, D. (2016). "Frontiers in neuroscience: biomarkers of traumatic brain injury and their relationship to pathology," in *Translational Research in Traumatic Brain Injury*, eds D. Laskowitz and G. Grant (Boca Raton, FL: CRC Press/Taylor and Francis Group), Chapter 12, 1–13.

Zhang, Z., Zhang, Z. Y., Wu, Y., and Schluesener, H. J. (2012). Immunolocalization of Toll-like receptors 2 and 4 as well as their endogenous ligand, heat shock protein 70, in rat traumatic brain injury. *Neuroimmunomodulation* 19, 10–19. doi: 10.1159/000326771

Ziebell, J. M., and Morganti-Kossmann, M. C. (2010). Involvement of pro- and anti-inflammatory cytokines and chemokines in the pathophysiology of traumatic brain injury. *Neurotherapeutics* 7, 22–30. doi: 10.1016/j.nurt.2009.10.016

Ziebell, J. M., Taylor, S. E., Cao, T., Harrison, J. L., and Lifshitz, J. (2012). Rod microglia: elongation, alignment, and coupling to form trains across the somatosensory cortex after experimental diffuse brain injury. *J. Neuroinflammat.* 9:247. doi: 10.1186/1742-2094-9-247

11

The Dual Role of Microglia in ALS: Mechanisms and Therapeutic Approaches

Maria Concetta Geloso [1]*, *Valentina Corvino* [1], *Elisa Marchese* [1], *Alessia Serrano* [1], *Fabrizio Michetti* [1,2] *and Nadia D'Ambrosi* [3]*

[1] *Institute of Anatomy and Cell Biology, Università Cattolica del Sacro Cuore, Rome, Italy,* [2] *IRCCS San Raffaele Scientific Institute, Università Vita-Salute San Raffaele, Milan, Italy,* [3] *Department of Biology, University of Rome Tor Vergata, Rome, Italy*

***Correspondence:**
Maria Concetta Geloso
mariaconcetta.geloso@unicatt.it
Nadia D'Ambrosi
nadia.dambrosi@uniroma2.it

Amyotrophic lateral sclerosis (ALS) is a neurodegenerative disease characterized by a non-cell autonomous motor neuron loss. While it is generally believed that the disease onset takes place inside motor neurons, different cell types mediating neuroinflammatory processes are considered deeply involved in the progression of the disease. On these grounds, many treatments have been tested on ALS animals with the aim of inhibiting or reducing the pro-inflammatory action of microglia and astrocytes and counteract the progression of the disease. Unfortunately, these anti-inflammatory therapies have been only modestly successful. The non-univocal role played by microglia during stress and injuries might explain this failure. Indeed, it is now well recognized that, during ALS, microglia displays different phenotypes, from surveillant in early stages, to activated states, M1 and M2, characterized by the expression of respectively harmful and protective genes in later phases of the disease. Consistently, the inhibition of microglial function seems to be a valid strategy only if the different stages of microglia polarization are taken into account, interfering with the reactivity of microglia specifically targeting only the harmful pathways and/or potentiating the trophic ones. In this review article, we will analyze the features and timing of microglia activation in the light of M1/M2 phenotypes in the main mice models of ALS. Moreover, we will also revise the results obtained by different anti-inflammatory therapies aimed to unbalance the M1/M2 ratio, shifting it towards a protective outcome.

Keywords: amyotrophic lateral sclerosis, M1/M2 microglia, neuroinflammation, anti-inflammatory drugs, genetic modifiers, mutant SOD1 mice

ALS AS A COMPOSITE DISEASE

Amyotrophic lateral sclerosis (ALS) is a multifactorial disease caused by genetic and non-inheritable components leading to motoneuron degeneration in the spinal cord, brain stem and primary motor cortex (Al-Chalabi and Hardiman, 2013). Most of ALS cases are sporadic (sALS), while 5%–20% report a familial history of the disease (fALS; Al-Chalabi et al., 2017). sALS and fALS share most neuropathological features and, from a clinical perspective, they appear very similar (Talbot, 2011). Pathological hallmarks characterizing degenerating motoneurons are cytoplasmic inclusions containing aggregated/ubiquitinated proteins as well as RNAs. Indeed, protein misfolding, with endoplasmic reticulum (ER) stress, impaired autophagy and damage to cytoskeleton are intracellular mechanisms involved in the pathogenesis of the disease (Taylor et al., 2016).

However, ALS appears as a composite syndrome where the aberrant cellular pathways may not derive solely from a conformational issue, but involve many aspects of cellular physiology: RNA processing and mitochondria homeostasis are compromised, oxidative stress is increased, excitotoxic pathways are enhanced, neurotrophic support is reduced, glial inflammatory response is oriented towards an harmful side (Rossi et al., 2016). Actually, more than 40 genes have been found mutated in ALS, affecting numerous cellular functions (Al-Chalabi et al., 2017), the most relevant of which are: a hexanucleotide repeat (GGGGCC) expansion in an intron of the C9orf72 gene (Dejesus-Hernandez et al., 2011; Renton et al., 2011), supposed to generate toxic RNA species, loss of protein and/or harmful dipeptide-repeats formation (Haeusler et al., 2016); superoxide dismutase 1 (SOD1; Rosen et al., 1993), forming toxic aggregates and interfering with mitochondrial functions and autophagy (Turner and Talbot, 2008). In this regard, transgenic SOD1 mice are so far the most widely used model to study ALS. Both active ($SOD1^{G93A}$, $SOD1^{G37R}$) and inactive ($SOD1^{G85R}$) mutants show a phenotype characterized by a progressive paralysis and death (at 5, 7 and 8.5 months, respectively), caused by degeneration of motoneurons (limited to 40% in $SOD1^{G85R}$ mice), and exhibit gliosis within the spinal cord, brain stem and cortex (Philips and Rothstein, 2015), suggesting that neurodegeneration relies on a gain of toxic function of the protein. Other mutated proteins are fused in sarcoma (FUS; Kwiatkowski et al., 2009; Vance et al., 2009) and TAR-DNA binding protein-43 (TDP-43; Neumann et al., 2006), involved in the maturation of mRNAs, found in cytoplasmic inclusions (Guerrero et al., 2016); proteins regulating cytoskeleton architecture, such as profiling-1 (Wu et al., 2012; Yang et al., 2016), and vesicle trafficking, as vesicle-associated membrane protein/synaptobrevin-associated membrane protein B (Nishimura et al., 2004; Tsuda et al., 2008); autophagy-linked proteins, among which sequestosome 1 (Teyssou et al., 2013), optineurin (Nakazawa et al., 2016) and TANK-binding protein kinase-1 (TBK-1; Cirulli et al., 2015; Freischmidt et al., 2015). Mutations in these genes also affect the function of cell types other than motoneurons. Indeed, ALS is non-cell autonomous, as astrocytes and microglia can participate to determine the disease phenotype by a local inflammatory response (neuroinflammation) and characterized by phenotypic transition, migration to the site of injury, proliferation and secretion of pro-inflammatory mediators (Philips and Rothstein, 2014). Glial activation leads to changes in the expression of a wide range of genes related to the production of soluble molecules, such as cytokines and chemokines, damage–associated molecular patterns (DAMPs), reactive nitrogen and oxygen species (ROS), giving rise to profound modifications in their interactions with neurons (Becher et al., 2017). Actually, a noticeable level of neuroinflammation has been detected in both sALS and fALS, as well as in transgenic models of the disease (Troost et al., 1989; Engelhardt and Appel, 1990; Schiffer et al., 1996; Hall et al., 1998; Henkel et al., 2004, 2006). Signs of microglia reactivity have been detected well before overt symptoms onset (Brites and Vaz, 2014; Tang and Le, 2016), concomitantly with loss of neuromuscular junctions (Gerber et al., 2012) and early motoneuron degeneration (Alexianu et al., 2001).

The role of microglia has been strengthened by recent studies opening new perspectives in the knowledge of the non-cell autonomous molecular pathways possibly contributing to ALS.

Lack of C9orf72 in a loss-of-function model of the disease produced no signs of motoneuron degeneration, but led to lysosomal accumulation and altered immune responses in macrophages and microglia (O'Rourke et al., 2016). Furthermore, the recently described ALS-susceptibility gene, TBK1, not only has a central function in autophagy processes, but is involved in innate immunity signaling pathways, regulating the production of interferon α (IFN α) and IFN β (Ahmad et al., 2016). A close relation between disruption of the autophagy machinery and microglial activation has been recently proposed (Plaza-Zabala et al., 2017): hence, an impaired autophagy linked to modifications in the response to pro-inflammatory stimuli and pathogen clearance by resident immune cells likely contributes to the etiopathology of the disease. Recent data show an earlier and more detrimental clinical course in $SOD1^{G93A}$ mice lacking telomerase (Linkus et al., 2016), evidencing therefore a possible aging effect on microglia priming in ALS. Indeed aged and mutant SOD1 (mSOD1)-expressing microglia display a common signature of gene expression, as well as specific patterns (Holtman et al., 2015).

In this review article, we therefore describe how the adaptive phenotypes of microglia participate to neurodegeneration in ALS, evidencing how the concept of a bipolar, protective vs. harmful, response of microglia has been rapidly changed in less than a decade. We also discuss how anti-inflammatory drugs have been used to polarize microglia towards a neuroprotective signature to control the extent of activation and if and how this has reached therapeutic benefits.

M1/M2 PHENOTYPE IN ALS

Overview

Microglia are largely considered as the brain's resident immune cell, which has been classically described to exist in two states, resting and activated (Cherry et al., 2014). In the adult healthy brain, two-photon imaging showed that the so called "resting" microglia is, in actual facts, a highly dynamic population (Nimmerjahn et al., 2005), which actively screen their microenvironment with motile processes, exerting a crucial role in maintaining homeostasis (Luo and Chen, 2012). It is indicated as "surveillant" microglia and participates to many physiological functions, including synaptic pruning, adult neurogenesis and modulation of neuronal networks (Walton et al., 2006; Kettenmann et al., 2013).

This highly specific interaction with the extracellular environment is tightly regulated (Nimmerjahn et al., 2005; Parisi et al., 2016b), therefore these cells rapidly react to abnormalities, adopting a less ramified/amoeboid phenotype, corresponding to activated microglia (Luo and Chen, 2012;

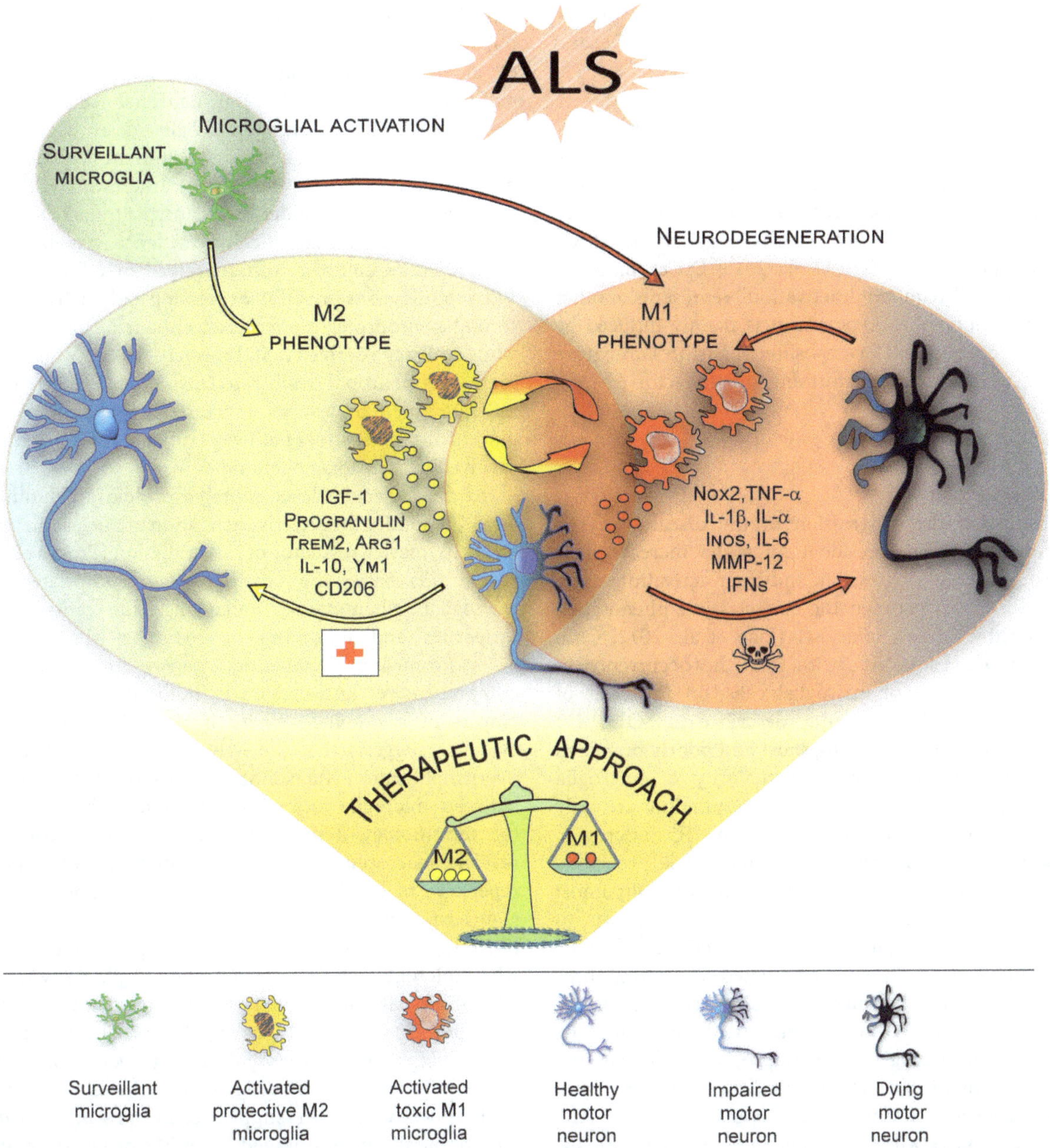

FIGURE 1 | M1/M2 microglia polarization during amyotrophic lateral sclerosis (ALS)-induced motor neuron degeneration. During ALS progression activated microglia represent a continuum between the neuroprotective M2 phenotype, which promotes tissue repair and supports neuron survival by releasing neuroprotective factors, vs. the toxic M1, which produces cytokines increasing inflammation and further supporting M1 polarization, thus contributing to neuronal death. Therapeutic approaches targeting microglia polarization and resulting in induction of the M2 phenotype are promising strategies to ameliorate local neurodegeneration and improve the clinical outcome of the disease (see **Table 1** for details).

Cherry et al., 2014). Similarly to peripheral macrophages, the term activation has been associated at least with two distinct phenotypes, M1 (toxic) and M2 (protective), in response to different microenvironmental signals, in turn involved in the production of a variety of effector molecules (Du et al., 2016). Microglia recognize pathogens via pattern recognition receptors, which interact with classes of DAMPs derived from exogenous microorganisms or endogenous cell types involved in immunity processes, respectively. The interaction triggers a downstream gene induction program aimed at initiating cellular defense mechanisms, including the release of inflammatory cytokines and chemokines (Colton, 2009; Kigerl et al., 2014).

In particular, in *in vitro* settings, lipopolysaccharide (LPS) or IFN-γ stimulate "classically activated" M1 microglia, which release pro-inflammatory mediators. They include pro-inflammatory cytokines (interleukin [IL]-1α, IL-1β, IL-6, IL-12, IL-23, tumor necrosis factor-α [TNF-α]), chemokines, prostaglandin E2, chemokine (C-C motif) ligand 2, ROS and inducible nitric oxide synthase (iNOS; Bagasra et al., 1995; Du et al., 2016; Orihuela et al., 2016).

In contrast, "alternatively activated" M2 phenotype, which is induced by anti-inflammatory cytokines IL-4, IL-10 or IL-13, suppresses inflammation, clears cellular debris through phagocytosis, promotes extracellular matrix reconstruction and supports neuron survival through the release of protective/trophic factors (Hu et al., 2015; Du et al., 2016; Tang and Le, 2016). "Acquired deactivation" represents another M2 anti-inflammatory phenotype and it is mainly induced by the uptake of apoptotic cells or exposure to anti-inflammatory cytokines, such as IL-10 and transforming growth factor-β (Tang and Le, 2016).

Microglia in ALS

Studies investigating the progression of the disease in ALS mice indicate that, *in vivo*, resident microglia increase their number during disease progression, and their activation states represent a continuum between the two classical phenotypes, i.e., neuroprotective M2 vs. toxic M1 (Liao et al., 2012; Chiu et al., 2013; **Figure 1**). In line with this, the occurrence of two different phenotypes of microglial cells, on the basis of their morphology, has been recently described in SOD1^{G93A} transgenic mice: type "R1", showing short and poorly branched processes, which represents the vast majority of microglia in the early-stage of the disease and corresponding to early transformation of surveillant microglia, and type "R3" microglia, exhibiting large cell bodies with short and thick processes, which are typical of end-stage phases of the disease (Ohgomori et al., 2016). Consistently, microglia have been shown to exhibit, at the pre-onset phase of SOD1-mediated disease, an anti-inflammatory profile with attenuated TLR2 responses to controlled immune challenge, and a overexpression of anti-inflammatory IL-10 (Gravel et al., 2016). Subsequently, at disease onset and during the slowly progressing phase, the prevalent expression of specific M2 markers, (e.g., Ym1 and CD206), was detected in the lumbar spinal cords of ALS mice (Beers et al., 2011a). Eventually, in end-stage animals, a microglial phenotype expressing high levels of NOX2, the subunit of nicotinamide-adenine-dinucleotide-phosphate oxidase expressed by macrophages considered M1 prototypic marker, appears to be prevalent (Beers et al., 2011b).

M1 ALS microglia appear hyper-reactive to inflammatory stimuli (D'Ambrosi et al., 2009) and the specific role of mutated proteins in driving this increased toxicity has been suggested by many studies (Beers et al., 2006; Xiao et al., 2007; Liao et al., 2012). Mutant forms of TDP-43 are able to activate microglia and upregulate the release of pro-inflammatory mediators, including NOX2, TNF-α and IL-1β (Zhao et al., 2015). Consistently, also the intracellular expression of high levels of TDP-43 underlies the occurrence of a more toxic microglial phenotype, when stimulated, *in vitro*, with LPS or ROS (Swarup et al., 2011).

Similarly, exogenous SOD1^{G93A} or SOD1^{G85R} induce, *in vitro*, morphological and functional activation of microglia, increasing their release of pro-inflammatory cytokines and ROS (Zhao et al., 2010). In chimeric mice with both normal and mSOD1-expressing cells, non-neuronal cells that do not express mSOD1, including microglia, delay degeneration and significantly extend survival of mutant protein-expressing motoneurons (Clement et al., 2003). Interestingly, also mSOD1-expressing microglia underlie phenotypic transformation during the disease. More specifically, evidence has been provided that, when co-culturing different-aged mSOD1 microglia with WT motoneurons, mSOD1-expressing early-activated microglia exhibit neuroprotective features, enhancing neuronal survival, while end-stage derived mSOD1 microglia show toxic properties, increasing neuronal death rate (Liao et al., 2012). Additionally, mSOD1 microglia shows increased expression of molecular players of the ER stress pathway (Ito et al., 2009), which may be involved in their toxic phenotype.

At the molecular level, mutated proteins, including TDP-43 and FUS, induce the selective activation of nuclear factor-kappa B (NF-kB), master regulator of inflammation (Frakes et al., 2014).

On this basis, the possibility to appropriately modulate microglial phenotypes, enhancing the anti-inflammatory properties and inhibiting or reducing M1 toxicity, could be a promising therapeutic strategy for ALS, therefore a comprehensive knowledge of both timing and molecular players of microglial activity is needed. However, emerging evidence suggests that the M1/M2 paradigm seems to be an oversimplification (Ransohoff, 2016) and substantial differences between microglia and peripheral macrophages, from which the terminology derives, should be carefully considered. As resident macrophages of the brain, microglia have an elaborate repertoire of brain specific functions, sustained by a peculiar gene expression profiling (Gautier et al., 2012). *In vitro*, phenotypic redirection is a feature of peripheral macrophages, while microglia exhibit a lower grade of plasticity (Parisi et al., 2016b). Coexistence of the two opposite phenotypes, more than transition from M2 to M1, during ALS progression has also been recently highlighted by several findings. For instance, beneficial components of inflammation, such as insulin growth factor-1 (IGF-1), whose release is suppressed in a pro-inflammatory (M1) environment but encouraged in an M2 protective environment (Suh et al., 2013), is overexpressed by SOD1^{G93A} microglia not only in pre-symptomatic stage, but also in end-stage (Chiu et al., 2008). Furthermore, a down-regulation of IL-6 over time, associated with an up-regulation of IL-1R antagonist, has been reported, suggesting the occurrence of an anti-inflammatory response (Chiu et al., 2008). Analysis of transcriptome changes of SOD1^{G93A} microglia essentially confirmed these observations. They also evidenced that the activation of genes involved in anti-inflammatory pathways, including, *Igf1*, *Progranulin* and *Trem2*, coexists with the upregulation of genes related to potentially neurotoxic factors, among which Matrix metalloproteinase-12 and classical proinflammatory cytokines, (Chiu et al., 2013). Interestingly, critical differences in gene expression profiling among M1/M2 macrophages, LPS-activated microglia and SOD1^{G93A} activated microglia

TABLE 1 | Preclinical approaches affecting microglia M1/M2 phenotype in transgenic mutant superoxide dismutase1 (mSOD1) mice.

Drug administered/Genes silenced	Action/Function	M1 modulation	M2 modulation	Outcomes
AMD3100 (Rabinovich-Nikitin et al., 2016)	CXCR4 antagonist	↓TNF-α, IL-6		Survival +10%, ↑onset, b.w., motor function
BBG (Apolloni et al., 2014)	P2X7 antagonist	↓NOX2, IL-1β; n.s.c. TNF-α, IL-6, iNOS	↑BDNF, IL-10	Survival n.s.c., ↑motor function
Bee venom (Yang et al., 2010)	anti-inflammation	TNF-α↓		Survival +18%, ↑onset, motor function
Celastrol (Kiaei et al., 2005b)		iNOS↓		Survival +13%, ↑onset, b.w., motor function
Celecoxib/Rofecoxib + Creatine (Klivenyi et al., 2004)	COX-2 inhibitor	PGE2↓		Survival +30%, ↑b.w., motor function
Clemastine (Apolloni et al., 2016b)	Antihistamine	↓CD68, gp91^{phox}	↑Arg1, BDNF	Survival n.c.s., ↑onset,
DL-NBP (Feng et al., 2012)	Neuroprotection	↓TNF-α		Survival +42%, ↑b.w., motor function
EGCG (Xu et al., 2006)	Neuroprotection	iNOS↓		Survival +10%, onset +9%,
hMSC (Zhou et al., 2013)	Stromal cells	↓TNF-α, iNOS		Survival +10%, onset +6%, ↑motor function
IL-1RA (Meissner et al., 2010)	IL-1R antagonist			Survival +4%, ↑motor function
Lenalidomide (Kiaei et al., 2006)	↓ TNF-α	↓TNF-α, IL-1α, IL-1β	↑TGF-β1	Survival +18%, ↑onset, b.w., motor function
*M-CSF (Gowing et al., 2009)	Cytokine	↑TNF-α, IL-1β;↓IL-6, NOX2	↓IL-4; ↑TGF-β1	Survival −3%
Minocycline (Kobayashi et al., 2013)	↓glia activation	↓TNF-α, IL-1β, INF-γ, CD86, CD68	n.s.c. CD206, Arg1, IL-4, IL-10, Ym1	Survival +54%, onset +15%
Nimesulide (Pompl et al., 2003)	COX-2 inhibitor	PGE2↓		Survival n.d., ↑onset, motor function
Pioglitazone (Kiaei et al., 2005a)	PPARγ agonist	↓iNOS, COX2		Survival +13%, ↑onset, b.w., motor function
R723 (Tada et al., 2014)	JAK2 inhibitor	↓CD11b, iNOS; n.s.c. TNF-α, IL6, IL-1β	n.s.c. Arg1, Ym1, IL-4	n.s.c.
scAAV9-VEGF (Wang et al., 2016)	↑ VEGF	↓TNF-α, CD68	↑Arg1, Ym1	Survival +10%, ↑b.w., motor function
Sulindac (Kiaei et al., 2005c)	COX inhibitor	COX2↓		Survival +10%, ↑b.w., motor function
Thalidomide (Kiaei et al., 2006)	↓ TNF-α	↓TNF-α; n.s.c. IL-1α, IL-1β	↑TGF-β1	Survival +12%, ↑onset, b.w., motor function
gp91^{phox-} (Wu et al., 2006)	NOX2 inhibition	IL-1β n.s.c.		Survival +11%
IL-1β$^{-/-}$ (Meissner et al., 2010)	IL-1β decrease	↓IL-1β$^{-/-}$		Survival +5%
iNOS$^{-/-}$ (Martin et al., 2007)	iNOS inhibition	↓iNOS		↑Survival
NOX2$^{-/-}$ (Marden et al., 2007)	NOX2 inhibition	↓NOX2		Survival +73%, ↑onset, b.w., motor function
**TNF-α$^{-/-}$ (Gowing et al., 2006)	TNF-α decrease	↓TNF-α		n.s.c.
*xCT$^{-/-}$ (Mesci et al., 2015)	↓ Glutamate release	Onset: ↑IL-1β, iNOS E.s.: ↓IL-1β, iNOS	Onset: ↓Arg1, Ym1 L.s.:↑Arg1, Ym1	Survival n.s.c., onset −9%, ↑b.w. (at l.s.), motor function

All trials were performed in SOD1^{G93A} mice except the cases indicated with asterisks (performed in SOD^{G37R} mice, ** performed both in SOD^{G93A} and SOD^{G37R} mice). The reported data refer to most effective results obtained in the cited article. Abbreviations: n.d., not described, n.s.c., non significant changes, ↑ increased, ↓ decreased; b.w., body weight, e.s., end stage, l.s., late symptomatic stage.*

emerge: while LPS-activated microglia show enriched in DNA replication-, cell cycle- and innate immune signaling-genes, $SOD1^{G93A}$ activated microglia are enriched in the transcripts of genes related to neurodegenerative diseases, e.g., AD, Huntington's and Parkinson's disease, suggesting a neurodegeneration-specific signature for ALS microglia. More interestingly, $SOD1^{G93A}$-expressing microglia do not display a significant prevalence of M1 or M2 phenotypes at any time point during disease progression (Chiu et al., 2013). In line with this results, an increased expression of both iNOS (M1 marker) and arginase 1 (Argl; M2 marker) has been shown to parallel the generalized increase of activated microglia in $SOD1^{G93A}$ mice (Lewis et al., 2014). Consistently, characteristics different from typical M1 or M2 phenotypes have been reported in end-stage $SOD1^{G93A}$ rats, which also show predominant microglial activation in most severely affected regions (lumbar spinal cord), as if several phenotypically different microglial subpopulations were present throughout differently affected regions of the CNS (Nikodemova et al., 2014).

MICROGLIAL SWITCH AND THERAPEUTIC APPROACHES IN ALS ANIMAL MODELS

Targeting the microglia has been the focus of neuroprotective strategies, based on pharmacological or genetic approaches, aimed at modulating microglia reactivity in the attempt to improve the clinical outcome in animal models of the disease (**Table 1**, **Figure 1**). In this regard, pioneer studies based on administration of minocycline, a tetracycline antibiotic that prevents microglial activation, showed that, when administered in both $SOD1^{G93A}$ and $SOD1^{G37R}$ mice before disease onset, it attenuates microglial activation and delays disease onset and mortality (Kriz et al., 2002; Van Den Bosch et al., 2002; Zhu et al., 2002). On the other hand, when administered after the onset of the disease, it fails to improve clinical and/or pathological features, even increasing microgliosis (Keller et al., 2011). Interestingly, recent findings obtained in $SOD1^{G37R}$ mice have shown that minocycline specifically attenuates the M1 phenotype, without influencing the expression of M2 markers (Kobayashi et al., 2013; **Table 1**), thus highlighting the crucial role exerted by the modulation of M1/M2 balance in the therapeutic effectiveness.

Hence, pharmacological modulation of molecular pathways related to microglial polarization has been explored. The hyperactivation of P2X7 receptors, strongly involved in neuroinflammatory response (Burnstock, 2008; Apolloni et al., 2009; Volonté et al., 2012; Sperlágh and Illes, 2014), has been described in microglia of both ALS patients and animal models (Yiangou et al., 2006; D'Ambrosi et al., 2009), where it is associated to the production of pro-inflammatory factors, including miR-125b (D'Ambrosi et al., 2009; Parisi et al., 2013, 2016a). Consistently, the administration of the P2X7 antagonist Brilliant Blue G (BBG), within a critical time frame, improves several features of the disease (Cervetto et al., 2013; Apolloni et al., 2014). BBG neuroprotection, obtained at late pre-onset administration, is supported by the upregulation of IL-10 and BDNF, associated to M2 phenotype, together with a reduction of NF-kB protein, NOX-2 and IL1β, markers of M1 polarization (**Table 1**). However, BBG administration at earlier phases fails to counteract disease progression. In this case, although it reduces M1 markers, it does not affect the expression of M2 mediators, whose neuroprotective properties seem to be essential to improve the clinical outcome (Apolloni et al., 2014).

Microglia-mediated neuroinflammation is also modulated by histamine (Ferreira et al., 2012; Volonté et al., 2015; Barata-Antunes et al., 2017). The antihistamine drug Clemastine, administered to $SOD1^{G93A}$ mice at the asymptomatic phase until the end-stage of disease, fails to improve clinical symptoms and lifespan, although it modulates the M1/M2 balance by reducing CD68, NOX2 and P2X7 expression and concomitantly up-regulating Argl (Apolloni et al., 2016b; **Table 1**). Conversely, when administered at the asymptomatic phase to the onset, it delays the disease onset and improves the motor functions and survival rate (Apolloni et al., 2016a). Clemastine also activates autophagy in $SOD1^{G93A}$ primary microglia, thus suggesting that targeting autophagy in microglia could be a promising therapeutic strategy (Apolloni et al., 2016a).

Alternative therapeutic strategies to shift the balance towards the M2 phenotype involve the use of trophic factors. Several findings showed that the delivery of viral vectors encoding growth factors, such as IGF-1, glial-derived neurotrophic factor, vascular endothelial growth factor (VEGF) extends lifespan and slows the progression of the disease in ALS animal models (Acsadi et al., 2002; Kaspar et al., 2003; Azzouz et al., 2004; Dodge et al., 2010; Wang et al., 2016). Interestingly, the intrathecal injection of self-complementary adeno-associated-virus (scAAV)9-VEGF at disease onset decreases TNF-α, IL-1β and CD68 levels and increases those of Arg-1 and Ym-1 (**Table 1**), showing that the modulation of M1/M2 balance could support the protective effects correlated to VEGF administration (Wang et al., 2016).

Further, the deletion of the cystine/glutamate-antiporter xCT/Slc7a11 (xCT), a critical glial transporter system involved in the excessive glutamate release from M1 microglia, has provided additional finding on this matter. Indeed, xCT deletion at the early-stages of the disease, in fact, increases the expression of M1 marker IL1β and concurrently reduces M2 marker Yml/Chil3, thus resulting in earlier disease onset. Conversely, lack of xCT, at the end-stage, increases Yml/Chil3 and Argl expression, which possibly sustains the delay of disease progression (Mesci et al., 2015; **Table 1**).

These data underline that the modulation of microglia-specific pathways may ameliorate local neurodegeneration. However, growing evidence suggests that a successful therapeutic strategy for ALS could be obtained only interfering with different pathways in different cell types. In light of this, it was recently demonstrated that microglial NF-κB suppression combined with mSOD1 reduction in astrocytes and motoneurons results not only in attenuated neuroinflammation and neurodegeneration, but also increases mice mean survival (Frakes et al., 2017), demonstrating that the redirection of microglia polarization may still be an effective strategy to counteract ALS when associated with the interception of other pathogenic mechanisms.

AUTHOR CONTRIBUTIONS

MCG and ND wrote respectively section 2 and 1 and conceived, designed and revised the manuscript; VC wrote section 3; EM prepared the artwork; AS created the table; FM revised the work.

ACKNOWLEDGMENTS

We thank Nando and Elsa Peretti Foundation (Fabrizio Michetti—Contract number NaEPF 2016-033) and Università Cattolica del Sacri Cuore (linea D.3.2 2015 to FM) for financial support.

REFERENCES

Acsadi, G., Anguelov, R. A., Yang, H., Toth, G., Thomas, R., Jani, A., et al. (2002). Increased survival and function of SOD1 mice after glial cell-derived neurotrophic factor gene therapy. *Hum. Gene Ther.* 13, 1047–1059. doi: 10.1089/104303402753812458

Ahmad, L., Zhang, S.-Y., Casanova, J.-L., and Sancho-Shimizu, V. (2016). Human TBK1: a gatekeeper of neuroinflammation. *Trends Mol. Med.* 22, 511–527. doi: 10.1016/j.molmed.2016.04.006

Al-Chalabi, A., and Hardiman, O. (2013). The epidemiology of ALS: a conspiracy of genes, environment and time. *Nat. Rev. Neurol.* 9, 617–628. doi: 10.1038/nrneurol.2013.203

Al-Chalabi, A., Van Den Berg, L. H., and Veldink, J. (2017). Gene discovery in amyotrophic lateral sclerosis: implications for clinical management. *Nat. Rev. Neurol.* 13, 96–104. doi: 10.1038/nrneurol.2016.182

Alexianu, M. E., Kozovska, M., and Appel, S. H. (2001). Immune reactivity in a mouse model of familial ALS correlates with disease progression. *Neurology* 57, 1282–1289. doi: 10.1212/wnl.57.7.1282

Apolloni, S., Amadio, S., Parisi, C., Matteucci, A., Potenza, R. L., Armida, M., et al. (2014). Spinal cord pathology is ameliorated by P2X7 antagonism in a SOD1-mutant mouse model of amyotrophic lateral sclerosis. *Dis. Model. Mech.* 7, 1101–1109. doi: 10.1242/dmm.017038

Apolloni, S., Fabbrizio, P., Amadio, S., and Volonté, C. (2016a). Actions of the antihistaminergic clemastine on presymptomatic SOD1-G93A mice ameliorate ALS disease progression. *J. Neuroinflammation* 13:191. doi: 10.1186/s12974-016-0658-8

Apolloni, S., Fabbrizio, P., Parisi, C., Amadio, S., and Volonte, C. (2016b). Clemastine confers neuroprotection and induces an anti-inflammatory phenotype in $SOD1^{G93A}$ mouse model of amyotrophic lateral sclerosis. *Mol. Neurobiol.* 53, 518–531. doi: 10.1007/s12035-014-9019-8

Apolloni, S., Montilli, C., Finocchi, P., and Amadio, S. (2009). Membrane compartments and purinergic signalling: P2X receptors in neurodegenerative and neuroinflammatory events. *FEBS J.* 276, 354–364. doi: 10.1111/j.1742-4658.2008.06796.x

Azzouz, M., Ralph, G. S., Storkebaum, E., Walmsley, L. E., Mitrophanous, K. A., Kingsman, S. M., et al. (2004). VEGF delivery with retrogradely transported lentivector prolongs survival in a mouse ALS model. *Nature* 429, 413–417. doi: 10.1038/nature02544

Bagasra, O., Michaels, F. H., Zheng, Y. M., Bobroski, L. E., Spitsin, S. V., Fu, Z. F., et al. (1995). Activation of the inducible form of nitric oxide synthase in the brains of patients with multiple sclerosis. *Proc. Natl. Acad. Sci. U S A* 92, 12041–12045. doi: 10.1073/pnas.92.26.12041

Barata-Antunes, S., Cristóvão, A. C., Pires, J., Rocha, S. M., and Bernardino, L. (2017). Dual role of histamine on microglia-induced neurodegeneration. *Biochim. Biophys. Acta* 1863, 764–769. doi: 10.1016/j.bbadis.2016.12.016

Becher, B., Spath, S., and Goverman, J. (2017). Cytokine networks in neuroinflammation. *Nat. Rev. Immunol.* 17, 49–59. doi: 10.1038/nri.2016.123

Beers, D. R., Henkel, J. S., Xiao, Q., Zhao, W., Wang, J., Yen, A. A., et al. (2006). Wild-type microglia extend survival in PU.1 knockout mice with familial amyotrophic lateral sclerosis. *Proc. Natl. Acad. Sci. U S A* 103, 16021–16026. doi: 10.1073/pnas.0607423103

Beers, D. R., Henkel, J. S., Zhao, W., Wang, J., Huang, A., Wen, S., et al. (2011a). Endogenous regulatory T lymphocytes ameliorate amyotrophic lateral sclerosis in mice and correlate with disease progression in patients with amyotrophic lateral sclerosis. *Brain* 134, 1293–1314. doi: 10.1093/brain/awr074

Beers, D. R., Zhao, W., Liao, B., Kano, O., Wang, J., Huang, A., et al. (2011b). Neuroinflammation modulates distinct regional and temporal clinical responses in ALS mice. *Brain Behav. Immun.* 25, 1025–1035. doi: 10.1016/j.bbi.2010.12.008

Brites, D., and Vaz, A. R. (2014). Microglia centered pathogenesis in ALS: insights in cell interconnectivity. *Front. Cell. Neurosci.* 8:117. doi: 10.3389/fncel.2014.00117

Burnstock, G. (2008). Purinergic signalling and disorders of the central nervous system. *Nat. Rev. Drug Discov.* 7, 575–590. doi: 10.1038/nrd2605

Cervetto, C., Frattaroli, D., Maura, G., and Marcoli, M. (2013). Motor neuron dysfunction in a mouse model of ALS: gender-dependent effect of P2X7 antagonism. *Toxicology* 311, 69–77. doi: 10.1016/j.tox.2013.04.004

Cherry, J. D., Olschowka, J. A., and O'Banion, M. K. (2014). Neuroinflammation and M2 microglia: the good, the bad, and the inflamed. *J. Neuroinflammation* 11:98. doi: 10.1186/1742-2094-11-98

Chiu, I. M., Chen, A., Zheng, Y., Kosaras, B., Tsiftsoglou, S. A., Vartanian, T. K., et al. (2008). T lymphocytes potentiate endogenous neuroprotective inflammation in a mouse model of ALS. *Proc. Natl. Acad. Sci. U S A* 105, 17913–17918. doi: 10.1073/pnas.0804610105

Chiu, I. M., Morimoto, E. T., Goodarzi, H., Liao, J. T., O'Keeffe, S., Phatnani, H. P., et al. (2013). A neurodegeneration-specific gene-expression signature of acutely isolated microglia from an amyotrophic lateral sclerosis mouse model. *Cell Rep.* 4, 385–401. doi: 10.1016/j.celrep.2013.06.018

Cirulli, E. T., Lasseigne, B. N., Petrovski, S., Sapp, P. C., Dion, P. A., Leblond, C. S., et al. (2015). Exome sequencing in amyotrophic lateral sclerosis identifies risk genes and pathways. *Science* 347, 1436–1441. doi: 10.1126/science.aaa3650

Clement, A. M., Nguyen, M. D., Roberts, E. A., Garcia, M. L., Boillée, S., Rule, M., et al. (2003). Wild-type nonneuronal cells extend survival of SOD1 mutant motor neurons in ALS mice. *Science* 302, 113–117. doi: 10.1126/science.1086071

Colton, C. A. (2009). Heterogeneity of microglial activation in the innate immune response in the brain. *J. Neuroimmune Pharmacol.* 4, 399–418. doi: 10.1007/s11481-009-9164-4

D'Ambrosi, N., Finocchi, P., Apolloni, S., Cozzolino, M., Ferri, A., Padovano, V., et al. (2009). The proinflammatory action of microglial P2 receptors is enhanced in SOD1 models for amyotrophic lateral sclerosis. *J. Immunol.* 183, 4648–4656. doi: 10.4049/jimmunol.0901212

Dejesus-Hernandez, M., Mackenzie, I. R., Boeve, B. F., Boxer, A. L., Baker, M., Rutherford, N. J., et al. (2011). Expanded GGGGCC hexanucleotide repeat in noncoding region of *C9ORF72* causes chromosome 9p-linked FTD and ALS. *Neuron* 72, 245–256. doi: 10.1016/j.neuron.2011.09.011

Dodge, J. C., Treleaven, C. M., Fidler, J. A., Hester, M., Haidet, A., Handy, C., et al. (2010). AAV4-mediated expression of IGF-1 and VEGF within cellular components of the ventricular system improves survival outcome in familial ALS mice. *Mol. Ther.* 18, 2075–2084. doi: 10.1038/mt.2010.206

Du, L., Zhang, Y., Chen, Y., Zhu, J., Yang, Y., and Zhang, H.-L. (2016). Role of microglia in neurological disorders and their potentials as a therapeutic target. *Mol. Neurobiol.* doi: 10.1007/s12035-016-0245-0 [Epub ahead of print].

Engelhardt, J. I., and Appel, S. H. (1990). IgG reactivity in the spinal cord and motor cortex in amyotrophic lateral sclerosis. *Arch. Neurol.* 47, 1210–1216. doi: 10.1001/archneur.1990.00530110068019

Feng, X., Peng, Y., Liu, M., and Cui, L. (2012). DL-3-n-butylphthalide extends survival by attenuating glial activation in a mouse model of amyotrophic lateral sclerosis. *Neuropharmacology* 62, 1004–1010. doi: 10.1016/j.neuropharm.2011.10.009

Ferreira, R., Santos, T., Gonçalves, J., Baltazar, G., Ferreira, L., Agasse, F., et al. (2012). Histamine modulates microglia function. *J. Neuroinflammation* 9:90. doi: 10.1186/1742-2094-9-90

Frakes, A. E., Braun, L., Ferraiuolo, L., Guttridge, D. C., and Kaspar, B. K. (2017). Additive amelioration of ALS by co-targeting independent pathogenic mechanisms. *Ann. Clin. Transl. Neurol.* 4, 76–86. doi: 10.1002/acn3.375

Frakes, A. E., Ferraiuolo, L., Haidet-Phillips, A. M., Schmelzer, L., Braun, L., Miranda, C. J., et al. (2014). Microglia induce motor neuron death via the classical NF-κB pathway in amyotrophic lateral sclerosis. *Neuron* 81, 1009–1023. doi: 10.1016/j.neuron.2014.01.013

Freischmidt, A., Wieland, T., Richter, B., Ruf, W., Schaeffer, V., Muller, K., et al. (2015). Haploinsufficiency of TBK1 causes familial ALS and fronto-temporal dementia. *Nat. Neurosci.* 18, 631–636. doi: 10.1038/nn.4000

Gautier, E. L., Shay, T., Miller, J., Greter, M., Jakubzick, C., Ivanov, S., et al. (2012). Gene-expression profiles and transcriptional regulatory pathways that underlie the identity and diversity of mouse tissue macrophages. *Nat. Immunol.* 13, 1118–1128. doi: 10.1038/ni.2419

Gerber, Y. N., Sabourin, J. C., Rabano, M., Vivanco, M., and Perrin, F. E. (2012). Early functional deficit and microglial disturbances in a mouse model of amyotrophic lateral sclerosis. *PLoS One* 7:e36000. doi: 10.1371/journal.pone.0036000

Gowing, G., Dequen, F., Soucy, G., and Julien, J. P. (2006). Absence of tumor necrosis factor-α does not affect motor neuron disease caused by superoxide dismutase 1 mutations. *J. Neurosci.* 26, 11397–11402. doi: 10.1523/jneurosci.0602-06.2006

Gowing, G., Lalancette-Hébert, M., Audet, J. N., Dequen, F., and Julien, J. P. (2009). Macrophage colony stimulating factor (M-CSF) exacerbates ALS disease in a mouse model through altered responses of microglia expressing mutant superoxide dismutase. *Exp. Neurol.* 220, 267–275. doi: 10.1016/j.expneurol.2009.08.021

Gravel, M., Béland, L. C., Soucy, G., Abdelhamid, E., Rahimian, R., Gravel, C., et al. (2016). IL-10 controls early microglial phenotypes and disease onset in ALS caused by misfolded superoxide dismutase 1. *J. Neurosci.* 36, 1031–1048. doi: 10.1523/JNEUROSCI.0854-15.2016

Guerrero, E. N., Wang, H., Mitra, J., Hegde, P. M., Stowell, S. E., Liachko, N. F., et al. (2016). TDP-43/FUS in motor neuron disease: complexity and challenges. *Prog. Neurobiol.* 145–146, 78–97. doi: 10.1016/j.pneurobio.2016.09.004

Haeusler, A. R., Donnelly, C. J., and Rothstein, J. D. (2016). The expanding biology of the *C9orf72* nucleotide repeat expansion in neurodegenerative disease. *Nat. Rev. Neurosci.* 17, 383–395. doi: 10.1038/nrn.2016.38

Hall, E. D., Oostveen, J. A., and Gurney, M. E. (1998). Relationship of microglial and astrocytic activation to disease onset and progression in a transgenic model of familial ALS. *Glia* 23, 249–256. doi: 10.1002/(sici)1098-1136(199807)23:3<249::aid-glia7>3.0.co;2-#

Henkel, J. S., Beers, D. R., Siklos, L., and Appel, S. H. (2006). The chemokine MCP-1 and the dendritic and myeloid cells it attracts are increased in the mSOD1 mouse model of ALS. *Mol. Cell. Neurosci.* 31, 427–437. doi: 10.1016/j.mcn.2005.10.016

Henkel, J. S., Engelhardt, J. I., Siklós, L., Simpson, E. P., Kim, S. H., Pan, T., et al. (2004). Presence of dendritic cells, MCP-1, and activated microglia/macrophages in amyotrophic lateral sclerosis spinal cord tissue. *Ann. Neurol.* 55, 221–235. doi: 10.1002/ana.10805

Holtman, I. R., Raj, D. D., Miller, J. A., Schaafsma, W., Yin, Z., Brouwer, N., et al. (2015). Induction of a common microglia gene expression signature by aging and neurodegenerative conditions: a co-expression meta-analysis. *Acta Neuropathol. Commun.* 3:31. doi: 10.1186/s40478-015-0203-5

Hu, X., Leak, R. K., Shi, Y., Suenaga, J., Gao, Y., Zheng, P., et al. (2015). Microglial and macrophage polarization-new prospects for brain repair. *Nat. Rev. Neurol.* 11, 56–64. doi: 10.1038/nrneurol.2014.207

Ito, Y., Yamada, M., Tanaka, H., Aida, K., Tsuruma, K., Shimazawa, M., et al. (2009). Involvement of CHOP, an ER-stress apoptotic mediator, in both human sporadic ALS and ALS model mice. *Neurobiol. Dis.* 36, 470–476. doi: 10.1016/j.nbd.2009.08.013

Kaspar, B. K., Lladó, J., Sherkat, N., Rothstein, J. D., and Gage, F. H. (2003). Retrograde viral delivery of IGF-1 prolongs survival in a mouse ALS model. *Science* 301, 839–842. doi: 10.1126/science.1086137

Keller, A. F., Gravel, M., and Kriz, J. (2011). Treatment with minocycline after disease onset alters astrocyte reactivity and increases microgliosis in SOD1 mutant mice. *Exp. Neurol.* 228, 69–79. doi: 10.1016/j.expneurol.2010.12.010

Kettenmann, H., Kirchhoff, F., and Verkhratsky, A. (2013). Microglia: new roles for the synaptic stripper. *Neuron* 77, 10–18. doi: 10.1016/j.neuron.2012.12.023

Kiaei, M., Kipiani, K., Chen, J., Calingasan, N. Y., and Beal, M. F. (2005a). Peroxisome proliferator-activated receptor-γ agonist extends survival in transgenic mouse model of amyotrophic lateral sclerosis. *Exp. Neurol.* 191, 331–336. doi: 10.1016/j.expneurol.2004.10.007

Kiaei, M., Kipiani, K., Petri, S., Chen, J., Calingasan, N. Y., and Beal, M. F. (2005b). Celastrol blocks neuronal cell death and extends life in transgenic mouse model of amyotrophic lateral sclerosis. *Neurodegener. Dis.* 2, 246–254. doi: 10.1159/000090364

Kiaei, M., Kipiani, K., Petri, S., Choi, D. K., Chen, J., Calingasan, N. Y., et al. (2005c). Integrative role of cPLA with COX-2 and the effect of non-steriodal anti-inflammatory drugs in a transgenic mouse model of amyotrophic lateral sclerosis. *J. Neurochem.* 93, 403–411. doi: 10.1111/j.1471-4159.2005.03024.x

Kiaei, M., Petri, S., Kipiani, K., Gardian, G., Choi, D. K., Chen, J., et al. (2006). Thalidomide and lenalidomide extend survival in a transgenic mouse model of amyotrophic lateral sclerosis. *J. Neurosci.* 26, 2467–2473. doi: 10.1523/JNEUROSCI.5253-05.2006

Kigerl, K. A., de Rivero Vaccari, J. P., Dietrich, W. D., Popovich, P. G., and Keane, R. W. (2014). Pattern recognition receptors and central nervous system repair. *Exp. Neurol.* 258, 5–16. doi: 10.1016/j.expneurol.2014.01.001

Klivenyi, P., Kiaei, M., Gardian, G., Calingasan, N. Y., and Beal, M. F. (2004). Additive neuroprotective effects of creatine and cyclooxygenase 2 inhibitors in a transgenic mouse model of amyotrophic lateral sclerosis. *J. Neurochem.* 88, 576–582. doi: 10.1046/j.1471-4159.2003.02160.x

Kobayashi, K., Imagama, S., Ohgomori, T., Hirano, K., Uchimura, K., Sakamoto, K., et al. (2013). Minocycline selectively inhibits M1 polarization of microglia. *Cell Death Dis.* 4:e525. doi: 10.1038/cddis.2013.54

Kriz, J., Nguyen, M. D., and Julien, J. P. (2002). Minocycline slows disease progression in a mouse model of amyotrophic lateral sclerosis. *Neurobiol. Dis.* 10, 268–278. doi: 10.1006/nbdi.2002.0487

Kwiatkowski, T. J. Jr., Bosco, D. A., Leclerc, A. L., Tamrazian, E., Vanderburg, C. R., Russ, C., et al. (2009). Mutations in the FUS/TLS gene on chromosome 16 cause familial amyotrophic lateral sclerosis. *Science* 323, 1205–1208. doi: 10.1126/science.1166066

Lewis, K. E., Rasmussen, A. L., Bennett, W., King, A., West, A. K., Chung, R. S., et al. (2014). Microglia and motor neurons during disease progression in the SOD1^{G93A} mouse model of amyotrophic lateral sclerosis: changes in arginase1 and inducible nitric oxide synthase. *J. Neuroinflammation* 11:55. doi: 10.1186/1742-2094-11-55

Liao, B., Zhao, W., Beers, D. R., Henkel, J. S., and Appel, S. H. (2012). Transformation from a neuroprotective to a neurotoxic microglial phenotype in a mouse model of ALS. *Exp. Neurol.* 237, 147–152. doi: 10.1016/j.expneurol.2012.06.011

Linkus, B., Wiesner, D., Meßner, M., Karabatsiakis, A., Scheffold, A., Rudolph, K. L., et al. (2016). Telomere shortening leads to earlier age of onset in ALS mice. *Aging (Albany NY)* 8, 382–393. doi: 10.18632/aging.100904

Luo, X. G., and Chen, S. D. (2012). The changing phenotype of microglia from homeostasis to disease. *Transl. Neurodegener.* 1:9. doi: 10.1186/2047-9158-1-9

Marden, J. J., Harraz, M. M., Williams, A. J., Nelson, K., Luo, M., Paulson, H., et al. (2007). Redox modifier genes in amyotrophic lateral sclerosis in mice. *J. Clin. Invest.* 117, 2913–2919. doi: 10.1172/jci31265

Martin, L. J., Liu, Z., Chen, K., Price, A. C., Pan, Y., Swaby, J. A., et al. (2007). Motor neuron degeneration in amyotrophic lateral sclerosis mutant superoxide dismutase-1 transgenic mice: mechanisms of mitochondriopathy and cell death. *J. Comp. Neurol.* 500, 20–46. doi: 10.1002/cne.21160

Meissner, F., Molawi, K., and Zychlinsky, A. (2010). Mutant superoxide dismutase 1-induced IL-1β accelerates ALS pathogenesis. *Proc. Natl. Acad. Sci. U S A* 107, 13046–13050. doi: 10.1073/pnas.1002396107

Mesci, P., Zaïdi, S., Lobsiger, C. S., Millecamps, S., Escartin, C., Seilhean, D., et al. (2015). System xC- is a mediator of microglial function and its deletion slows symptoms in amyotrophic lateral sclerosis mice. *Brain* 138, 53–68. doi: 10.1093/brain/awu312

Nakazawa, S., Oikawa, D., Ishii, R., Ayaki, T., Takahashi, H., Takeda, H., et al. (2016). Linear ubiquitination is involved in the pathogenesis of optineurin-associated amyotrophic lateral sclerosis. *Nat. Commun.* 7:12547. doi: 10.1038/ncomms12547

Neumann, M., Sampathu, D. M., Kwong, L. K., Truax, A. C., Micsenyi, M. C., Chou, T. T., et al. (2006). Ubiquitinated TDP-43 in frontotemporal lobar degeneration and amyotrophic lateral sclerosis. *Science* 314, 130–133. doi: 10.1126/science.1134108

Nikodemova, M., Small, A. L., Smith, S. M., Mitchell, G. S., and Watters, J. J. (2014). Spinal but not cortical microglia acquire an atypical phenotype with high VEGF, galectin-3 and osteopontin and blunted inflammatory responses in ALS rats. *Neurobiol. Dis.* 69, 43–53. doi: 10.1016/j.nbd.2013.11.009

Nimmerjahn, A., Kirchhoff, F., and Helmchen, F. (2005). Resting microglial cells are highly dynamic surveillants of brain parenchyma *in vivo*. *Science* 308, 1314–1318. doi: 10.1126/science.1110647

Nishimura, A. L., Mitne-Neto, M., Silva, H. C., Richieri-Costa, A., Middleton, S., Cascio, D., et al. (2004). A mutation in the vesicle-trafficking protein VAPB causes late-onset spinal muscular atrophy and amyotrophic lateral sclerosis. *Am. J. Hum. Genet.* 75, 822–831. doi: 10.1086/425287

Ohgomori, T., Yamada, J., Takeuchi, H., Kadomatsu, K., and Jinno, S. (2016). Comparative morphometric analysis of microglia in the spinal cord of SOD1 ^{G93A} transgenic mouse model of amyotrophic lateral sclerosis. *Eur. J. Neurosci.* 43, 1340–1351. doi: 10.1111/ejn.13227

Orihuela, R., McPherson, C. A., and Harry, G. J. (2016). Microglial M1/M2 polarization and metabolic states. *Br. J. Pharmacol.* 173, 649–665. doi: 10.1111/bph.13139

O'Rourke, J. G., Bogdanik, L., Yáñez, A., Lall, D., Wolf, A. J., Muhammad, A. K., et al. (2016). *C9orf72* is required for proper macrophage and microglial function in mice. *Science* 351, 1324–1329. doi: 10.1126/science.aaf1064

Parisi, C., Arisi, I., D'Ambrosi, N., Storti, A. E., Brandi, R., D'Onofrio, M., et al. (2013). Dysregulated microRNAs in amyotrophic lateral sclerosis microglia modulate genes linked to neuroinflammation. *Cell Death Dis.* 4:e959. doi: 10.1038/cddis.2013.491

Parisi, C., Napoli, G., Amadio, S., Spalloni, A., Apolloni, S., Longone, P., et al. (2016a). MicroRNA-125b regulates microglia activation and motor neuron death in ALS. *Cell Death Differ.* 23, 531–541. doi: 10.1038/cdd.2015.153

Parisi, C., Napoli, G., Pelegrin, P., and Volonté, C. (2016b). M1 and M2 functional imprinting of primary microglia: role of P2X7 activation and miR-125b. *Mediators Inflamm.* 2016:2989548. doi: 10.1155/2016/2989548

Philips, T., and Rothstein, J. D. (2014). Glial cells in amyotrophic lateral sclerosis. *Exp. Neurol.* 262, 111–120. doi: 10.1016/j.expneurol.2014.05.015

Philips, T., and Rothstein, J. D. (2015). Rodent models of amyotrophic lateral sclerosis. *Curr. Protoc. Pharmacol.* 69, 5.67.1–5.67.21. doi: 10.1002/0471141755.ph0567s69

Plaza-Zabala, A., Sierra-Torre, V., and Sierra, A. (2017). Autophagy and microglia: novel partners in neurodegeneration and aging. *Int. J. Mol. Sci.* 18:e598. doi: 10.3390/ijms18030598

Pompl, P. N., Ho, L., Bianchi, M., McManus, T., Qin, W., and Pasinetti, G. M. (2003). A therapeutic role for cyclooxygenase-2 inhibitors in a transgenic mouse model of amyotrophic lateral sclerosis. *FASEB J.* 17, 725–727. doi: 10.1096/fj.02-0876fje

Rabinovich-Nikitin, I., Ezra, A., Barbiro, B., Rabinovich-Toidman, P., and Solomon, B. (2016). Chronic administration of AMD3100 increases survival and alleviates pathology in SOD1^{G93A} mice model of ALS. *J. Neuroinflammation* 13:123. doi: 10.1186/s12974-016-0587-6

Ransohoff, R. M. (2016). A polarizing question: do M1 and M2 microglia exist? *Nat. Neurosci.* 19, 987–991. doi: 10.1038/nn.4338

Renton, A. E., Majounie, E., Waite, A., Simón-Sánchez, J., Rollinson, S., Gibbs, J. R., et al. (2011). A hexanucleotide repeat expansion in *C9ORF72* is the cause of chromosome 9p21-linked ALS-FTD. *Neuron* 72, 257–268. doi: 10.1016/j.neuron.2011.09.010

Rosen, D. R., Siddique, T., Patterson, D., Figlewicz, D. A., Sapp, P., Hentati, A., et al. (1993). Mutations in Cu/Zn superoxide dismutase gene are associated with familial amyotrophic lateral sclerosis. *Nature* 362, 59–62. doi: 10.1038/362059a0

Rossi, S., Cozzolino, M., and Carrì, M. T. (2016). Old versus new mechanisms in the pathogenesis of ALS. *Brain Pathol.* 26, 276–286. doi: 10.1111/bpa.12355

Schiffer, D., Cordera, S., Cavalla, P., and Migheli, A. (1996). Reactive astrogliosis of the spinal cord in amyotrophic lateral sclerosis. *J. Neurol. Sci.* 139, 27–33. doi: 10.1016/0022-510x(96)00073-1

Sperlágh, B., and Illes, P. (2014). P2X7 receptor: an emerging target in central nervous system diseases. *Trends Pharmacol. Sci.* 35, 537–547. doi: 10.1016/j.tips.2014.08.002

Suh, H. S., Zhao, M. L., Derico, L., Choi, N., and Lee, S. C. (2013). Insulin-like growth factor 1 and 2 (IGF1, IGF2) expression in human microglia: differential regulation by inflammatory mediators. *J. Neuroinflammation* 10:37. doi: 10.1186/1742-2094-10-37

Swarup, V., Phaneuf, D., Dupre, N., Petri, S., Strong, M., Kriz, J., et al. (2011). Deregulation of TDP-43 in amyotrophic lateral sclerosis triggers nuclear factor κB-mediated pathogenic pathways. *J. Exp. Med.* 208, 2429–2447. doi: 10.1084/jem.20111313

Tada, S., Okuno, T., Hitoshi, Y., Yasui, T., Honorat, J. A., Takata, K., et al. (2014). Partial suppression of M1 microglia by Janus kinase 2 inhibitor does not protect against neurodegeneration in animal models of amyotrophic lateral sclerosis. *J. Neuroinflammation* 11:179. doi: 10.1186/s12974-014-0179-2

Talbot, K. (2011). Familial versus sporadic amyotrophic lateral sclerosis—a false dichotomy? *Brain* 134, 3429–3431. doi: 10.1093/brain/awr296

Tang, Y., and Le, W. (2016). Differential roles of M1 and M2 microglia in neurodegenerative diseases. *Mol. Neurobiol.* 53, 1181–1194. doi: 10.1007/s12035-014-9070-5

Taylor, A. A., Fournier, C., Polak, M., Wang, L., Zach, N., Keymer, M., et al. (2016). Predicting disease progression in amyotrophic lateral sclerosis. *Ann. Clin. Transl. Neurol.* 3, 866–875. doi: 10.1002/acn3.348

Teyssou, E., Takeda, T., Lebon, V., Boillée, S., Doukouré, B., Bataillon, G., et al. (2013). Mutations in SQSTM1 encoding p62 in amyotrophic lateral sclerosis: genetics and neuropathology. *Acta Neuropathol.* 125, 511–522. doi: 10.1007/s00401-013-1090-0

Troost, D., van den Oord, J. J., de Jong, J. M., and Swaab, D. F. (1989). Lymphocytic infiltration in the spinal cord of patients with amyotrophic lateral sclerosis. *Clin. Neuropathol.* 8, 289–294.

Tsuda, H., Han, S. M., Yang, Y., Tong, C., Lin, Y. Q., Mohan, K., et al. (2008). The amyotrophic lateral sclerosis 8 protein VAPB is cleaved, secreted, and acts as a ligand for Eph receptors. *Cell* 133, 963–977. doi: 10.1016/j.cell.2008.04.039

Turner, B. J., and Talbot, K. (2008). Transgenics, toxicity and therapeutics in rodent models of mutant SOD1-mediated familial ALS. *Prog. Neurobiol.* 85, 94–134. doi: 10.1016/j.pneurobio.2008.01.001

Vance, C., Rogelj, B., Hortobágyi, T., De Vos, K. J., Nishimura, A. L., Sreedharan, J., et al. (2009). Mutations in FUS, an RNA processing protein, cause familial amyotrophic lateral sclerosis type 6. *Science* 323, 1208–1211. doi: 10.1126/science.1165942

Van Den Bosch, L., Tilkin, P., Lemmens, G., and Robberecht, W. (2002). Minocycline delays disease onset and mortality in a transgenic model of ALS. *Neuroreport* 13, 1067–1070. doi: 10.1097/00001756-200206120-00018

Volonté, C., Apolloni, S., Skaper, S. D., and Burnstock, G. (2012). P2X7 receptors: channels, pores and more. *CNS Neurol. Disord. Drug Targets* 11, 705–721. doi: 10.2174/187152712803581137

Volonté, C., Parisi, C., and Apolloni, S. (2015). New kid on the block: does histamine get along with inflammation in amyotrophic lateral sclerosis? *CNS Neurol. Disord. Drug Targets* 14, 677–686. doi: 10.2174/1871527314666150225143921

Walton, N. M., Sutter, B. M., Laywell, E. D., Levkoff, L. H., Kearns, S. M., Marshall, G. P., et al. (2006). Microglia instruct subventricular zone neurogenesis. *Glia* 54, 815–825. doi: 10.1002/glia.20419

Wang, Y., Duan, W., Wang, W., Di, W., Liu, Y., Liu, Y., et al. (2016). scAAV9-VEGF prolongs the survival of transgenic ALS mice by promoting activation of M2 microglia and the PI3K/Akt pathway. *Brain Res.* 1648, 1–10. doi: 10.1016/j.brainres.2016.06.043

Wu, C. H., Fallini, C., Ticozzi, N., Keagle, P. J., Sapp, P. C., Piotrowska, K., et al. (2012). Mutations in the profilin 1 gene cause familial amyotrophic lateral sclerosis. *Nature* 488, 499–503. doi: 10.1038/nature11280

Wu, D. C., Ré, D. B., Nagai, M., Ischiropoulos, H., and Przedborski, S. (2006). The inflammatory NADPH oxidase enzyme modulates motor neuron degeneration in amyotrophic lateral sclerosis mice. *Proc. Natl. Acad. Sci. U S A* 103, 12132–12137. doi: 10.1073/pnas.0603670103

Xiao, Q., Zhao, W., Beers, D. R., Yen, A. A., Xie, W., Henkel, J. S., et al. (2007). Mutant SOD1^{G93A} microglia are more neurotoxic relative to wild-type microglia. *J. Neurochem.* 102, 2008–2019. doi: 10.1111/j.1471-4159.2007.04677.x

Xu, Z., Chen, S., Li, X., Luo, G., Li, L., and Le, W. (2006). Neuroprotective effects of (−)-epigallocatechin-3-gallate in a transgenic mouse model of amyotrophic lateral sclerosis. *Neurochem. Res.* 31, 1263–1269. doi: 10.1007/s11064-006-9166-z

Yang, C., Danielson, E. W., Qiao, T., Metterville, J., Brown, R. H. Jr., Landers, J. E., et al. (2016). Mutant PFN1 causes ALS phenotypes and progressive motor neuron degeneration in mice by a gain of toxicity. *Proc. Natl. Acad. Sci. U S A* 113, E6209–E6218. doi: 10.1073/pnas.1605964113

Yang, E. J., Jiang, J. H., Lee, S. M., Yang, S. C., Hwang, H. S., Lee, M. S., et al. (2010). Bee venom attenuates neuroinflammatory events and extends survival in amyotrophic lateral sclerosis models. *J. Neuroinflammation* 7:69. doi: 10.1186/1742-2094-7-69

Yiangou, Y., Facer, P., Durrenberger, P., Chessell, I. P., Naylor, A., Bountra, C., et al. (2006). COX-2, CB2 and P2X7-immunoreactivities are increased in activated microglial cells/macrophages of multiple sclerosis and amyotrophic lateral sclerosis spinal cord. *BMC Neurol.* 6:12. doi: 10.1186/1471-2377-6-12

Zhao, W., Beers, D. R., Bell, S., Wang, J., Wen, S., Baloh, R. H., et al. (2015). TDP-43 activates microglia through NF-κB and NLRP3 inflammasome. *Exp. Neurol.* 273, 24–35. doi: 10.1016/j.expneurol.2015.07.019

Zhao, W., Beers, D. R., Henkel, J. S., Zhang, W., Urushitani, M., Julien, J. P., et al. (2010). Extracellular mutant SOD1 induces microglial-mediated motoneuron injury. *Glia* 58, 231–243. doi: 10.1002/glia.20919

Zhou, C., Zhang, C., Zhao, R., Chi, S., Ge, P., and Zhang, C. (2013). Human marrow stromal cells reduce microglial activation to protect motor neurons in a transgenic mouse model of amyotrophic lateral sclerosis. *J. Neuroinflammation* 10:52. doi: 10.1186/1742-2094-10-52

Zhu, S., Stavrovskaya, I. G., Drozda, M., Kim, B. Y., Ona, V., Li, M., et al. (2002). Minocycline inhibits cytochrome c release and delays progression of amyotrophic lateral sclerosis in mice. *Nature* 417, 74–78. doi: 10.1038/417074a

12

Role of Atypical Chemokine Receptors in Microglial Activation and Polarization

Valentina Salvi[1†], *Francesca Sozio*[1,2†], *Silvano Sozzani*[1,2*‡] *and Annalisa Del Prete*[1,2‡]

[1]*Department of Molecular and Translational Medicine, University of Brescia, Brescia, Italy,* [2]*IRCCS-Humanitas Clinical and Research Center, Rozzano-Milano, Italy*

***Correspondence:**
Silvano Sozzani
silvano.sozzani@unibs.it

[†]*Shared first authorship.*
[‡]*Shared last authorship.*

Inflammatory reactions occurring in the central nervous system (CNS), known as neuroinflammation, are key components of the pathogenic mechanisms underlying several neurological diseases. The chemokine system plays a crucial role in the recruitment and activation of immune and non-immune cells in the brain, as well as in the regulation of microglia phenotype and function. Chemokines belong to a heterogeneous family of chemotactic agonists that signal through the interaction with G protein-coupled receptors (GPCRs). Recently, a small subset of chemokine receptors, now identified as "atypical chemokine receptors" (ACKRs), has been described. These receptors lack classic GPCR signaling and chemotactic activity and are believed to limit inflammation through their ability to scavenge chemokines at the inflammatory sites. Recent studies have highlighted a role for ACKRs in neuroinflammation. However, in the CNS, the role of ACKRs seems to be more complex than the simple control of inflammation. For instance, CXCR7/ACKR3 was shown to control T cell trafficking through the regulation of CXCL12 internalization at CNS endothelial barriers. Furthermore, D6/ACKR2 KO mice were protected in a model of experimental autoimmune encephalomyelitis (EAE). D6/ACKR2 KO showed an abnormal accumulation of dendritic cells at the immunization and a subsequent impairment in T cell priming. Finally, CCRL2, an ACKR-related protein, was shown to play a role in the control of the resolution phase of EAE. Indeed, CCRL2 KO mice showed exacerbated, non-resolving disease with protracted inflammation and increased demyelination. This phenotype was associated with increased microglia and macrophage activation markers and imbalanced M1 vs. M2 polarization. This review will summarize the current knowledge on the role of the ACKRs in neuroinflammation with a particular attention to their role in microglial polarization and function.

Keywords: chemokine receptors, neuroinflammation, microglia, atypical chemokine receptors, CCRL2

INTRODUCTION

The central nervous system (CNS) degeneration, which characterizes several chronic neurodegenerative diseases, such as Alzheimer's disease (AD), Parkinson's disease (PD), amyotrophic lateral sclerosis (ALS) and multiple sclerosis (MS), is closely linked to immune activation occurring in the CNS called neuroinflammation (Ransohoff, 2016a). Regardless the triggering mechanisms that can include viral infections, immune-mediate disorders and neuron damage, the immune activation involves microglia and astrocytes (Sofroniew and Vinters, 2010; Perry and Teeling, 2013). These cells represent immune cells resident in the CNS, which regulate CNS homeostasis from the development of brain to the adult life and aging (Schwartz et al., 2013). In particular, any insult is followed by activation of microglia, which culminates with the production of a series of pro-inflammatory mediators that alter brain-blood barrier permeability and induce infiltration of circulating leukocytes inside the CNS (Noh et al., 2014). This effect is regulated by the chemokine system which plays an important role in the control of immune surveillance in the brain (Takeshita and Ransohoff, 2012). The inflammatory response is usually self-limiting and culminates with tissue repair and resolution mechanisms, which mostly involve M2 polarized microglia. However, when this process persists and become chronic, the long-standing activation state of microglia sustains the release of detrimental inflammatory mediators and neurotoxic products which contribute to neurodegenerative sequelae (González et al., 2014; Ransohoff, 2016a).

This review article will focus on the mechanisms involved in the tight regulation of local immune responses occurring during CNS inflammatory process, with particular attention to the role of the chemokine system and atypical chemokine receptors (ACKRs) in microglial activation and polarization.

MICROGLIAL ACTIVATION AND POLARIZATION

Microglia are tissue-resident macrophages of the brain and spinal cord, derived from primitive myeloid progenitors in the yolk sac that invade the brain parenchyma during embryonic development (Ginhoux et al., 2010). As mononuclear phagocytes of the CNS, microglia play an important role in maintaining normal brain functions in both physiological and pathological conditions (Wolf et al., 2017). In CNS development, microglia regulate neurogenesis by phagocyting apoptotic newborn cells in the sub-granular zone (Sierra et al., 2010) and support neuronal survival by accumulating around axons and secreting trophic factors like IGF-1 (Ueno et al., 2013). In addition, microglia actively remove the excess of synaptic connections and play a major role in synaptic pruning during postnatal development in mice (Paolicelli et al., 2011). In physiological conditions microglia are responsible to eliminate and remodel synapses and support myelin turnover by phagocytosis of axon terminals and dendritic spines also in adult brain (Tremblay, 2011). Morphology of microglia reveals the different activation states of these cells. In healthy brain, microglia have a ramified shape with extensively branched processes in contact with neurons, astrocytes and blood vessels, that continually survey and monitor changes in the local milieu (Nimmerjahn et al., 2005). Once activated by tissue damage, viral or bacterial insults or pro-inflammatory stimuli these cells develop ameboid morphology characterized by cell body enlargement, shortened cell processes and the presence of numerous cytoplasmic vacuoles, associated with phagocytosis and pro-inflammatory functions (Djukic et al., 2006; Colonna and Butovsky, 2017).

Microglia like macrophages are plastic cells able to acquire distinct functional phenotypes according to the nature of the local microenvironment (**Figure 1**). In addition to morphological differentiation, these cells express different surface markers such as Toll-like receptors, NOD-like receptors, nucleotide-binding oligomerization domain and scavenger receptors. In response to pro-inflammatory stimuli, like LPS, IFNγ and TNF-α, microglial cells produce inflammatory cytokines such as IL-1α/β, IL-6, IL-12, IL-23, TNF-α, iNOS, CCL5 and express Fc receptors CD16, CD32, CD64 and CD68. This pro-inflammatory polarization corresponds to the "classical" M1 activation state (Boche et al., 2013; Cherry et al., 2014). On the other hand, anti-inflammatory stimuli such as IL-4, IL-10, IL-13, TGF-β and glucocorticoids polarize microglia in the "alternative" M2 phenotype that promotes resolution of inflammation and restoring of homeostasis. M2 polarized cells produce anti-inflammatory molecules like arginase-1 (Arg-1), that contributes to matrix deposition and wound healing, growth factors like IGF-1, chitinase 3-like 3 (Ym-1) and FIZZ1 which promote deposition of extracellular matrix and express characteristic receptors of M2 phagocytes such as mannose receptor (CD206) and TREM2 (Raes et al., 2002; Orihuela et al., 2016). Activation of microglial cells strongly influence the pathogenesis of neuroinflammatory and neurodegenerative diseases such as PD, ALS, MS, AD, traumatic brain injuries, stroke and brain tumors (Wolf et al., 2017). However, the concept of microglia polarization is now debated, since M1/M2 paradigm may represent an oversimplification of *in vivo* activation. Transcriptomic and proteomic analysis will help to define the heterogeneity of microglial phenotype associated to different pathological contexts (Ransohoff, 2016b).

CHEMOKINE SYSTEM IN NEUROINFLAMMATION

Chemokines are small, secreted chemotactic cytokines involved in leukocyte trafficking both in homeostatic and inflammatory conditions. Chemokines play their functional role by the engagement of the cognate G protein-coupled receptors (GPCRs), which results in the receptor activation and the triggering of intracellular signaling cascade that regulates several cell activities such as migration, adhesion, phagocytosis, cytokine secretion, proliferation and apoptosis (Bachelerie et al., 2014a). More than 50 different chemokines and about 20 chemokine receptors have been discovered (Bachelerie et al., 2014a). Chemokines are divided into CC, CXC, XC and CX3C subfamilies according to the specific nature of the cysteine motif (Zlotnik and Yoshie, 2000). The chemokine system displays promiscuity features in ligand binding and chemokine receptor expression on different leukocytes (Bachelerie et al., 2014a).

In CNS, chemokines play a role in physiological conditions being involved in neuronal migration, cell proliferation and synaptic activities. During neuroinflammation, in addition to their primary role in leukocytes recruitment, they can also have direct effects on neuronal cells and mediate the cross

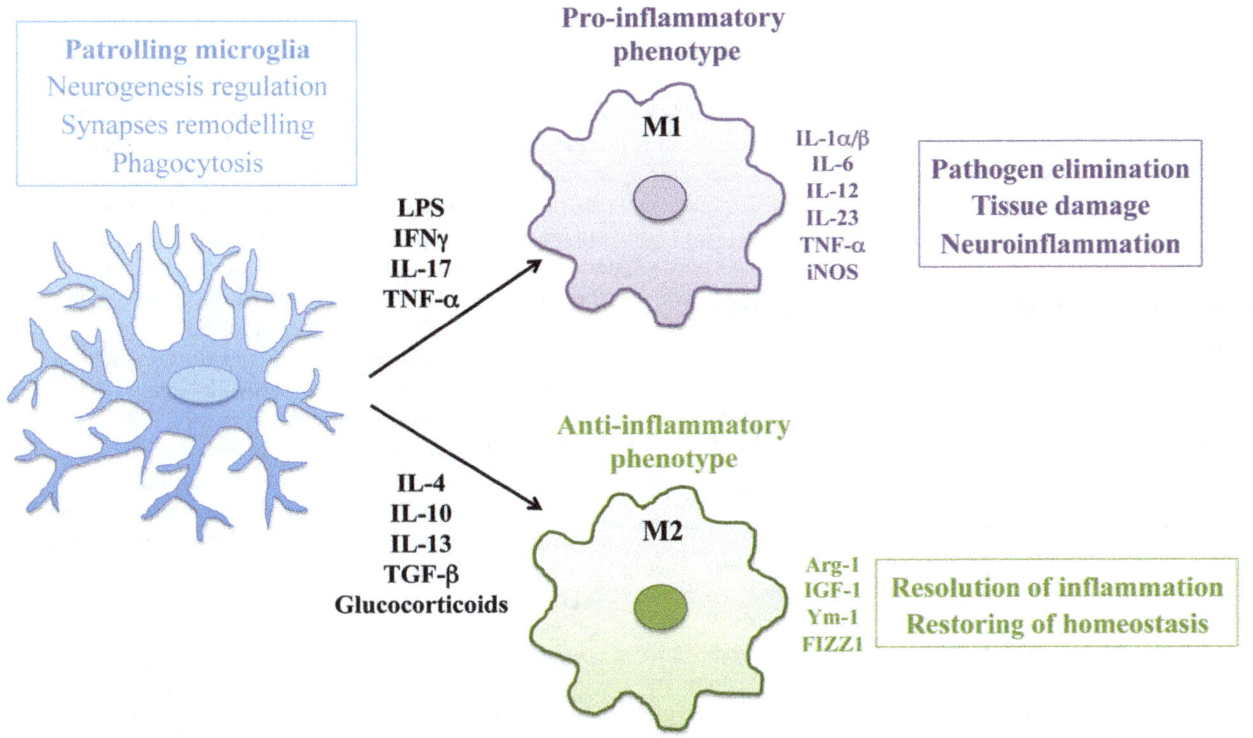

FIGURE 1 | Activation and polarization of microglia in resting conditions and during neuroinflammation. The morphology and the phenotype associated with different functional states of microglia are represented. In physiological conditions patrolling microglia regulate central nervous system (CNS) homeostasis. In neuroinflammation microglia assume ameboid morphology and acquire classical M1 or alternative M2 phenotype according to the nature of local milieu.

talk between neurons and inflammatory cells (Cartier et al., 2005). Chemokines can exert neuroprotective role. For instance, CCL2 was described to play a role as a protective agent against the toxic effects of glutamate and HIV-tat-induced apoptosis (Eugenin et al., 2003). In addition, the signaling of the neuronal CX3CL1 and its receptor CX3CR1 were shown to reduce the levels of neurotoxic substances such as TNF-α and nitric oxide in activated microglia during neuroinflammation (Mattison et al., 2013). On the contrary, chemokines can directly induce neuronal death or indirectly through the activation of microglia killing mechanisms (Sui et al., 2006; Yang et al., 2011). A new role for chemokines in the modulation of the release of neuropeptides and neurotransmitters was also proposed (Rostène et al., 2007, 2011), as shown by the effect of CXCL12 in tuning the firing pattern of vasopressin neurons (Callewaere et al., 2006).

In active MS patients, the pathogenic Th1 axis, involving CXCL10, CCL3, CCL4, CCL5 and the receptors CXCR3 and CCR5, is activated in blood and cerebrospinal fluid (Uzawa et al., 2010). On the contrary, the Th2 receptors CCR4 and CCR3 and the ligand CCL2 play a protective role (Nakajima et al., 2004). Th17 are recruited by CCR6/CCL20 axis expressed by epithelial cells of choroid plexus as shown in the experimental autoimmune encephalomyelitis (EAE) model (Reboldi et al., 2009; Cao et al., 2015). CXCL12 acts as double edge sword since it is responsible for the recruitment of monocytes in the CNS during MS (Azin et al., 2012) and, at the same time, contributes to remyelination and neuroprotection processes (Khorramdelazad et al., 2016). Moreover, in MS, CXCL13 secreted by microglia has been shown to be involved in the recruitment of CXCR5 expressing Th1, Th17 and B cells (Huber and Irani, 2015).

The dysregulation of the CX3CL1-CX3CR1 communications between neurons and microglia has been investigated in AD patients showing opposite effects. In one study CX3CR1 deficiency was reported to reduce beta-amyloid deposition in AD experimental model (Lee et al., 2010). Other work showed different contribution of the soluble vs. the membrane-bound forms of CX3CL1 in the regulation of microglial phagocytosis of plaques (Cho et al., 2011; Lee et al., 2014). CX3CL1 gene expression was upregulated in the brain of AD patient (Strobel et al., 2015). Other chemokines, such as CCL3, CXCL10 and CCL2 were implicated in the regulation of glial activity involved in neuroinflammation and neurotoxic environment during the AD development (Xia et al., 2000; Galimberti et al., 2006; Meyer-Luehmann et al., 2008; Dos Passos et al., 2016). A relevant role of glial activation in the development of neuroinflammation associated with damage of the nigro-striatal dopaminergic system was suggested in PD (Przedborski, 2010). The CXCL12 and CXCR4 expression is increased and can promote apoptosis of dopamine neurons (Shimoji et al., 2009). On the contrary, CX3CL1 exerts a neuroprotective effect during PD development (Pabon et al., 2011).

Overall, neuroinflammation is a complex process involved in several CNS diseases ranging from autoimmune to degenerative pathologies and chemokine system plays key role in immune surveillance, in microglial activation and functions, in neurocommunications among several CNS cell types and can orchestrate both neuroprotective and detrimental effects.

ATYPICAL CHEMOKINE RECEPTORS IN NEUROINFLAMMATION

ACKRs represent a small subset of proteins expressing high degree of homology with chemokine receptors. Since ACKRs lack structural domains required for proper $G\alpha_i$ signaling, they are unable to activate canonical G protein-dependent receptor signaling and chemotactic functions (Bachelerie et al., 2014a,b). At the moment, the ACKR family includes four proteins, namely ACKR1, ACKR2, ACKR3 and ACKR4. Other two proteins, namely CCRL2 and PITPNM3 have been provisionally included with the name of "Ackr5" and "Ackr6", respectively, but they still need formal approval (Bachelerie et al., 2014b). In the last few years, the role of ACKRs is gradually clarifying since they were shown to regulate inflammation acting as scavenger receptors, promoting chemokine transcytosis or regulating chemokine gradient formation (Mantovani et al., 2001; Nibbs and Graham, 2013; Bachelerie et al., 2014a,b; Bonecchi and Graham, 2016). The role of ACKRs in neuroinflammation is described below and summarized in **Table 1**.

ACKR1

ACKR1 binds, with high affinity over 20 inflammatory chemokines belonging to the CC and CXC families (Novitzky-Basso and Rot, 2012). ACKR1 is expressed on erythrocytes, cerebellar Purkinje cells, postcapillary venules and capillary endothelial cells. Depending on its cellular expression, the biological functions of ACKR1 are quite different. Indeed, ACKR1 expressed by erythrocytes regulates the bioavailability of circulating chemokines by binding them with high affinity (Schnabel et al., 2010), while endothelial ACKR1 induces chemokine internalization and transcytosis from the basolateral to the luminal side of endothelium, where the chemokines are immobilized and contribute to leukocyte extravasation *in vivo* (Pruenster et al., 2009). In neuroinflammation, ACKR1 is upregulated on endothelial cells in CNS microvessels during EAE and in MS where it mediates the abluminal to luminal transport of inflammatory chemokines across the blood-brain barrier and contributes to EAE pathogenesis (Minten et al., 2014). In bone marrow chimera experiments, ACKR1 expression in erythrocytes was shown to be responsible for the increased plasma levels of inflammatory chemokines observed during EAE. However, for the full development of the disease, the expression of ACKR1 was necessary also on endothelial cells (Minten et al., 2014).

ACKR2

ACKR2 binds a broad panel of inflammatory CC chemokines and is expressed by lymphatic endothelial cells, trophoblasts, keratinocytes and some leukocyte subsets, mostly innate-like B cells (Lee et al., 2013). ACKR2 binds and internalizes its ligands and target them for lysosomal degradation. Therefore, ACKR2 is a chemokine-scavenging receptor, aiding the resolution of inflammatory reactions (Graham, 2009). Studies in EAE model suggested that ACKR2 functions may be context-dependent. Indeed, ACKR2 KO mice are unexpectedly resistant to the induction of EAE due to impaired encephalitogenic responses (Liu et al., 2006). This observation is ascribed to defective T-cell priming resulting by the suppression of dendritic cells migration to the lymph nodes caused by excessive inflammation at the immunization site (Liu et al., 2006). In contrast, ACKR2 deficiency was recently associated with an exacerbated EAE phenotype when mice were immunized with the entire protein but not the MOG peptide, suggesting a regulatory role for ACKR2 mediated by T cell polarization (Hansell et al., 2015).

ACKR3

ACKR3 binds two chemokines, namely CXCL12 and CXCL11. ACKR3 is expressed by endothelial cells, some hematopoietic cells, mesenchymal cells, neurons and astrocytes. ACKR3 is able to internalize CXCL12 and modulate CXCR4 expression and signaling by forming heterodimers with CXCR4 (Levoye et al., 2009; Décaillot et al., 2011). Thus, ACKR3 can control chemokine responsiveness by regulating CXCR4 protein levels and CXCL12 scavenging activity as shown in migrating cortical interneurons (Sánchez-Alcañiz et al., 2011; Abe et al., 2014). Loss of CXCL12, a chemokine that restricts the CNS entry of CXCR4-expressing leukocytes from abluminal surfaces of blood-brain barriers, has been described in MS. During EAE, ACKR3 expression on endothelial barriers is increased at sites of inflammatory infiltration (Cruz-Orengo et al., 2011b) and its activation, by scavenging CXCL12, is essential for leukocyte entry via endothelial barriers into the CNS parenchyma (Cruz-Orengo et al., 2011b). Administration of ACKR3 specific antagonist CCX771 increases abluminal levels of CXCL12 at the blood-brain barrier, preventing the pathological entry of immune cells into CNS parenchyma, thus improving clinical signs of EAE disease (Cruz-Orengo et al., 2011b). In addition, ACKR3 antagonism during EAE helps preserving axonal integrity (Cruz-Orengo et al., 2011a). In mice with EAE, ACKR3 is also upregulated in migrating oligodendrocytes progenitors, important cells for the remyelination process, in the subventricular zone (Banisadr et al., 2016). More recently, it was reported that ACKR3 expression is responsible for the migration of activated microglia and positively correlated with the clinical severity of EAE (Bao et al., 2016). Indeed, an ACKR3 neutralizing antibody modulates microglial chemotaxis and ameliorates EAE symptoms (Bao et al., 2016).

ACKR4

ACKR4 binds the homeostatic CC chemokines CCL19, CCL21, CCL25 and with lower affinity CXCL13. ACKR4 is expressed by

TABLE 1 | Atypical chemokine receptors (ACKRs) and their role in neuroinflammation.

Receptor name	Alternative names	Sites of expression	Role in neuroinflammation	References
ACKR1	Duffy antigen receptor for chemokines (DARC), CD234	Erythrocytes Vascular endothelial cells Purkinje cells	On erythrocyte it acts as chemokine reservoir On endothelium it contributes to EAE pathogenesis	Minten et al. (2014)
ACKR2	CCBP2, D6, CMKBR9	Lymphatic endothelial cells Innate-like B cells Keratinocytes Trophoblasts	It is required for generating T cell responses in EAE It suppresses Th17 responses in EAE	Liu et al. (2006), Hansell et al. (2015)
ACKR3	RDC1, CXCR7, CMKOR1	Endothelial cells Hematopoietic cells, Mesenchymal cells Neurons Astrocytes	It contributes to EAE pathogenesis It mediates chemotaxis of activated microglia during EAE	Cruz-Orengo et al. (2011b); Bao et al. (2016)
ACKR4	CCRL1, CCXCKR, CCR11	Thymic epithelial cells Keratinocytes Lymphatic endothelial cells	It delays the onset of EAE and reduces disease severity	Comerford et al. (2010)

thymic epithelial cells, keratinocytes and lymphatic endothelial cells. After chemokine binding ACKR4 internalizes and drives its ligand to degradation (Comerford et al., 2006), thus representing the homeostatic counterpart of the inflammatory CC chemokine scavenger receptor ACKR2. In an EAE model, ACKR4 deficient mice developed the disease earlier and with more severity compared to wild type mice. This earlier onset was associated with an enhanced splenic Th17-type response, an elevated expression of IL-23 transcript, and an increase in CCL21 in the CNS (Comerford et al., 2010).

ROLE OF CCRL2 IN MICROGLIAL POLARIZATION

CCRL2 is a seven transmembrane protein that shares some structural and functional aspects with ACKRs, such as the lack of conventional GPCR signaling and the inability to induce cell migration (Zabel et al., 2008; Del Prete et al., 2013; Bachelerie et al., 2014a; De Henau et al., 2016). Some authors described binding and/or functional activation of CCRL2 in response to chemokines CCL2, CCL5, CCL7, CCL8 and CCL19 (Biber et al., 2003; Catusse et al., 2010; Leick et al., 2010). However, these results were not subsequently confirmed by other groups (Del Prete et al., 2013; De Henau et al., 2016). CCRL2 binds and presents chemerin, a non-chemokine chemotactic protein, to adjacent cells expressing the functional chemerin receptor ChemR23, and acts as regulator of chemerin bioavailability (Zabel et al., 2008; Gonzalvo-Feo et al., 2014). Neither internalization nor calcium mobilization was described upon chemerin binding (Zabel et al., 2008). CCRL2 is expressed by endothelial and epithelial cells, and by a variety of leukocytes, including macrophages, dendritic cells, mast cells and neutrophils and its expression is increased by pro-inflammatory stimuli (Galligan et al., 2004; Zabel et al., 2008; Otero et al., 2010; Monnier et al., 2012; Del Prete et al., 2013; Gonzalvo-Feo et al., 2014). In particular, CCRL2 was described to play a non-redundant role in the regulation of dendritic cell migration during airway inflammation (Otero et al., 2010). Moreover, *in vitro* and *in vivo* studies showed CCRL2 expression in mouse microglia and astrocytes and upregulation in macrophages in the EAE model (Zuurman et al., 2003; Brouwer et al., 2004). To better understand the role of CCRL2 in CNS physiopathology, our group studied the role of CCRL2 deficiency in EAE model (Mazzon et al., 2016).

CCRL2 expression was found upregulated following $MOG_{aa35-55}$ immunization and paralleled the kinetics of the clinical symptoms, reaching the peak induction at the acme of the disease and declining thereafter (Mazzon et al., 2016). During the development of EAE, the upregulation of CCRL2 was associated with increased levels of chemerin (Graham et al., 2009; Mazzon et al., 2016), mimicking the regulation of ACKR3 and its ligand CXCL12 (Banisadr et al., 2016). CCRL2 deficient mice showed exacerbated EAE clinical phenotype, in terms of increased mortality, higher maximum and cumulative clinical score. The histopathological analysis revealed an intense and persistent inflammatory reaction associated with increased demyelination in CCRL2 deficient spinal cords at the recovery phase of the disease. These observations were paralleled by the increase in T cell infiltration in CCRL2 deficient mice. In addition, in CCRL2 KO mice, the macrophage/microglia activation markers, namely Iba-1, CD68, and TREM2 remained elevated during the recovery phase of the disease. An unbalanced M1/M2 polarization, with a persistent predominance of the M1 markers was also observed during the recovery phase of the disease. This was in contrast to control mice that developed all the signs of resolution of inflammation including the M2 phenotype characterizing the CNS regenerative response. These results candidate CCRL2 as an important player in EAE-associated inflammatory reactions and suggest the tuning of microglial activation and polarization as an additional mechanism used by ACKRs to regulate CNS inflammatory responses.

CONCLUSIONS

Neuroinflammation is a key component of neurodegenerative diseases. This process involves the effector components of both innate and adaptive immunity. In the CNS, microglia represent the resident immune component involved in tissue homeostasis. Being an immune sensor of altered homeostasis, microglia accumulate in response to neuron injury and after the entry of foreign substances in the CNS. The way microglia become activated represents a crucial element in the regulation of neuroinflammation and may be associated with either beneficial or detrimental effects resulting in neuroprotection or neurotoxicity. The chemokine system plays multiple roles in the modulation of this multifaceted process. Our growing understanding on the functions of the ACKRs increases the level of complexity of this scenario and provides new potential targets to be exploited in the control of neuroinflammation.

AUTHOR CONTRIBUTIONS

VS and FS wrote and edited the manuscript and prepared the Table and Figure. SS and ADP contributed in writing and supervised the final version of the manuscript.

ACKNOWLEDGMENTS

This work was supported by Associazione Italiana Ricerca sul Cancro (AIRC); Interuniversity Attraction Poles (IAP) 7-40 program.

REFERENCES

Abe, P., Mueller, W., Schütz, D., MacKay, F., Thelen, M., Zhang, P., et al. (2014). CXCR7 prevents excessive CXCL12-mediated downregulation of CXCR4 in migrating cortical interneurons. *Development* 141, 1857–1863. doi: 10.1242/dev.104224

Azin, H., Vazirinejad, R., Ahmadabadi, B. N., Khorramdelazad, H., Zarandi, E. R., Arababadi, M. K., et al. (2012). The SDF-1 3′a genetic variation of the chemokine SDF-1α (CXCL12) in parallel with its increased circulating levels is associated with susceptibility to MS: a study on Iranian multiple sclerosis patients. *J. Mol. Neurosci.* 47, 431–436. doi: 10.1007/s12031-011-9672-6

Bachelerie, F., Ben-Baruch, A., Burkhardt, A. M., Combadiere, C., Farber, J. M., Graham, G. J., et al. (2014a). International union of basic and clinical pharmacology. LXXXIX. Update on the extended family of chemokine receptors and introducing a new nomenclature for atypical chemokine receptors. *Pharmacol. Rev.* 66, 1–79. doi: 10.1124/pr.113.007724

Bachelerie, F., Graham, G. J., Locati, M., Mantovani, A., Murphy, P. M., Nibbs, R., et al. (2014b). New nomenclature for atypical chemokine receptors. *Nat. Immunol.* 15, 207–208. doi: 10.1038/ni.2812

Banisadr, G., Podojil, J. R., Miller, S. D., and Miller, R. J. (2016). Pattern of CXCR7 gene expression in mouse brain under normal and inflammatory conditions. *J. Neuroimmune Pharmacol.* 11, 26–35. doi: 10.1007/s11481-015-9616-y

Bao, J., Zhu, J., Luo, S., Cheng, Y., and Zhou, S. (2016). CXCR7 suppression modulates microglial chemotaxis to ameliorate experimentally-induced autoimmune encephalomyelitis. *Biochem. Biophys. Res. Commun.* 469, 1–7. doi: 10.1016/j.bbrc.2015.11.059

Biber, K., Zuurman, M. W., Homan, H., and Boddeke, H. W. (2003). Expression of L-CCR in HEK 293 cells reveals functional responses to CCL2, CCL5, CCL7, and CCL8. *J. Leukoc. Biol.* 74, 243–251. doi: 10.1189/jlb.0802415

Boche, D., Perry, V. H., and Nicoll, J. A. (2013). Review: activation patterns of microglia and their identification in the human brain. *Neuropathol. Appl. Neurobiol.* 39, 3–18. doi: 10.1111/nan.12011

Bonecchi, R., and Graham, G. J. (2016). Atypical chemokine receptors and their roles in the resolution of the inflammatory response. *Front. Immunol.* 7:224. doi: 10.3389/fimmu.2016.00224

Brouwer, N., Zuurman, M. W., Wei, T., Ransohoff, R. M., Boddeke, H. W., and Biber, K. (2004). Induction of glial L-CCR mRNA expression in spinal cord and brain in experimental autoimmune encephalomyelitis. *Glia* 46, 84–94. doi: 10.1002/glia.10352

Callewaere, C., Banisadr, G., Desarménien, M. G., Mechighel, P., Kitabgi, P., Rostène, W. H., et al. (2006). The chemokine SDF-1/CXCL12 modulates the firing pattern of vasopressin neurons and counteracts induced vasopressin release through CXCR4. *Proc. Natl. Acad. Sci. U S A* 103, 8221–8226. doi: 10.1073/pnas.0602620103

Cao, Y., Goods, B. A., Raddassi, K., Nepom, G. T., Kwok, W. W., Love, J. C., et al. (2015). Functional inflammatory profiles distinguish myelin-reactive T cells from patients with multiple sclerosis. *Sci. Transl. Med.* 7:287ra274. doi: 10.1126/scitranslmed.aaa8038

Cartier, L., Hartley, O., Dubois-Dauphin, M., and Krause, K. H. (2005). Chemokine receptors in the central nervous system: role in brain inflammation and neurodegenerative diseases. *Brain Res. Rev.* 48, 16–42. doi: 10.1016/j.brainresrev.2004.07.021

Catusse, J., Leick, M., Groch, M., Clark, D. J., Buchner, M. V., Zirlik, K., et al. (2010). Role of the atypical chemoattractant receptor CRAM in regulating CCL19 induced CCR7 responses in B-cell chronic lymphocytic leukemia. *Mol. Cancer* 9:297. doi: 10.1186/1476-4598-9-297

Cherry, J. D., Olschowka, J. A., and O'Banion, M. K. (2014). Neuroinflammation and M2 microglia: the good, the bad, and the inflamed. *J. Neuroinflammation* 11:98. doi: 10.1186/1742-2094-11-98

Cho, S. H., Sun, B., Zhou, Y., Kauppinen, T. M., Halabisky, B., Wes, P., et al. (2011). CX3CR1 protein signaling modulates microglial activation and protects against plaque-independent cognitive deficits in a mouse model of Alzheimer disease. *J. Biol. Chem.* 286, 32713–32722. doi: 10.1074/jbc.M111.254268

Colonna, M., and Butovsky, O. (2017). Microglia function in the central nervous system during health and neurodegeneration. *Annu. Rev. Immunol.* 35, 441–468. doi: 10.1146/annurev-immunol-051116-052358

Comerford, I., Milasta, S., Morrow, V., Milligan, G., and Nibbs, R. (2006). The chemokine receptor CCX-CKR mediates effective scavenging of CCL19 *in vitro*. *Eur. J. Immunol.* 36, 1904–1916. doi: 10.1002/eji.2005 35716

Comerford, I., Nibbs, R. J., Litchfield, W., Bunting, M., Harata-Lee, Y., Haylock-Jacobs, S., et al. (2010). The atypical chemokine receptor CCX-CKR scavenges homeostatic chemokines in circulation and tissues and suppresses Th17 responses. *Blood* 116, 4130–4140. doi: 10.1182/blood-2010-01-264390

Cruz-Orengo, L., Chen, Y. J., Kim, J. H., Dorsey, D., Song, S. K., and Klein, R. S. (2011a). CXCR7 antagonism prevents axonal injury during experimental autoimmune encephalomyelitis as revealed by *in vivo* axial diffusivity. *J. Neuroinflammation* 8:170. doi: 10.1186/1742-2094-8-170

Cruz-Orengo, L., Holman, D. W., Dorsey, D., Zhou, L., Zhang, P., Wright, M., et al. (2011b). CXCR7 influences leukocyte entry into the CNS parenchyma by controlling abluminal CXCL12 abundance during autoimmunity. *J. Exp. Med.* 208, 327–339. doi: 10.1084/jem.20102010

De Henau, O., Degroot, G. N., Imbault, V., Robert, V., De Poorter, C., McHeik, S., et al. (2016). Signaling properties of chemerin receptors CMKLR1, GPR1 and CCRL2. *PLoS One* 11:e0164179. doi: 10.1371/journal.pone.0164179

Décaillot, F. M., Kazmi, M. A., Lin, Y., Ray-Saha, S., Sakmar, T. P., and Sachdev, P. (2011). CXCR7/CXCR4 heterodimer constitutively recruits β-arrestin to enhance cell migration. *J. Biol. Chem.* 286, 32188–32197. doi: 10.1074/jbc.M111.277038

Del Prete, A., Bonecchi, R., Vecchi, A., Mantovani, A., and Sozzani, S. (2013). CCRL2, a fringe member of the atypical chemoattractant receptor family. *Eur. J. Immunol.* 43, 1418–1422. doi: 10.1002/eji.201243179

Djukic, M., Mildner, A., Schmidt, H., Czesnik, D., Brück, W., Priller, J., et al. (2006). Circulating monocytes engraft in the brain, differentiate into microglia and contribute to the pathology following meningitis in mice. *Brain* 129, 2394–2403. doi: 10.1093/brain/awl206

Dos Passos, G. R., Sato, D. K., Becker, J., and Fujihara, K. (2016). Th17 cells pathways in multiple sclerosis and neuromyelitis optica spectrum disorders: pathophysiological and therapeutic implications. *Mediators Inflamm.* 2016:5314541. doi: 10.1155/2016/5314541

Eugenin, E. A., D'Aversa, T. G., Lopez, L., Calderon, T. M., and Berman, J. W. (2003). MCP-1 (CCL2) protects human neurons and astrocytes from NMDA or HIV-tat-induced apoptosis. *J. Neurochem.* 85, 1299–1311. doi: 10.1046/j.1471-4159.2003.01775.x

Galimberti, D., Fenoglio, C., Lovati, C., Venturelli, E., Guidi, I., Corrà, B., et al. (2006). Serum MCP-1 levels are increased in mild cognitive impairment and mild Alzheimer's disease. *Neurobiol. Aging* 27, 1763–1768. doi: 10.1016/j.neurobiolaging.2005.10.007

Galligan, C. L., Matsuyama, W., Matsukawa, A., Mizuta, H., Hodge, D. R., Howard, O. M., et al. (2004). Up-regulated expression and activation of the orphan chemokine receptor, CCRL2, in rheumatoid arthritis. *Arthritis Rheum.* 50, 1806–1814. doi: 10.1002/art.20275

Ginhoux, F., Greter, M., Leboeuf, M., Nandi, S., See, P., Gokhan, S., et al. (2010). Fate mapping analysis reveals that adult microglia derive from primitive macrophages. *Science* 330, 841–845. doi: 10.1126/science.1194637

González, H., Elgueta, D., Montoya, A., and Pacheco, R. (2014). Neuroimmune regulation of microglial activity involved in neuroinflammation and neurodegenerative diseases. *J. Neuroimmunol.* 274, 1–13. doi: 10.1016/j.jneuroim.2014.07.012

Gonzalvo-Feo, S., Del Prete, A., Pruenster, M., Salvi, V., Wang, L., Sironi, M., et al. (2014). Endothelial cell-derived chemerin promotes dendritic cell transmigration. *J. Immunol.* 192, 2366–2373. doi: 10.4049/jimmunol.1302028

Graham, G. J. (2009). D6 and the atypical chemokine receptor family: novel regulators of immune and inflammatory processes. *Eur. J. Immunol.* 39, 342–351. doi: 10.1002/eji.200838858

Graham, K. L., Zabel, B. A., Loghavi, S., Zuniga, L. A., Ho, P. P., Sobel, R. A., et al. (2009). Chemokine-like receptor-1 expression by central nervous system-infiltrating leukocytes and involvement in a model of autoimmune demyelinating disease. *J. Immunol.* 183, 6717–6723. doi: 10.4049/jimmunol.080343

Hansell, C. A., MacLellan, L. M., Oldham, R. S., Doonan, J., Chapple, K. J., Anderson, E. J., et al. (2015). The atypical chemokine receptor ACKR2 suppresses Th17 responses to protein autoantigens. *Immunol. Cell Biol.* 93, 167–176. doi: 10.1038/icb.2014.90

Huber, A. K., and Irani, D. N. (2015). Targeting CXCL13 during neuroinflammation. *Adv. Neuroimmune. Biol.* 6, 1–8. doi: 10.3233/nib-150101

Khorramdelazad, H., Bagheri, V., Hassanshahi, G., Zeinali, M., and Vakilian, A. (2016). New insights into the role of stromal cell-derived factor 1 (SDF-1/CXCL12) in the pathophysiology of multiple sclerosis. *J. Neuroimmunol.* 290, 70–75. doi: 10.1016/j.jneuroim.2015.11.021

Lee, K. M., Nibbs, R. J., and Graham, G. J. (2013). D6: the 'crowd controller' at the immune gateway. *Trends Immunol.* 34, 7–12. doi: 10.1016/j.it.2012.08.001

Lee, S., Varvel, N. H., Konerth, M. E., Xu, G., Cardona, A. E., Ransohoff, R. M., et al. (2010). CX3CR1 deficiency alters microglial activation and reduces β-amyloid deposition in two Alzheimer's disease mouse models. *Am. J. Pathol.* 177, 2549–2562. doi: 10.2353/ajpath.2010.100265

Lee, S., Xu, G., Jay, T. R., Bhatta, S., Kim, K. W., Jung, S., et al. (2014). Opposing effects of membrane-anchored CX3CL1 on amyloid and tau pathologies via the p38 MAPK pathway. *J. Neurosci.* 34, 12538–12546. doi: 10.1523/JNEUROSCI.0853-14.2014

Leick, M., Catusse, J., Follo, M., Nibbs, R. J., Hartmann, T. N., Veelken, H., et al. (2010). CCL19 is a specific ligand of the constitutively recycling atypical human chemokine receptor CRAM-B. *Immunology* 129, 536–546. doi: 10.1111/j.1365-2567.2009.03209.x

Levoye, A., Balabanian, K., Baleux, F., Bachelerie, F., and Lagane, B. (2009). CXCR7 heterodimerizes with CXCR4 and regulates CXCL12-mediated G protein signaling. *Blood* 113, 6085–6093. doi: 10.1182/blood-2008-12-196618

Liu, L., Graham, G. J., Damodaran, A., Hu, T., Lira, S. A., Sasse, M., et al. (2006). Cutting edge: the silent chemokine receptor D6 is required for generating T cell responses that mediate experimental autoimmune encephalomyelitis. *J. Immunol.* 177, 17–21. doi: 10.4049/jimmunol.177.1.17

Mantovani, A., Locati, M., Vecchi, A., Sozzani, S., and Allavena, P. (2001). Decoy receptors: a strategy to regulate inflammatory cytokines and chemokines. *Trends Immunol.* 22, 328–336. doi: 10.1016/s1471-4906(01)01941-x

Mattison, H. A., Nie, H., Gao, H., Zhou, H., Hong, J. S., and Zhang, J. (2013). Suppressed pro-inflammatory response of microglia in CX3CR1 knockout mice. *J. Neuroimmunol.* 257, 110–115. doi: 10.1016/j.jneuroim.2013.02.008

Mazzon, C., Zanotti, L., Wang, L., Del Prete, A., Fontana, E., Salvi, V., et al. (2016). CCRL2 regulates M1/M2 polarization during EAE recovery phase. *J. Leukoc. Biol.* 99, 1027–1033. doi: 10.1189/jlb.3ma0915-444RR

Meyer-Luehmann, M., Spires-Jones, T. L., Prada, C., Garcia-Alloza, M., de Calignon, A., Rozkalne, A., et al. (2008). Rapid appearance and local toxicity of amyloid-β plaques in a mouse model of Alzheimer's disease. *Nature* 451, 720–724. doi: 10.1038/nature06616

Minten, C., Alt, C., Gentner, M., Frei, E., Deutsch, U., Lyck, R., et al. (2014). DARC shuttles inflammatory chemokines across the blood-brain barrier during autoimmune central nervous system inflammation. *Brain* 137, 1454–1469. doi: 10.1093/brain/awu045

Monnier, J., Lewén, S., OéHara, E., Huang, K., Tu, H., Butcher, E. C., et al. (2012). Expression, regulation, and function of atypical chemerin receptor CCRL2 on endothelial cells. *J. Immunol.* 189, 956–967. doi: 10.4049/jimmunol.1102871

Nakajima, H., Fukuda, K., Doi, Y., Sugino, M., Kimura, F., Hanafusa, T., et al. (2004). Expression of TH1/TH2-related chemokine receptors on peripheral T cells and correlation with clinical disease activity in patients with multiple sclerosis. *Eur. Neurol.* 52, 162–168. doi: 10.1159/000081856

Nibbs, R. J., and Graham, G. J. (2013). Immune regulation by atypical chemokine receptors. *Nat Rev Immunol* 13, 815–829. doi: 10.1038/nri3544

Nimmerjahn, A., Kirchhoff, F., and Helmchen, F. (2005). Resting microglial cells are highly dynamic surveillants of brain parenchyma *in vivo*. *Science* 308, 1314–1318. doi: 10.1126/science.1110647

Noh, H., Jeon, J., and Seo, H. (2014). Systemic injection of LPS induces region-specific neuroinflammation and mitochondrial dysfunction in normal mouse brain. *Neurochem. Int.* 69, 35–40. doi: 10.1016/j.neuint.2014.02.008

Novitzky-Basso, I., and Rot, A. (2012). Duffy antigen receptor for chemokines and its involvement in patterning and control of inflammatory chemokines. *Front. Immunol.* 3:266. doi: 10.3389/fimmu.2012.00266

Orihuela, R., McPherson, C. A., and Harry, G. J. (2016). Microglial M1/M2 polarization and metabolic states. *Br. J. Pharmacol.* 173, 649–665. doi: 10.1111/bph.13139

Otero, K., Vecchi, A., Hirsch, E., Kearley, J., Vermi, W., Del Prete, A., et al. (2010). Nonredundant role of CCRL2 in lung dendritic cell trafficking. *Blood* 116, 2942–2949. doi: 10.1182/blood-2009-12-259903

Pabon, M. M., Bachstetter, A. D., Hudson, C. E., Gemma, C., and Bickford, P. C. (2011). CX3CL1 reduces neurotoxicity and microglial activation in a rat model of Parkinson's disease. *J. Neuroinflammation* 8:9. doi: 10.1186/1742-2094-8-9

Paolicelli, R. C., Bolasco, G., Pagani, F., Maggi, L., Scianni, M., Panzanelli, P., et al. (2011). Synaptic pruning by microglia is necessary for normal brain development. *Science* 333, 1456–1458. doi: 10.1126/science.1202529

Perry, V. H., and Teeling, J. (2013). Microglia and macrophages of the central nervous system: the contribution of microglia priming and systemic inflammation to chronic neurodegeneration. *Semin. Immunopathol.* 35, 601–612. doi: 10.1007/s00281-013-0382-8

Pruenster, M., Mudde, L., Bombosi, P., Dimitrova, S., Zsak, M., Middleton, J., et al. (2009). The Duffy antigen receptor for chemokines transports chemokines and supports their promigratory activity. *Nat. Immunol.* 10, 101–108. doi: 10.1038/ni.1675

Przedborski, S. (2010). Inflammation and Parkinson's disease pathogenesis. *Mov. Disord.* 25, S55–S57. doi: 10.1002/mds.22638

Raes, G., Noel, W., Beschin, A., Brys, L., de Baetselier, P., and Hassanzadeh, G. H. (2002). FIZZ1 and Ym as tools to discriminate between differentially activated macrophages. *Dev. Immunol.* 9, 151–159. doi: 10.1080/1044667031000137629

Ransohoff, R. M. (2016a). How neuroinflammation contributes to neurodegeneration. *Science* 353, 777–783. doi: 10.1126/science.aag2590

Ransohoff, R. M. (2016b). A polarizing question: do M1 and M2 microglia exist? *Nat. Neurosci.* 19, 987–991. doi: 10.1038/nn.4338

Reboldi, A., Coisne, C., Baumjohann, D., Benvenuto, F., Bottinelli, D., Lira, S., et al. (2009). C-C chemokine receptor 6-regulated entry of TH-17 cells into the CNS through the choroid plexus is required for the initiation of EAE. *Nat. Immunol.* 10, 514–523. doi: 10.1038/ni.1716

Rostène, W., Dansereau, M.-A., Godefroy, D., Van Steenwinckel, J., Reaux-Le Goazigo, A., Mélik-Parsadaniantz, S., et al. (2011). Neurochemokines: a menage a trois providing new insights on the functions of chemokines in the central nervous system. *J. Neurochem.* 118, 680–694. doi: 10.1111/j.1471-4159.2011.07371.x

Rostène, W., Kitabgi, P., and Parsadaniantz, S. M. (2007). Chemokines: a new class of neuromodulator? *Nat. Rev. Neurosci.* 8, 895–903. doi: 10.1038/nrn2255

Sánchez-Alcañiz, J. A., Haege, S., Mueller, W., Pla, R., Mackay, F., Schulz, S., et al. (2011). Cxcr7 controls neuronal migration by regulating chemokine responsiveness. *Neuron* 69, 77–90. doi: 10.1016/j.neuron.2010.12.006

Schnabel, R. B., Baumert, J., Barbalic, M., Dupuis, J., Ellinor, P. T., Durda, P., et al. (2010). Duffy antigen receptor for chemokines (Darc) polymorphism regulates circulating concentrations of monocyte chemoattractant protein-1 and other inflammatory mediators. *Blood* 115, 5289–5299. doi: 10.1182/blood-2009-05-221382

Schwartz, M., Kipnis, J., Rivest, S., and Prat, A. (2013). How do immune cells support and shape the brain in health, disease, and aging? *J. Neurosci.* 33, 17587–17596. doi: 10.1523/JNEUROSCI.3241-13.2013

Shimoji, M., Pagan, F., Healton, E. B., and Mocchetti, I. (2009). CXCR4 and CXCL12 expression is increased in the nigro-striatal system of Parkinson's disease. *Neurotox. Res.* 16, 318–328. doi: 10.1007/s12640-009-9076-3

Sierra, A., Encinas, J. M., Deudero, J. J., Chancey, J. H., Enikolopov, G., Overstreet-Wadiche, L. S., et al. (2010). Microglia shape adult hippocampal neurogenesis through apoptosis-coupled phagocytosis. *Cell Stem Cell* 7, 483–495. doi: 10.1016/j.stem.2010.08.014

Sofroniew, M. V., and Vinters, H. V. (2010). Astrocytes: biology and pathology. *Acta Neuropathol.* 119, 7–35. doi: 10.1007/s00401-009-0619-8

Strobel, S., Grunblatt, E., Riederer, P., Heinsen, H., Arzberger, T., Al-Sarraj, S., et al. (2015). Changes in the expression of genes related to neuroinflammation over the course of sporadic Alzheimer's disease progression: CX3CL1, TREM2, and PPARγ. *J. Neural Transm.* 122, 1069–1076. doi: 10.1007/s00702-015-1369-5

Sui, Y., Stehno-Bittel, L., Li, S., Loganathan, R., Dhillon, N. K., Pinson, D., et al. (2006). CXCL10-induced cell death in neurons: role of calcium dysregulation. *Eur. J. Neurosci.* 23, 957–964. doi: 10.1111/j.1460-9568.2006.04631.x

Takeshita, Y., and Ransohoff, R. M. (2012). Inflammatory cell trafficking across the blood-brain barrier: chemokine regulation and *in vitro* models. *Immunol. Rev.* 248, 228–239. doi: 10.1111/j.1600-065x.2012.01127.x

Tremblay, M. È. (2011). The role of microglia at synapses in the healthy CNS: novel insights from recent imaging studies. *Neuron Glia Biol.* 7, 67–76. doi: 10.1017/s1740925x12000038

Ueno, M., Fujita, Y., Tanaka, T., Nakamura, Y., Kikuta, J., Ishii, M., et al. (2013). Layer V cortical neurons require microglial support for survival during postnatal development. *Nat. Neurosci.* 16, 543–551. doi: 10.1038/nn.3358

Uzawa, A., Mori, M., Hayakawa, S., Masuda, S., Nomura, F., and Kuwabara, S. (2010). Expression of chemokine receptors on peripheral blood lymphocytes in multiple sclerosis and neuromyelitis optica. *BMC Neurol.* 10:113. doi: 10.1186/1471-2377-10-113

Wolf, S. A., Boddeke, H. W., and Kettenmann, H. (2017). Microglia in physiology and disease. *Annu. Rev. Physiol.* 79, 619–643. doi: 10.1146/annurev-physiol-022516-034406

Xia, M. Q., Bacskai, B. J., Knowles, R. B., Qin, S. X., and Hyman, B. T. (2000). Expression of the chemokine receptor CXCR3 on neurons and the elevated expression of its ligand IP-10 in reactive astrocytes: *in vitro* ERK1/2 activation and role in Alzheimer's disease. *J. Neuroimmunol.* 108, 227–235. doi: 10.1016/s0165-5728(00)00285-x

Yang, G., Meng, Y., Li, W., Yong, Y., Fan, Z., Ding, H., et al. (2011). Neuronal MCP-1 mediates microglia recruitment and neurodegeneration induced by the mild impairment of oxidative metabolism. *Brain Pathol.* 21, 279–297. doi: 10.1111/j.1750-3639.2010.00445.x

Zabel, B. A., Nakae, S., Zuniga, L., Kim, J. Y., Ohyama, T., Alt, C., et al. (2008). Mast cell-expressed orphan receptor CCRL2 binds chemerin and is required for optimal induction of IgE-mediated passive cutaneous anaphylaxis. *J. Exp. Med.* 205, 2207–2220. doi: 10.1084/jem.20080300

Zlotnik, A., and Yoshie, O. (2000). Chemokines: a new classification system and their role in immunity. *Immunity* 12, 121–127. doi: 10.1016/S1074-7613(00)80165-X

Zuurman, M. W., Heeroma, J., Brouwer, N., Boddeke, H. W., and Biber, K. (2003). LPS-induced expression of a novel chemokine receptor (L-CCR) in mouse glial cells *in vitro* and *in vivo*. *Glia* 41, 327–336. doi: 10.1002/glia.10156

13

Lessons Learned about Neurodegeneration from Microglia and Monocyte Depletion Studies

*Harald Lund, Melanie Pieber and Robert A. Harris**

Department of Clinical Neuroscience, Karolinska Institutet, Centre for Molecular Medicine, Karolinska Hospital at Solna, Solna, Sweden

***Correspondence:**
Robert A. Harris
robert.harris@ki.se

While bone marrow-derived Ly6C^{hi} monocytes can infiltrate the central nervous system (CNS) they are developmentally and functionally distinct from resident microglia. Our understanding of the relative importance of these two populations in the distinct processes of pathogenesis and resolution of inflammation during neurodegenerative disorders was limited by a lack of tools to specifically manipulate each cell type. During recent years, the development of experimental cell-specific depletion models has enabled this issue to be addressed. Herein we compare and contrast the different depletion approaches that have been used, focusing on the respective functionalities of microglia and monocyte-derived macrophages in a range of neurodegenerative disease states, and discuss their prospects for immunotherapy.

Keywords: microglia, monocyte, neurodegeneration, depletion, experimental models in neuroscience

PERIPHERAL AND RESIDENT MYELOID CELL POPULATIONS

"Myeloid cell" is a collective term that encompasses many innate immune cells including macrophages and monocytes. Resident macrophages are specialized subsets defined by their organ location (e.g., central nervous system (CNS) microglia, liver Kupffer cells), having been differentiated in these specialized microenvironments during development from (in the majority of cases) embryonic precursors. They primarily conduct homeostatic functions in the tissues, but their numbers and properties can change during a local inflammatory process, and they can proliferate within tissues in order to maintain homeostasis. In contrast, circulating monocytes are derived from hematopoietic stem cells in the bone marrow and are generally divided into two subsets in the blood of mice based on their expression of Ly6C. Ly6C^{low} monocytes have endothelium patrolling and scavenging functions whereas Ly6C^{hi} monocytes infiltrate tissue in response to inflammation and differentiate into macrophages. Monocytes are constantly turned over and generally have limited life spans in the circulation.

MICROGLIA DEPLETION MODELS

Depletion of CNS-resident or infiltrating microglia/macrophage cell populations has been used to dissect the role of these cell types during neurodegenerative disorders. The major advances in developing microglia/macrophage depletion tools are summarized below, but for a more detailed review the reader is referred to Waisman et al. (2015), Wieghofer et al. (2015) and Jäkel and Dimou (2017). Depletion of macrophage populations first became a readily available technique through the development of clodronate-encapsulated liposomes in the 1980s (van Rooijen, 1989). Intravenous administration efficiently depleted circulating monocytes (Sunderkötter et al., 2004) and since they did not pass the blood brain barrier this technique could be used to ablate circulating monocytes without affecting CNS-resident macrophage populations (Zattoni et al., 2011). More specific targeting of $Ly6C^{hi}$ monocytes can be accomplished by antibody-mediated depletion (Mack et al., 2001), or by the use of $CCR2^{-/-}$ mice in which $Ly6C^{hi}$ monocytes are unable to leave the bone marrow (Serbina and Pamer, 2006). Intracerebroventricular (i.c.v) delivery of clodronate liposomes has also been used to deplete microglia (Lee et al., 2012; Hanafy, 2013; Asai et al., 2015). In addition, i.c.v injection of mannosylated liposomes is an established technique to specifically target mannose receptor (CD206)-expressing perivascular macrophages without affecting resident microglia numbers in both rats (Polfliet et al., 2001; Newman et al., 2005) and mice (Galea et al., 2005; Hawkes and McLaurin, 2009).

A major breakthrough in the development of efficient microglia depletion tools was the development of mice expressing the herpes-simplex virus encoded suicide-gene thymidine kinase (HSVTK) under the CD11b-promoter (Heppner et al., 2005). Administration of ganciclovir via an osmotic pump-connected i.c.v cannula resulted in up to 95% depletion of microglia (Grathwohl et al., 2009) with the only drawback being that drug administration became toxic after extended delivery, thereby limiting this approach to a period of 4 weeks. In subsequent studies, it was demonstrated that cessation of ganciclovir delivery resulted in complete exchange of the microglial pool by peripheral myeloid cells (Varvel et al., 2012, 2015; Prokop et al., 2015). A major step forward in achieving more specific microglia targeting was the development of $CX3CR1^{CreER}$ mice (Goldmann et al., 2013; Parkhurst et al., 2013). When bred with $Rosa26^{DTR}$ mice and subsequent to peripheral administration of the drug tamoxifen followed by diphtheria toxin, efficient depletion of microglia resulted without affecting bone marrow-derived $CX3CR1^{+}$ cells (Parkhurst et al., 2013; Bruttger et al., 2015). Since other CNS-associated (perivascular, meningeal and choroid plexus) macrophages also express CX3CR1 (Goldmann et al., 2016), these cells are most likely also depleted in $CX3CR1^{CreER}Rosa26^{DTR}$ mice. Transcriptional profiling has revealed genes uniquely expressed by microglia such as *Sall1*, and this has been successfully utilized in $Sall1^{CreER}$ mice which target microglia while sparing both peripheral and CNS-associated macrophage populations (Buttgereit et al., 2016). However, $Sall1^{CreER}$ mice have currently not been used to deplete microglia.

Microglia require CSF1R during development, since $CSF1R^{-/-}$ mice completely lack microglia (Ginhoux et al., 2010). Microglia can use both ligands of CSF1R for their survival (CSF1 and IL-34) since mice mutant for either cytokine display reduction but not complete loss of microglia (Ginhoux et al., 2010; Greter et al., 2012; Wang et al., 2012). Elmore et al. (2014) recently demonstrated that microglia remain dependent on CSF1R for survival in adult animals. Pharmacological inhibition of CSF1R yields complete ablation (>99%) of microglia within 21 days. This approach is practical because it requires no mouse breeding and microglial depletion can be maintained as long as the drug is administered. Depletion of the microglial pool disturbs CNS homeostasis, and while neurons do not regenerate, microglia have significant potential to self-renew through proliferation. The incomplete depletion (80%) accomplished in $CX3CR1^{CreER}Rosa26^{DTR}$ mice is quickly recuperated by hyper-proliferation of surviving microglia (Bruttger et al., 2015). Even more efficient depletion (99%) using the CSF1R-inhibitor is followed by such rapid repopulation that the existence of a microglia-progenitor has been suggested (Elmore et al., 2014). A recent report, however, demonstrates the relatively high turnover of microglia in the steady-state, arguing against the existence of a microglia progenitor (Tay et al., 2017). Conversely, using the CD11b-HSVTK model repopulation occurs from peripheral myeloid cells (Varvel et al., 2012; Prokop et al., 2015).

Given this historic perspective of microglia depletion research, we review below the lessons learned using these different strategies, focusing on models of neuroinflammation (experimental autoimmune encephalomyelitis, EAE), acute neurodegeneration (stroke, toxin-induced neurodegeneration) or chronic neurodegeneration (Amyotrophic Lateral Sclerosis (ALS), Alzheimer's disease, Prion disease). We do not review the role of microglia in development or homeostasis and refer the reader to separate reviews addressing these areas of research (Greter and Merad, 2012; Nayak et al., 2014).

AMYOTROPHIC LATERAL SCLEROSIS

ALS is a generally fatal neurodegenerative disease characterized by progressive paralysis of skeletal muscles associated with motor neuron death and glial activation in the lumbar spinal cord. The most commonly used mouse model of ALS is based on the over-expression of human SOD1 carrying the G93A mutation (mSOD1 mice). Mice accumulate mutant SOD1 aggregates in the spinal cord, leading to motor neuron death and recapitulation of the central aspects of ALS pathology including an age-dependent accumulation of $CD11b^{+}$ (Alexianu et al., 2001; Gowing et al., 2008), $CD68^{+}$ (Henkel et al., 2006; Beers et al., 2011), MHC II^{+} (Hall et al., 1998), $CD11c^{+}$ (Beers et al., 2011) microglia/macrophages in the spinal cord of mSOD1 mice.

That mutant SOD1 expression in microglia/macrophages contribute to disease progression has been convincingly demonstrated in the slow progressing SOD1G37R line in which CD11b-Cre-mediated removal of SOD1 from myeloid cells slowed progression of disease and extended survival (Boillée et al., 2006). Similarly, repopulating the empty microglial niche in mSOD1/$PU.1^{-/-}$ mice with wildtype bone marrow extends survival compared to mice transplanted with mSOD1 bone marrow (Beers et al., 2006; Lee et al., 2012). It should be noted that one study reported no increase in motorneuron loss following partial (40%) elimination of microglia/macrophages during the symptomatic disease stage in CD11b-TK/mSOD1 mice (Gowing et al., 2008; **Table 1**).

Whether microglia or monocytes make up the majority of the activated macrophage population in the spinal cord is a matter of controversy. One elegant study using parabiotically connected GFP^{+} and mSOD1 mice recorded no parenchymal

TABLE 1 | Chronic neurodegeneration models.

Disease setting	Depletion model	Effect	References
Amyotrophic lateral sclerosis	$SOD1^{G93A}/PU.1^{-/-}$ repopulated with WT bone marrow	Repopulation of empty microglial niche with WT extends survival compared to mice transplanted with $mSOD^{G93A}$ bone marrow	Beers et al. (2006)
Amyotrophic lateral sclerosis	Gangciclovir to the spinal cord via osmotic pump in CD11b-HSVTK:$SOD1^{G93A}$ mice	40% microglia reduction did not affect motor neuron loss	Gowing et al. (2008)
Amyotrophic lateral sclerosis	Clodronate depletion i.c.v in $SOD1^{G93A}$ mice with WT repopulation	Microglial depletion significantly slowed disease progression and prolonged survival of the ALS mice but did not affect disease onset.	Lee et al. (2012)
Amyotrophic lateral sclerosis	α-Ly6C antibody in $SOD1^{G93A}$ mice from symptom onset	Depletion of $Ly6C^{hi}$ monocytes improved rotarod performance and extended survival	Butovsky et al. (2012)
Alzheimer's disease	Clodronate i.c.v in 4-month old TgCRND8 mice	Depletion of perivascular macrophages reduced cerebrovascular amyloid deposition.	Hawkes and McLaurin (2009)
Alzheimer's disease	Oral gangciclovir in 5-month old CD11b-HSVTK/APPPS1 mice	Microglial depletion affected neither amyloid plaque formation and maintenance or amyloid-associated neuritic dystrophy.	Grathwohl et al. (2009)
Alzheimer's disease	Chimera using cytotoxic drugs and transplantation of $Nr4a1^{-/-}$ bone marrow to APPPS1 mice	Depletion of $Ly6C^{low}$ monocytes increased plaque load in cortex and hippocampus.	Michaud et al. (2013)
Alzheimer's disease	Gangciclovir i.c.v via osmotic pump in CD11b-HSVTK/APPPS1 or CD11b-HSVTK/APP23 mice	Microglial depletion and repopulation from bone marrow in 3-month old amyloid-depositing mice had no effect on amyloid pathology after 3 months	Varvel et al. (2015)
Alzheimer's disease	Gangciclovir i.c.v via osmotic pump in CD11b-HSVTK/APPPS1 mice	Microglial depletion and repopulation with bone marrow myeloid cells results in no net effect on amyloid beta pathology after 1 month.	Prokop et al. (2015)
Alzheimer's disease	Clodronate depletion i.c.v or PLX3397 CSF1R inhibition (chow) in AAV-GFP/tau mice	Microglial depletion suppressed the propagation of tau and reduced excitability in the dentate gyrus	Asai et al. (2015)
Alzheimer's disease	PLX3397 CSF1R inhibition (chow) for 28 days	In 10-month old mice a 90% reduction in non-plaque associated microglia and 50% reduction in plaque-associated microglia resulted in prevention of neuronal loss and improved memory. No effect on amyloid beta load. In 1.5-month old mice, no effect on amyloid pathology.	Spangenberg et al. (2016)
Prion disease	GW2580 CSF1R inhibition orally in mice injected with scrapie (ME7)	Microglial inhibition slowed the progression of chronic neurodegeneration and prevented development of the hyperactive behavioral deficits	Gómez-Nicola et al. (2013)
Prion disease	$CCR2^{-/-}$ mice injected with scrapie (ME7)	Monocyte loss does not affect neuropathology or disease course	Gómez-Nicola et al. (2014)
Prion disease	Ganciclovir i.c.v via osmotic pump in CD11b-HSVTK and $IL\text{-}34^{-/-}$ mice injected with scrapie (RML6)	Microglial depletion accelerated prion disease and reduced survival	Zhu et al. (2016)
Experimental autoimmune encephalomyelitis	Clodronate i.v in guinea pig spinal cord homogenate immunized pre-onset in Lewis rats	Macrophage depletion led to reduced clinical symptoms.	Huitinga et al. (1990)
Experimental autoimmune encephalomyelitis	Clodronate i.v MBP T cell adoptive transfer pre-onset in Lewis rats	Macrophage depletion led to reduced clinical symptoms and CNS inflammation.	Huitinga et al. (1995)
Experimental autoimmune encephalomyelitis	Clodronate i.v MBP T cell adoptive transfer pre-onset in SJL/J mice	Macrophage depletion led to reduced clinical symptoms and CNS inflammation.	Tran et al. (1998)
Experimental autoimmune encephalomyelitis	Ganciclovir i.p in CD11b-HSVTK mice pre-induction for MOG_{35-55} peptide EAE	Conditional paralysis of microglia delayed disease onset and in repression of clinical EAE signs through	Heppner et al. (2005)
Experimental autoimmune encephalomyelitis	α-CCR2 antibody i.p in $CX3CR1^{GFP/+}$ mice pre-induction for MOG_{35-55} EAE	Depletion of $CCR2^{+}Ly\text{-}6C^{hi}$ monocytes strongly reduced central nervous system autoimmunity	Mildner et al. (2009)
Experimental autoimmune encephalomyelitis	Clodronate i.v at onset in C57BL/6 mice for MOG_{35-55} EAE	Long-term depletion of monocytes prevents worsening of neurological deficits and long-term axonal loss	Moreno et al. (2016)
Experimental autoimmune encephalomyelitis	CD169-DTR mice pre-onset for MOG_{35-55} EAE	Depletion of $CD169^{+}$ cells markedly reduced neuroinflammation and ameliorated disease symptoms in EAE-affected mice.	Bogie et al. (2017)

$GFP^+Iba\text{-}1^+$ cells in the spinal cord at the late stage of disease when microgliosis is extensive (Ajami et al., 2007). Similarly, a more recent study did not detect any $Ly6C^+$ cells within the $CD11b^+CD45^+$ "microglial" compartment (Chiu et al., 2013). However, Butovsky et al. (2012) reported that $Ly6C^{hi}$ monocytes progressively accumulate in the spinal cord (but not brain) of mSOD1 mice, reaching as much as 30% of the $CD11b^+$ compartment in late stage animals, and that their antibody-mediated depletion attenuated motor neuron death and delayed disease onset and mortality. Such monocyte-specific contribution to disease progression is very interesting, since most previous studies have used targeting systems that do not discriminate between microglia and monocytes. However, this study would benefit from confirmation in other laboratories since the presence of spinal cord monocyte-derived macrophages is contradicted by parabiosis experiments (Ajami et al., 2007).

ALZHEIMER'S DISEASE

Alzheimer's disease is the most prevalent form of neurodegeneration and is characterized by the presence of amyloid beta plaques and neurofibrillary tangles. The recognition of a glial reaction as a hallmark of Alzheimer's disease neuropathology was, despite being described by Alois Alzheimer himself (Alzheimer et al., 1995) long disregarded as an epiphenomenon. However, the recent discoveries that several immune and microglia/myeloid-expressed genes (i.e., CD33, CR1, TREM2) are genetically linked to Alzheimer's disease has established the role of microglia in disease progression (Lambert et al., 2009; Griciuc et al., 2013; Guerreiro et al., 2013; Jonsson et al., 2013).

Amyloid Beta

The *in vivo* microglial response to amyloid beta has been well characterized in amyloid-depositing mouse models. Microglia rapidly migrate to newly formed plaques (Meyer-Luehmann et al., 2008) where they display an altered morphology (Frautschy et al., 1998; Stalder et al., 1999) and upregulate a vast array of surface molecules (Bornemann et al., 2001; Frank et al., 2008). Whether microglia actively internalize amyloid beta fibrils in naive APP mice has been a matter of debate (Stalder et al., 2001; Bolmont et al., 2008), but the increasing amyloid load observed with age indicates that microglia are ultimately unable to control the amyloid burden. Direct proof that microglia do not limit either amyloid plaque formation or growth was provided by Grathwohl et al. (2009) who demonstrated that complete ablation of microglia for 4 weeks in either young or aged APPPS1 mice resulted in no net effect on amyloid beta burden or plaque-associated neuritic pathology (**Table 1**). This finding was replicated in the 5XFAD disease model using CSF1R inhibition to deplete microglia, which resulted in no difference in amyloid pathology in either young or old 5XFAD mice. Interestingly, however, this model is characterized by development of substantial neuronal loss with age and microglial depletion both prevented this neuronal loss and improved contextual memory. Microglial depletion was also accompanied by an attenuation of disease-driven inflammatory gene expression (Spangenberg et al., 2016).

These studies are important because they explain the observation that amyloid deposits progressively increase in APP mice despite the association of microglia. This is supported by evidence that microglia in the vicinity of amyloid beta plaques progressively lose phagocytic capacity (Hickman et al., 2008; Krabbe et al., 2013). However, it is important to understand that microglia can be stimulated into removing existing amyloid plaques by a variety of means (Boissonneault et al., 2009; Leinenga and Götz, 2015; Iaccarino et al., 2016; Daria et al., 2017).

Whether monocytes take part in the response to amyloid deposits is a matter of long-standing debate. Previous studies claimed that monocytes/peripheral myeloid cells possessed superior ability to remove amyloid deposits compared to microglia (Malm et al., 2005; Stalder et al., 2005; Simard et al., 2006; Butovsky et al., 2007). However, these studies were all based on whole body irradiation chimeras and exposure of the brain to irradiation has subsequently been elucidated to condition the brain for monocyte infiltration (Mildner et al., 2007). More recent studies using brain-protected irradiation chimeras (Mildner et al., 2011) or chemotherapy-induced myeloablation (Lampron et al., 2012; Michaud et al., 2013) have demonstrated very little engraftment of monocytes during disease progression in amyloid-depositing mice. Furthermore, complete exchange of the microglial compartment with peripheral monocytic cells did not affect amyloid beta burden (Prokop et al., 2015; Varvel et al., 2015), which was final proof that monocytes do not confer better amyloid beta removal ability than do microglia.

The possibility remains that monocytes take part in the removal of amyloid deposits in the cerebrovasculature, so-called cerebral amyloid angiopathy. Using two-photon *in vivo* imaging patrolling $Ly6C^{low}$ monocytes have been observed to actively crawl on amyloid beta-laden cerebral blood vessels (Michaud et al., 2013). $Ly6C^{low}$ monocytes are dependent on the transcription factor Nr4a1 for their survival (Hanna et al., 2012) and specific elimination of $Ly6C^{low}$ monocytes by transplanting $Nr4a1^{-/-}$ bone marrow into chemotherapy-myeloablated APP/PS1 mice significantly increased the build up of amyloid deposits (Michaud et al., 2013).

Lack of $Ly6C^{low}$ monocytes could also explain why $CCR2^{-/-}$APP mice have increased levels of amyloid deposition in cerebral blood vessels (El Khoury et al., 2007; Mildner et al., 2011). While the authors attributed increased amyloid buildup to loss of CCR2 in the perivascular myeloid compartment, involvement of $Ly6C^{low}$ monocytes cannot be excluded. In fact, perivascular macrophages are not lost in $CCR2^{-/-}$ mice (Goldmann et al., 2016), in contrast to $Ly6C^{low}$ monocytes which are directly derived from $Ly6C^{hi}$ monocytes and therefore are also significantly reduced in $CCR2^{-/-}$ mice (Yona et al., 2013). Another study has attempted to more specifically address the role of perivascular macrophages in buildup of vascular amyloid deposits through i.c.v injection of clodronate to deplete

$CD163^+$ perivascular macrophages while sparing parenchymal Iba-1^+ microglia, this procedure resulting in a 5-fold increase in cerebral amyloid angiopathy load (Hawkes and McLaurin, 2009).

Tau

Microtubule-associated protein tau (MAPT, tau) is a microtubule-stabilizing protein that during the course of AD becomes hyperphosphorylated, a process leading to dissociation from microtubules and aggregation into paired helical filaments and formation of neurofibrillary tangles (Wang and Mandelkow, 2016). Tau aggregates follow a predictable pattern of neuron-to-neuron spreading in the brain (Braak et al., 2011) and a recent study addressed the possible role of microglia in this process. Asai et al. (2015) developed a simple but elegant model of tau propagation in wildtype mice by injecting tau-expressing adeno-associated virus into the entorhinal cortex and observed how tau aggregates spread to the nearby hippocampus in only 4 weeks. Depletion of microglia using either clodronate liposomes or CSF1R inhibition dramatically halted the propagation of tau into the hippocampus. Similar results were obtained by inhibiting exosome synthesis, suggesting microglia could seed tauopathy (Asai et al., 2015).

There is also evidence that microgliosis can precede deposition of insoluble tau in transgenic mice (Yoshiyama et al., 2007; Maphis et al., 2015), indicating that microglia could drive spatiotemporal tau propagation through production of neuroinflammatory mediators. Loss of CX3CR1 amplifies tau pathology in hTau mice in an IL-1β-dependent manner (Bhaskar et al., 2010) and tau hyperphosphorylation could be induced in wildtype mice by intracerebral transplantation of $CX3CR1^{-/-}$ hTau microglia (Maphis et al., 2015). This was the proof-of-concept that reactive microglia could drive tau pathology.

PRION DISEASE

Prion disease is a transmissible neurodegenerative disorder affecting both animals and humans. The contribution of myeloid subsets to disease progression has been characterized using mouse models in which prion disease is produced by intracerebral inoculation of scrapie protein strains. While microglial proliferation and activation occurs irrespective of the inoculated prion strain (Cunningham et al., 2005) and correlates with onset of neurological deficits (Boche et al., 2006) there is little evidence of monocyte infiltration during disease progression. Preventing monocytes from entering the circulation using $CCR2^{-/-}$ mice does not exacerbate neuropathology or disease course in prion-infected mice (Gómez-Nicola et al., 2014; **Table 1**). Whether microglial proliferation observed during prion disease is beneficial or deleterious is a matter of conflicting data. Using a CSF1R inhibitor Gómez-Nicola et al. (2013) limited microglial proliferation which prevented neurodegeneration, improved behavioral impairments and extended survival in prion mice. Conversely, Zhu et al. (2016) reported that microglial depletion (CD11b-HSVTK) or reduction (IL-$34^{-/-}$) exacerbated prion disease and reduced survival, suggesting a neuroprotective role for microglia. Since the two studies have used different scrapie strains, different strategies to limit the microglial response and different timing of the microglial targeting, it is difficult to consolidate the data sets. However, it could indicate strain-specific microglial responses or suggest that microglia possess neuroprotective and neurotoxic reactions to prions at different time points during the disease course.

EXPERIMENTAL AUTOIMMUNE ENCEPHALOMYELITIS

The development of demyelinating lesions that is characteristic of multiple sclerosis (MS) and its mouse model EAE is initiated by autoreactive, myelin-specific $CD4^+$ T cells. These are reactivated within the CNS (Goverman, 2009), secreting factors that open the blood-brain barrier and recruit a heterogeneous population of myeloid cells that drive demyelination. The primary importance of myeloid cells in pathogenesis is indicated by the strong genetic association of MHC II and MS (Sawcer et al., 2011). While infiltrating monocyte-derived macrophages drive disease pathogenesis (as detailed below), the contribution of resident microglia during the different disease phases is still not completely understood.

It has been demonstrated that EAE severity correlates with numbers of monocytes infiltrating the spinal cord and that prevention of this infiltration protects against EAE development (Fife et al., 2000; Mildner et al., 2009; Ajami et al., 2011). Importantly, the presence of the infiltrating cells in the CNS is transient, their numbers decreasing significantly during the remission phase of EAE (Hesske et al., 2010; Ajami et al., 2011), leaving the niche occupied by resident microglia. It is evident from our review (**Table 1**), that the majority of depletion studies in EAE have focused on preventing monocyte infiltration into the CNS from the periphery, with EAE pathology and symptoms being abrogated irrespective of the manner in which this is accomplished. Compared to infiltrating monocytes, microglia display low levels of MHCII and co-stimulatory molecules during EAE (Vainchtein et al., 2014) and their MHCII expression is dispensable for EAE induction (Greter et al., 2005). While preventing microglial expansion (referred to as microglial paralysis) has been demonstrated to substantially ameliorate the clinical signs of EAE and to strongly reduce CNS inflammation (Heppner et al., 2005), recent data indicate an alternative role of microglia compared to monocytes. Using electron-microscopy to study microglia and macrophage-specific interactions with axons, monocytes were shown to initiate demyelination at nodes of Ranvier, whereas microglia appeared to scavenge myelin debris (Yamasaki et al., 2014).

Given that EAE is primarily a disease state caused by infiltrating monocytes, the role of microglia in driving pathogenesis is not major. However, the role of microglia in restoring CNS during remission (healing) phases, or their lack of achieving this role during chronic disease states, warrants further investigation.

STROKE

Stroke is caused by severe occlusion or stenosis of a cerebral artery and is the second leading cause of death and disability worldwide. Brain resident microglia become activated by various cytokines and damage-associated molecular patterns which are released by necrotic or apoptotic tissues (Shichita et al., 2012). An inflammatory response is triggered during the early stages of brain injury, leading to an influx of peripheral immune cells including macrophages and neutrophils (Tanaka et al., 2003; Gelderblom et al., 2009). Different studies have been performed to characterize the role of resident microglia and infiltrating peripheral macrophages in various mouse and rat models of stroke, but their roles are still under debate and vary depending on the experimental model employed (**Table 2**).

Using macrophage depletion via clodronate liposomes, Gliem et al. (2012) reported that the early influx of peripheral macrophages prevents hemorrhagic infarct transformation in a model of middle cerebral artery occlusion (MCAO), with mice treated at early time points having increased peri-lesional hemorrhage. Similar results were obtained using CD11b-DTR mice for macrophage depletion in the same study. In contrast, Ma et al. (2016) demonstrated a positive effect of peripheral macrophage depletion on the stroke lesion following clodronate treatment, with decreased myelin damage and microglial activation as well as decreased brain atrophy and increased neurological recovery following MCAO. Likewise, antibody blockade of CCR2-infiltrating macrophages reduced early motor deficits following intracerebral hemorrhage (Hammond et al., 2014), again indicating a negative role of myeloid cells in this model. Yet another recently published study contradicts all the aforementioned studies and concludes that targeting monocytes/macrophages (using clodronate, anti-CCR2 antibody or M1/M2 transfer) had no therapeutic value in acute ischemic stroke but only on mortality (Schmidt et al., 2017). The discrepancies in these studies, even though the same disease model was used, can be explained due to the different time points of monocyte depletion. Both studies that reported a detrimental effect of monocyte depletion (Hammond et al., 2014; Ma et al., 2016) depleted monocytes before inducing MCAO whereas in the first study (Gliem et al., 2012) monocyte depletion was performed after stroke induction, suggesting a differing role of monocytes during the course of disease.

Numerous stroke studies have been performed using selective depletion of microglia instead of peripheral monocytes. Microglia seem to have a supporting role in various models of stroke, as exemplified by studies of neonatal focal arterial stroke. The i.c.v injection of clodronate liposomes before induction of the lesion yielded specific microglia depletion without affecting the periphery, resulting in increased local inflammation and injury severity as well as reduced vessel coverage that triggers hemorrhages in the injured brain regions (Faustino et al., 2011; Fernández-López et al., 2016). Microglia are therefore thought to contribute to the endogenous protection mechanisms of the brain during early stages after injury in neonates. Similarly, depletion of proliferating microglia using adult CD11b-HSVTK mice resulted in exacerbation of the stroke lesion, increased neuronal death and pro-inflammatory cytokine levels (Lalancette-Hébert et al., 2007). Depletion of microglia using a CSF1R inhibitor prior and subsequent to MCAO also exacerbated brain infarction and neurological deficits by promoting leukocyte infiltration into the brain and increased inflammatory cytokine levels in the area of the lesion, supporting the beneficial role of microglia in MCAO (Jin et al., 2017). Interestingly, using the same depletion method in the intracerebral hemorrhage model, microglia were concluded to have the completely opposite role in that model of brain injury. Depletion of microglia thus led to reduced lesion size, brain edema and neurodeficits, a lack of microglia attenuated leukocyte infiltration, decreased inflammatory cytokine levels and preserved the integrity of the blood brain barrier (Li et al., 2017). Most studies to date have focused on the effect of microglia/monocyte depletion during the acute phase of brain injury. However, the roles of microglia/monocytes can differ at various time points and between injury models, underlining the many potential roles of inflammatory monocytes and microglia in the pathogenic and regenerative CNS (Hammond et al., 2014).

TOXIN-INDUCED NEURODEGENERATION

Microglia can have multiple roles during acute hippocampal neurodegeneration (**Table 3**), as demonstrated using a model of diphtheria toxin-inducible neuronal loss. Microglia numbers increase dramatically after lesion formation, without evidence of peripheral myeloid infiltration. Elimination of microglia during this procedure exacerbated neuronal loss (Rice et al., 2015). However, elimination subsequent to lesion formation improved cognitive recovery and reduced inflammatory signaling (Rice et al., 2015), demonstrating a deleterious response of microglia *after* as opposed to *during* lesion formation, again stressing how important accurate timing in microglia depletion studies is to obtain comparable results between studies. In a subsequent study, the elimination and repopulation of microglia after the procedure was reported to similarly reduce neuroinflammation, improve behavioral recovery and synaptic densities (Rice et al., 2017). The role of microglia in these toxin-induced models appears to be time-dependent, with an acute pathogenic role becoming a return-to-homeostasis (healing) role at later timepoints.

While partial depletion of circulating monocytes did not affect MPTP-induced neuronal loss in the basal ganglia (Côté et al., 2015; a model of Parkinson's disease), LPS-induced striatal neurodegeneration in gerbils was attenuated by similar means (Zito et al., 2001). Kainic acid- or pilocarpine-induced eplieptic seizures in mice provoke microglial activation in the hippocampus and a delayed entry of monocytes into the parenchyma (Varvel et al., 2016). Varvel et al. (2016) elegantly showed that monocytopenic $CCR2^{-/-}$ mice developed less hippocampal neurodegeneration, suggesting a detrimental role of monocytes. However, peripheral clodronate administration reduced accumulation of CNS-infiltrating

TABLE 2 | Acute neurodegeneration models—stroke and related conditions.

Disease setting	Depletion model	Effect	References
Subarachnoid hemorrhage	Post-operative clodronate i.c.v in C57BL/6 mice injected with autologous blood	Reduced neuronal apoptosis d7 after surgery but not d15. Reduced vasospasm d7 and d15	Hanafy (2013)
Intra-cerebral hemorrhage	α-CCR2 antibody i.p in C57BL/6 mice and Ccr2$^{-/-}$ BM chimeras pre- injection with autologous blood	Ly6C^{hi} monocyte depleted animals displayed a significantly less severe left hemiparesis	Hammond et al. (2014)
Aneurysmal subarachnoid hemorrhage by filament perforation	Ganciclovir i.c.v in CD11b-HSVTK mice post-ASH	Microglial depletion resulted in significantly reduce neuronal death	Schneider et al. (2015)
Intracerebral hemorrhage	PLX3397 oral gavage CSF1R inhibition by 21 days prior to injection of collagenase or autologous blood in C57BL/6 mice	Reduced leukocyte infiltration in the brain and improved blood–brain barrier integrity	Li et al. (2017)
Neonatal focal arterial stroke	Clodronate i.c.v in neonatal rats or CCR2$^{RFP+/-}$CX3CR1$^{GFP+/-}$ mice	Microglial depletion exacerbated injury and induced hemorrhages at 24 h	Fernández-López et al. (2016)
MCAO ischemic inflammation and brain injury	Ganciclovir i.p in CD11b-HSVTK mice pre-stroke	Selective ablation of proliferating microglial cells exacerbates ischemic injury in the brain.	Lalancette-Hébert et al. (2007)
MCAO ischemic inflammation and brain injury	Mac-1-saporin i.c.v in Wistar rats pre- or post-stroke	Microglial depletion did not affect the number of neuroblasts exiting the SVZ or their migration in the striatum	Heldmann et al. (2011)
MCAO ischemic inflammation and brain injury	Clodronate i.c.v in neonatal Sprague-Dawley rats pre-stroke	Lack of microglia increased brain levels of several cytokines and chemokines already elevated by ischemia–reperfusion, and increased the severity and volume of injury	Faustino et al. (2011)
Transient MCAO or photothrombosis	CD11b-DTR mice or CCR2$^{-/-}$ chimeric mice	Early depletion of monocytes dramatically increases rate of hemorrhages in both stroke models and worse performance in rotarod	Gliem et al. (2012)
MCAO ischemic inflammation and brain injury	Human umbilical cord blood (HUCB) mononuclear cell transplantation i.v post-stroke in Sprague-Dawley rats	Monocyte depletion prevented HUCB cell treatment from reducing infarct size while monocyte enrichment was sufficient to reduce infarct size	Womble et al. (2014)
MCAO ischemic inflammation and brain injury	Clodronate i.p in ICR mice pre-challenge	Peripheral macrophage depletion reduced the myelin damage and microglia activation, enhanced microvessel density in the peri-infarct region, attenuated brain atrophy, and promoted neurological recovery	Ma et al. (2016)
MCAO ischemic inflammation and brain injury	PLX3397 (chow) CSF1R inhibition in C57BL/6 mice post-challenge	Microglial depletion exacerbated neurodeficits and brain infarction	Jin et al. (2017)
MCAO remote filament brain injury	PLX3397 (chow) CSF1R inhibition in Cx3Cr1$^{GFP/+}$ mice	Microglia depletion leads to dysregulated neuronal calcium responses, calcium overload and increased neuronal death	Szalay et al. (2016)
MCAO ischemic inflammation and brain injury	Clodronate i.p or α-CCR2 antibody	Depletion of Ly6C^{hi} monocytes increased mortality in monocyte-depleted mice likely due to clodronate toxicity. Specific Ly6C^{hi} depletion did not influence mortality nor infarct volume or rotarod performance	Schmidt et al. (2017)

TABLE 3 | Acute neurodegeneration models—toxin-induced neurodegeneration.

Disease setting	Depletion model	Effect	References
Diptheria Toxin-induced hippocampal lesion	PLX3397 CSF1R inhibition (drinking water) in CaM/Tet-DTA mice post-lesion or during lesion	Post-lesion microglial depletion improves behavior (elevated-plus maze and morris-water maze) and reverses lesion-induced increase in inflammatory signaling. Microglial depletion during lesion exacerbates neuronal loss in hippocampus	Rice et al. (2015)
Diptheria Toxin-induced hippocampal lesion	PLX5622 CSF1R inhibition (chow) in CaM/Tet-DTA mouse post-lesion	Microglial elimination and repopulation, largely resolves chronic neuroinflammatory responses and improved behavioral abilities	Rice et al. (2017)
LPS-induced striatal neurodegeneration	Clodronate depletion i.v in gerbils	Attenuated striatal macrophage infiltration reduced the severity of LPS-induced neurodegeneration	Zito et al. (2001)
Parkinson's disease	Clodronate i.v in MPTP (i.p) model of PD in C57BL/6	Partial depletion of peripheral Ly6C^{hi} monocytes does not affect basal ganglia TH$^+$ neuronal loss but protected against loss of TH$^+$ neurons in the myenteric plexus (enteric nervous system)	Côté et al. (2015)
Kainic-acid induced epilepsy	Clodronate i.p. in C57BL/6	Depletion of F4/80$^+$ cells in hippocampus reduces survival of dentate gyrus granule neurons.	Zattoni et al. (2011)
Pilocarpine-induced epilepsy	Pilocarpine-induced epileptic seizures in CCR2$^{-/-}$ mice	CCR2$^{-/-}$ and WT mice develop similar seizure severity but CCR2$^{-/-}$ mice develop less hippocampal neurodegeneration	Varvel et al. (2016)

F4/80$^+$ macrophages and reduced survival of dentate gyrus granule cells (Zattoni et al., 2011) indicating a beneficial role of monocytes.

INJURY

Acute injury can be inflicted on the CNS in different ways, be it by crush or cut in the spinal cord, or traumatic brain injury (**Table 4**) as typified by traffic accidents and more recently by professional American sportsmen (Cherry et al., 2016). What is often characteristic of these injuries is a chronic state of neuroinflammation that can be experienced years after the initial injury, and this is associated with permanent microglial dysfunction. Despite this variation in the type of injury model and in the method of microglial depletion that have been reported there are few effects of reduced microglia numbers during the responses in these settings.

Thus in a model of repetitive brain concussion microglia did not contribute to acute axon degeneration after multiple concussive injuries, although there is still a possibility of longer-term effects on axon functionality (Bennett and Brody, 2014). However, in a mouse model of spine transection, resident microglia and peripheral monocytes were concluded to act synergistically to initiate hypersensitivity and to promote the transition from acute to chronic pain following peripheral nerve injury (Peng et al., 2016).

It is possible that the severity of the extensive trauma in many of these models affects too large an area to make the microglial loss significantly synergistic, or alternatively that the ensuing chronic microglial dysfunction only gradually develops over time.

OTHER *IN VIVO* AND *IN VITRO* MODELS OF DEPLETION

Given the proven propensity of pharmacological agents to efficiently deplete microglia and macrophages, it is not surprising that these have been applied in additional *in vivo* and *in vitro* settings (**Table 5**). It is apparent that clinical cognitive decline is a long-term condition induced by both cranial irradiation (Acharya et al., 2016) and peripheral surgery (Degos et al., 2013), and in both settings the depletion of myeloid cells increases cognitive ability. While in the former setting an effect on microglia would be expected, and has recently been reported to differ depending on the age of the mice (Han et al., 2016), the latter is intriguing as a peripheral skeletal injury is seemingly a long distance away from the CNS. The interplay between peripheral macrophages and CNS-resident microglia is thus probably more intricate and extensive than we currently understand. Organotypic CNS slice cultures provide an alternative to live mice for study of CNS homeostasis and disease, and microglia depletion agents can be applied to these.

Generally the findings suggest that tissues devoid of microglia have less ability to protect neurons.

POINTS OF PERSPECTIVE

Given the vast expansion in the field of microglia research during recent years it will be important to build on previous interpretations in the light of new knowledge. For example, the absence of any effect on amyloid beta burden by microglia depletion in Alzheimer's disease models could be explained by recent results suggesting that the key function of amyloid plaque-associated microglia is to form a barrier around it (to compact the amyloid fibrils into a dense plaque) rather than solely their previously perceived role in amyloid phagocytosis (Yuan et al., 2016).

It has proven difficult to permanently deplete microglia in a specific manner and there are caveats with all the depletion models employed. The nature of the cell death of depleted microglia within the CNS is also an issue that has not been addressed, and this might not only vary between depletion systems, but might also trigger downstream (e.g.,

TABLE 4 | Acute neurodegeneration models—injury.

Disease setting	Depletion model	Effect	References
Partial sciatic nerve ligation	Mac-1-saporin i.t in C57BL/6 mice pre-ligation	Acute depletion of spinal cord microglia had no effect on mechanical or thermal activity nor on allodynia following PSNL injury	Yao et al. (2016)
Neuropathic pain in spinal nerve transection	$CX3CR1^{CreER}R26^{DTR}$ mice pre-injury	Depletion of microglia delayed but did not reverse neuropathic hypersensitivity after peripheral nerve injury	Peng et al. (2016)
Repetitive concussive traumatic brain injury	Valganciclovir i.c.v in CD11b-HSVTK mice pre-TBI	Microglial depletion did not affect the rate of neuronal death	Bennett and Brody (2014)
Spinal cord injury	Clodronate i.p/i.v in $LysM^{EGFP}$ mice pre-acute compression injury	Macrophage depletion did not affect the extent of the microglial-based inflammatory response in the lesion	Mawhinney et al. (2012)
Spinal cord injury	Clodronate i.p in $LysM^{tdTom}$ > $CX3CR1^{GFP}$ chimeric mice post-mid-thoracic (T8) contusive injury	Macrophage depletion resulted in changes in multiple cytokines that make the injury site less fibrotic and more conducive to axonal growth	Zhu et al. (2015)

TABLE 5 | Other *in vivo* and *in vitro* models.

Disease setting	Depletion model	Effect	References
Cranial irradiation	PLX5622 CSF1R inhibition (chow) in C57BL/6 mice	Elimination of microglia ameliorates radiation-induced cognitive deficits (novel object recognition, object in place, fear conditioning) but has no effect in non-irradiated mice	Acharya et al. (2016)
Post-operative cognitive decline	Clodronate i.p in $CCR2^{RFP/+}$ $CX3CR1^{GFP/+}$ mice with stabilized tibial fracture	Depletion of macrophages prevents hippocampal neuroinflammation and memory dysfunction	Degos et al. (2013)
NMDA-induced excitotoxic lesion in organotypic hippocampal slice cultures	Clodronate depletion in Wistar rat tissues	Microglial depletion increases the number of degenerating neurons after excitotoxic lesions	Kallendrusch et al. (2013)
Mixed neuronal cultures	Deoxyglucose-induced death in cell culture	Microglia death via inhibition of glycolysis and ATP depletion, inducing microglial necrosis and their phagocytosis by other microglia	Vilalta and Brown (2014)
Organotypic spinal cord slice culture	Clodronate depletion in Sprague-Dawley rat tissues co-cultured with neural progenitor cells	Depletion of microglia decreased the apoptotic rate of NPCs, more NPCs differentiated into neurons, and glial differentiation was impaired	Liu et al. (2013)

epigenetic) programmes that we are currently unaware of but which have significant bearing on the interpretation of the studies.

The enormous propensity of the CNS to repopulate with myeloid cells, be they surviving microglia colonies that hyperproliferate, or CNS-adapted infiltrating monocytes that fill up the available niche, indicates that a myeloid-deficient CNS is a highly non-physiological condition. While the infiltrating monocytes co-occupy the CNS and begin to express microglia-specific proteins, it still remains to be proven if they develop *full* microglial functionality. Exactly how the CNS regulates the repopulation process and senses when the niche is replenished are important unanswered questions.

What is clear from our review is that there is some disparity between the results of different microglia depletion systems in the same disease model. Discerning the underlying molecular mechanisms that lead to these different outcomes will serve to further our knowledge of the pathogenesis that we wish to target therapeutically. In particular, the relative timing of microglial depletion in relation to the insult might explain some of the disparity, and deserves further consideration.

While the homeostatic functions of microglia are well understood, these cells always having activity in surveying the CNS, the molecular basis for these functions are less well characterized. TGFβ appears to be a key cytokine in preventing microglia and other infiltrating myeloid cells from pro-inflammatory (pathogenic) activation (Buttgereit et al., 2016; Parsa et al., 2016). The existence of sub-populations in different regions of the CNS has been demonstrated (Grabert et al., 2016), and so it is plausible that even homeostatic microglia function varies between different CNS microenvironments (Harris, 2014). A very recent study using a novel fate-mapping strategy has described such regional differences of self-organization of mature microglial subpopulations during both health and disease in the CNS (Tay et al., 2017). If and when subpopulation-specific microglial markers can be defined then it might even be possible to deplete individual subpopulations in the future. The more refined our understanding of these issues becomes, the more likely we will be able to design efficient therapeutic paradigms.

As it is clear that microglia are implicated as a part of all the neurodegenerative diseases described in this review article, modulation of microglial functionality (suppression of pro-inflammatory, pathogenic properties) or replacement with CNS-adapting macrophages are intriguing prospects for immunotherapy. We have previously reported that immunosuppressive macrophages can down-modulate pro-inflammatory macrophage and T cell activities in settings of experimental MS (Zhang et al., 2014), indicating that immunomodulation with favorable clinical outcome is possible. With the knowledge that monocytes can become CNS-adapted during repopulation of a microglia depleted CNS, further effort in manipulating this phenomenon to a therapeutic end is warranted.

AUTHOR CONTRIBUTIONS

All authors have had similar roles in defining the literature to be reviewed, preparing individual sections of the text and working up the final version of the manuscript.

FUNDING

Funding provided by the Swedish Medical Research Council, AlzheimerFond and Karolinska Institutet (KID).

REFERENCES

Acharya, M. M., Green, K. N., Allen, B. D., Najafi, A. R., Syage, A., Minasyan, H., et al. (2016). Elimination of microglia improves cognitive function following cranial irradiation. *Sci. Rep.* 6:31545. doi: 10.1038/srep31545

Ajami, B., Bennett, J. L., Krieger, C., McNagny, K. M., and Rossi, F. M. V. (2011). Infiltrating monocytes trigger EAE progression, but do not contribute to the resident microglia pool. *Nat. Neurosci.* 14, 1142–1149. doi: 10.1038/nn.2887

Ajami, B., Bennett, J. L., Krieger, C., Tetzlaff, W., and Rossi, F. M. V. (2007). Local self-renewal can sustain CNS microglia maintenance and function throughout adult life. *Nat. Neurosci.* 10, 1538–1543. doi: 10.1038/nn2014

Alexianu, M. E., Kozovska, M., and Appel, S. H. (2001). Immune reactivity in a mouse model of familial ALS correlates with disease progression. *Neurology* 57, 1282–1289. doi: 10.1212/wnl.57.7.1282

Alzheimer, A., Stelzmann, R. A., Schnitzlein, H. N., and Murtagh, F. R. (1995). An English translation of Alzheimer's 1907 paper, "Über eine eigenartige Erkankung der Hirnrinde". *Clin. Anat.* 8, 429–431. doi: 10.1002/ca.980080612

Asai, H., Ikezu, S., Tsunoda, S., Medalla, M., Luebke, J., Haydar, T., et al. (2015). Depletion of microglia and inhibition of exosome synthesis halt tau propagation. *Nat. Neurosci.* 18, 1584–1593. doi: 10.1038/nn.4132

Beers, D. R., Henkel, J. S., Xiao, Q., Zhao, W., Wang, J., Yen, A. A., et al. (2006). Wild-type microglia extend survival in PU.1 knockout mice with familial amyotrophic lateral sclerosis. *Proc. Natl. Acad. Sci. U S A* 103, 16021–16026. doi: 10.1073/pnas.0607423103

Beers, D. R., Zhao, W., Liao, B., Kano, O., Wang, J., Huang, A., et al. (2011). Neuroinflammation modulates distinct regional and temporal clinical responses in ALS mice. *Brain Behav. Immun.* 25, 1025–1035. doi: 10.1016/j.bbi.2010.12.008

Bennett, R. E., and Brody, D. L. (2014). Acute reduction of microglia does not alter axonal injury in a mouse model of repetitive concussive traumatic brain injury. *J. Neurotrauma* 31, 1647–1663. doi: 10.1089/neu.2013.3320

Bhaskar, K., Konerth, M., Kokiko-Cochran, O. N., Cardona, A., Ransohoff, R. M., and Lamb, B. T. (2010). Regulation of tau pathology by the microglial fractalkine receptor. *Neuron* 68, 19–31. doi: 10.1016/j.neuron.2010.08.023

Boche, D., Cunningham, C., Docagne, F., Scott, H., and Perry, V. H. (2006). TGFβ1 regulates the inflammatory response during chronic neurodegeneration. *Neurobiol. Dis.* 22, 638–650. doi: 10.1016/j.nbd.2006.01.004

Bogie, J. F., Boelen, E., Louagie, E., Delputte, P., Elewaut, D., van Horssen, J., et al. (2017). CD169 is a marker for highly pathogenic phagocytes in multiple sclerosis. *Mult. Scler.* 101:1352458517698759. doi: 10.1177/1352458517698759 [Epub ahead of print].

Boillée, S., Yamanaka, K., Lobsiger, C. S., Copeland, N. G., Jenkins, N. A., Kassiotis, G., et al. (2006). Onset and progression in inherited ALS determined by motor neurons and microglia. *Science* 312, 1389–1392. doi: 10.1126/science.1123511

Boissonneault, V., Filali, M., Lessard, M., Relton, J., Wong, G., and Rivest, S. (2009). Powerful beneficial effects of macrophage colony-stimulating factor on β-amyloid deposition and cognitive impairment in Alzheimer's disease. *Brain* 132, 1078–1092. doi: 10.1093/brain/awn331

Bolmont, T., Haiss, F., Eicke, D., Radde, R., Mathis, C. A., Klunk, W. E., et al. (2008). Dynamics of the microglial/amyloid interaction indicate a role in plaque maintenance. *J. Neurosci.* 28, 4283–4292. doi: 10.1523/jneurosci.4814-07.2008

Bornemann, K. D., Wiederhold, K.-H., Pauli, C., Ermini, F., Stalder, M., Schnell, L., et al. (2001). Aβ-induced inflammatory processes in microglia cells of APP23 transgenic mice. *Am. J. Pathol.* 158, 63–73. doi: 10.1016/s0002-9440(10)63945-4

Braak, H., Thal, D. R., Ghebremedhin, E., and Del Tredici, K. (2011). Stages of the pathologic process in Alzheimer disease: age categories from 1 to 100 years. *J. Neuropathol. Exp. Neurol.* 70, 960–969. doi: 10.1097/NEN.0b013e318232a379

Bruttger, J., Karram, K., Wörtge, S., Regen, T., Marini, F., Hoppmann, N., et al. (2015). Genetic cell ablation reveals clusters of local self-renewing microglia in the mammalian central nervous system. *Immunity* 43, 92–106. doi: 10.1016/j.immuni.2015.06.012

Butovsky, O., Kunis, G., Koronyo-Hamaoui, M., and Schwartz, M. (2007). Selective ablation of bone marrow-derived dendritic cells increases amyloid plaques in a mouse Alzheimer's disease model. *Eur. J. Neurosci.* 26, 413–416. doi: 10.1111/j.1460-9568.2007.05652.x

Butovsky, O., Siddiqui, S., Gabriely, G., Lanser, A. J., Dake, B., Murugaiyan, G., et al. (2012). Modulating inflammatory monocytes with a unique microRNA gene signature ameliorates murine ALS. *J. Clin. Invest.* 122, 3063–3087. doi: 10.1172/jci62636

Buttgereit, A., Lelios, I., Yu, X., Vrohlings, M., Krakoski, N. R., Gautier, E. L., et al. (2016). Sall1 is a transcriptional regulator defining microglia identity and function. *Nat. Immunol.* 17, 1397–1406. doi: 10.1038/ni.3585

Cherry, J. D., Tripodis, Y., Alvarez, V. E., Huber, B., Kiernan, P. T., Daneshvar, D. H., et al. (2016). Microglial neuroinflammation contributes to tau accumulation in chronic traumatic encephalopathy. *Acta Neuropathol. Commun.* 4:112. doi: 10.1186/s40478-016-0382-8

Chiu, I. M., Morimoto, E. T. A., Goodarzi, H., Liao, J. T., O'Keeffe, S., Phatnani, H. P., et al. (2013). A neurodegeneration-specific gene-expression signature of acutely isolated microglia from an amyotrophic lateral sclerosis mouse model. *Cell Rep.* 4, 385–401. doi: 10.1016/j.celrep.2013.06.018

Côté, M., Poirier, A. A., Aubé, B., Jobin, C., Lacroix, S., and Soulet, D. (2015). Partial depletion of the proinflammatory monocyte population is neuroprotective in the myenteric plexus but not in the basal ganglia in a MPTP mouse model of Parkinson's disease. *Brain Behav. Immun.* 46, 154–167. doi: 10.1016/j.bbi.2015.01.009

Cunningham, C., Deacon, R. M. J., Chan, K., Boche, D., Rawlins, J. N. P., and Perry, V. H. (2005). Neuropathologically distinct prion strains give rise to similar temporal profiles of behavioral deficits. *Neurobiol. Dis.* 18, 258–269. doi: 10.1016/j.nbd.2004.08.015

Daria, A., Colombo, A., Llovera, G., Hampel, H., Willem, M., Liesz, A., et al. (2017). Young microglia restore amyloid plaque clearance of aged microglia. *EMBO J.* 36, 583–603. doi: 10.15252/embj.201694591

Degos, V., Vacas, S., Han, Z., Van Rooijen, N., Gressens, P., Su, H., et al. (2013). Depletion of bone marrow-derived macrophages perturbs the innate immune response to surgery and reduces postoperative memory dysfunction. *Anesthesiology* 118, 527–536. doi: 10.1097/aln.0b013e3182834d94

El Khoury, J., Toft, M., Hickman, S. E., Means, T. K., Terada, K., Geula, C., et al. (2007). *Ccr2* deficiency impairs microglial accumulation and accelerates progression of Alzheimer-like disease. *Nat. Med.* 13, 432–438. doi: 10.1038/nm1555

Elmore, M. R. P., Najafi, A. R., Koike, M. A., Dagher, N. N., Spangenberg, E. E., Rice, R. A., et al. (2014). Colony-stimulating factor 1 receptor signaling is necessary for microglia viability, unmasking a microglia progenitor cell in the adult brain. *Neuron* 82, 380–397. doi: 10.1016/j.neuron.2014.02.040

Faustino, J. V., Wang, X., Johnson, C. E., Klibanov, A., Derugin, N., Wendland, M. F., et al. (2011). Microglial cells contribute to endogenous brain defenses after acute neonatal focal stroke. *J. Neurosci.* 31, 12992–13001. doi: 10.1523/jneurosci.2102-11.2011

Fernández-López, D., Faustino, J., Klibanov, A. L., Derugin, N., Blanchard, E., Simon, F., et al. (2016). Microglial cells prevent hemorrhage in neonatal focal arterial stroke. *J. Neurosci.* 36, 2881–2893. doi: 10.1523/jneurosci.0140-15.2016

Fife, B. T., Huffnagle, G. B., Kuziel, W. A., and Karpus, W. J. (2000). CC chemokine receptor 2 is critical for induction of experimental autoimmune encephalomyelitis. *J. Exp. Med.* 192, 899–906. doi: 10.1084/jem.192.6.899

Frank, S., Burbach, G. J., Bonin, M., Walter, M., Streit, W., Bechmann, I., et al. (2008). TREM2 is upregulated in amyloid plaque-associated microglia in aged APP23 transgenic mice. *Glia* 56, 1438–1447. doi: 10.1002/glia.20710

Frautschy, S. A., Yang, F., Irrizarry, M., Hyman, B., Saido, T. C., Hsiao, K., et al. (1998). Microglial response to amyloid plaques in APPsw transgenic mice. *Am. J. Pathol.* 152, 307–317.

Galea, I., Palin, K., Newman, T. A., Van Rooijen, N., Perry, V. H., and Boche, D. (2005). Mannose receptor expression specifically reveals perivascular macrophages in normal, injured, and diseased mouse brain. *Glia* 49, 375–384. doi: 10.1002/glia.20124

Gelderblom, M., Leypoldt, F., Steinbach, K., Behrens, D., Choe, C.-U., Siler, D. A., et al. (2009). Temporal and spatial dynamics of cerebral immune cell accumulation in stroke. *Stroke* 40, 1849–1857. doi: 10.1161/strokeaha.108.534503

Ginhoux, F., Greter, M., Leboeuf, M., Nandi, S., See, P., Gokhan, S., et al. (2010). Fate mapping analysis reveals that adult microglia derive from primitive macrophages. *Science* 330, 841–845. doi: 10.1126/science.1194637

Gliem, M., Mausberg, A. K., Lee, J.-I., Simiantonakis, I., van Rooijen, N., Hartung, H.-P., et al. (2012). Macrophages prevent hemorrhagic infarct transformation in murine stroke models. *Ann. Neurol.* 71, 743–752. doi: 10.1002/ana.23529

Goldmann, T., Wieghofer, P., Jordão, M. J. C., Prutek, F., Hagemeyer, N., Frenzel, K., et al. (2016). Origin, fate and dynamics of macrophages at central nervous system interfaces. *Nat. Immunol.* 17, 797–805. doi: 10.1038/ni.3423

Goldmann, T., Wieghofer, P., Müller, P. F., Wolf, Y., Varol, D., Yona, S., et al. (2013). A new type of microglia gene targeting shows TAK1 to be pivotal in CNS autoimmune inflammation. *Nat. Neurosci.* 16, 1618–1626. doi: 10.1038/nn.3531

Gómez-Nicola, D., Fransen, N. L., Suzzi, S., and Perry, V. H. (2013). Regulation of microglial proliferation during chronic neurodegeneration. *J. Neurosci.* 33, 2481–2493. doi: 10.1523/JNEUROSCI.4440-12.2013

Gómez-Nicola, D., Schetters, S. T. T., and Perry, V. H. (2014). Differential role of CCR2 in the dynamics of microglia and perivascular macrophages during prion disease. *Glia* 62, 1041–1052. doi: 10.1002/glia.22660

Goverman, J. (2009). Autoimmune T cell responses in the central nervous system. *Nat. Rev. Immunol.* 9, 393–407. doi: 10.1038/nri2550

Gowing, G., Philips, T., Van Wijmeersch, B., Audet, J. N., Dewil, M., Van Den Bosch, L., et al. (2008). Ablation of proliferating microglia does not affect motor neuron degeneration in amyotrophic lateral sclerosis caused by mutant superoxide dismutase. *J. Neurosci.* 28, 10234–10244. doi: 10.1523/JNEUROSCI.3494-08.2008

Grabert, K., Michoel, T., Karavolos, M. H., Clohisey, S., Baillie, J. K., Stevens, M. P., et al. (2016). Microglial brain region-dependent diversity and selective regional sensitivities to aging. *Nat. Neurosci.* 19, 504–516. doi: 10.1038/nn.4222

Grathwohl, S. A., Kälin, R. E., Bolmont, T., Prokop, S., Winkelmann, G., Kaeser, S. A., et al. (2009). Formation and maintenance of Alzheimer's disease β-amyloid plaques in the absence of microglia. *Nat. Neurosci.* 12, 1361–1363. doi: 10.1038/nn.2432

Greter, M., Heppner, F. L., Lemos, M. P., Odermatt, B. M., Goebels, N., Laufer, T., et al. (2005). Dendritic cells permit immune invasion of the CNS in an animal model of multiple sclerosis. *Nat. Med.* 11, 328–334. doi: 10.1038/nm1197

Greter, M., Lelios, I., Pelczar, P., Hoeffel, G., Price, J., Leboeuf, M., et al. (2012). Stroma-derived interleukin-34 controls the development and maintenance of langerhans cells and the maintenance of microglia. *Immunity* 37, 1050–1060. doi: 10.1016/j.immuni.2012.11.001

Greter, M., and Merad, M. (2012). Regulation of microglia development and homeostasis. *Glia* 61, 121–127. doi: 10.1002/glia.22408

Griciuc, A., Serrano-Pozo, A., Parrado, A. R., Lesinski, A. N., Asselin, C. N., Mullin, K., et al. (2013). Alzheimer's disease risk gene *CD33* inhibits microglial uptake of amyloid β. *Neuron* 78, 631–643. doi: 10.1016/j.neuron.2013.04.014

Guerreiro, R., Wojtas, A., Bras, J., Carrasquillo, M., Rogaeva, E., Majounie, E., et al. (2013). TREM2 variants in Alzheimer's disease. *N. Engl. J. Med.* 368, 117–127. doi: 10.1056/NEJMoa1211851

Hall, E. D., Oostveen, J. A., and Gurney, M. E. (1998). Relationship of microglial and astrocytic activation to disease onset and progression in a transgenic model of familial ALS. *Glia* 23, 249–256. doi: 10.1002/(SICI)1098-1136(199807)23:3<249::AID-GLIA7>3.0.CO;2-#

Hammond, M. D., Taylor, R. A., Mullen, M. T., Ai, Y., Aguila, H. L., Mack, M., et al. (2014). $CCR2^{+}Ly6C^{hi}$ inflammatory monocyte recruitment exacerbates acute disability following intracerebral hemorrhage. *J. Neurosci.* 34, 3901–3909. doi: 10.1523/JNEUROSCI.4070-13.2014

Han, W., Umekawa, T., Zhou, K., Zhang, X.-M., Ohshima, M., Dominguez, C. A., et al. (2016). Cranial irradiation induces transient microglia accumulation, followed by long-lasting inflammation and loss of microglia. *Oncotarget* 7, 82305–82323. doi: 10.18632/oncotarget.12929

Hanafy, K. A. (2013). The role of microglia and the TLR4 pathway in neuronal apoptosis and vasospasm after subarachnoid hemorrhage. *J. Neuroinflammation* 10:83. doi: 10.1186/1742-2094-10-83

Hanna, R. N., Shaked, I., Hubbeling, H. G., Punt, J. A., Wu, R., Herrley, E., et al. (2012). NR4A1 (Nur77) deletion polarizes macrophages toward an inflammatory phenotype and increases atherosclerosis. *Circ. Res.* 110, 416–427. doi: 10.1161/CIRCRESAHA.111.253377

Harris, R. A. (2014). Spatial, temporal, and functional aspects of macrophages during "the good, the bad, and the ugly" phases of inflammation. *Front. Immunol.* 5:612. doi: 10.3389/fimmu.2014.00612

Hawkes, C. A., and McLaurin, J. (2009). Selective targeting of perivascular macrophages for clearance of β-amyloid in cerebral amyloid angiopathy. *Proc. Natl. Acad. Sci. U S A* 106, 1261–1266. doi: 10.1073/pnas.0805453106

Heldmann, U., Mine, Y., Kokaia, Z., Ekdahl, C. T., and Lindvall, O. (2011). Selective depletion of Mac-1-expressing microglia in rat subventricular zone does not alter neurogenic response early after stroke. *Exp. Neurol.* 229, 391–398. doi: 10.1016/j.expneurol.2011.03.005

Henkel, J. S., Beers, D. R., Siklós, L., and Appel, S. H. (2006). The chemokine MCP-1 and the dendritic and myeloid cells it attracts are increased in the mSOD1 mouse model of ALS. *Mol. Cell. Neurosci.* 31, 427–437. doi: 10.1016/j.mcn.2005.10.016

Heppner, F. L., Greter, M., Marino, D., Falsig, J., Raivich, G., Hövelmeyer, N., et al. (2005). Experimental autoimmune encephalomyelitis repressed by microglial paralysis. *Nat. Med.* 11, 146–152. doi: 10.1038/nm1177

Hesske, L., Vincenzetti, C., Heikenwalder, M., Prinz, M., Reith, W., Fontana, A., et al. (2010). Induction of inhibitory central nervous system-derived and stimulatory blood-derived dendritic cells suggests a dual role for granulocyte-macrophage colony-stimulating factor in central nervous system inflammation. *Brain* 133, 1637–1654. doi: 10.1093/brain/awq081

Hickman, S. E., Allison, E. K., and El Khoury, J. (2008). Microglial dysfunction and defective -amyloid clearance pathways in aging alzheimer's disease mice. *J. Neurosci.* 28, 8354–8360. doi: 10.1523/JNEUROSCI.0616-08.2008

Huitinga, I., Ruuls, S. R., Jung, S., Van Rooijen, N., Hartung, H. P., and Dijkstra, C. D. (1995). Macrophages in T cell line-mediated, demyelinating, and chronic relapsing experimental autoimmune encephalomyelitis in Lewis rats. *Clin. Exp. Immunol.* 100, 344–351. doi: 10.1111/j.1365-2249.1995.tb03675.x

Huitinga, I., van Rooijen, N., de Groot, C. J., Uitdehaag, B. M., and Dijkstra, C. D. (1990). Suppression of experimental allergic encephalomyelitis in Lewis rats after elimination of macrophages. *J. Exp. Med.* 172, 1025–1033. doi: 10.1084/jem.172.4.1025

Iaccarino, H. F., Singer, A. C., Martorell, A. J., Rudenko, A., Gao, F., Gillingham, T. Z., et al. (2016). Gamma frequency entrainment attenuates amyloid load and modifies microglia. *Nature* 540, 230–235. doi: 10.1038/nature20587

Jäkel, S., and Dimou, L. (2017). Glial cells and their function in the adult brain: a journey through the history of their ablation. *Front. Cell. Neurosci.* 11:81. doi: 10.3389/fncel.2017.00024

Jin, W.-N., Shi, S. X.-Y., Li, Z., Li, M., Wood, K., Gonzales, R. J., et al. (2017). Depletion of microglia exacerbates postischemic inflammation and brain injury. *J. Cereb. Blood Flow Metab.* 37, 2224–2236. doi: 10.1177/0271678x17694185

Jonsson, T., Stefansson, H., Steinberg, S., Jonsdottir, I., Jonsson, P. V., Snaedal, J., et al. (2013). Variant of TREM2 associated with the risk of Alzheimer's disease. *N. Engl. J. Med.* 368, 107–116. doi: 10.1056/NEJMoa1211103

Kallendrusch, S., Kremzow, S., Nowicki, M., Grabiec, U., Winkelmann, R., Benz, A., et al. (2013). The G protein-coupled receptor 55 ligand l-α-lysophosphatidylinositol exerts microglia-dependent neuroprotection after excitotoxic lesion. *Glia* 61, 1822–1831. doi: 10.1002/glia.22560

Krabbe, G., Halle, A., Matyash, V., Rinnenthal, J. L., Eom, G. D., Bernhardt, U., et al. (2013). Functional impairment of microglia coincides with beta-amyloid deposition in mice with Alzheimer-like pathology. *PLoS One* 8:e60921. doi: 10.1371/journal.pone.0060921

Lalancette-Hébert, M., Gowing, G., Simard, A., Weng, Y. C., and Kriz, J. (2007). Selective ablation of proliferating microglial cells exacerbates ischemic injury in the brain. *J. Neurosci.* 27, 2596–2605. doi: 10.1523/JNEUROSCI.5360-06.2007

Lambert, J.-C., Heath, S., Even, G., Campion, D., Sleegers, K., Hiltunen, M., et al. (2009). Genome-wide association study identifies variants at CLU and CR1 associated with Alzheimer's disease. *Nat. Genet.* 41, 1094–1099. doi: 10.1038/ng.439

Lampron, A., Lessard, M., and Rivest, S. (2012). Effects of myeloablation, peripheral chimerism, and whole-body irradiation on the entry of bone marrow-derived cells into the brain. *Cell Transplant.* 21, 1149–1159. doi: 10.3727/096368911x593154

Lee, J. C., Seong, J., Kim, S. H., Lee, S. J., Cho, Y. J., An, J., et al. (2012). Replacement of microglial cells using Clodronate liposome and bone marrow transplantation in the central nervous system of $SOD1^{G93A}$ transgenic mice as an *in vivo* model of amyotrophic lateral sclerosis. *Biochem. Biophys. Res. Commun.* 418, 359–365. doi: 10.1016/j.bbrc.2012.01.026

Leinenga, G., and Götz, J. (2015). Scanning ultrasound removes amyloid-β and restores memory in an Alzheimer's disease mouse model. *Sci. Transl. Med.* 7:278ra33. doi: 10.1126/scitranslmed.aaa2512

Li, M., Li, Z., Ren, H., Jin, W.-N., Wood, K., Liu, Q., et al. (2017). Colony stimulating factor 1 receptor inhibition eliminates microglia and attenuates brain injury after intracerebral hemorrhage. *J. Cereb. Blood Flow Metab.* 37, 2383–2395. doi: 10.1177/0271678x16666551

Liu, X., Chu, T.-H., Su, H., Guo, A., and Wu, W. (2013). Neural progenitor cell apoptosis and differentiation were affected by activated microglia in spinal cord slice culture. *Neurol. Sci.* 35, 415–419. doi: 10.1007/s10072-013-1532-4

Ma, Y., Li, Y., Jiang, L., Wang, L., Jiang, Z., Wang, Y., et al. (2016). Macrophage depletion reduced brain injury following middle cerebral artery occlusion in mice. *J. Neuroinflammation* 13:38. doi: 10.1186/s12974-016-0504-z

Mack, M., Cihak, J., Simonis, C., Luckow, B., Proudfoot, A. E., Plachý, J., et al. (2001). Expression and characterization of the chemokine receptors CCR2 and CCR5 in mice. *J. Immunol.* 166, 4697–4704. doi: 10.4049/jimmunol.166.7.4697

Malm, T. M., Koistinaho, M., Pärepalo, M., Vatanen, T., Ooka, A., Karlsson, S., et al. (2005). Bone-marrow-derived cells contribute to the recruitment of microglial cells in response to β-amyloid deposition in APP/PS1 double transgenic Alzheimer mice. *Neurobiol. Dis.* 18, 134–142. doi: 10.1016/j.nbd.2004.09.009

Maphis, N., Xu, G., Kokiko-Cochran, O. N., Jiang, S., Cardona, A., Ransohoff, R. M., et al. (2015). Reactive microglia drive tau pathology and contribute to the spreading of pathological tau in the brain. *Brain* 138, 1738–1755. doi: 10.1093/brain/awv081

Mawhinney, L. A., Thawer, S. G., Lu, W.-Y., Rooijen, N. V., Weaver, L. C., Brown, A., et al. (2012). Differential detection and distribution of microglial and hematogenous macrophage populations in the injured spinal cord of lys-EGFP-ki transgenic mice. *J. Neuropathol. Exp. Neurol.* 71, 180–197. doi: 10.1097/NEN.0b013e3182479b41

Meyer-Luehmann, M., Spires-Jones, T. L., Prada, C., Garcia-Alloza, M., de Calignon, A., Rozkalne, A., et al. (2008). Rapid appearance and local toxicity of amyloid-β plaques in a mouse model of Alzheimer's disease. *Nature* 451, 720–724. doi: 10.1038/nature06616

Michaud, J.-P., Bellavance, M.-A., Préfontaine, P., and Rivest, S. (2013). Real-time *in vivo* imaging reveals the ability of monocytes to clear vascular amyloid beta. *Cell Rep.* 5, 646–653. doi: 10.1016/j.celrep.2013.10.010

Mildner, A., Mack, M., Schmidt, H., Brück, W., Djukic, M., Zabel, M. D., et al. (2009). $CCR2^{+}Ly\text{-}6C^{hi}$ monocytes are crucial for the effector phase of autoimmunity in the central nervous system. *Brain* 132, 2487–2500. doi: 10.1093/brain/awp144

Mildner, A., Schlevogt, B., Kierdorf, K., Bottcher, C., Erny, D., Kummer, M. P., et al. (2011). Distinct and non-redundant roles of microglia and myeloid subsets in mouse models of Alzheimer's disease. *J. Neurosci.* 31, 11159–11171. doi: 10.1523/JNEUROSCI.6209-10.2011

Mildner, A., Schmidt, H., Nitsche, M., Merkler, D., Hanisch, U.-K., Mack, M., et al. (2007). Microglia in the adult brain arise from $Ly\text{-}6C^{hi}CCR2^{+}$ monocytes only under defined host conditions. *Nat. Neurosci.* 10, 1544–1553. doi: 10.1038/nn2015

Moreno, M. A., Burns, T., Yao, P., Miers, L., Pleasure, D., and Soulika, A. M. (2016). Therapeutic depletion of monocyte-derived cells protects from long-term axonal loss in experimental autoimmune encephalomyelitis. *J. Neuroimmunol.* 290, 36–46. doi: 10.1016/j.jneuroim.2015.11.004

Nayak, D., Roth, T. L., and McGavern, D. B. (2014). Microglia development and function. *Annu. Rev. Immunol.* 32, 367–402. doi: 10.1146/annurev-immunol-032713-120240

Newman, T. A., Galea, I., van Rooijen, N., and Perry, V. H. (2005). Blood-derived dendritic cells in an acute brain injury. *J. Neuroimmunol.* 166, 167–172. doi: 10.1016/j.jneuroim.2005.04.026

Parkhurst, C. N., Yang, G., Ninan, I., Savas, J. N., Yates, J. R. III, Lafaille, J. J., et al. (2013). Microglia promote learning-dependent synapse formation through brain-derived neurotrophic factor. *Cell* 155, 1596–1609. doi: 10.1016/j.cell.2013.11.030

Parsa, R., Lund, H., Tosevski, I., Zhang, X.-M., Malipiero, U., Beckervordersandforth, J., et al. (2016). TGFβ regulates persistent neuroinflammation by controlling Th1 polarization and ROS production via monocyte-derived dendritic cells. *Glia* 64, 1925–1937. doi: 10.1002/glia.23033

Peng, J., Gu, N., Zhou, L., B Eyo, U., Murugan, M., Gan, W.-B., et al. (2016). Microglia and monocytes synergistically promote the transition from acute to chronic pain after nerve injury. *Nat. Commun.* 7:12029. doi: 10.1038/ncomms12029

Polfliet, M. M., Goede, P. H., van Kesteren-Hendrikx, E. M., van Rooijen, N., Dijkstra, C. D., and van den Berg, T. K. (2001). A method for the selective depletion of perivascular and meningeal macrophages in the central nervous system. *J. Neuroimmunol.* 116, 188–195. doi: 10.1016/s0165-5728(01)00282-x

Prokop, S., Miller, K. R., Drost, N., Handrick, S., Mathur, V., Luo, J., et al. (2015). Impact of peripheral myeloid cells on amyloid-β pathology in Alzheimer's disease-like mice. *J. Exp. Med.* 212, 1811–1818. doi: 10.1084/jem.20150479

Rice, R. A., Pham, J., Lee, R. J., Najafi, A. R., West, B. L., and Green, K. N. (2017). Microglial repopulation resolves inflammation and promotes brain recovery after injury. *Glia* 65, 931–944. doi: 10.1002/glia.23135

Rice, R. A., Spangenberg, E. E., Yamate-Morgan, H., Lee, R. J., Arora, R. P. S., Hernandez, M. X., et al. (2015). Elimination of microglia improves functional outcomes following extensive neuronal loss in the hippocampus. *J. Neurosci.* 35, 9977–9989. doi: 10.1523/JNEUROSCI.0336-15.2015

Sawcer, S., Hellenthal, G., Pirinen, M., Spencer, C. C. A., Patsopoulos, N. A., Moutsianas, L., et al. (2011). Genetic risk and a primary role for cell-mediated immune mechanisms in multiple sclerosis. *Nature* 476, 214–219. doi: 10.1038/nature10251

Schmidt, A., Strecker, J.-K., Hucke, S., Bruckmann, N.-M., Herold, M., Mack, M., et al. (2017). Targeting different monocyte/macrophage subsets has no impact on outcome in experimental stroke. *Stroke* 48, 1061–1069. doi: 10.1161/STROKEAHA.116.015577

Schneider, U. C., Davids, A.-M., Brandenburg, S., Müller, A., Elke, A., Magrini, S., et al. (2015). Microglia inflict delayed brain injury after subarachnoid hemorrhage. *Acta Neuropathol.* 130, 215–231. doi: 10.1007/s00401-015-1440-1

Serbina, N. V., and Pamer, E. G. (2006). Monocyte emigration from bone marrow during bacterial infection requires signals mediated by chemokine receptor CCR2. *Nat. Immunol.* 7, 311–317. doi: 10.1038/ni1309

Shichita, T., Sakaguchi, R., Suzuki, M., and Yoshimura, A. (2012). Post-ischemic inflammation in the brain. *Front. Immunol.* 3:132. doi: 10.3389/fimmu.2012.00132

Simard, A. R., Soulet, D., Gowing, G., Julien, J.-P., and Rivest, S. (2006). Bone marrow-derived microglia play a critical role in restricting senile plaque formation in Alzheimer's disease. *Neuron* 49, 489–502. doi: 10.1016/j.neuron.2006.01.022

Spangenberg, E. E., Lee, R. J., Najafi, A. R., Rice, R. A., Elmore, M. R. P., Blurton-Jones, M., et al. (2016). Eliminating microglia in Alzheimer's mice prevents neuronal loss without modulating amyloid-β pathology. *Brain* 139, 1265–1281. doi: 10.1093/brain/aww016

Stalder, M., Deller, T., Staufenbiel, M., and Jucker, M. (2001). 3D-reconstruction of microglia and amyloid in APP23 transgenic mice: no evidence of intracellular amyloid. *Neurobiol. Aging* 22, 427–434. doi: 10.1016/s0197-4580(01)00209-3

Stalder, A. K., Ermini, F., Bondolfi, L., Krenger, W., Burbach, G. J., Deller, T., et al. (2005). Invasion of hematopoietic cells into the brain of amyloid precursor protein transgenic mice. *J. Neurosci.* 25, 11125–11132. doi: 10.1523/JNEUROSCI.2545-05.2005

Stalder, M., Phinney, A., Probst, A., Sommer, B., Staufenbiel, M., and Jucker, M. (1999). Association of microglia with amyloid plaques in brains of APP23 transgenic mice. *Am. J. Pathol.* 154, 1673–1684. doi: 10.1016/s0002-9440(10)65423-5

Sunderkötter, C., Nikolic, T., Dillon, M. J., Van Rooijen, N., Stehling, M., Drevets, D. A., et al. (2004). Subpopulations of mouse blood monocytes differ in maturation stage and inflammatory response. *J. Immunol.* 172, 4410–4417. doi: 10.4049/jimmunol.172.7.4410

Szalay, G., Martinecz, B., Lénárt, N., Környei, Z., Orsolits, B., Judák, L., et al. (2016). Microglia protect against brain injury and their selective elimination dysregulates neuronal network activity after stroke. *Nat. Commun.* 7:11499. doi: 10.1038/ncomms11499

Tanaka, R., Komine-Kobayashi, M., Mochizuki, H., Yamada, M., Furuya, T., Migita, M., et al. (2003). Migration of enhanced green fluorescent protein expressing bone marrow-derived microglia/macrophage into the mouse brain following permanent focal ischemia. *Neuroscience* 117, 531–539. doi: 10.1016/s0306-4522(02)00954-5

Tay, T. L., Mai, D., Dautzenberg, J., Fernández-Klett, F., Lin, G., Sagar, et al. (2017). A new fate mapping system reveals context-dependent random or clonal expansion of microglia. *Nat. Neurosci.* 20, 793–803. doi: 10.1038/nn.4547

Tran, E. H., Hoekstra, K., van Rooijen, N., Dijkstra, C. D., and Owens, T. (1998). Immune invasion of the central nervous system parenchyma and experimental allergic encephalomyelitis, but not leukocyte extravasation from blood, are prevented in macrophage-depleted mice. *J. Immunol.* 161, 3767–3775.

Vainchtein, I. D., Vinet, J., Brouwer, N., Brendecke, S., Biagini, G., Biber, K., et al. (2014). In acute experimental autoimmune encephalomyelitis, infiltrating macrophages are immune activated, whereas microglia remain immune suppressed. *Glia* 62, 1724–1735. doi: 10.1002/glia.22711

van Rooijen, N. (1989). The liposome-mediated macrophage "suicide" technique. *J. Immunol. Methods* 124, 1–6. doi: 10.1016/0022-1759(89)90178-6

Varvel, N. H., Grathwohl, S. A., Baumann, F., Liebig, C., Bosch, A., Brawek, B., et al. (2012). Microglial repopulation model reveals a robust homeostatic process for replacing CNS myeloid cells. *Proc. Natl. Acad. Sci. U S A* 109, 18150–18155. doi: 10.1073/pnas.1210150109

Varvel, N. H., Grathwohl, S. A., Degenhardt, K., Resch, C., Bosch, A., Jucker, M., et al. (2015). Replacement of brain-resident myeloid cells does not alter cerebral amyloid-β deposition in mouse models of Alzheimer's disease. *J. Exp. Med.* 212, 1803–1809. doi: 10.1084/jem.20150478

Varvel, N. H., Neher, J. J., Bosch, A., Wang, W., Ransohoff, R. M., Miller, R. J., et al. (2016). Infiltrating monocytes promote brain inflammation and exacerbate neuronal damage after status epilepticus. *Proc. Natl. Acad. Sci. U S A* 113, E5665–E5674. doi: 10.1073/pnas.1604263113

Vilalta, A., and Brown, G. C. (2014). Deoxyglucose prevents neurodegeneration in culture by eliminating microglia. *J. Neuroinflammation* 11:58. doi: 10.1186/1742-2094-11-58

Waisman, A., Ginhoux, F., Greter, M., and Bruttger, J. (2015). Homeostasis of microglia in the adult brain: review of novel microglia depletion systems. *Trends Immunol.* 36, 625–636. doi: 10.1016/j.it.2015.08.005

Wang, Y., and Mandelkow, E. (2016). Tau in physiology and pathology. *Nat. Rev. Neurosci.* 17, 5–21. doi: 10.1038/nrn.2015.1

Wang, Y., Szretter, K. J., Vermi, W., Gilfillan, S., Rossini, C., Cella, M., et al. (2012). IL-34 is a tissue-restricted ligand of CSF1R required for the development of Langerhans cells and microglia. *Nat. Immunol.* 13, 753–760. doi: 10.1038/ni.2360

Wieghofer, P., Knobeloch, K.-P., and Prinz, M. (2015). Genetic targeting of microglia. *Glia* 63, 1–22. doi: 10.1002/glia.22727

Womble, T. A., Green, S., Shahaduzzaman, M., Grieco, J., Sanberg, P. R., Pennypacker, K. R., et al. (2014). Monocytes are essential for the neuroprotective effect of human cord blood cells following middle cerebral artery occlusion in rat. *Mol. Cell. Neurosci.* 59, 76–84. doi: 10.1016/j.mcn.2014.01.004

Yamasaki, R., Lu, H., Butovsky, O., Ohno, N., Rietsch, A. M., Cialic, R., et al. (2014). Differential roles of microglia and monocytes in the inflamed central nervous system. *J. Exp. Med.* 211, 1533–1549. doi: 10.1084/jem.20132477

Yao, Y., Echeverry, S., Shi, X. Q., Yang, M., Yang, Q. Z., Wang, G. Y. F., et al. (2016). Dynamics of spinal microglia repopulation following an acute depletion. *Sci. Rep.* 6:22839. doi: 10.1038/srep22839

Yona, S., Kim, K.-W., Wolf, Y., Mildner, A., Varol, D., Breker, M., et al. (2013). Fate mapping reveals origins and dynamics of monocytes and tissue macrophages under homeostasis. *Immunity* 38, 79–91. doi: 10.1016/j.immuni.2012.12.001

Yoshiyama, Y., Higuchi, M., Zhang, B., Huang, S.-M., Iwata, N., Saido, T. C., et al. (2007). Synapse loss and microglial activation precede tangles in a P301S tauopathy mouse model. *Neuron* 53, 337–351. doi: 10.1016/j.neuron.2007.01.010

Yuan, P., Condello, C., Keene, C. D., Wang, Y., Bird, T. D., Paul, S. M., et al. (2016). TREM2 haplodeficiency in mice and humans impairs the microglia barrier function leading to decreased amyloid compaction and severe axonal dystrophy. *Neuron* 92, 252–264. doi: 10.1016/j.neuron.2016.09.016

Zattoni, M., Mura, M. L., Deprez, F., Schwendener, R. A., Engelhardt, B., Frei, K., et al. (2011). Brain infiltration of leukocytes contributes to the pathophysiology of temporal lobe epilepsy. *J. Neurosci.* 31, 4037–4050. doi: 10.1523/JNEUROSCI.6210-10.2011

Zhang, X.-M., Lund, H., Mia, S., Parsa, R., and Harris, R. A. (2014). Adoptive transfer of cytokine-induced immunomodulatory adult microglia attenuates experimental autoimmune encephalomyelitis in DBA/1 mice. *Glia* 62, 804–817. doi: 10.1002/glia.22643

Zhu, C., Herrmann, U. S., Falsig, J., Abakumova, I., Nuvolone, M., Schwarz, P., et al. (2016). A neuroprotective role for microglia in prion diseases. *J. Exp. Med.* 213, 1047–1059. doi: 10.1083/jcb.2134oia109

Zhu, Y., Soderblom, C., Krishnan, V., Ashbaugh, J., Bethea, J. R., and Lee, J. K. (2015). Hematogenous macrophage depletion reduces the fibrotic scar and increases axonal growth after spinal cord injury. *Neurobiol. Dis.* 74, 114–125. doi: 10.1016/j.nbd.2014.10.024

Zito, M. A., Koennecke, L. A., McAuliffe, M. J., McNally, B., Van Rooijen, N., and Heyes, M. P. (2001). Depletion of systemic macrophages by liposome-encapsulated clodronate attenuates striatal macrophage invasion and neurodegeneration following local endotoxin infusion in gerbils. *Brain Res.* 892, 13–26. doi: 10.1016/s0006-8993(00)03135-8

14

Targeting Microglial Activation States as a Therapeutic Avenue in Parkinson's Disease

*Sudhakar R. Subramaniam and Howard J. Federoff**

Department of Neurology, University of California, Irvine, Irvine, CA, United States

***Correspondence:**
Howard J. Federoff
federoff@uci.edu

Parkinson's disease (PD) is a chronic and progressive disorder characterized neuropathologically by loss of dopamine neurons in the substantia nigra, intracellular proteinaceous inclusions, reduction of dopaminergic terminals in the striatum, and increased neuroinflammatory cells. The consequent reduction of dopamine in the basal ganglia results in the classical parkinsonian motor phenotype. A growing body of evidence suggest that neuroinflammation mediated by microglia, the resident macrophage-like immune cells in the brain, play a contributory role in PD pathogenesis. Microglia participate in both physiological and pathological conditions. In the former, microglia restore the integrity of the central nervous system and, in the latter, they promote disease progression. Microglia acquire different activation states to modulate these cellular functions. Upon activation to the M1 phenotype, microglia elaborate pro-inflammatory cytokines and neurotoxic molecules promoting inflammation and cytotoxic responses. In contrast, when adopting the M2 phenotype microglia secrete anti-inflammatory gene products and trophic factors that promote repair, regeneration, and restore homeostasis. Relatively little is known about the different microglial activation states in PD and a better understanding is essential for developing putative neuroprotective agents. Targeting microglial activation states by suppressing their deleterious pro-inflammatory neurotoxicity and/or simultaneously enhancing their beneficial anti-inflammatory protective functions appear as a valid therapeutic approach for PD treatment. In this review, we summarize microglial functions and, their dual neurotoxic and neuroprotective role in PD. We also review molecules that modulate microglial activation states as a therapeutic option for PD treatment.

Keywords: Parkinson's disease, microglia, therapeutics, neuroinflammation, polarization

INTRODUCTION

Parkinson's disease (PD) is a common movement disorder and the second most prevalent neurodegenerative disorder worldwide, that affects nearly 2% of the elderly population. PD is characterized by loss of dopaminergic neurons in the substantia nigra pars compacta (SNpc) and consequently reduced dopamine (DA) levels in the basal ganglia, causing motor dysfunction (**Figure 1**). Lewy bodies, intracellular proteinaceous inclusions, are the pathological hallmark within PD brains. Lewy bodies contain fibrillar α-synuclein among other proteins (Spillantini et al., 1997). It is evident that the immune system is involved in PD risk by genome-wide association

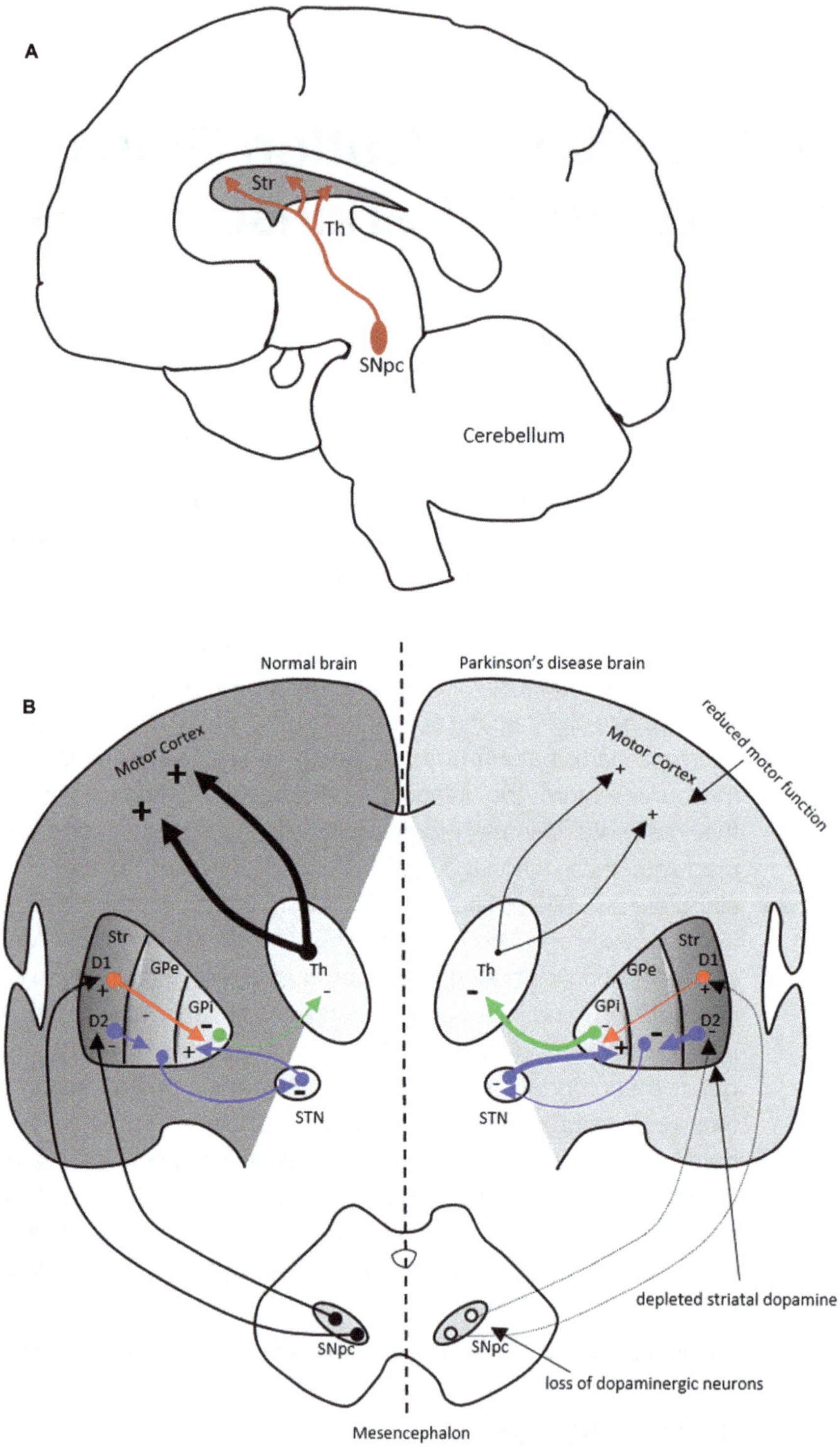

FIGURE 1 | The nigrostriatal dopaminergic pathway and motor basal ganglia circuitry in Parkinson's disease (PD) brain. **(A)** In the nigrostriatal pathway, the striatum, Str (caudate nucleus and putamen), receives dopaminergic innervation from the substantia nigra pars compacta (SNpc) in the midbrain. **(B)** A schematic showing normal motor basal ganglia circuitry (left side) and its irregularities in PD brain (right side), adapted from (Bjarkam and Sorensen, 2004). *Normal brain (left)*: The dopaminergic afferent neurons from the SN synapse with GABAergic neurons which display either D1 or D2 dopaminergic receptors. These GABAergic populations project directly (red arrows) or indirectly (blue arrows; through globus pallidus externa, GPe, and subthalamic nucleus, STN) to globus pallidus interna (GPi). The output from the GPi (green arrows) to the thalamus is inhibitory and modulates normal motor function. *PD brain (right)*: The loss of dopaminergic neurons in the SN and depletion of striatal dopamine leads to elevated inhibitory output from the GPi to the thalamus causing reduction in normal motor function. Inhibitory and excitatory inputs are marked as (–) and (+), respectively. The intensity of the inputs is marked with thickness of lines. Str, striatum; Th, thalamus.

studies (GWAS), implicating the human leukocyte antigen (HLA) locus with sporadic PD (Hamza et al., 2010) and, as well, by the neuropathology in PD brains demonstrating highly activated microglial and T-cells (McGeer et al., 1988; Imamura et al., 2003). Several inflammatory markers have been identified in SNpc of PD brains including cytokines and neurotrophins (Nagatsu et al., 2000; Hunot and Hirsch, 2003). Also, widespread microglial activation is a concomitant in PD neuropathology (Gerhard et al., 2006). A meta-analysis of anti-inflammatory drug trials revealed an association between non-steroidal anti-inflammatory drugs (NSAIDs) use and reduced risk for developing PD possibly implicating neuroinflammatory processes in the disease (Gagne and Power, 2010). Evidence supports the conclusion that microglia, the brain resident macrophage-like immune cells, participate in the inflammatory response of the disease (Qian and Flood, 2008; Long-Smith et al., 2009; Moehle and West, 2015). In addition, other observations implicate peripheral immune cells in PD (Saunders et al., 2012; Funk et al., 2013; Chen et al., 2015). Together these data indicate that inflammation and microglial activation contribute to the in pathogenesis of PD. Hence, immunomodulation might be a possible therapeutic avenue for PD.

The distribution of microglial M1/M2 phenotypes depends on the stage and severity of the disease. Understanding stage-specific switching of microglial phenotypes and the capacity to manipulate these transitions within appropriate time windows might be beneficial for PD therapy. In this review, we will outline different microglial activation states and provide evidence of M1/M2 activation states in PD. We will also discuss how manipulation of M1/M2 activation may be of potential therapeutic value.

MICROGLIA FUNCTIONS

In the central nervous system (CNS), the innate immune response is predominantly mediated by microglia and astrocytes. Microglia play a vital role in both physiological and pathological conditions. Tissue-specific macrophages can be found in most tissues of the body, whereas microglia are present distinctly in the brain. Microglia are derived from primitive yolk sac myeloid progenitors that seed the developing brain parenchyma (Alliot et al., 1999; Ginhoux and Jung, 2014). Microglia represent 10–15% of the total population of cells within the brain and manifest different morphologies across anatomic regions (Lawson et al., 1990; Mittelbronn et al., 2001). Microglia appear to be involved in several regulatory processes in the brain that are crucial for tissue development, maintenance of the neural environment and, response to injury and promoting repair. Similar to peripheral macrophages, microglia directly respond to pathogens and maintain cellular homeostasis by purging said pathogens, as well as dead cells and pathological gene products (Gehrmann et al., 1995; Bruce-Keller, 1999; Stevens et al., 2007; Tremblay et al., 2010; Olah et al., 2011; Paolicelli et al., 2011). In addition, microglial function can be altered by interactions with neurons, astrocytes, migrating T-cells, and the blood–brain barrier itself (Gonzalez et al., 2014).

Under physiological conditions, microglia acquire a neural-specific, relatively inactive phenotype (Schmid et al., 2009) where they sample and inspect the local environment and other brain cells types (Davalos et al., 2005; Nimmerjahn et al., 2005). In a healthy brain, resting quiescent microglia exhibit a ramified morphology, with relatively long cytoplasmic protrusions, a stable cell body and little or no movement (**Figure 2**). Quiescent microglia extend processes into their surrounding environment (Nimmerjahn et al., 2005). This resting stage is partly maintained by signals conveyed by neuronal and astrocyte-derived factors (Neumann et al., 2009; Ransohoff and Cardona, 2010). The maintenance of this inactive state is regulated by several intrinsic factors like Runx1 (Runt-related transcription factor 1) and Irf8 (Interferon regulatory factor 8), and extrinsic factors such as TREM2 (triggering receptor also expressed on myeloid cells-2), chemokine CX3CR1 and CD200R (Kierdorf and Prinz, 2013). In the normal CNS environment, healthy neurons provide signals to microglia via secreted and membrane bound factors, such as CX3CL1, neurotransmitters, neurotrophins and CD22 (Sunnemark et al., 2005; Frank et al., 2006; Lyons et al., 2007; Pocock and Kettenmann, 2007). In addition, microglia express elevated levels of microRNA-124 which in turn reduces CD46, MHC-II (major histocompatibility complex II) and CD11b, to maintain the quiescent state (Conrad and Dittel, 2011).

MICROGLIAL ACTIVATION: THE DUAL ROLES OF MICROGLIA

As peripheral macrophages respond to endogenous stimuli promoting both pathogenic and protective functions, so do microglia. Upon exposure to endogenous stimuli microglia become activated. Among the gene products released by microglia are various substances including pro-inflammatory cytokines, neurotoxic proteins, chemokines, anti-inflammatory cytokines, and neurotrophic factors (Mahad and Ransohoff, 2003; Block et al., 2007; Benarroch, 2013; Nakagawa and Chiba, 2015). Microglia also display signaling immunoreceptors such as Toll-like receptors (TLRs), scavenger receptors (SRs), nucleotide binding oligomerization domains (NODs) and NOD-like receptors (Ransohoff and Brown, 2012). Fundamentally, the two polar states of microglia, the M1 and M2 phenotypes are associated phenomenologically with injury and homeostasis, respectively (as described below). Differential states of microglial activation within an injured tissue evolve during an inflammatory epoch (Graeber, 2010).

M1 Polarization State

When classically activated, microglia acquire the M1 phenotype, characterized by pro-inflammatory and pro-killing functions that serve as the first line of defense. In M1 microglial activation state both secreted factors and cellular markers are dysregulated (**Table 1**). During M1 polarization (driving from another, often resting state), microglia release pro-inflammatory cytokines: interleukin-1β (IL-1β), IL-6, IL-12, IL-17, IL-18, IL-23, tumor necrosis factor-α (TNF-α), interferon-γ (IFN-γ) and

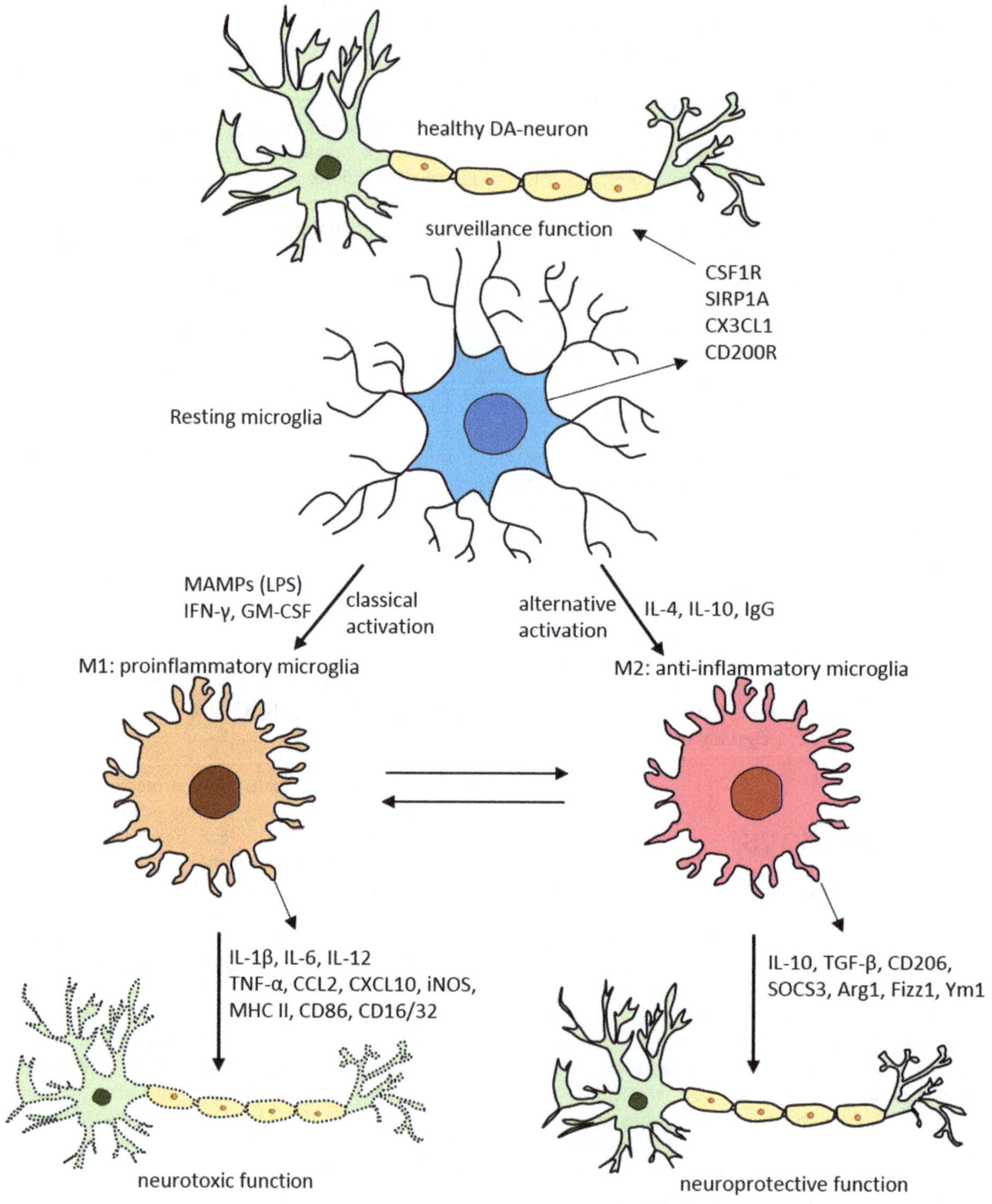

FIGURE 2 | Schematic of microglial polarization states and function. In normal physiological conditions microglia acquire the surveillance phenotype to maintain all CNS cell types including neurons. To maintain this surveillance state, microglia secrete several factors including colony stimulating factor 1 receptor (CSF1R), signal regulatory protein CD172 (SIRP1A), chemokine CX3CL1 and CD200R. Upon classical activation when triggered by LPS, IFN-γ, or GM-CSF microglia acquire M1 pro-inflammatory phenotype leading to neurotoxicity by secreting several pro-inflammatory substances (for detailed list, see **Table 1**). When activated alternatively by IL-1, IgG, or IL-10 microglia attain M2 anti-inflammatory state prompting neuroprotection through secretion of variety of substances (for detailed list, see **Table 1**). Arg1, arginase 1; CCL, chemokine (C-C motif) ligand; CD, cluster of differentiation; CSF1R, colony stimulating factor 1 receptor; CXCL, chemokine (C-X-C motif) ligand; Fizz1, found in inflammatory zone; IL, interleukin; GM-CSF, granulocyte-macrophage colony-stimulating factor; IFN-γ, interferon-γ; iNOS, inducible nitric oxide synthase; LPS, lipopolysaccharide; MAMPs, microbe-associated molecular patterns; MHC-II, major histocompatibility complex II; SIRP1A, signal regulatory protein CD172; SOCS3, suppressor of cytokine signaling-3; TNF-α, tumor necrosis factor-α; Ym1, chitinase-like protein.

TABLE 1 | Microglial polarization states and substances produced.

Activation type/function	Source	Substances produced	Reference
M1 (classical activation): pro-inflammatory and pro-killing	LPS, IFN-γ	*Cytokines*: IL-1β, IL-6, IL-12, IL-17, IL-18, IL-23, TNF-α *Markers*: CD86, MHC-II *Chemokines*: CCL2 *Metabolic enzyme/redox molecules*: iNOS, COX-2, reactive oxygen species and reactive nitrogen species prostaglandin E2	Mahad and Ransohoff, 2003; Kawanokuchi et al., 2006 Kawanokuchi et al., 2008; Loane and Byrnes, 2010; Benarroch, 2013; Chhor et al., 2013; Franco and Fernandez-Suarez, 2015; Nakagawa and Chiba, 2015
M2a (alternative activation): tissue repair and phagocytosis	IL-4, IL-13	*Cytokines*: IL-10 *Markers*: CD206, SR-A1, SR-B1, Arg1, Ym1, Fizz1 *Others*: extracellular matrix proteins, PPAR	Mahad and Ransohoff, 2003; Loane and Byrnes, 2010, Benarroch, 2013; Chhor et al., 2013; Franco and Fernandez-Suarez, 2015; Nakagawa and Chiba, 2015
M2b (alternative activation): recruitment of regulatory T cells	Fcγ receptors, TLRs and immune complexes (IgG)	*Cytokines*: IL-1β, IL-6, IL-10, TNF-α *Markers*: CD86, MHC-II *Others*: SOCS3, COX-2, Sphk	
M2c (alternative activation): anti-inflammatory and healing	IL-10, TGF-β and glucocorticoids	*Cytokines*: IL-10, TGF-β *Markers*: CD163	

Arg1, arginase 1; CCL, chemokine (C-C motif) ligand; CD, cluster of differentiation; COX-2, cyclooxygenase-2; Fizz1, found in inflammatory zone; IFN-γ, interferon-γ; IL, interleukin; iNOS, inducible nitric oxide synthase; MHC-II, major histocompatibility complex II; SOCS3, suppressor of cytokine signaling-3; Sphk, sphingosine kinase; SR-A1, scavenger receptor class A1; SR-B1, scavenger receptor class B1; TGF, transforming growth factor; TNF-α, tumor necrosis factor-α; Ym1, chitinase-like protein.

nitric oxide, and chemokines: CCL2 (Mahad and Ransohoff, 2003; Kawanokuchi et al., 2006, 2008; Loane and Byrnes, 2010; Benarroch, 2013; Nakagawa and Chiba, 2015). Also upon M1 activation microglia appear to present phenotypic markers: inducible nitric oxide synthase (iNOS), cyclooxygenase-2 (COX-2), MHC-II, and CD86 (cluster of differentiation marker 86) (Chhor et al., 2013; Franco and Fernandez-Suarez, 2015) and, other substances including reactive oxygen species (ROS), reactive nitrogen species, and prostaglandin E2 (Benarroch, 2013; Nakagawa and Chiba, 2015). These orchestrated processes are to purge foreign pathogens and polarize T-cells to elicit an adaptive immune response.

The M1 phenotype of microglia can be induced in experimental models using microbe-associated molecular pattern molecules such as lipopolysaccharide (LPS), an endotoxin present in the cell membranes of Gram-negative bacteria, or others related to infections such as IFN-γ (**Figure 3**; Loane and Byrnes, 2010; Boche et al., 2013). Similarly, an aseptic inflammatory response also occurs after exposure to trauma or ischemia-reperfusion injury or chemical injury.

IFN-γ utilizes the JAK/STAT (Janus kinase/signal transducer and activator of transcription) signaling pathway to activate the M1 phenotype. M1 activation by IFN-γ occurs through activation of IFN-γ receptors 1 and 2 (IFN-γR1/2) leading to JAK1/2 activation, phosphorylation and the nuclear translocation of STAT1 along with interferon regulatory factors (IRFs). This signaling cascade promotes expression of M1-associated cytokines, chemokines, and other genes (Hu and Ivashkiv, 2009; Boche et al., 2013).

LPS induces M1 activation via TLRs, which recognize specific patterns of microbial macromolecules. LPS binds to TLR4 on the cell surface that is coupled to MD2 (myeloid differentiation protein 2) (TLR/MD2) with participation of co-receptors CD14 and LBP (LPS-binding protein). LPS binding to TLR4 results in activation through MyD88 (myeloid differentiation primary response protein 88) and TRIF (TIR domain-containing adaptor inducing IFN-β), and transcription factors such as NF-κB (nuclear factor kappa B), STAT5, and IRFs (Takeda and Akira, 2004). This causes transcriptional upregulation of M1-associated cytokines, chemokines and other genes. Alternative M1 activation stimulation through granulocyte-macrophage colony-stimulating factor (GM-CSF) has been demonstrated recently (Lacey et al., 2012). However, unlike LPS and IFN-γ, GM-CSF is reported to instigate pleomorphic activation states that shows characteristics of both M1 and M2 phenotypes (Weisser et al., 2013). **Figure 3** (left side) provides further details on M1 activation.

M2 Polarization State

The alternative M2 microglial activation state is involved in various events including immunoregulation, inflammation dampening, and repair and injury resolution. M2 microglia is morphologically characterized by enlarged cell bodies (**Figure 2**). M2 microglial activation produces an array of mediators such as anti-inflammatory cytokines, extracellular matrix proteins, glucocorticoids, and other substances.

Presently, the mechanism of M2 activation in microglia is poorly understood compared to macrophages. It is believed that microglia can develop diverse M2 phenotypes similar to macrophages (Morgan et al., 2005; Herber et al., 2006; Schwartz et al., 2006). The characteristics of M2 polarization of microglia parallel that of the macrophages (Chhor et al., 2013; Freilich et al., 2013) producing IL-4 and IL-10 stimulation through Argl (arginase 1), Yml (chitinase-like protein), Fizzl (found in inflammatory zone), and PPAR (peroxisome proliferator-activated receptor) (Michelucci et al., 2009). M2 macrophage activation is sub-classified into M2a, M2b, and M2c, and these

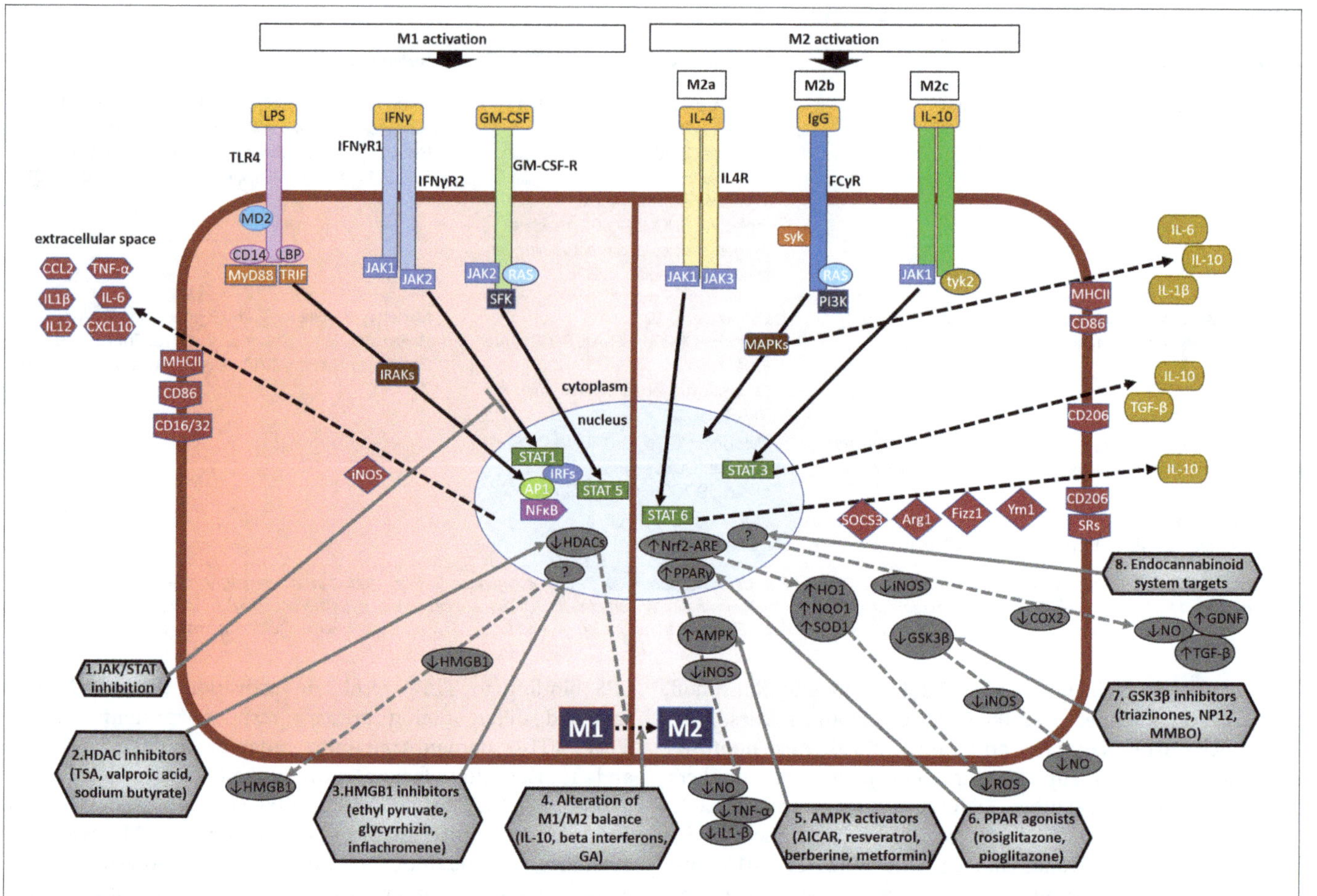

FIGURE 3 | Overview of microglial M1 and M2 signaling in neurodegeneration, and potential targets for neuroprotection. The left side of the figure compartment shows M1 microglial phenotype and its major signaling pathways. LPS binds to TLR4 on the cell surface which is coupled to MD2 (TLR/MD2) with participation of co-receptors CD14 and LBP (LPS-binding protein), activates interleukin-1 receptor-associated kinases (IRAKs) through MyD88 and TRIF that causes translocation of transcription factors such as NF-κB, STAT5, activator protein-1 (AP1), and interferon regulatory factors (IRFs) to the nucleus. M1 activation by IFN-γ occurs through IFN-γ receptors 1 and 2 (IFN-γR1/2) leading to the recruitment of Janus kinase 1 and 2 (JAK1/2) that phosphorylate and translocate STAT1 and IRFs to the nucleus. M1 activation stimulation through granulocyte-macrophage colony-stimulating factor (GM-CSF) occurs when GM-CSF binds to its receptor GM-CSF-R, which activates rat sarcoma oncoproteins (RAS), JAK2, and SFK, and causes translocation of STAT5 to the nucleus. The translocation of NF-κB, STAT1, STAT5, AP1, and IRFs to the nucleus causes upregulation of intracellular iNOS and cell surface markers (CD86, CD16/32, MHC-II). M1 stimulation also causes transcriptional upregulation of M1-associated pro-inflammatory cytokines (IL-1β, IL-6, IL-12, TNF-α) and chemokines (CCL2, CXCL10). The right side of the figure compartment shows various M2 microglial phenotypes and major signaling pathways involved. M2 activation can be classified into M2a, M2b, and M2c. M2a state is induced mainly by IL-4. IL-4 binds to IL-4R, which stimulates JAK1 or JAK3 that causes translocation of STAT6 to the nucleus leading to transcription of M2a-associated genes including IL-10, cell surface markers (CD206, scavenger receptors, SRs), and intracellular components such as suppressor of cytokine signaling 3 (SOCS3), Ym1 (chitinase-like protein) and Fizz1 (found in inflammatory zone). The M2b activation state, which has some M1 response characteristics, is stimulated when TLRs fuse Fcγ receptors, which then bind to IgG (B cells) to derive the M2b phenotype. M2b activation results in secretion of IL-10 and, cell surface markers (CD86, MHC-II). M2c activation is induced by IL-10 which stimulates the IL-10 Receptor 1 and 2 subunits that activates JAK1 leading to the translocation of STAT3 to the nucleus. STAT3 translocation inhibits M1-associated pro-inflammatory cytokines and upregulation of IL-10, TGF-β and the cell surface marker CD206. M2c state plays an important role in immunoregulation, matrix deposition and tissue remodeling. The bottom half of the figure shows potential therapeutic microglial targets for neuroprotection. (1) JAK/STAT inhibition: M1 phenotype is induced via the JAK/STAT signaling pathway and inhibition of this pathway may suppress the downstream M1-associated pro-inflammatory genes. (2) Histone deacetylase (HDAC) inhibitors: Histone acetylation is increased in M1 state that may lead to the expression and release of pro-inflammatory cytokines. HDAC inhibitors prevent neurodegeneration by shifting microglia toward protective M2 phenotype and anti-inflammatory mechanisms. (3) Microglia-produced high-mobility group box-1 (HMGB1) inhibitors: HMGB1 is a pro-inflammatory cytokine released by microglia which is toxic to neurons. HMGB1 inhibitors show neuroprotection by binding to HMGB1 and inhibiting its cytokine-like activity. (4) Alteration of M1/M2 balance: These agents promote the shift M1 pro-inflammatory phenotype toward protective M2 phenotype, and also exhibit neuroprotection by counteracting excessive pro-inflammatory M1 cytokines. (5) Adenosine monophosphate-activated protein kinase (AMPK) activators: AMPK activators act by inhibiting the expression of pro-inflammatory cytokines and iNOS by reducing NF-κB activation. (6) Peroxisome proliferator-activated receptor (PPAR) agonists: PPAR agonists exhibit neuroprotection by upregulating AMPK and protective genes, reducing oxidative damage, maintaining mitochondrial function and anti-inflammatory mechanisms. (7) Glycogen synthase kinase-3 β (GSK3β) inhibitors: GSK3β regulate microglial migration, inflammation, and neurotoxicity through astrocytes. GSK3β inhibitors decrease inflammation by reducing iNOS expression and release of nitric oxide (NO). (8) Endocannabinoid system targets: Agents that target the endogenous cannabinoid ligands anandamide and 2-arachidonoylglycerol (2-AG) increase TGF-β, arginase 1 and glial cell line-derived neurotrophic factor (GDNF), and reduce iNOS and COX-2, expression. AICAR, 5-amino-4-imidazole carboxamide riboside; GA, glatiramer acetate; HO-1, heme oxygenase 1; MMBO, 2-methyl-5-methylsulfinylphenyl-1-benzofuranyl-1,3,4-oxadiazole; NP-12, tideglusib; NQO1, NAD(P)H quinone dehydrogenase 1; Nrf2, nuclear erythroid 2-related factor 2; ARE, antioxidant response element; SOD1, superoxide dismutase 1; TSA, trichostatin A.

activation states may be envisaged to microglia (Boche et al., 2013; **Figure 3** and **Table 1**). The M2a state is induced by IL-4 or IL-13 and, is associated with tissue repair and phagocytosis. IL-4 binds to different receptor pairs, which stimulate JAK1 or JAK3 and activates STAT6 leading to transcription of M2a-associated genes including CD206, suppressor of cytokine signaling 3 (SOCS3) and SRs. The M2b activation state is stimulated by engagement of TLRs and the IL-1 receptor, and is involved in the recruitment of regulatory T cells. Activated TLRs fuse Fcγ receptors, which then bind to IgG (B cells) to derive the M2b phenotype. M2b activation results in secretion of IL-10, CD86 (on cell surface) and MHC-II. M2c activation state is induced by IL-10 and glucocorticoid hormones, and is involved in anti-inflammatory and healing functions. IL-10 stimulates the IL-10R1 and IL-10R2 which activate JAK1 leading to the translocation of STAT3 into the nucleus. STAT3 translocation suppresses most of the M1-associated pro-inflammatory cytokines (Franco and Fernandez-Suarez, 2015; Michell-Robinson et al., 2015). Overall, it is considered that the M2 activation promotes healing and tissue repair whereas the M1 activation state is the first line of defense with pro-killing functions. Please see **Figure 3** (right side) for details on M2 activation.

Polarization Transitions

The transition from the M1 pro-inflammatory state to the regulatory or anti-inflammatory M2 phenotype is thought to assist improved functional outcomes and restore homeostasis (Orihuela et al., 2016). Recently, histone H3K27me3 demethylase Jumonji was shown to be essential for M2 polarization and down-regulation of the M1 phenotype (Tang et al., 2014). The induction of M1 phenotype is a relatively standard response during injury. For peripheral immune cells it is thought that M1 polarization is terminal and the cells die during the inflammatory response (Orihuela et al., 2016). Although a shift from M1 to the M2 phenotype is considered rare for peripheral immune cells, the microglia *can shift* from M1 to M2 phenotype when exposed to IL-10, glatiramer acetate, beta interferons, PPARγ agonists and other molecules discussed in the later section. Although, the M1 and M2 microglial phenotypes vastly differ in their function, different subpopulations in an injury environment may express specific phenotypes resulting in concurrent expression of M1- and M2-related factors or mixed M1/M2 phenotypes (Ziegler-Heitbrock et al., 2010; Pettersen et al., 2011; Vogel et al., 2013). The potential to pharmacologically promote a microglial M1 to M2 shift may have therapeutic implications in the setting of neurodegenerative diseases associated with neuroinflammation.

MICROGLIA-MEDIATED INFLAMMATION IN PD

The involvement of innate immunity in PD was first proposed by McGeer et al. (1988) when brain from PD patients showed high levels of reactive microglia that were positive for human leukocyte antigen-D related (HLA-DR) in the substantia nigra and putamen. GWAS indicate that variants in the HLA region are linked to sporadic PD (Hamza et al., 2010; Hill-Burns et al., 2011). Activated microglia in PD brain appear responsible for exacerbating neurodegeneration (McGeer and McGeer, 2004), and the exposure of human neuromelanin discharged from dead DA neurons cause chemotaxis and increases the pro-inflammatory substances in microglial cultures (Wilms et al., 2007). M1 activation-associated inflammatory markers such as MHC-II (Imamura et al., 2003), TNF-α and IL-6 (Boka et al., 1994; Imamura et al., 2003) have been reported in patients with PD. Recent positron emission tomography (PET) studies show that PD patients have cortical microglial activation and lower brain glucose metabolism early in the disease, and imply that microglial activation may be a contributing factor in the disease progression (Edison et al., 2013). PET with inflammatory ligands show elevation in several areas of the basal ganglia involved in PD pathology (Gerhard et al., 2006; Edison et al., 2013; Iannaccone et al., 2013). TLR2 is increased in postmortem PD brain tissue, which correlates with pathological α-synuclein deposition. The neuronal TLR2 rather than glial expression of TLR2 is significantly elevated in PD brain and correlates with disease progression. In addition, TLR2 is strongly localized in α-synuclein positive Lewy bodies (Dzamko et al., 2017). These observations highlight the crucial role of neuroinflammation in PD pathogenesis.

PERIPHERAL INFLAMMATION IN PD

"The dual hit theory" of PD development states that a neurotropic pathogen enters the brain by nasal and/or gastric route by axonal transport, the latter via the vagus nerve (Braak et al., 2003; Hawkes et al., 2009). There is evidence that some forms of α-synuclein can be transmitted from the gut to the brain (Pan-Montojo et al., 2010; Ulusoy et al., 2013; Holmqvist et al., 2014). Instillation of rotenone into the rodent stomach exhibits progressive pathological α-synuclein inclusions in the enteric nervous system, the vagus nerve and subsequently in the brain stem (Pan-Montojo et al., 2010). Vagotomy prevents transport of pathological proteins from the gut to CNS (Phillips et al., 2008; Pan-Montojo et al., 2012). A recent study in Danish patients reveals that those who underwent full truncal vagotomy had lower risk for PD, suggesting that the vagus nerve might be critically involved in PD pathogenesis (Svensson et al., 2015). Another clinical study reports that serum levels of the pro-inflammatory cytokine IL-1β discriminated asymptomatic LRRK2-G2019S carriers from controls and suggests that peripheral inflammation is greater in a percentage of subjects carrying LRRK2-G2019S mutation (Dzamko et al., 2016).

The major peripheral immune cells, T-lymphocytes and B-lymphocytes, are not found in the CNS in normal biological conditions. However, with peripheral inflammation such as infection or injury, blood monocytes, and tissue-resident immune cells are activated and secrete variety of pro-inflammatory mediators including TNF-α, IL-6, and

IL-1β. These pro-inflammatory mediators cross the blood–brain barrier leading to the activation of brain resident microglia, which then triggers a neuroinflammatory cascade. The blood–brain barrier is considered to be impermeable to external pathogens and circulating macrophages, hence serving as an additional line of defense to the CNS. Nevertheless, damage to the integrity of the blood–brain barrier renders the brain vulnerable. PET studies on patients with PD reveal dysfunctional blood–brain barrier (Kortekaas et al., 2005). Damage to the blood–brain barrier in rats induce degeneration of dopaminergic neurons in the substantia nigra and activate glial cells (Rite et al., 2007). $CD8^+$ and $CD4^+$ T cells are observed in the postmortem human PD brain and MPTP (1-methyl-4-phenyl-1,2,3,6-tetrahydropyridine) mouse model of PD during its neurodegenerative phase suggesting T cell-mediated dopaminergic toxicity as a putative mechanism (Brochard et al., 2009). Moreover, rats with ulcerative colitis are more susceptible to LPS-induced dopaminergic neuron loss, blood–brain barrier permeability, microglial activation, and generation of pro-inflammatory mediators suggesting that peripheral inflammation may increase the risk of PD (Villaran et al., 2010). A recent study in the acute MPTP mouse model where nigrostriatal pathologies are not robust show that administration of chemokines [regulated on activation, normal T cell expressed and secreted (RANTES) and eotaxin] that facilitate T cell trafficking can lead to marked nigral α-synuclein pathology, loss of dopaminergic neurons and striatal neurotransmitter depletion, glial-associated inflammation, and motor impairments. However, systemic administration of pro-inflammatory cytokines, TNF-α and IL-1β, did not induce such disease pathologies in this acute MPTP model (Chandra et al., 2017). Taken together these studies suggest a more direct link between peripheral inflammation and, potential to elicit and affect the timing of PD onset.

GENETIC FACTORS LINKED TO INFLAMMATION IN PD

Mutations in leucine-rich repeat kinase (LRRK2, PARK8) are linked with autosomal dominantly inherited PD and is the greatest known genetic contributor to PD. LRRK2-G2019S mutation in the kinase domain is the most common mutation in both familial and sporadic form of the disease (Goldwurm et al., 2005). GWAS show that the genetic locus containing the LRRK2 gene presents a risk factor for sporadic PD (Singleton and Hardy, 2011). Interestingly, GWAS implicate LRRK2 as a major susceptibility gene in inflammatory bowel diseases that involve chronic inflammation (Barrett et al., 2008; Liu and Lenardo, 2012). LRRK2 is reported to be a target gene for IFN-γ, a M1-activation-associated pro-inflammatory cytokine. LRRK2 expression is elevated in human intestinal tissue of patients with Crohn's disease inflammation (Gardet et al., 2010). LRRK2 shows high expression in immune cells including microglia and inhibition of LRRK2 function reduces M1-associated inflammation and PD neurodegeneration (Moehle et al., 2012; Daher et al., 2014, 2015; Russo et al., 2015). Collectively, these studies point toward the importance of LRRK2 function in M1-activation responses in PD animal models (Moehle and West, 2015).

Three different missense mutations (A530T, A30P, and E46K) within the open reading frame or duplication or triplication of the wild type α-synuclein gene (SNCA, PARK1) are associated with autosomal dominant PD (Polymeropoulos et al., 1997; Kruger et al., 1998; Singleton et al., 2003; Zarranz et al., 2004). Fibrillar forms of α-synuclein are a major component of the Lewy bodies in both sporadic and familial PD. α-Synuclein, a cytoplasmic protein, can be expressed in microglia and may be involve modulation and pre-sensitization of microglial activation (Barkholt et al., 2012; Roodveldt et al., 2013; Zhang et al., 2017). Most activated microglia in PD patient brains are associated with α-synuclein-positive Lewy neurites (Imamura et al., 2003), and there is significant correlation between the expression of M1 activation-associated marker MHC-II and α-synuclein deposition in the substantia nigra of PD patients (Croisier et al., 2005). Previous studies by our group and others using *in vitro* and animal models show that both wild type and mutant α-synuclein can modulate microglial activation leading to neuroinflammation. Our previous work shows that α-synuclein activates microglia in a dose-dependent manner in cultured cells and an early microglial activation event occurs in mice overexpressing wild type α-synuclein (Su et al., 2008). Another study reveals that mutant α-synuclein can directly interact with cultured microglia releasing pro-inflammatory substances and mice overexpressing mutant α-synuclein exhibit microglial activation at a very early age (Su et al., 2009). In addition, we show that misfolded α-synuclein induces microglial activation and the release of pro-inflammatory cytokines in BV2 microglial cells (Beraud et al., 2013). Overexpression of α-synuclein in BV2 microglial cells increase pro-inflammatory mediators (TNF-α, IL-6, nitric oxide, COX-2) and induce a reactive microglial phenotype (Rojanathammanee et al., 2011). Interestingly, TLR4, which is activated by LPS to induce microglial M1-phenotype, is reported to mediate α-synuclein-induced microglial phagocytosis, upregulation of pro-inflammatory cytokine expression and ROS generation in primary microglial cultures (Fellner et al., 2013). In addition, α-synuclein is reported to play a crucial role in modulating microglial activation states in postnatal brain derived microglial cultures (Austin et al., 2006). Moreover, neuroinflammation with activated microglia and increased pro-inflammatory cytokines (TNF-α, IL-1β, IFN-γ) precedes α-synuclein-mediated neuronal cell death in rats delivered with mutant A53T human α-synuclein (Chung et al., 2009). There is a rich literature on the role of α-synuclein in the progression of PD by inducing microglia activation and neuroinflammation which is reviewed elsewhere (Zhang et al., 2017).

In addition, genes linked to familial recessive PD including phosphatase and tensin homolog (PTEN)-induced kinase 1 (PINK1, PARK6) and DJ-1 (PARK7) are strongly associated with neuroinflammation. Deletion of PINK1 or DJ-1 causes aberrant expression of genes involved in p38 MAP kinase/NF-κB signaling pathways that regulate innate immune responses in disease models (Cornejo Castro et al., 2010; Akundi et al., 2011).

INFLAMMATION IN PD ANIMAL MODELS

LPS, a bacterial endotoxin from cell wall of Gram-negative bacteria, induces M1-polarization of microglia through activation the pattern recognition TLR4. LPS administration into rodent brains recapitulate certain characteristics of sporadic PD including progressive degeneration of nigrostriatal dopaminergic pathway and motor anomalies. A single injection or 2-week infusion of LPS in the supranigral region in rat brain causes rapid microglia activation followed by dose and time-dependent degeneration of nigrostriatal dopaminergic circuitry (Castano et al., 1998; Gao et al., 2002; Liu, 2006; Dutta et al., 2008). Direct injection of LPS shows dopaminergic neuron loss specifically in SNpc but not in ventral tegmental area which also houses dopaminergic neurons (Kim et al., 2000). This specific neurotoxicity in SNpc may be attributed to the high proportion of microglia in SNpc compared with other brain regions (Lawson et al., 1990), that may trigger inflammatory events leading to the degeneration of nigrostriatal pathway. Moreover, injection of a TLR3 agonist in the substantia nigra of adult rats induces a sustained inflammatory reaction in the substantia nigra (SN) and dorsolateral striatum, and also increases the vulnerability of midbrain dopaminergic neurons to a subsequent neurotoxic trigger (Deleidi et al., 2010).

A transgenic mouse PD model that overexpresses human wild type α-synuclein, Thy1-aSyn (line 61) (Chesselet et al., 2012), shows microglial activation as early as 1 month and persists until 14 months of age (Watson et al., 2012). Increased levels of TNF-α, TLRs (TLR1, TLR2, TLR4, and TLR8), MHC-II, CD4, and CD8 are observed in Thy1-aSyn mice at different ages. This study also reveals that despite expression of α-synuclein globally in the brain only the regions containing cell bodies and axon terminals of nigrostriatal pathway show early inflammatory response. Another transgenic rodent model overexpressing doubly mutated (A53T and A30P) human α-synuclein show glial mitochondria alterations (Schmidt et al., 2011). In a PD mouse model that overexpresses human α-synuclein by recombinant adeno-associated virus vector, serotype 2 (rAAV2)-mediated transduction in the SNpc, inflammatory responses such as microglial activation and greater infiltration of B and T lymphocytes are observed in addition to dopaminergic neurodegeneration (Theodore et al., 2008). These studies show that animal models overexpressing human or mutant α-synuclein exhibit microglial activation and neuroinflammation.

MPTP, a meperidine analog byproduct, is a neurotoxin that causes acute and irreversible human parkinsonism (Davis et al., 1979; Langston et al., 1983). MPTP is a lipophilic compound that can actively cross the blood–brain barrier and gets oxidized by monoamine oxidase to the toxic cation, MPP^+ (1-methyl-4-phenylpyridinium) in the glial cells (Langston et al., 1984; Markey et al., 1984). MPP^+ utilizes the DA transporter (DAT) to get into the dopaminergic neurons. MPP^+ accumulates in the mitochondria and inhibits the mitochondrial complex I in the electron transport chain (ETC) (Nicklas et al., 1985; Ramsay et al., 1986) resulting in reduced ATP levels and production of ROS (Hasegawa et al., 1990; Chan et al., 1991; Hantraye et al., 1996; Przedborski et al., 1996; Fabre et al., 1999; Pennathur et al., 1999). In animal models, MPTP induces inflammatory responses that lead to neurodegeneration. MPTP causes microglial activation and an increase in M1-associated pro-inflammatory cytokines such as IL-6, IFN-γ and TNF-α. The glial response to MPTP is reported to peak before dopaminergic neuron loss (Czlonkowska et al., 1996; Smeyne and Jackson-Lewis, 2005). In support of these findings, it is reported that mice lacking IFN-γ or TNF-α signaling show resistance to MPTP-induced neurodegeneration (Sriram et al., 2002; Mount et al., 2007). Mice treated with MPTP show T-cell ($CD4^+$) infiltration into the substantia nigra and the MPTP-induced dopaminergic neuron loss is attenuated in T-cell deficient mice suggesting a pro-inflammatory role for T-cells ($CD4^+$) in MPTP neurotoxicity (Brochard et al., 2009). In addition, treatment with anti-inflammatory agents such as minocycline (Du et al., 2001), ibuprofen (Swiatkiewicz et al., 2013), flavonoid pycnogenol (Khan et al., 2013) and peptide carnosine (Tsai et al., 2010) and inhibition of pro-inflammatory mediators (Watanabe et al., 2004; Zhao et al., 2007), reduce inflammation and prevent neurodegeneration in MPTP animal models.

REGULATORS OF MICROGLIAL ACTIVATION STATES

Microglial activation, astrogliosis and invasion of activated peripheral immune cells trigger deleterious events in the brain that lead to neuronal loss and progression of PD (Hirsch and Hunot, 2009). These observations led to several animal studies and clinical trials to test a variety of established anti-inflammatory molecules (see **Table 2**). Acetylsalicylic acid, a COX-1/COX-2 inhibitor, exhibits neuroprotective effects in *in vitro* and in MPTP animal models of PD (Teismann and Ferger, 2001). A prospective clinical study shows that consumption of non-aspirin NSAIDs may delay or prevent the onset of PD (Chen et al., 2003). A Cochrane collaboration study which analyzed several prevention trials and observational anti-inflammatory studies reveals that while ibuprofen use might reduce the risk of developing PD, there is no existing evidence that supports NSAID use in PD prevention (Rees et al., 2011). A clinical study in PD cases shows an association between use of ibuprofen and lesser PD risk. However, this association is not shared by other NSAIDs studied (Gao et al., 2011). Similarly, minocycline, a tetracycline antibiotic that showed promising anti-inflammatory properties in PD animal models (Du et al., 2001; He et al., 2001; Wu et al., 2002), did not provide any symptomatic improvement in PD patients (Ninds Net-Pd Investigators, 2008). See **Table 2** for the list of anti-inflammatory agents studied in PD. Hence, NSAID use appears to provide benefits in PD susceptibility in some cases (Wahner et al., 2007; Samii et al., 2009; Gagne and Power, 2010; Steurer, 2011), however, this beneficial effect of NSAIDs were not replicated in several other studies (Shaunak et al., 1995; Bornebroek et al., 2007; Samii et al., 2009; Becker et al., 2011). One study even suggests that anti-inflammatory drug treatment may be detrimental if given at the later stage of the

TABLE 2 | NSAIDs and other anti-inflammatory agents in PD models and clinical trials.

Molecule	PD model	Mechanism	Response	Reference
Ibuprofen	Mouse MPTP	Anti-inflammatory	Prevent striatal-TH loss	Swiatkiewicz et al., 2013
	Clinical trial	Anti-inflammatory	Reduce PD risk	Gao et al., 2011
Acetylsalicylic acid	Mouse MPTP	COX-1/COX-2 inhibitor	Attenuate loss of nigral DA-neurons, striatal dopamine and locomotor activity	Teismann and Ferger, 2001
NSAIDs	Clinical trials	Anti-inflammatory	Delay or prevent onset of PD	Chen et al., 2003; Wahner et al., 2007; Samii et al., 2009; Gagne and Power, 2010; Steurer, 2011
	Clinical trials	Anti-inflammatory	Exacerbate PD symptoms/Does NOT improve PD risk	Shaunak et al., 1995; Bornebroek et al., 2007; Samii et al., 2009; Becker et al., 2011
Minocycline	Mouse MPTP Mouse 6-OHDA	Anti-inflammatory Anti-inflammatory	Attenuate loss of nigral DA-neurons and striatal dopamine Protect TH-positive cells	Du et al., 2001; Wu et al., 2002; He et al., 2001
	Clinical trial	Anti-inflammatory	Does NOT improve PD symptoms	Ninds Net-Pd Investigators, 2008

COX, cyclooxygenase; DA, dopamine; MPTP, 1-methyl-4-phenyl-1,2,3,6-tetrahydropyridine; NSAIDs, non-steroidal anti-inflammatory drugs; TH, tyrosine hydroxylase.

disease (Keller et al., 2011). This therapeutic approach aiming to counteract general neuroinflammation has failed in several disease therapies as reviewed elsewhere (Pena-Altamira et al., 2016). Collectively, these studies indicate that the non-specific inflammatory blockade is unlikely to be beneficial for the disease treatment. Concurrently, the data on the dual role of microglial activation has led to the emergence of the novel therapeutic strategy in other inflammatory diseases such as rheumatoid arthritis, ankylosing spondylitis, and multiple sclerosis (MS) (Rau, 2002; Braun et al., 2007; Wilms et al., 2010; Noda et al., 2013). This approach of the M1 to the M2 phenotype shift might be beneficial in neuroprotection compared to completely blocking microglial activation through anti-inflammatory drugs. Hence, a more reasonable approach of more specific treatment related to the M1/M2 activation stage by inhibiting the M1 responses and/or promoting the shift of M1 to M2 phenotypic responses is necessary in PD.

Targeting M1 Polarization State: Inhibition of Pro-inflammatory M1 Phenotype

M1 activation of microglia results in a pro-inflammatory and pro-killing output. To inhibit the pro-inflammatory damage through M1 activation of microglia, its downstream signaling pathways could be targeted. M1 phenotype is induced by IFN-γ via the JAK/STAT signaling pathway and targeting this pathway may arrest M1 activation. In fact, studies show that inhibition of the JAK/STAT pathway leads to suppression of the downstream M1-associated genes in several disease models including experimental allergic encephalomyelitis models and myeloproliferative neoplasms (Liu et al., 2014; Mascarenhas et al., 2014). Another approach to suppress M1 activation would be to target the pro-inflammatory cytokines such as TNF-α, IL-1β and IFN-γ, and decrease its ability to interact with its receptors on other cell types. TNF has been targeted through different approaches in PD animal models to suppress M1-associated toxicity. A single injection of lentivirus-expressing dominant negative TNF (DN-TNF) into the rat substantia nigra concomitantly with 6-hydroxydopamine (6-OHDA) lesion in the striatum attenuates dopaminergic neuron loss and behavioral anomalies in rats (McCoy et al., 2008). In another study intended to examine the role of TNF in delayed and progressive neurodegeneration model, rats administered with DN-TNF in the substantia nigra 2 weeks after the 6-OHDA lesion show no further dopaminergic neuron loss even after 5 weeks of 6-OHDA suggesting that TNF is an essential mediator of inflammation and hence a promising therapeutic target in PD (Harms et al., 2011). In addition, adeno-associated virus (AAV)-mediated transduction of dopaminergic neurons with human ras homolog enriched in brain with S16H mutation, [hRheb(S16H)], attenuates nigrostriatal toxicity in 6-OHDA rat model of PD (Kim et al., 2011, 2012). This protective effect is mediated by the production of cAMP response element-binding protein (p-CREB), glial cell line-derived neurotrophic factor (GDNF), and brain-derived neurotrophic factor (BDNF) in unilateral MPP^+ neurotoxin PD model (Nam et al., 2015).

PPARs are actively involved in microglial activation and inflammatory pathways. PPAR agonists are postulated to be beneficial for PD and other neurodegenerative diseases (Agarwal et al., 2017). The administration of a PPARγ agonist, rosiglitazone, arrests degeneration in both striatum and SNpc by decreasing TNF-α production and modulating microglial polarization in MPTPp (MPTP + probenecid) progressive mouse model of PD (Carta et al., 2011; Pisanu et al., 2014). Pioglitazone, a PPARγ agonist, prevents tyrosine hydroxylase (TH)-positive neuron loss in substantia nigra and partially averts striatal DA loss in MPTP mice model of PD. Pioglitazone treatment decreases microglial activation, iNOS production and nitric oxide-mediated toxicity in both striatum and substantia nigra (Dehmer et al., 2004). However, a recent clinical trial concluded that pioglitazone did not modify progression in early PD (Ninds Exploratory Trials in Parkinson Disease (Net-Pd) Fs-Zone Investigators, 2015). On the other hand, pioglitazone and rosiglitazone are currently being evaluated in clinical trials for its potential to reduce progression of AD. In addition, treatment of LPS/IFN-γ-activated neuronal and glial cultures with a PPARγ endogenous ligand, 15-deoxy-$\Delta^{12,14}$-prostaglandin J_2, inhibits pro-inflammatory response through the CD200-CD200R1 dependent mechanism (Dentesano et al., 2014). Unpublished data from our group show that administration of a PPAR agonist protects dopaminergic neurons in SNpc and neurites in striatum in MPTP mouse model of PD. This PPAR agonist reduces LPS-induced M1-associated pro-inflammatory cytokine IL-1β in BV2 cells and primary astrocytes in a PPARα-independent manner. Thus, PPAR agonists are potential molecules for curing PD through their property to inhibit M1 microglia-induced neuroinflammation.

Alterations in expression of cannabinoid receptors and endocannabinoid concentrations are illustrated in PD pathogenesis (Garcia et al., 2015). The endocannabinoid system includes the cannabinoid receptors CB1 and CB2, the endogenous ligands (anandamide and 2-arachidonoylglycerol, 2-AG), and their regulatory enzymes. CB1 receptors are abundant in neurons whereas CB2 receptors are most specifically expressed in glia (Onaivi, 2006; Lanciego et al., 2011; Fernandez-Suarez et al., 2014; Sierra et al., 2015). The expression of CB2 receptors significantly increases during microglial activation (Maresz et al., 2005; Yiangou et al., 2006) and CB2 receptors are reported to be localized in substantia nigra, and significantly downregulated in PD patients (Garcia et al., 2015). A naturally occurring CB2 receptor agonist, β-caryophyllene (BCP), prevented nigral DA-neuron and striatal-TH loss, reduced glial activation and inhibited pro-inflammatory cytokines in rat rotenone model of PD (Javed et al., 2016). Another study shows that a non-selective cannabinoid agonist protects loss of DA-neurons in the substantia nigra and DA in the striatum of MPTP intoxicated mice. In addition, this cannabinoid agonist also reduces MPTP-induced motor deficits and microglial activation (Price et al., 2009). Modification of the endocannabinoid system, to reduce pro-inflammatory toxicity, may provide a novel therapeutic avenue for PD treatment.

Tanshinone-I, a bioactive flavonoid, reduces the production of M1-pro-inflammatory mediators (nitric oxide, TNF-α, IL-6 and IL-1β) and, inhibits G-CSF and NF-κB expression after LPS-induced inflammation in BV2 microglial cell lines. In the MPTP mouse model of PD, Tanshinone-I prevents dopaminergic neurotoxicity, improves motor deficits and striatal neurotransmitters (Wang et al., 2015). Ghrelin, a stomach-derived endogenous ligand for growth hormone secretagogue receptor 1a (GHS-R1a), prevents loss of nigral dopaminergic neurons and striatal neurites, and improves motor performance in MPTP mouse model of PD. Ghrelin reduces toxicant-induced microglial activation, production of pro-inflammatory cytokines (IL-1β, TNF-α) and iNOS levels in MPTP mice (Jiang et al., 2008; Moon et al., 2009). Piperine, a naturally occurring bioactive molecule, attenuates the loss of TH-positive neurons in the substantia nigra and MPTP-induced motor anomalies. In addition, piperine decreases MPTP-induced microglial activation, pro-inflammatory IL-1β expression and apoptosis in these mice (Yang et al., 2015). See **Table 3** for the summary of other potential molecules that act by inhibiting M1 activation in PD models.

Targeting M2 Polarization State

The molecules with the capability to activate the anti-inflammatory M2 phenotype or promote the transition of pro-inflammatory M1 phenotype to anti-inflammatory M2 could be useful in the treatment of PD. Anti-inflammatory molecules such as IL-10 and beta interferons produce neuroprotection by altering the M1 and M2 balance. Cerebral infusion of AAV-expressing human IL-10 in a MPTP mouse model of PD decreases the expression of pro-inflammatory iNOS and importantly enhances the levels of anti-inflammatory mediators including IFN-γ and transforming growth factor-β (TGF-β). Infusion of AAV-expressing human IL-10 prevents the loss of striatal DA and reduces TH transcriptome levels suggesting neuroprotection in MPTP intoxicated mice (Schwenkgrub et al., 2013; Joniec-Maciejak et al., 2014).

Treatment with pioglitazone, a PPARγ agonist, causes a phenotypic conversion of microglia from the pro-inflammatory M1 state to the anti-inflammatory M2 state. This conversion is strongly linked to increase in phagocytosis of misfolded protein deposits resulting in the reduction of amyloid levels and an associated reversal of contextual memory deficits in AD mice (Mandrekar-Colucci et al., 2012). As mentioned before, pioglitazone treatment decreases microglial activation, iNOS production and NO-mediated nigrostriatal toxicity in MPTP mouse model (Dehmer et al., 2004).

The endocannabinoid system is implicated in PD pathogenesis (Garcia et al., 2015). In a chronic MPTPp model of PD, the administration of an inhibitor that prevents degradation of 2-AG (JZL184), an endocannabinoid ligand, prevents MPTPp-induced motor impairment and protects the nigrostriatal pathway (Fernandez-Suarez et al., 2014). MPTPp mice treated with JZL184 exhibits microglial phenotypic changes and restorative microglial activation along with increased TGF-β and GDNF levels.

Glatiramer acetate is a Food and Drug Administration (FDA) approved drug for MS treatment (English and Aloi, 2015) and its neuroprotective effect is mediated by activation of the microglial M2 phenotype (Giunti et al., 2014). Glatiramer acetate protects dopaminergic neurons in a MPTP mouse model by helping the recruitment of T lymphocytes in the SN, while inhibiting microglial activation and upregulation of GDNF expression (Benner et al., 2004; Burger et al., 2009). Glatiramer acetate also exhibits neuroprotection in Alzheimer's disease animal models where its treatment induces microglial co-localization with amyloid fibrils and a switch in microglial phenotype that produces insulin like growth factor 1 (Butovsky et al., 2006). Dimethyl fumarate (DMF), an approved drug for MS treatment, protects against the depletion of striatal DA and its transporters and, reduces MPTP-induced increase in IL-1β and COX-2 activity in MPTP mouse model of PD. DMF also modulates microglial activation states and restores nerve growth factor levels to provide neuroprotection in MPTP-intoxicated mice (Campolo et al., 2017). Other molecules that are reported to possess neuroprotective properties by inducing M2 microglial activation are listed in **Table 3**.

TABLE 3 | Molecules targeting microglia activation in PD animal models and clinical trials.

Molecule	PD model	Mechanism	Response	Reference
Pioglitazone	Mouse MPTP	Inhibit M1 phenotype	Prevent loss of nigral DA-neurons and partial striatal neurites	Dehmer et al., 2004
	Clinical trial	Inhibit M1 phenotype	Does NOT modify progression in early PD	Investigators, 2015
Rosiglitazone	Mouse MPTPp (MPTP + probenecid)	Inhibit M1 phenotype and induce M2 phenotype	Prevent loss of nigral DA-neurons and striatal neurites	Carta et al., 2011; Pisanu et al., 2014
Lentivirus-expressing dominant negative TNF (DN-TNF)	Rat 6-OHDA (concomitant model)	Inhibit M1-TNF	Prevent nigral DA-neuron loss and behavior deficits	McCoy et al., 2008
Lentivirus-expressing DN-TNF	Rat 6-OHDA (delayed model)	Inhibit M1-TNF	Prevent progressive nigral DA-neuron loss	Harms et al., 2011
AAV-expressing human IL-10	Mouse MPTP	Induce M2 phenotype	Prevent loss of striatal dopamine and TH	Schwenkgrub et al., 2013; Joniec-Maciejak et al., 2014
Glatiramer acetate	Mouse MPTP	Induce M2 phenotype	Prevent loss of nigral DA-neurons	Benner et al., 2004; Burger et al., 2009
Endocannabinoid ligand 2-AG enhancer	Mouse MPTPp	Induce M2 phenotype	Prevent loss of striatal dopamine and TH	Fernandez-Suarez et al., 2014
Tanshinone-I	Mouse MPTP	Inhibit M1 phenotype	Prevent nigral DA-neuron loss and motor deficits	Wang et al., 2015
β-Caryophyllene	Rat-rotenone	Inhibit M1 phenotype	Prevent loss of nigral DA-neurons and striatal neurites	Javed et al., 2016
Atractylenolide-I	Mouse MPTP	Inhibit M1 phenotype	Attenuate loss of nigral DA-neurons and behavior deficits	More and Choi, 2017
Loganin	Mouse MPTP	Inhibit M1 phenotype	Prevent loss of striatal dopamine and TH	Xu et al., 2017
α-Asarone	Mouse MPTP	Inhibit M1 phenotype	Attenuate behavior deficits	Kim et al., 2015
Capsaicin	Mouse MPTP	Inhibit M1 phenotype	Attenuate loss of nigral DA-neurons, striatal dopamine, and behavioral deficits	Chung et al., 2017
Isobavachalcone	Mouse MPTP	Inhibit M1 phenotype	Attenuate behavior deficits and neuronal necrosis	Jing et al., 2017
Vitamin-D	Mouse MPTP	Inhibit M1 phenotype and induce M2 phenotype	Prevent loss of TH-positive neurons	Calvello et al., 2017
Mitoapocynin	Mouse MPTP	Inhibit M1 phenotype	Attenuate loss of nigral DA-neurons, striatal dopamine and behavioral deficits	Ghosh et al., 2016
Ginsenoside Rg1	Mouse MPTPp	Inhibit M1 phenotype	Attenuate loss of nigral DA-neurons and behavior deficits	Heng et al., 2016

AAV, adeno-associated virus; DA, dopamine; IL, interleukin; MPTP, 1-methyl-4-phenyl-1,2,3,6-tetrahydropyridine; 6-OHDA, 6-hydroxydopamine; TH, tyrosine hydroxylase; TNF, tumor necrosis factor.

NOVEL MICROGLIAL TARGETS

Other novel potential microglial targets for immunomodulation are reviewed elsewhere (Pena-Altamira et al., 2016). These approaches include the following targets: (1) 5′ adenosine monophosphate-activated protein kinase (AMPK): a critical enzyme in cellular energy homeostasis, (2) microglia-produced high-mobility group box-1 (HMGB1): an early released pro-inflammatory cytokine, (3) glycogen synthase kinase-3β (GSK3β): an enzyme that mediates microglial migration and inflammation-induced neurotoxicity, and (4) histone deacetylases (HDACs).

CONCLUDING REMARKS AND FUTURE DIRECTIONS

The critical role of microglia in most neurodegenerative pathologies including PD is increasingly documented through many studies. Until recently, microglial activation in pathological conditions was considered to be detrimental to neuronal survival in the substantia nigra of PD brains. Recent findings highlight the crucial physiological and neuroprotective role of microglia and other glial cells in neuropathological conditions. Studies on anti-inflammatory treatments targeting neuroinflammation in PD and other diseases by delaying or blocking microglial activation failed in many trials due to the lack of a specific treatment approach, possibly the stage of disease and an incorrect understanding of mechanisms underlying microglial activation. With the updated knowledge on different microglial activation states, drugs that can shift microglia from a pro-inflammatory M1 state to anti-inflammatory M2 state could be beneficial for PD. The M1 and M2 microglial phenotypes probably need further characterization, particularly in PD pathological conditions for better therapeutic targeting. We support targeting of microglial cells by modulating their activation states as a novel therapeutic approach for PD.

AUTHOR CONTRIBUTIONS

HF conceived of the project, SS and HF wrote the manuscript.

REFERENCES

Agarwal, S., Yadav, A., and Chaturvedi, R. K. (2017). Peroxisome proliferator-activated receptors (PPARs) as therapeutic target in neurodegenerative disorders. *Biochem. Biophys. Res. Commun.* 483, 1166–1177. doi: 10.1016/j.bbrc.2016.08.043

Akundi, R. S., Huang, Z., Eason, J., Pandya, J. D., Zhi, L., Cass, W. A., et al. (2011). Increased mitochondrial calcium sensitivity and abnormal expression of innate immunity genes precede dopaminergic defects in Pink1-deficient mice. *PLoS ONE* 6:e16038. doi: 10.1371/journal.pone.0016038

Alliot, F., Godin, I., and Pessac, B. (1999). Microglia derive from progenitors, originating from the yolk sac, and which proliferate in the brain. *Brain Res. Dev. Brain Res.* 117, 145–152. doi: 10.1016/S0165-3806(99)00113-3

Austin, S. A., Floden, A. M., Murphy, E. J., and Combs, C. K. (2006). Alpha-synuclein expression modulates microglial activation phenotype. *J. Neurosci.* 26, 10558–10563. doi: 10.1523/JNEUROSCI.1799-06.2006

Barkholt, P., Sanchez-Guajardo, V., Kirik, D., and Romero-Ramos, M. (2012). Long-term polarization of microglia upon alpha-synuclein overexpression in nonhuman primates. *Neuroscience* 208, 85–96. doi: 10.1016/j.neuroscience.2012.02.004

Barrett, J. C., Hansoul, S., Nicolae, D. L., Cho, J. H., Duerr, R. H., Rioux, J. D., et al. (2008). Genome-wide association defines more than 30 distinct susceptibility loci for Crohn's disease. *Nat. Genet.* 40, 955–962. doi: 10.1038/ng.175

Becker, C., Jick, S. S., and Meier, C. R. (2011). NSAID use and risk of Parkinson disease: a population-based case-control study. *Eur. J. Neurol.* 18, 1336–1342. doi: 10.1111/j.1468-1331.2011.03399.x

Benarroch, E. E. (2013). Microglia: multiple roles in surveillance, circuit shaping, and response to injury. *Neurology* 81, 1079–1088. doi: 10.1212/WNL.0b013e3182a4a577

Benner, E. J., Mosley, R. L., Destache, C. J., Lewis, T. B., Jackson-Lewis, V., Gorantla, S., et al. (2004). Therapeutic immunization protects dopaminergic neurons in a mouse model of Parkinson's disease. *Proc. Natl. Acad. Sci. U.S.A.* 101, 9435–9440. doi: 10.1073/pnas.0400569101

Beraud, D., Hathaway, H. A., Trecki, J., Chasovskikh, S., Johnson, D. A., Johnson, J. A., et al. (2013). Microglial activation and antioxidant responses induced by the Parkinson's disease protein alpha-synuclein. *J. Neuroimmune Pharmacol.* 8, 94–117. doi: 10.1007/s11481-012-9401-0

Bjarkam, C. R., and Sorensen, J. C. (2004). Therapeutic strategies for neurodegenerative disorders: emerging clues from Parkinson's disease. *Biol. Psychiatry* 56, 213–216. doi: 10.1016/j.biopsych.2003.12.025

Block, M. L., Zecca, L., and Hong, J. S. (2007). Microglia-mediated neurotoxicity: uncovering the molecular mechanisms. *Nat. Rev. Neurosci.* 8, 57–69. doi: 10.1038/nrn2038

Boche, D., Perry, V. H., and Nicoll, J. A. (2013). Review: activation patterns of microglia and their identification in the human brain. *Neuropathol. Appl. Neurobiol.* 39, 3–18. doi: 10.1111/nan.12011

Boka, G., Anglade, P., Wallach, D., Javoy-Agid, F., Agid, Y., and Hirsch, E. C. (1994). Immunocytochemical analysis of tumor necrosis factor and its receptors in Parkinson's disease. *Neurosci. Lett.* 172, 151–154. doi: 10.1016/0304-3940(94)90684-X

Bornebroek, M., de Lau, L. M., Haag, M. D., Koudstaal, P. J., Hofman, A., Stricker, B. H., et al. (2007). Nonsteroidal anti-inflammatory drugs and the risk of Parkinson disease. *Neuroepidemiology* 28, 193–196. doi: 10.1159/000108110

Braak, H., Rub, U., Gai, W. P., and Del Tredici, K. (2003). Idiopathic Parkinson's disease: possible routes by which vulnerable neuronal types may be subject to neuroinvasion by an unknown pathogen. *J. Neural Transm.* 110, 517–536. doi: 10.1007/s00702-002-0808-2

Braun, J., McHugh, N., Singh, A., Wajdula, J. S., and Sato, R. (2007). Improvement in patient-reported outcomes for patients with ankylosing spondylitis treated with etanercept 50 mg once-weekly and 25 mg twice-weekly. *Rheumatology* 46, 999–1004. doi: 10.1093/rheumatology/kem069

Brochard, V., Combadiere, B., Prigent, A., Laouar, Y., Perrin, A., Beray-Berthat, V., et al. (2009). Infiltration of CD4+ lymphocytes into the brain contributes to neurodegeneration in a mouse model of Parkinson disease. *J. Clin. Invest.* 119, 182–192. doi: 10.1172/JCI36470

Bruce-Keller, A. J. (1999). Microglial-neuronal interactions in synaptic damage and recovery. *J. Neurosci. Res.* 58, 191–201. doi: 10.1002/(SICI)1097-4547(19991001)58:1<191::AID-JNR17>3.0.CO;2-E

Burger, D., Molnarfi, N., Weber, M. S., Brandt, K. J., Benkhoucha, M., Gruaz, L., et al. (2009). Glatiramer acetate increases IL-1 receptor antagonist but decreases T cell-induced IL-1beta in human monocytes and multiple sclerosis. *Proc. Natl. Acad. Sci. U.S.A.* 106, 4355–4359. doi: 10.1073/pnas.0812183106

Butovsky, O., Koronyo-Hamaoui, M., Kunis, G., Ophir, E., Landa, G., Cohen, H., et al. (2006). Glatiramer acetate fights against Alzheimer's disease by inducing dendritic-like microglia expressing insulin-like growth factor 1. *Proc. Natl. Acad. Sci. U.S.A.* 103, 11784–11789. doi: 10.1073/pnas.0604681103

Calvello, R., Cianciulli, A., Nicolardi, G., De Nuccio, F., Giannotti, L., Salvatore, R., et al. (2017). Vitamin D treatment attenuates neuroinflammation and dopaminergic neurodegeneration in an animal model of Parkinson's disease, shifting M1 to M2 microglia responses. *J. Neuroimmune Pharmacol.* 12, 327–339. doi: 10.1007/s11481-016-9720-7

Campolo, M., Casili, G., Biundo, F., Crupi, R., Cordaro, M., Cuzzocrea, S., et al. (2017). The neuroprotective effect of dimethyl fumarate in an MPTP-mouse model of Parkinson's disease: involvement of reactive oxygen species/nuclear factor-kappaB/nuclear transcription factor related to NF-E2. *Antioxid. Redox Signal.* doi: 10.1089/ars.2016.6800 [Epub ahead of print].

Carta, A. R., Frau, L., Pisanu, A., Wardas, J., Spiga, S., and Carboni, E. (2011). Rosiglitazone decreases peroxisome proliferator receptor-gamma levels in microglia and inhibits TNF-alpha production: new evidences on neuroprotection in a progressive Parkinson's disease model. *Neuroscience* 194, 250–261. doi: 10.1016/j.neuroscience.2011.07.046

Castano, A., Herrera, A. J., Cano, J., and Machado, A. (1998). Lipopolysaccharide intranigral injection induces inflammatory reaction and damage in nigrostriatal dopaminergic system. *J. Neurochem.* 70, 1584–1592. doi: 10.1046/j.1471-4159.1998.70041584.x

Chan, P., DeLanney, L. E., Irwin, I., Langston, J. W., and Di Monte, D. (1991). Rapid ATP loss caused by 1-methyl-4-phenyl-1,2,3,6-tetrahydropyridine in mouse brain. *J. Neurochem.* 57, 348–351. doi: 10.1111/j.1471-4159.1991.tb02134.x

Chandra, G., Roy, A., Rangasamy, S. B., and Pahan, K. (2017). Induction of adaptive immunity leads to nigrostriatal disease progression in MPTP mouse model of Parkinson's disease. *J. Immunol.* doi: 10.4049/jimmunol.1700149 [Epub ahead of print].

Chen, H., Zhang, S. M., Hernan, M. A., Schwarzschild, M. A., Willett, W. C., Colditz, G. A., et al. (2003). Nonsteroidal anti-inflammatory drugs and the risk of Parkinson disease. *Arch. Neurol.* 60, 1059–1064. doi: 10.1001/archneur.60.8.1059

Chen, Y., Qi, B., Xu, W., Ma, B., Li, L., Chen, Q., et al. (2015). Clinical correlation of peripheral CD4+cell subsets, their imbalance and Parkinson's disease. *Mol. Med. Rep.* 12, 6105–6111. doi: 10.3892/mmr.2015.4136

Chesselet, M. F., Richter, F., Zhu, C., Magen, I., Watson, M. B., and Subramaniam, S. R. (2012). A progressive mouse model of Parkinson's disease: the Thy1-aSyn ("Line 61") mice. *Neurotherapeutics* 9, 297–314. doi: 10.1007/s13311-012-0104-2

Chhor, V., Le Charpentier, T., Lebon, S., Ore, M. V., Celador, I. L., Josserand, J., et al. (2013). Characterization of phenotype markers and neuronotoxic potential of polarised primary microglia in vitro. *Brain Behav. Immun.* 32, 70–85. doi: 10.1016/j.bbi.2013.02.005

Chung, C. Y., Koprich, J. B., Siddiqi, H., and Isacson, O. (2009). Dynamic changes in presynaptic and axonal transport proteins combined with striatal neuroinflammation precede dopaminergic neuronal loss in a rat model of AAV alpha-synucleinopathy. *J. Neurosci.* 29, 3365–3373. doi: 10.1523/JNEUROSCI.5427-08.2009

Chung, Y. C., Baek, J. Y., Kim, S. R., Ko, H. W., Bok, E., Shin, W. H., et al. (2017). Capsaicin prevents degeneration of dopamine neurons by inhibiting glial activation and oxidative stress in the MPTP model of Parkinson's disease. *Exp. Mol. Med.* 49, e298. doi: 10.1038/emm.2016.159

Conrad, A. T., and Dittel, B. N. (2011). Taming of macrophage and microglial cell activation by microRNA-124. *Cell Res.* 21, 213–216. doi: 10.1038/cr.2011.9

Cornejo Castro, E. M., Waak, J., Weber, S. S., Fiesel, F. C., Oberhettinger, P., Schutz, M., et al. (2010). Parkinson's disease-associated DJ-1 modulates innate immunity signaling in *Caenorhabditis elegans*. *J. Neural Transm.* 117, 599–604. doi: 10.1007/s00702-010-0397-4

Croisier, E., Moran, L. B., Dexter, D. T., Pearce, R. K., and Graeber, M. B. (2005). Microglial inflammation in the parkinsonian substantia nigra: relationship to alpha-synuclein deposition. *J. Neuroinflammation* 2, 14.

Czlonkowska, A., Kohutnicka, M., Kurkowska-Jastrzebska, I., and Czlonkowski, A. (1996). Microglial reaction in MPTP (1-methyl-4-phenyl-1,2,3,6-tetrahydropyridine) induced Parkinson's disease mice model. *Neurodegeneration* 5, 137–143. doi: 10.1006/neur.1996.0020

Daher, J. P., Abdelmotilib, H. A., Hu, X., Volpicelli-Daley, L. A., Moehle, M. S., Fraser, K. B., et al. (2015). Leucine-rich repeat kinase 2 (LRRK2) Pharmacological inhibition abates alpha-synuclein gene-induced neurodegeneration. *J. Biol. Chem.* 290, 19433–19444. doi: 10.1074/jbc.M115.660001

Daher, J. P., Volpicelli-Daley, L. A., Blackburn, J. P., Moehle, M. S., and West, A. B. (2014). Abrogation of alpha-synuclein-mediated dopaminergic neurodegeneration in LRRK2-deficient rats. *Proc. Natl. Acad. Sci. U.S.A.* 111, 9289–9294. doi: 10.1073/pnas.1403215111

Davalos, D., Grutzendler, J., Yang, G., Kim, J. V., Zuo, Y., Jung, S., et al. (2005). ATP mediates rapid microglial response to local brain injury in vivo. *Nat. Neurosci.* 8, 752–758. doi: 10.1038/nn1472

Davis, G. C., Williams, A. C., Markey, S. P., Ebert, M. H., Caine, E. D., Reichert, C. M., et al. (1979). Chronic Parkinsonism secondary to intravenous injection of meperidine analogues. *Psychiatry Res.* 1, 249–254. doi: 10.1016/0165-1781(79)90006-4

Dehmer, T., Heneka, M. T., Sastre, M., Dichgans, J., and Schulz, J. B. (2004). Protection by pioglitazone in the MPTP model of Parkinson's disease correlates with I kappa B alpha induction and block of NF kappa B and iNOS activation. *J. Neurochem.* 88, 494–501. doi: 10.1046/j.1471-4159.2003.02210.x

Deleidi, M., Hallett, P. J., Koprich, J. B., Chung, C. Y., and Isacson, O. (2010). The Toll-like receptor-3 agonist polyinosinic: polycytidylic acid triggers nigrostriatal dopaminergic degeneration. *J. Neurosci.* 30, 16091–16101. doi: 10.1523/JNEUROSCI.2400-10.2010

Dentesano, G., Serratosa, J., Tusell, J. M., Ramon, P., Valente, T., Saura, J., et al. (2014). CD200R1 and CD200 expression are regulated by PPAR-gamma in activated glial cells. *Glia* 62, 982–998. doi: 10.1002/glia.22656

Du, Y., Ma, Z., Lin, S., Dodel, R. C., Gao, F., Bales, K. R., et al. (2001). Minocycline prevents nigrostriatal dopaminergic neurodegeneration in the MPTP model of Parkinson's disease. *Proc. Natl. Acad. Sci. U.S.A.* 98, 14669–14674. doi: 10.1073/pnas.251341998

Dutta, G., Zhang, P., and Liu, B. (2008). The lipopolysaccharide Parkinson's disease animal model: mechanistic studies and drug discovery. *Fundam. Clin. Pharmacol.* 22, 453–464. doi: 10.1111/j.1472-8206.2008.00616.x

Dzamko, N., Gysbers, A., Perera, G., Bahar, A., Shankar, A., Gao, J., et al. (2017). Toll-like receptor 2 is increased in neurons in Parkinson's disease brain and may contribute to alpha-synuclein pathology. *Acta Neuropathol.* 133, 303–319. doi: 10.1007/s00401-016-1648-8

Dzamko, N., Rowe, D. B., and Halliday, G. M. (2016). Increased peripheral inflammation in asymptomatic leucine-rich repeat kinase 2 mutation carriers. *Mov. Disord.* 31, 889–897. doi: 10.1002/mds.26529

Edison, P., Ahmed, I., Fan, Z., Hinz, R., Gelosa, G., Ray Chaudhuri, K., et al. (2013). Microglia, amyloid, and glucose metabolism in Parkinson's disease with and without dementia. *Neuropsychopharmacology* 38, 938–949. doi: 10.1038/npp.2012.255

English, C., and Aloi, J. J. (2015). New FDA-approved disease-modifying therapies for multiple sclerosis. *Clin. Ther.* 37, 691–715. doi: 10.1016/j.clinthera.2015.03.001

Fabre, E., Monserrat, J., Herrero, A., Barja, G., and Leret, M. L. (1999). Effect of MPTP on brain mitochondrial H2O2 and ATP production and on dopamine and DOPAC in the striatum. *J. Physiol. Biochem.* 55, 325–331.

Fellner, L., Irschick, R., Schanda, K., Reindl, M., Klimaschewski, L., Poewe, W., et al. (2013). Toll-like receptor 4 is required for alpha-synuclein dependent activation of microglia and astroglia. *Glia* 61, 349–360. doi: 10.1002/glia.22437

Fernandez-Suarez, D., Celorrio, M., Riezu-Boj, J. I., Ugarte, A., Pacheco, R., Gonzalez, H., et al. (2014). Monoacylglycerol lipase inhibitor JZL184 is neuroprotective and alters glial cell phenotype in the chronic MPTP mouse model. *Neurobiol. Aging* 35, 2603–2616. doi: 10.1016/j.neurobiolaging.2014.05.021

Franco, R., and Fernandez-Suarez, D. (2015). Alternatively activated microglia and macrophages in the central nervous system. *Prog. Neurobiol.* 131, 65–86. doi: 10.1016/j.pneurobio.2015.05.003

Frank, M. G., Barrientos, R. M., Biedenkapp, J. C., Rudy, J. W., Watkins, L. R., and Maier, S. F. (2006). mRNA up-regulation of MHC II and pivotal pro-inflammatory genes in normal brain aging. *Neurobiol. Aging* 27, 717–722. doi: 10.1016/j.neurobiolaging.2005.03.013

Freilich, R. W., Woodbury, M. E., and Ikezu, T. (2013). Integrated expression profiles of mRNA and miRNA in polarized primary murine microglia. *PLoS ONE* 8:e79416. doi: 10.1371/journal.pone.0079416

Funk, N., Wieghofer, P., Grimm, S., Schaefer, R., Buhring, H. J., Gasser, T., et al. (2013). Characterization of peripheral hematopoietic stem cells and monocytes in Parkinson's disease. *Mov. Disord.* 28, 392–395. doi: 10.1002/mds.25300

Gagne, J. J., and Power, M. C. (2010). Anti-inflammatory drugs and risk of Parkinson disease: a meta-analysis. *Neurology* 74, 995–1002. doi: 10.1212/WNL.0b013e3181d5a4a3

Gao, H. M., Jiang, J., Wilson, B., Zhang, W., Hong, J. S., and Liu, B. (2002). Microglial activation-mediated delayed and progressive degeneration of rat nigral dopaminergic neurons: relevance to Parkinson's disease. *J. Neurochem.* 81, 1285–1297. doi: 10.1046/j.1471-4159.2002.00928.x

Gao, X., Chen, H., Schwarzschild, M. A., and Ascherio, A. (2011). Use of ibuprofen and risk of Parkinson disease. *Neurology* 76, 863–869. doi: 10.1212/WNL.0b013e31820f2d79

Garcia, M. C., Cinquina, V., Palomo-Garo, C., Rabano, A., and Fernandez-Ruiz, J. (2015). Identification of CB(2) receptors in human nigral neurons that degenerate in Parkinson's disease. *Neurosci. Lett.* 587, 1–4. doi: 10.1016/j.neulet.2014.12.003

Gardet, A., Benita, Y., Li, C., Sands, B. E., Ballester, I., Stevens, C., et al. (2010). LRRK2 is involved in the IFN-gamma response and host response to pathogens. *J. Immunol.* 185, 5577–5585. doi: 10.4049/jimmunol.1000548

Gehrmann, J., Matsumoto, Y., and Kreutzberg, G. W. (1995). Microglia: intrinsic immuneffector cell of the brain. *Brain Res. Brain Res. Rev.* 20, 269–287. doi: 10.1016/0165-0173(94)00015-H

Gerhard, A., Pavese, N., Hotton, G., Turkheimer, F., Es, M., Hammers, A., et al. (2006). In vivo imaging of microglial activation with [11C](R)-PK11195 PET in idiopathic Parkinson's disease. *Neurobiol. Dis.* 21, 404–412. doi: 10.1016/j.nbd.2005.08.002

Ghosh, A., Langley, M. R., Harischandra, D. S., Neal, M. L., Jin, H., Anantharam, V., et al. (2016). Mitoapocynin treatment protects against neuroinflammation and dopaminergic neurodegeneration in a preclinical animal model of Parkinson's disease. *J. Neuroimmune Pharmacol.* 11, 259–278. doi: 10.1007/s11481-016-9650-4

Ginhoux, F., and Jung, S. (2014). Monocytes and macrophages: developmental pathways and tissue homeostasis. *Nat. Rev. Immunol.* 14, 392–404. doi: 10.1038/nri3671

Giunti, D., Parodi, B., Cordano, C., Uccelli, A., and Kerlero de Rosbo, N. (2014). Can we switch microglia's phenotype to foster neuroprotection? Focus on multiple sclerosis. *Immunology* 141, 328–339. doi: 10.1111/imm.12177

Goldwurm, S., Di Fonzo, A., Simons, E. J., Rohe, C. F., Zini, M., Canesi, M., et al. (2005). The G6055A (G2019S) mutation in LRRK2 is frequent in both early and late onset Parkinson's disease and originates from a common ancestor. *J. Med. Genet.* 42, e65. doi: 10.1136/jmg.2005.035568

Gonzalez, H., Elgueta, D., Montoya, A., and Pacheco, R. (2014). Neuroimmune regulation of microglial activity involved in neuroinflammation and neurodegenerative diseases. *J. Neuroimmunol.* 274, 1–13. doi: 10.1016/j.jneuroim.2014.07.012

Graeber, M. B. (2010). Changing face of microglia. *Science* 330, 783–788. doi: 10.1126/science.1190929

Hamza, T. H., Zabetian, C. P., Tenesa, A., Laederach, A., Montimurro, J., Yearout, D., et al. (2010). Common genetic variation in the HLA region is associated with late-onset sporadic Parkinson's disease. *Nat. Genet.* 42, 781–785. doi: 10.1038/ng.642

Hantraye, P., Brouillet, E., Ferrante, R., Palfi, S., Dolan, R., Matthews, R. T., et al. (1996). Inhibition of neuronal nitric oxide synthase prevents MPTP-induced parkinsonism in baboons. *Nat. Med.* 2, 1017–1021. doi: 10.1038/nm0996-1017

Harms, A. S., Barnum, C. J., Ruhn, K. A., Varghese, S., Trevino, I., Blesch, A., et al. (2011). Delayed dominant-negative TNF gene therapy halts progressive loss of nigral dopaminergic neurons in a rat model of Parkinson's disease. *Mol. Ther.* 19, 46–52. doi: 10.1038/mt.2010.217

Hasegawa, E., Takeshige, K., Oishi, T., Murai, Y., and Minakami, S. (1990). 1-Methyl-4-phenylpyridinium (MPP+) induces NADH-dependent superoxide formation and enhances NADH-dependent lipid peroxidation in bovine heart submitochondrial particles. *Biochem. Biophys. Res. Commun.* 170, 1049–1055. doi: 10.1016/0006-291X(90)90498-C

Hawkes, C. H., Del Tredici, K., and Braak, H. (2009). Parkinson's disease: the dual hit theory revisited. *Ann. N. Y. Acad. Sci.* 1170, 615–622. doi: 10.1111/j.1749-6632.2009.04365.x

He, Y., Appel, S., and Le, W. (2001). Minocycline inhibits microglial activation and protects nigral cells after 6-hydroxydopamine injection into mouse striatum. *Brain Res.* 909, 187–193. doi: 10.1016/S0006-8993(01)02681-6

Heng, Y., Zhang, Q. S., Mu, Z., Hu, J. F., Yuan, Y. H., and Chen, N. H. (2016). Ginsenoside Rg1 attenuates motor impairment and neuroinflammation in the MPTP-probenecid-induced parkinsonism mouse model by targeting alpha-synuclein abnormalities in the substantia nigra. *Toxicol. Lett.* 243, 7–21. doi: 10.1016/j.toxlet.2015.12.005

Herber, D. L., Maloney, J. L., Roth, L. M., Freeman, M. J., Morgan, D., and Gordon, M. N. (2006). Diverse microglial responses after intrahippocampal administration of lipopolysaccharide. *Glia* 53, 382–391. doi: 10.1002/glia.20272

Hill-Burns, E. M., Factor, S. A., Zabetian, C. P., Thomson, G., and Payami, H. (2011). Evidence for more than one Parkinson's disease-associated variant within the HLA region. *PLoS ONE* 6:e27109. doi: 10.1371/journal.pone.0027109

Hirsch, E. C., and Hunot, S. (2009). Neuroinflammation in Parkinson's disease: a target for neuroprotection? *Lancet Neurol.* 8, 382–397. doi: 10.1016/S1474-4422(09)70062-6

Holmqvist, S., Chutna, O., Bousset, L., Aldrin-Kirk, P., Li, W., Bjorklund, T., et al. (2014). Direct evidence of Parkinson pathology spread from the gastrointestinal tract to the brain in rats. *Acta Neuropathol.* 128, 805–820. doi: 10.1007/s00401-014-1343-6

Hu, X., and Ivashkiv, L. B. (2009). Cross-regulation of signaling pathways by interferon-gamma: implications for immune responses and autoimmune diseases. *Immunity* 31, 539–550. doi: 10.1016/j.immuni.2009.09.002

Hunot, S., and Hirsch, E. C. (2003). Neuroinflammatory processes in Parkinson's disease. *Ann. Neurol.* 53(Suppl. 3), S49–S58. doi: 10.1002/ana.10481

Iannaccone, S., Cerami, C., Alessio, M., Garibotto, V., Panzacchi, A., Olivieri, S., et al. (2013). In vivo microglia activation in very early dementia with Lewy bodies, comparison with Parkinson's disease. *Parkinsonism Relat. Disord.* 19, 47–52. doi: 10.1016/j.parkreldis.2012.07.002

Imamura, K., Hishikawa, N., Sawada, M., Nagatsu, T., Yoshida, M., and Hashizume, Y. (2003). Distribution of major histocompatibility complex class II-positive microglia and cytokine profile of Parkinson's disease brains. *Acta Neuropathol.* 106, 518–526. doi: 10.1007/s00401-003-0766-2

Javed, H., Azimullah, S., Haque, M. E., and Ojha, S. K. (2016). Cannabinoid type 2 (CB2) receptors activation protects against oxidative stress and neuroinflammation associated dopaminergic neurodegeneration in rotenone model of Parkinson's disease. *Front. Neurosci.* 10:321. doi: 10.3389/fnins.2016.00321

Jiang, H., Li, L. J., Wang, J., and Xie, J. X. (2008). Ghrelin antagonizes MPTP-induced neurotoxicity to the dopaminergic neurons in mouse substantia nigra. *Exp. Neurol.* 212, 532–537. doi: 10.1016/j.expneurol.2008.05.006

Jing, H., Wang, S., Wang, M., Fu, W., Zhang, C., and Xu, D. (2017). Isobavachalcone attenuates MPTP-induced Parkinson's disease in mice by inhibition of microglial activation through NF-kappaB pathway. *PLoS ONE* 12:e0169560. doi: 10.1371/journal.pone.0169560

Joniec-Maciejak, I., Ciesielska, A., Wawer, A., Sznejder-Pacholek, A., Schwenkgrub, J., Cudna, A., et al. (2014). The influence of AAV2-mediated gene transfer of human IL-10 on neurodegeneration and immune response in a murine model of Parkinson's disease. *Pharmacol. Rep.* 66, 660–669. doi: 10.1016/j.pharep.2014.03.008

Kawanokuchi, J., Mizuno, T., Takeuchi, H., Kato, H., Wang, J., Mitsuma, N., et al. (2006). Production of interferon-gamma by microglia. *Mult. Scler.* 12, 558–564. doi: 10.1177/1352458506070763

Kawanokuchi, J., Shimizu, K., Nitta, A., Yamada, K., Mizuno, T., Takeuchi, H., et al. (2008). Production and functions of IL-17 in microglia. *J. Neuroimmunol.* 194, 54–61. doi: 10.1016/j.jneuroim.2007.11.006

Keller, A. F., Gravel, M., and Kriz, J. (2011). Treatment with minocycline after disease onset alters astrocyte reactivity and increases microgliosis in SOD1 mutant mice. *Exp. Neurol.* 228, 69–79. doi: 10.1016/j.expneurol.2010.12.010

Khan, M. M., Kempuraj, D., Thangavel, R., and Zaheer, A. (2013). Protection of MPTP-induced neuroinflammation and neurodegeneration by Pycnogenol. *Neurochem. Int.* 62, 379–388. doi: 10.1016/j.neuint.2013.01.029

Kierdorf, K., and Prinz, M. (2013). Factors regulating microglia activation. *Front. Cell Neurosci.* 7:44. doi: 10.3389/fncel.2013.00044

Kim, B. W., Koppula, S., Kumar, H., Park, J. Y., Kim, I. W., More, S. V., et al. (2015). alpha-Asarone attenuates microglia-mediated neuroinflammation by inhibiting NF kappa B activation and mitigates MPTP-induced behavioral deficits in a mouse model of Parkinson's disease. *Neuropharmacology* 97, 46–57. doi: 10.1016/j.neuropharm.2015.04.037

Kim, S. R., Chen, X., Oo, T. F., Kareva, T., Yarygina, O., Wang, C., et al. (2011). Dopaminergic pathway reconstruction by Akt/Rheb-induced axon regeneration. *Ann. Neurol.* 70, 110–120. doi: 10.1002/ana.22383

Kim, S. R., Kareva, T., Yarygina, O., Kholodilov, N., and Burke, R. E. (2012). AAV transduction of dopamine neurons with constitutively active Rheb protects from neurodegeneration and mediates axon regrowth. *Mol. Ther.* 20, 275–286. doi: 10.1038/mt.2011.213

Kim, W. G., Mohney, R. P., Wilson, B., Jeohn, G. H., Liu, B., and Hong, J. S. (2000). Regional difference in susceptibility to lipopolysaccharide-induced neurotoxicity in the rat brain: role of microglia. *J. Neurosci.* 20, 6309–6316.

Kortekaas, R., Leenders, K. L., van Oostrom, J. C., Vaalburg, W., Bart, J., Willemsen, A. T., et al. (2005). Blood-brain barrier dysfunction in parkinsonian midbrain in vivo. *Ann. Neurol.* 57, 176–179. doi: 10.1002/ana.20369

Kruger, R., Kuhn, W., Muller, T., Woitalla, D., Graeber, M., Kosel, S., et al. (1998). Ala30Pro mutation in the gene encoding alpha-synuclein in Parkinson's disease. *Nat. Genet.* 18, 106–108. doi: 10.1038/ng0298-106

Lacey, D. C., Achuthan, A., Fleetwood, A. J., Dinh, H., Roiniotis, J., Scholz, G. M., et al. (2012). Defining GM-CSF- and macrophage-CSF-dependent macrophage responses by in vitro models. *J. Immunol.* 188, 5752–5765. doi: 10.4049/jimmunol.1103426

Lanciego, J. L., Barroso-Chinea, P., Rico, A. J., Conte-Perales, L., Callen, L., Roda, E., et al. (2011). Expression of the mRNA coding the cannabinoid receptor 2 in the pallidal complex of Macaca fascicularis. *J. Psychopharmacol.* 25, 97–104. doi: 10.1177/0269881110367732

Langston, J. W., Ballard, P., Tetrud, J. W., and Irwin, I. (1983). Chronic Parkinsonism in humans due to a product of meperidine-analog synthesis. *Science* 219, 979–980. doi: 10.1126/science.6823561

Langston, J. W., Irwin, I., Langston, E. B., and Forno, L. S. (1984). 1-Methyl-4-phenylpyridinium ion (MPP+): identification of a metabolite of MPTP, a toxin selective to the substantia nigra. *Neurosci. Lett.* 48, 87–92. doi: 10.1016/0304-3940(84)90293-3

Lawson, L. J., Perry, V. H., Dri, P., and Gordon, S. (1990). Heterogeneity in the distribution and morphology of microglia in the normal adult mouse brain. *Neuroscience* 39, 151–170. doi: 10.1016/0306-4522(90)90229-W

Liu, B. (2006). Modulation of microglial pro-inflammatory and neurotoxic activity for the treatment of Parkinson's disease. *AAPS J.* 8, E606–E621. doi: 10.1208/aapsj080369

Liu, Y., Holdbrooks, A. T., De Sarno, P., Rowse, A. L., Yanagisawa, L. L., McFarland, B. C., et al. (2014). Therapeutic efficacy of suppressing the Jak/STAT pathway in multiple models of experimental autoimmune encephalomyelitis. *J. Immunol.* 192, 59–72. doi: 10.4049/jimmunol.1301513

Liu, Z., and Lenardo, M. J. (2012). The role of LRRK2 in inflammatory bowel disease. *Cell Res.* 22, 1092–1094. doi: 10.1038/cr.2012.42

Loane, D. J., and Byrnes, K. R. (2010). Role of microglia in neurotrauma. *Neurotherapeutics* 7, 366–377. doi: 10.1016/j.nurt.2010.07.002

Long-Smith, C. M., Sullivan, A. M., and Nolan, Y. M. (2009). The influence of microglia on the pathogenesis of Parkinson's disease. *Prog. Neurobiol.* 89, 277–287. doi: 10.1016/j.pneurobio.2009.08.001

Lyons, A., Downer, E. J., Crotty, S., Nolan, Y. M., Mills, K. H., and Lynch, M. A. (2007). CD200 ligand receptor interaction modulates microglial activation in vivo and in vitro: a role for IL-4. *J. Neurosci.* 27, 8309–8313. doi: 10.1523/JNEUROSCI.1781-07.2007

Mahad, D. J., and Ransohoff, R. M. (2003). The role of MCP-1 (CCL2) and CCR2 in multiple sclerosis and experimental autoimmune encephalomyelitis (EAE). *Semin. Immunol.* 15, 23–32. doi: 10.1016/S1044-5323(02)00125-2

Mandrekar-Colucci, S., Karlo, J. C., and Landreth, G. E. (2012). Mechanisms underlying the rapid peroxisome proliferator-activated receptor-gamma-mediated amyloid clearance and reversal of cognitive deficits in a murine model of Alzheimer's disease. *J. Neurosci.* 32, 10117–10128. doi: 10.1523/JNEUROSCI.5268-11.2012

Maresz, K., Carrier, E. J., Ponomarev, E. D., Hillard, C. J., and Dittel, B. N. (2005). Modulation of the cannabinoid CB2 receptor in microglial cells in response to inflammatory stimuli. *J. Neurochem.* 95, 437–445. doi: 10.1111/j.1471-4159.2005.03380.x

Markey, S. P., Johannessen, J. N., Chiueh, C. C., Burns, R. S., and Herkenham, M. A. (1984). Intraneuronal generation of a pyridinium metabolite may cause drug-induced parkinsonism. *Nature* 311, 464–467. doi: 10.1038/311464a0

Mascarenhas, J. O., Cross, N. C., and Mesa, R. A. (2014). The future of JAK inhibition in myelofibrosis and beyond. *Blood Rev.* 28, 189–196. doi: 10.1016/j.blre.2014.06.002

McCoy, M. K., Ruhn, K. A., Martinez, T. N., McAlpine, F. E., Blesch, A., and Tansey, M. G. (2008). Intranigral lentiviral delivery of dominant-negative TNF attenuates neurodegeneration and behavioral deficits in hemiparkinsonian rats. *Mol. Ther.* 16, 1572–1579. doi: 10.1038/mt.2008.146

McGeer, P. L., Itagaki, S., Boyes, B. E., and McGeer, E. G. (1988). Reactive microglia are positive for HLA-DR in the substantia nigra of Parkinson's and Alzheimer's disease brains. *Neurology* 38, 1285–1291. doi: 10.1212/WNL.38.8.1285

McGeer, P. L., and McGeer, E. G. (2004). Inflammation and neurodegeneration in Parkinson's disease. *Parkinsonism Relat. Disord.* 10(Suppl. 1), S3–S7. doi: 10.1016/j.parkreldis.2004.01.005

Michell-Robinson, M. A., Touil, H., Healy, L. M., Owen, D. R., Durafourt, B. A., Bar-Or, A., et al. (2015). Roles of microglia in brain development, tissue maintenance and repair. *Brain* 138, 1138–1159. doi: 10.1093/brain/awv066

Michelucci, A., Heurtaux, T., Grandbarbe, L., Morga, E., and Heuschling, P. (2009). Characterization of the microglial phenotype under specific pro-inflammatory and anti-inflammatory conditions: effects of oligomeric and fibrillar amyloid-beta. *J. Neuroimmunol.* 210, 3–12. doi: 10.1016/j.jneuroim.2009.02.003

Mittelbronn, M., Dietz, K., Schluesener, H. J., and Meyermann, R. (2001). Local distribution of microglia in the normal adult human central nervous system differs by up to one order of magnitude. *Acta Neuropathol.* 101, 249–255.

Moehle, M. S., Webber, P. J., Tse, T., Sukar, N., Standaert, D. G., DeSilva, T. M., et al. (2012). LRRK2 inhibition attenuates microglial inflammatory responses. *J. Neurosci.* 32, 1602–1611. doi: 10.1523/JNEUROSCI.5601-11.2012

Moehle, M. S., and West, A. B. (2015). M1 and M2 immune activation in Parkinson's disease: foe and ally? *Neuroscience* 302, 59–73. doi: 10.1016/j.neuroscience.2014.11.018

Moon, M., Kim, H. G., Hwang, L., Seo, J. H., Kim, S., Hwang, S., et al. (2009). Neuroprotective effect of ghrelin in the 1-methyl-4-phenyl-1,2,3,6-tetrahydropyridine mouse model of Parkinson's disease by blocking microglial activation. *Neurotox. Res.* 15, 332–347. doi: 10.1007/s12640-009-9037-x

More, S., and Choi, D. K. (2017). Neuroprotective role of atractylenolide-I in an in vitro and in vivo model of Parkinson's disease. *Nutrients* 9, E451. doi: 10.3390/nu9050451

Morgan, D., Gordon, M. N., Tan, J., Wilcock, D., and Rojiani, A. M. (2005). Dynamic complexity of the microglial activation response in transgenic models of amyloid deposition: implications for Alzheimer therapeutics. *J. Neuropathol. Exp. Neurol.* 64, 743–753. doi: 10.1097/01.jnen.0000178444.33972.e0

Mount, M. P., Lira, A., Grimes, D., Smith, P. D., Faucher, S., Slack, R., et al. (2007). Involvement of interferon-gamma in microglial-mediated loss of dopaminergic neurons. *J. Neurosci.* 27, 3328–3337. doi: 10.1523/JNEUROSCI.5321-06.2007

Nagatsu, T., Mogi, M., Ichinose, H., and Togari, A. (2000). Changes in cytokines and neurotrophins in Parkinson's disease. *J. Neural Transm. Suppl.* 60, 277–290. doi: 10.1007/978-3-7091-6301-6_19

Nakagawa, Y., and Chiba, K. (2015). Diversity and plasticity of microglial cells in psychiatric and neurological disorders. *Pharmacol. Ther.* 154, 21–35. doi: 10.1016/j.pharmthera.2015.06.010

Nam, J. H., Leem, E., Jeon, M. T., Jeong, K. H., Park, J. W., Jung, U. J., et al. (2015). Induction of GDNF and BDNF by hRheb(S16H) transduction of SNpc neurons: neuroprotective mechanisms of hRheb(S16H) in a model of Parkinson's disease. *Mol. Neurobiol.* 51, 487–499. doi: 10.1007/s12035-014-8729-2

Neumann, H., Kotter, M. R., and Franklin, R. J. (2009). Debris clearance by microglia: an essential link between degeneration and regeneration. *Brain* 132, 288–295. doi: 10.1093/brain/awn109

Nicklas, W. J., Vyas, I., and Heikkila, R. E. (1985). Inhibition of NADH-linked oxidation in brain mitochondria by 1-methyl-4-phenyl-pyridine, a metabolite of the neurotoxin, 1-methyl-4-phenyl-1,2,5,6-tetrahydropyridine. *Life Sci.* 36, 2503–2508. doi: 10.1016/0024-3205(85)90146-8

Nimmerjahn, A., Kirchhoff, F., and Helmchen, F. (2005). Resting microglial cells are highly dynamic surveillants of brain parenchyma in vivo. *Science* 308, 1314–1318. doi: 10.1126/science.1110647

Ninds Exploratory Trials in Parkinson Disease (Net-Pd) Fs-Zone Investigators (2015). Pioglitazone in early Parkinson's disease: a phase 2, multicentre, double-blind, randomised trial. *Lancet Neurol.* 14, 795–803. doi: 10.1016/S1474-4422(15)00144-1

Ninds Net-Pd Investigators (2008). A pilot clinical trial of creatine and minocycline in early Parkinson disease: 18-month results. *Clin. Neuropharmacol.* 31, 141–150. doi: 10.1097/WNF.0b013e3181342f32

Noda, H., Takeuchi, H., Mizuno, T., and Suzumura, A. (2013). Fingolimod phosphate promotes the neuroprotective effects of microglia. *J. Neuroimmunol.* 256, 13–18. doi: 10.1016/j.jneuroim.2012.12.005

Olah, M., Biber, K., Vinet, J., and Boddeke, H. W. (2011). Microglia phenotype diversity. *CNS Neurol. Disord. Drug Targets* 10, 108–118. doi: 10.2174/187152711794488575

Onaivi, E. S. (2006). Neuropsychobiological evidence for the functional presence and expression of cannabinoid CB2 receptors in the brain. *Neuropsychobiology* 54, 231–246. doi: 10.1159/000100778

Orihuela, R., McPherson, C. A., and Harry, G. J. (2016). Microglial M1/M2 polarization and metabolic states. *Br. J. Pharmacol.* 173, 649–665. doi: 10.1111/bph.13139

Pan-Montojo, F., Anichtchik, O., Dening, Y., Knels, L., Pursche, S., Jung, R., et al. (2010). Progression of Parkinson's disease pathology is reproduced by intragastric administration of rotenone in mice. *PLoS ONE* 5:e8762. doi: 10.1371/journal.pone.0008762

Pan-Montojo, F., Schwarz, M., Winkler, C., Arnhold, M., O'Sullivan, G. A., Pal, A., et al. (2012). Environmental toxins trigger PD-like progression via increased alpha-synuclein release from enteric neurons in mice. *Sci. Rep.* 2:898. doi: 10.1038/srep00898

Paolicelli, R. C., Bolasco, G., Pagani, F., Maggi, L., Scianni, M., Panzanelli, P., et al. (2011). Synaptic pruning by microglia is necessary for normal brain development. *Science* 333, 1456–1458. doi: 10.1126/science.1202529

Pena-Altamira, E., Prati, F., Massenzio, F., Virgili, M., Contestabile, A., Bolognesi, M. L., et al. (2016). Changing paradigm to target microglia in neurodegenerative diseases: from anti-inflammatory strategy to active immunomodulation. *Expert Opin. Ther. Targets* 20, 627–640. doi: 10.1517/14728222.2016.1121237

Pennathur, S., Jackson-Lewis, V., Przedborski, S., and Heinecke, J. W. (1999). Mass spectrometric quantification of 3-nitrotyrosine, ortho-tyrosine, and o,o′-dityrosine in brain tissue of 1-methyl-4-phenyl-1,2,3, 6-tetrahydropyridine-treated mice, a model of oxidative stress in Parkinson's disease. *J. Biol. Chem.* 274, 34621–34628. doi: 10.1074/jbc.274.49.34621

Pettersen, J. S., Fuentes-Duculan, J., Suarez-Farinas, M., Pierson, K. C., Pitts-Kiefer, A., Fan, L., et al. (2011). Tumor-associated macrophages in the cutaneous SCC microenvironment are heterogeneously activated. *J. Invest. Dermatol.* 131, 1322–1330. doi: 10.103/jid.2011.9

Phillips, R. J., Walter, G. C., Wilder, S. L., Baronowsky, E. A., and Powley, T. L. (2008). Alpha-synuclein-immunopositive myenteric neurons and vagal preganglionic terminals: autonomic pathway implicated in Parkinson's disease? *Neuroscience* 153, 733–750. doi: 10.1016/j.neuroscience.2008.02.074

Pisanu, A., Lecca, D., Mulas, G., Wardas, J., Simbula, G., Spiga, S., et al. (2014). Dynamic changes in pro- and anti-inflammatory cytokines in microglia after PPAR-gamma agonist neuroprotective treatment in the MPTPp mouse model of progressive Parkinson's disease. *Neurobiol. Dis.* 71, 280–291. doi: 10.1016/j.nbd.2014.08.011

Pocock, J. M., and Kettenmann, H. (2007). Neurotransmitter receptors on microglia. *Trends Neurosci.* 30, 527–535. doi: 10.1016/j.tins.2007.07.007

Polymeropoulos, M. H., Lavedan, C., Leroy, E., Ide, S. E., Dehejia, A., Dutra, A., et al. (1997). Mutation in the alpha-synuclein gene identified in families with Parkinson's disease. *Science* 276, 2045–2047. doi: 10.1126/science.276.5321.2045

Price, D. A., Martinez, A. A., Seillier, A., Koek, W., Acosta, Y., Fernandez, E., et al. (2009). WIN55,212-2, a cannabinoid receptor agonist, protects against nigrostriatal cell loss in the 1-methyl-4-phenyl-1,2,3,6-tetrahydropyridine mouse model of Parkinson's disease. *Eur. J. Neurosci.* 29, 2177–2186. doi: 10.1111/j.1460-9568.2009.06764.x

Przedborski, S., Jackson-Lewis, V., Yokoyama, R., Shibata, T., Dawson, V. L., and Dawson, T. M. (1996). Role of neuronal nitric oxide in 1-methyl-4-phenyl-1,2,3,6-tetrahydropyridine (MPTP)-induced dopaminergic neurotoxicity. *Proc. Natl. Acad. Sci. U.S.A.* 93, 4565–4571. doi: 10.1073/pnas.93.10.4565

Qian, L., and Flood, P. M. (2008). Microglial cells and Parkinson's disease. *Immunol. Res.* 41, 155–164. doi: 10.1007/s12026-008-8018-0

Ramsay, R. R., Salach, J. I., Dadgar, J., and Singer, T. P. (1986). Inhibition of mitochondrial NADH dehydrogenase by pyridine derivatives and its possible relation to experimental and idiopathic parkinsonism. *Biochem. Biophys. Res. Commun.* 135, 269–275. doi: 10.1016/0006-291X(86)90972-1

Ransohoff, R. M., and Brown, M. A. (2012). Innate immunity in the central nervous system. *J. Clin. Invest.* 122, 1164–1171. doi: 10.1172/JCI58644

Ransohoff, R. M., and Cardona, A. E. (2010). The myeloid cells of the central nervous system parenchyma. *Nature* 468, 253–262. doi: 10.1038/nature 09615

Rau, R. (2002). Adalimumab (a fully human anti-tumour necrosis factor alpha monoclonal antibody) in the treatment of active rheumatoid arthritis: the initial results of five trials. *Ann. Rheum. Dis.* 61(Suppl. 2), ii70–ii73. doi: 10.1136/ard.61.suppl_2.ii70

Rees, K., Stowe, R., Patel, S., Ives, N., Breen, K., Clarke, C. E., et al. (2011). Non-steroidal anti-inflammatory drugs as disease-modifying agents for Parkinson's disease: evidence from observational studies. *Cochrane Database Syst. Rev.* 11, CD008454. doi: 10.1002/14651858.cd008454.pub2

Rite, I., Machado, A., Cano, J., and Venero, J. L. (2007). Blood-brain barrier disruption induces in vivo degeneration of nigral dopaminergic neurons. *J. Neurochem.* 101, 1567–1582. doi: 10.1111/j.1471-4159.2007.04567.x

Rojanathammanee, L., Murphy, E. J., and Combs, C. K. (2011). Expression of mutant alpha-synuclein modulates microglial phenotype in vitro. *J. Neuroinflammation* 8:44. doi: 10.1186/1742-2094-8-44

Roodveldt, C., Labrador-Garrido, A., Gonzalez-Rey, E., Lachaud, C. C., Guilliams, T., Fernandez-Montesinos, R., et al. (2013). Preconditioning of microglia by alpha-synuclein strongly affects the response induced by toll-like receptor (TLR) stimulation. *PLoS ONE* 8:e79160. doi: 10.1371/journal.pone.0079160

Russo, I., Berti, G., Plotegher, N., Bernardo, G., Filograna, R., Bubacco, L., et al. (2015). Leucine-rich repeat kinase 2 positively regulates inflammation and down-regulates NF-kappaB p50 signaling in cultured microglia cells. *J. Neuroinflammation* 12, 230. doi: 10.1186/s12974-015-0449-7

Samii, A., Etminan, M., Wiens, M. O., and Jafari, S. (2009). NSAID use and the risk of Parkinson's disease: systematic review and meta-analysis of observational studies. *Drugs Aging* 26, 769–779. doi: 10.2165/11316780-000000000-00000

Saunders, J. A., Estes, K. A., Kosloski, L. M., Allen, H. E., Dempsey, K. M., Torres-Russotto, D. R., et al. (2012). CD4+ regulatory and effector/memory T cell subsets profile motor dysfunction in Parkinson's disease. *J. Neuroimmune Pharmacol.* 7, 927–938. doi: 10.1007/s11481-012-9402-z

Schmid, C. D., Melchior, B., Masek, K., Puntambekar, S. S., Danielson, P. E., Lo, D. D., et al. (2009). Differential gene expression in LPS/IFNgamma activated microglia and macrophages: in vitro versus in vivo. *J. Neurochem.* 109(Suppl. 1), 117–125. doi: 10.1111/j.1471-4159.2009.05984.x

Schmidt, S., Linnartz, B., Mendritzki, S., Sczepan, T., Lubbert, M., Stichel, C. C., et al. (2011). Genetic mouse models for Parkinson's disease display severe pathology in glial cell mitochondria. *Hum. Mol. Genet.* 20, 1197–1211. doi: 10.1093/hmg/ddq564

Schwartz, M., Butovsky, O., Bruck, W., and Hanisch, U. K. (2006). Microglial phenotype: is the commitment reversible? *Trends Neurosci.* 29, 68–74.

Schwenkgrub, J., Joniec-Maciejak, I., Sznejder-Pacholek, A., Wawer, A., Ciesielska, A., Bankiewicz, K., et al. (2013). Effect of human interleukin-10 on the expression of nitric oxide synthases in the MPTP-based model of Parkinson's disease. *Pharmacol. Rep.* 65, 44–49. doi: 10.1016/S1734-1140(13)70962-9

Shaunak, S., Brown, P., and Morgan-Hughes, J. A. (1995). Exacerbation of idiopathic Parkinson's disease by naproxen. *BMJ* 311, 422. doi: 10.1136/bmj.311.7002.422b

Sierra, S., Luquin, N., Rico, A. J., Gomez-Bautista, V., Roda, E., Dopeso-Reyes, I. G., et al. (2015). Detection of cannabinoid receptors CB1 and CB2 within basal ganglia output neurons in macaques: changes following experimental parkinsonism. *Brain Struct. Funct.* 220, 2721–2738. doi: 10.1007/s00429-014-0823-8

Singleton, A., and Hardy, J. (2011). A generalizable hypothesis for the genetic architecture of disease: pleomorphic risk loci. *Hum. Mol. Genet.* 20, R158–R162. doi: 10.1093/hmg/ddr358

Singleton, A. B., Farrer, M., Johnson, J., Singleton, A., Hague, S., Kachergus, J., et al. (2003). alpha-Synuclein locus triplication causes Parkinson's disease. *Science* 302, 841. doi: 10.1126/science.1090278

Smeyne, R. J., and Jackson-Lewis, V. (2005). The MPTP model of Parkinson's disease. *Brain Res. Mol. Brain Res.* 134, 57–66. doi: 10.1016/j.molbrainres.2004.09.017

Spillantini, M. G., Schmidt, M. L., Lee, V. M., Trojanowski, J. Q., Jakes, R., and Goedert, M. (1997). Alpha-synuclein in lewy bodies. *Nature* 388, 839–840. doi: 10.1038/42166

Sriram, K., Matheson, J. M., Benkovic, S. A., Miller, D. B., Luster, M. I., and O'Callaghan, J. P. (2002). Mice deficient in TNF receptors are protected against dopaminergic neurotoxicity: implications for Parkinson's disease. *FASEB J.* 16, 1474–1476. doi: 10.1096/fj.02-0216fje

Steurer, J. (2011). [Nonsteroidal analgesics have a protective effect against Parkinson disease]. *Praxis* 100, 617–618. doi: 10.1024/1661-8157/a000535

Stevens, B., Allen, N. J., Vazquez, L. E., Howell, G. R., Christopherson, K. S., Nouri, N., et al. (2007). The classical complement cascade mediates CNS synapse elimination. *Cell* 131, 1164–1178. doi: 10.1016/j.cell.2007.10.036

Su, X., Federoff, H. J., and Maguire-Zeiss, K. A. (2009). Mutant alpha-synuclein overexpression mediates early proinflammatory activity. *Neurotox. Res.* 16, 238–254. doi: 10.1007/s12640-009-9053-x

Su, X., Maguire-Zeiss, K. A., Giuliano, R., Prifti, L., Venkatesh, K., and Federoff, H. J. (2008). Synuclein activates microglia in a model of Parkinson's disease. *Neurobiol. Aging* 29, 1690–1701. doi: 10.1016/j.neurobiolaging.2007.04.006

Sunnemark, D., Eltayeb, S., Nilsson, M., Wallstrom, E., Lassmann, H., Olsson, T., et al. (2005). CX3CL1 (fractalkine) and CX3CR1 expression in myelin oligodendrocyte glycoprotein-induced experimental autoimmune encephalomyelitis: kinetics and cellular origin. *J. Neuroinflammation* 2, 17.

Svensson, E., Horvath-Puho, E., Thomsen, R. W., Djurhuus, J. C., Pedersen, L., Borghammer, P., et al. (2015). Vagotomy and subsequent risk of Parkinson's disease. *Ann. Neurol.* 78, 522–529. doi: 10.1002/ana.24448

Swiatkiewicz, M., Zaremba, M., Joniec, I., Czlonkowski, A., and Kurkowska-Jastrzebska, I. (2013). Potential neuroprotective effect of ibuprofen, insights from the mice model of Parkinson's disease. *Pharmacol. Rep.* 65, 1227–1236. doi: 10.1016/S1734-1140(13)71480-4

Takeda, K., and Akira, S. (2004). TLR signaling pathways. *Semin. Immunol.* 16, 3–9. doi: 10.1016/j.smim.2003.10.003

Tang, Y., Li, T., Li, J., Yang, J., Liu, H., Zhang, X. J., et al. (2014). Jmjd3 is essential for the epigenetic modulation of microglia phenotypes in the immune pathogenesis of Parkinson's disease. *Cell Death Differ.* 21, 369–380. doi: 10.1038/cdd.2013.159

Teismann, P., and Ferger, B. (2001). Inhibition of the cyclooxygenase isoenzymes COX-1 and COX-2 provide neuroprotection in the MPTP-mouse model of Parkinson's disease. *Synapse* 39, 167–174. doi: 10.1002/1098-2396(200102)39:2<167::AID-SYN8>3.0.CO;2-U

Theodore, S., Cao, S., McLean, P. J., and Standaert, D. G. (2008). Targeted overexpression of human alpha-synuclein triggers microglial activation and an adaptive immune response in a mouse model of Parkinson disease. *J. Neuropathol. Exp. Neurol.* 67, 1149–1158. doi: 10.1097/NEN.0b013e31818e5e99

Tremblay, M. E., Lowery, R. L., and Majewska, A. K. (2010). Microglial interactions with synapses are modulated by visual experience. *PLoS Biol.* 8:e1000527. doi: 10.1371/journal.pbio.1000527

Tsai, S. J., Kuo, W. W., Liu, W. H., and Yin, M. C. (2010). Antioxidative and anti-inflammatory protection from carnosine in the striatum of MPTP-treated mice. *J. Agric. Food Chem.* 58, 11510–11516. doi: 10.1021/jf103258p

Ulusoy, A., Rusconi, R., Perez-Revuelta, B. I., Musgrove, R. E., Helwig, M., Winzen-Reichert, B., et al. (2013). Caudo-rostral brain spreading of alpha-synuclein through vagal connections. *EMBO Mol. Med.* 5, 1051–1059. doi: 10.1002/emmm.201302475

Villaran, R. F., Espinosa-Oliva, A. M., Sarmiento, M., De Pablos, R. M., Arguelles, S., Delgado-Cortes, M. J., et al. (2010). Ulcerative colitis exacerbates lipopolysaccharide-induced damage to the nigral dopaminergic system: potential risk factor in Parkinson's disease. *J. Neurochem.* 114, 1687–1700. doi: 10.1111/j.1471-4159.2010.06879.x

Vogel, D. Y., Vereyken, E. J., Glim, J. E., Heijnen, P. D., Moeton, M., van der Valk, P., et al. (2013). Macrophages in inflammatory multiple sclerosis lesions have an intermediate activation status. *J. Neuroinflammation* 10:35. doi: 10.1186/1742-2094-10-35

Wahner, A. D., Bronstein, J. M., Bordelon, Y. M., and Ritz, B. (2007). Nonsteroidal anti-inflammatory drugs may protect against Parkinson disease. *Neurology* 69, 1836–1842. doi: 10.1212/01.wnl.0000279519.99344.ad

Wang, S., Jing, H., Yang, H., Liu, Z., Guo, H., Chai, L., et al. (2015). Tanshinone I selectively suppresses pro-inflammatory genes expression in activated microglia and prevents nigrostriatal dopaminergic neurodegeneration in a mouse model of Parkinson's disease. *J. Ethnopharmacol.* 164, 247–255. doi: 10.1016/j.jep.2015.01.042

Watanabe, H., Muramatsu, Y., Kurosaki, R., Michimata, M., Matsubara, M., Imai, Y., et al. (2004). Protective effects of neuronal nitric oxide synthase inhibitor in mouse brain against MPTP neurotoxicity: an immunohistological study. *Eur. Neuropsychopharmacol.* 14, 93–104. doi: 10.1016/S0924-977X(03)00065-8

Watson, M. B., Richter, F., Lee, S. K., Gabby, L., Wu, J., Masliah, E., et al. (2012). Regionally-specific microglial activation in young mice over-expressing human wildtype alpha-synuclein. *Exp. Neurol.* 237, 318–334. doi: 10.1016/j.expneurol.2012.06.025

Weisser, S. B., McLarren, K. W., Kuroda, E., and Sly, L. M. (2013). Generation and characterization of murine alternatively activated macrophages. *Methods Mol. Biol.* 946, 225–239. doi: 10.1007/978-1-62703-128-8_14

Wilms, H., Sievers, J., Rickert, U., Rostami-Yazdi, M., Mrowietz, U., and Lucius, R. (2010). Dimethylfumarate inhibits microglial and astrocytic inflammation by suppressing the synthesis of nitric oxide, IL-1beta, TNF-alpha and IL-6 in an in-vitro model of brain inflammation. *J. Neuroinflammation* 7:30. doi: 10.1186/1742-2094-7-30

Wilms, H., Zecca, L., Rosenstiel, P., Sievers, J., Deuschl, G., and Lucius, R. (2007). Inflammation in Parkinson's diseases and other neurodegenerative diseases: cause and therapeutic implications. *Curr. Pharm. Des.* 13, 1925–1928. doi: 10.2174/138161207780858429

Wu, D. C., Jackson-Lewis, V., Vila, M., Tieu, K., Teismann, P., Vadseth, C., et al. (2002). Blockade of microglial activation is neuroprotective in the 1-methyl-4-phenyl-1,2,3,6-tetrahydropyridine mouse model of Parkinson disease. *J. Neurosci.* 22, 1763–1771.

Xu, Y. D., Cui, C., Sun, M. F., Zhu, Y. L., Chu, M., Shi, Y. W., et al. (2017). Neuroprotective effects of loganin on MPTP-induced Parkinson's disease mice: neurochemistry, glial reaction and autophagy studies. *J. Cell. Biochem.* [Epub ahead of print], doi: 10.1002/jcb.26010

Yang, W., Chen, Y. H., Liu, H., and Qu, H. D. (2015). Neuroprotective effects of piperine on the 1-methyl-4-phenyl-1,2,3,6-tetrahydropyridine-induced Parkinson's disease mouse model. *Int. J. Mol. Med.* 36, 1369–1376. doi: 10.3892/ijmm.2015.2356

Yiangou, Y., Facer, P., Durrenberger, P., Chessell, I. P., Naylor, A., Bountra, C., et al. (2006). COX-2, CB2 and P2X7-immunoreactivities are increased in activated microglial cells/macrophages of multiple sclerosis and amyotrophic lateral sclerosis spinal cord. *BMC Neurol.* 6:12. doi: 10.1186/1471-2377-6-12

Zarranz, J. J., Alegre, J., Gomez-Esteban, J. C., Lezcano, E., Ros, R., Ampuero, I., et al. (2004). The new mutation, E46K, of alpha-synuclein causes Parkinson and Lewy body dementia. *Ann. Neurol.* 55, 164–173. doi: 10.1002/ana.10795

Zhang, Q. S., Heng, Y., Yuan, Y. H., and Chen, N. H. (2017). Pathological alpha-synuclein exacerbates the progression of Parkinson's disease through microglial activation. *Toxicol. Lett.* 265, 30–37. doi: 10.1016/j.toxlet.2016.11.002

Zhao, C., Ling, Z., Newman, M. B., Bhatia, A., and Carvey, P. M. (2007). TNF-alpha knockout and minocycline treatment attenuates blood-brain barrier leakage in MPTP-treated mice. *Neurobiol. Dis.* 26, 36–46. doi: 10.1016/j.nbd.2006.11.012

Ziegler-Heitbrock, L., Ancuta, P., Crowe, S., Dalod, M., Grau, V., Hart, D. N., et al. (2010). Nomenclature of monocytes and dendritic cells in blood. *Blood* 116, e74–e80. doi: 10.1182/blood-2010-02-258558

15

The Role of Microglia in Retinal Neurodegeneration: Alzheimer's Disease, Parkinson and Glaucoma

Ana I. Ramirez [1,2], *Rosa de Hoz* [1,2], *Elena Salobrar-Garcia* [1,3], *Juan J. Salazar* [1,2], *Blanca Rojas* [1,3], *Daniel Ajoy* [1], *Inés López-Cuenca* [1], *Pilar Rojas* [1,4], *Alberto Triviño* [1,3] and *José M. Ramírez* [1,3]*

[1] *Instituto de Investigaciones Oftalmológicas Ramón Castroviejo. Universidad Complutense de Madrid, Madrid, Spain,* [2] *Departamento de Oftalmología y ORL, Facultad de Óptica y Optometría, Universidad Complutense de Madrid (UCM), Madrid, Spain,* [3] *Departamento de Oftalmología y ORL, Facultad de Medicina, Universidad Complutense de Madrid (UCM), Madrid, Spain,* [4] *Servicio de Oftalmología, Hospital Gregorio Marañón, Madrid, Spain*

Correspondence:
José M. Ramírez
ramirezs@med.ucm.es

Microglia, the immunocompetent cells of the central nervous system (CNS), act as neuropathology sensors and are neuroprotective under physiological conditions. Microglia react to injury and degeneration with immune-phenotypic and morphological changes, proliferation, migration, and inflammatory cytokine production. An uncontrolled microglial response secondary to sustained CNS damage can put neuronal survival at risk due to excessive inflammation. A neuroinflammatory response is considered among the etiological factors of the major aged-related neurodegenerative diseases of the CNS, and microglial cells are key players in these neurodegenerative lesions. The retina is an extension of the brain and therefore the inflammatory response in the brain can occur in the retina. The brain and retina are affected in several neurodegenerative diseases, including Alzheimer's disease (AD), Parkinson's disease (PD), and glaucoma. AD is an age-related neurodegeneration of the CNS characterized by neuronal and synaptic loss in the cerebral cortex, resulting in cognitive deficit and dementia. The extracellular deposits of beta-amyloid (Aβ) and intraneuronal accumulations of hyperphosphorylated tau protein (pTau) are the hallmarks of this disease. These deposits are also found in the retina and optic nerve. PD is a neurodegenerative locomotor disorder with the progressive loss of dopaminergic neurons in the substantia nigra. This is accompanied by Lewy body inclusion composed of α-synuclein (α-syn) aggregates. PD also involves retinal dopaminergic cell degeneration. Glaucoma is a multifactorial neurodegenerative disease of the optic nerve, characterized by retinal ganglion cell loss. In this pathology, deposition of Aβ, synuclein, and pTau has also been detected in retina. These neurodegenerative diseases share a common pathogenic mechanism, the neuroinflammation, in which microglia play an important role. Microglial activation has been reported in AD, PD, and glaucoma in relation to protein aggregates and degenerated neurons. The activated microglia can release pro-inflammatory cytokines which can aggravate and propagate neuroinflammation, thereby degenerating neurons and impairing brain as well as retinal function. The aim of the present review is to describe the contribution in retina to microglial-mediated neuroinflammation in AD, PD, and glaucomatous neurodegeneration.

Keywords: microglia, neuroinflammation, Alzheimer's Disease, Parkinson, glaucoma, retina, beta-amyloid, synuclein

INTRODUCTION

Alzheimer's Disease (AD) and Parkinson's Disease (PD) are the most common neurodegenerative disorders (de Lau and Breteler, 2006). AD involves progressive memory loss and dementia (Sharma and Lipincott, 2017), while the PD is a chronic and progressive movement disorder (Orr et al., 2002). Glaucoma, a neurodegenerative disease of the optic nerve, is characterized by death of retinal ganglion cells (RGCs) (de Hoz et al., 2016). Recently, neurodegenerative lesions have been detected in the intracranial optic nerve, the lateral geniculate nucleus, and the visual cortex (Gupta et al., 2006, 2007), suggesting that this pathology could be grouped as a neurodegenerative disease (Yucel et al., 2003).

AD is a neurodegenerative disorder related to age, in which neuronal and synaptic losses in the cerebral cortex lead to cognitive impairment, behavioral deficits and dementia (Ghiso et al., 2013). The major pathology related to AD is the extracellular deposit of β-amyloid (Aβ) in the form of parenchymal plaques and cerebral amyloid angiopathy co-existing with intraneuronal accumulations of hyperphosphorylated tau (pTau) (neurofribillary tangles) (Ghiso et al., 2013).These deposits can induce neuronal death by apoptosis (Garcia-Ospina et al., 2003). Initially, it was thought that age was the main risk factor for this disease. However, it is now known to have a multifactorial origin and it seems to result from a complex interaction of multiple environmental and genetic factors (Wostyn et al., 2010). AD has been related to genetic mutations, among them in the gene encoding the Aβ precursor protein peptide, mutations in the presenilins genes (Calabrese et al., 2001) and the presence of the APOE ε4 allele (Martínez-Lazcano et al., 2010). In addition, AD is frequently associated with vascular dysfunctions and inflammation (Dudvarski Stankovic et al., 2016).

PD is characterized by the progressive loss of dopaminergic neurons in the substantia nigra pars compacta and the nerve terminals in the striatum (Dauer and Przedborski, 2003). The clinical symptoms of PD are mainly motor problems, including bradykinesia, rigidity, tremors, and postural instability. In addition, PD presents non-motor symptoms including disorganized speech and altered moods (Fakhoury, 2016). The loss of neurons is accompanied by abnormal intracytoplasmic filamentous aggregates called Lewy bodies. These aggregates (deposited in somas and axons) are constituted by α-syn, parkin, phosphorylated neurofilament and components of the protheosomic-ubiquitin pathway (Orr et al., 2002). The main etiological factors proposed for PD are aging, environmental toxins, and genetic factors. Neurodegeneration could be due to exposure to dopaminergic neurotoxins e.g., herbicides (MPTP), insecticides (Rotenone), and metals (Hernández-Montiel, 2006). Genetic factors include mutations in α-syn (Olanow and Tatton, 1999; Pérez and Arancibia, 2007), while mitochondrial dysfunction and oxidative stress may also act by causing the accumulation of misfolded proteins (Dauer and Przedborski, 2003).

Glaucoma is an age-related multifactorial neurodegenerative disease of the optic nerve, with an irreversible decrease in RGCs, causing a visual-field loss and cupping of the optic nerve head (Quigley et al., 1988). In glaucoma, increased intraocular pressure (IOP), vascular dysregulation, and the immune system activation can trigger several changes in retina and optic nerve including: disrupted axonal transport and neurofilament accumulation, microvascular abnormalities, extracellular matrix remodeling, and glial cell activation. These alterations can lead to secondary damage such as, excitotoxicity, neurotrophin deprivation, oxidative damage, mitochondrial dysfunction, and eventually RGC death (Nickells, 1999; Gallego et al., 2012). In addition, there is a dendritic atrophy of the lateral geniculate nucleus, the site to which the RGC axons project (Gupta et al., 2007; Park and Ou, 2013).

The AD, PD and glaucoma share certain biological features, for example: (i) they are slow and chronic neurodegenerative disorders with a strong age-related incidence; (ii) they have similar mechanisms of cell injury and deposition of protein aggregates in specific anatomical areas (Wostyn et al., 2010; Kaarniranta et al., 2011; Ghiso et al., 2013); and (iii) death occurs in one or more populations of neurons (RGCs in glaucoma, hippocampal and cortical neurons in AD and nigrostriatal dopaminergic neurons in PD) (Mattson, 2000). Although the exact mechanism bringing about this neuronal death remains unknown, these neurodegenerative disorders seem to have pathogenic mechanisms in common. These mechanisms include: oxidative stress (Uttara et al., 2009), mitochondrial dysfunction (Lee et al., 2011; Lascaratos et al., 2012; Chrysostomou et al., 2013), alterations in the ubiquitin-proteasome system (Campello et al., 2013), abnormal accumulation of misfolded proteins, glutamate excitotoxicity (Gazulla and Cavero-Nagore, 2006; Guimaraes et al., 2009), and glial activation and inflammation (Verkhratsky et al., 2014; Brown and Vilalta, 2015). These mechanisms could act individually or synergistically (Ghiso et al., 2013).

Inflammation is a defensive process of the body against damage that seeks to restore tissue integrity. Neuroinflammation, the inflammation of central nervous system (CNS), is essential to protect the tissue. However, uncontrolled and prolonged neuroinflammation is potentially harmful and can cause cellular damage. The astrocytes and microglia could play a major role in the neuroinflammation associated with neurodegenerative diseases (Cherry et al., 2014). The presence of reactive astrocytes, the microglial activation, and the release of inflammatory mediators such as cytokines, reactive oxygen species (ROS), nitric oxide (NO), and Tumor Necrosis Factor-α (TNF-α) could cause a state of chronic inflammation that may exert neurotoxic effects (Cuenca et al., 2014).

The neuroinflammatory process occurs not only in the brain, but also in the retina, which is a projection of the CNS. The retina and brain are associated over a range of neurological and neurovascular conditions of varying etiologies, because the retina and brain are similar, and respond similarly to disease. Thus, it has been described that the retina is a "window to the brain," and the manifestation of disease in the brain is the same as in the retina (MacCormick et al., 2015). The neuroinflammatory changes could be observed using optical coherence tomography (OCT), a routinely diagnostic techniques used in ophthalmology. This technique provides anatomic detail of pathological changes in the retina and optic nerve. Changes in OCT measurements have been used to study the course of particular neurologic diseases such AD (Garcia-Martin et al., 2014; Maldonado et al., 2015; Salobrar-Garcia et al., 2015, 2016a,b), PD (Yu et al., 2014; Stemplewitz et al., 2015; Boeke et al., 2016; Satue et al., 2017), and glaucoma (Leung, 2016; Fallon et al., 2017), suggesting that the data compiled may be useful as a biomarker in diagnosing and treating neurodegenerative disease.

The aforementioned data underline the importance of knowing the function of inflammatory processes in the retina of neurodegenerative diseases (AD, PD, and glaucoma), especially the contribution to microglial-mediated neuroinflammation.

MICROGLIAL ACTIVATION

In neurodegenerative diseases, neuroinflammation constitutes a fundamental process in which microglial cells play a key role (Glass et al., 2010). Microglial cells are CNS resident immune cells which have sensor and effector functions as well as phagocytic capacity (Streit et al., 2005). In the developing of CNS these cells enter from the bloodstream, develop from monocytes, and differentiate into microglia. Thus, they maintain numerous cellular antigens present in macrophages and monocytes (Ransohoff and Cardona, 2010). Microglia express CD11b/c, D45^{low}, and the chemokine fractalkine receptor (CX3CR1) (Dudvarski Stankovic et al., 2016). These cells survey the CNS in order to detect homeostasis alteration and they respond accordingly, combining a defensive service with neuroprotective functions (Verkhratsky and Butt, 2013).

In addition to the immune functions, microglia have an essential role in the physiology and survival of neurons. Fractalkine, involved in indirect neuroprotection, is released by neurons and the receptor is expressed by microglia, their interactions constituting a neuron-microglial signaling system (Ransohoff and El Khoury, 2015). The fractalkine expressed by neurons can induce adenosine release from microglia. This adenosine (via adenosine A1 receptor) can activate survival pathways in neurons sensitive to excitotoxicity challenge (Lauro et al., 2008, 2010). The signaling mediated by CX3CR1 could regulate microglial behavior in the neurodegenerative diseases.

The presence of protein aggregates in the CNS is a common feature of most neurodegenerative disorders. These aggregates are identified by the Toll-like receptors (TLRs) which are danger-signal sensors. Microglial cells express these receptors (TLR1-TLR9) and their co-receptors, which promote microglial activation (Gonzalez et al., 2014). Concretely, TLR4 and TLR2 are associated with both neuro-inflammation and clearance of protein aggregates in neurodegenerative disorders (Jack et al., 2005).

Microglia constitute the first line of immune defense in CNS. After injury these cells become activated and in this state change their morphology, proliferate, migrate to the damage sites, modify the expression of enzymes and receptors, and release a variety of inflammatory factors, such as NO, tumor necrosis factor (TNF-α), interleukin (IL-6) among others (Magni et al., 2012). The morphology of activated microglia includes a retraction of processes, enlargement of the soma, and increased expression of myeloid cell markers (Ransohoff and Cardona, 2010). In their state of high activation, microglial cells acquire an amoeboid morphology and act like macrophages, engulfing debris (Brown and Neher, 2014). Excessive microglia activation might prompt the release of cytotoxic factors, causing neuronal damage, which could accelerate the progression of some CNS diseases.

Microglial cells may undergo two different kinds of activation in response to infections or injuries. The first is a neurotoxic phenotype called M1-like. This phenotype generates a massive inflammatory response releasing interleukin-1β (IL-1β), IL-12, TNF-α and inducible nitric oxide synthase (iNOS). M1 microglial cells present amoeboid morphology as well as high phagocytic capacity and motility (Varnum and Ikezu, 2012; Gonzalez et al., 2014; Jones and Bouvier, 2014). However, in certain circumstances, the neuroinflammation can help stimulate myelin repair or remove toxic aggregated proteins and cell debris from CNS (Ding et al., 2004; Simard et al., 2006; Glezer et al., 2007). After this acute M1 activation, microglial cells can suffer an uncontrolled activation leading to a state of chronic inflammation. In this state, microglia release neurotoxic inflammatory factors (TNF-α, IL-1α, IL-1β, IL-6, NO, hydrogen peroxide, superoxide anion, chemokines, and glutamate), which lead to neuronal death (Block et al., 2007; Lull and Block, 2010; Burguillos et al., 2011; Kettenmann et al., 2011; Gordon et al., 2012).

The second microglial phenotype, M2-like, secrete anti-inflammatory mediators and neurotrophic factors, thus inducing a supportive microenvironment for neurons (Kettenmann et al., 2011). The M2 microglial cells are characterized by thin cellular bodies and ramified processes (Menzies et al., 2010; Komori et al., 2011; Varnum and Ikezu, 2012; Jones and Bouvier, 2014; Zhou et al., 2014). These cells can release anti-inflammatory cytokines including IL-4, IL-13, IL-10, TGF-β and neurotrophic factors, such as insulin-like growth factor 1 (IGF-1) to assist inflammation resolution and promote neuron survival (Suh et al., 2013; Tang and Le, 2016). M2 microglia are the major effector cells with the potential to dampen pro-inflammatory immune responses and promote the expression of repair genes (Tang and Le, 2016). The change of microglia between M1 and M2 phenotypes is a dynamic process and microglial activation can switch from M2 to M1 phenotype during the course of disease (Cherry et al., 2014).

Recently, it has been reported that microglia release extracellular microvesicles (Evs) by exocytosis. These microvesicles are involved in all immune activities and can be protective or detrimental, affecting some pathologies of the CNS. EVs have a heterogeneous molecular composition, including receptors, integrins and cytokines, bioactive lipids, miRNA, mRNA, DNA, and organelles, being similar to their parental cells. They can be detected in the plasma and other biological fluids such as the cerebral spinal fluid (CSF). The microglial EVs representing a "liquid biopsy" of their parental cells, and could provide information on the functional phenotype (protective or damaging) of microglial cells over the course of neurodegeneration (Nigro et al., 2016).

Microglia and astrocytes are the main innate immune effector cells in the CNS (da Fonseca et al., 2014). Under pathological conditions, astrocytes and microglia can collaborate to induce an inflammatory response. After injury, astrocytes produce cytokines and chemokines (CCL2, CXCL1, CXCL10, GM-CSF, and IL-6), which activate microglia and recruit peripheral immune cells to the CNS. By contrast, a recent report has described an astrocyte subtype A1 that is abundant in AD and PD and other human neurodegenerative diseases. Activated microglia can induce A1 astrocytes by secreting IL-1α, TNF, and C1q, and this type of astrocyte contribute to the death of neurons in the neurodegenerative disorders and could be analog to the M1-like phenotype microglia (Liddelow et al., 2017).

Microglia, together with endothelial cells, pericytes, and astrocytes, form the functional blood-brain barrier (BBB) that selectively separates the brain parenchyma from blood circulation. In this perivascular location, the microglia survey the influx of blood-borne components entering the CNS. The activated microglia can induce the dysfunction of the BBB, being correlated with the disruption of the BBB in the neurodegenerative diseases (Dudvarski Stankovic et al., 2016). During inflammatory conditions, innate immune cells (DCs, neutrophils, monocytes, and natural killer cells) and adaptive immune cells (activated B cells together with CD4+ and CD8+ T cells) are recruited by chemoattractants to cross the BBB from the periphery. The presence of this cellular infiltrate in the CNS can directly or indirectly provoke neuroinflammation by producing pro-inflammatory cytokines/chemokines. All this could generate oxidative stress, which leads to neuronal death. In addition, activated microglia are capable of upregulating CD11c, MHC I, and MHC II to act as antigen-presenting cells, which activate T cells. This activation would in turn damage the nervous system (Xu et al., 2016).

As mentioned above, during the inflammatory process, there is a are released of cytokines. Cytokines bind to receptors in the microglia and activate the JAK/STAT signaling pathway (Yan et al., 2016). This pathway plays a critical role in the initiation and regulation of innate immune responses and adaptive immunity (Yan et al., 2016). Although the same JAK/STAT components are used, the gene expression in response to a specific cytokine, depending on the cell type (van Boxel-Dezaire et al., 2006). This pathway constitutes a pattern-recognition system by which microglial cells respond to foreign antigens and inflammation in the CNS (Hanisch and Kettenmann, 2007).

In microglial cells, other receptors called the "triggering-receptors-expressed-on-myeloid-cells" (TREM) are thought to play a central role in the immune-system regulation and inflammation. The signaling pathway TREM2 regulates apoptosis, the immune response, and phagocytic activity. Brain homeostasis without inflammation depends on eliminating extracellular aggregates and apoptotic debris, this being mediated by the TREM2/DAP12 receptor complex (Han et al., 2017). The signaling pathway TREM2 regulates the apoptosis, the immune response, and the phagocytic activity. This pathway, induced in the microglial cells by anti-inflammatory cytokines, is modulated by CD33 and is down-regulated by agonists of TLR2, 4, and 9, as well as by inflammatory stimuli such as lipopolysaccharides and RNA interference. An overexpression of TREM2 promotes phagocytosis and reduces the pro-inflammatory response (Han et al., 2017). This receptor is a critical regulator of microglia and macrophage phenotype and is involved in neurodegenerative diseases (Andreasson et al., 2016).

After damage, microglia transform into active phagocytes. These cells migrate to the damaged area and adopt an amoeboid morphology, releasing both pro- and anti-inflammatory molecules. They also have the capacity to remove apoptotic cells and debris. As mentioned above, for phagocytosis to occur the expression of specific receptors on the microglial surface is necessary. The principal receptors are the TLRs, which have high affinity for pathogens, and TREM2, which recognizes apoptotic cellular substances (Hsieh et al., 2009). In addition, other receptors also participate in cell-debris clearance (Fc receptors, complement receptors, scavenger receptors (SR), pyrimidinergic receptors P2Y, G-protein coupled,6 (P2RY6), macrophage antigen complex 2 (MAC-2), mannose receptor, and low-density lipoprotein receptor-related protein (LRP) (Fu et al., 2014).

Although microglia are the main agents responsible for phagocytosis of cell debris in the CNS, the complement system can play a primordial role in removing damaged and apoptotic cells (Fakhoury, 2016). Microglial cells can activate the complement by local secretion of the complement component from both the classical and the alternative pathway and also express C3 and C5 (Luo et al., 2011). The complement also participates in the physiological process, termed synaptic pruning. The synapses and axons have to be labeled by complement components C1q and C3 before being phagocytosed, which prompts their selective recognition by microglial cells (Paolicelli et al., 2011; Linnartz et al., 2012; Schafer et al., 2012).

Given the central role of microglial cells in neurodegeneration, the evaluation of activated microglia *in vivo* is an important approach. Positron emission tomography (PET) is the most widely used *in vivo* method for detecting microglial activation (Owen and Matthews, 2011; Mirzaei et al., 2016).

It has been found that activated microglia and astrocytes overexpress mitochondrial translocator protein (TSPO) within or surrounding senile plaques. Thus, it has been proposed that neuroimaging of TSPO using PET is a good marker of neuroinflammation (Cosenza-Nashat et al., 2009; Pasqualetti et al., 2015).

AD AND MICROGLIA

The primary pathogenic process in AD is the accumulation of Aβ protein. This protein aggregates into extracellular amyloid plaques, which are the hallmark of this pathology (Southam et al., 2016). The amyloid hypothesis for AD is based on a linear, quantitative, centered neuron model. This model postulates that the initial deposition of Aβ triggers mechanisms that progressively lead to Tau pathology, synaptic dysfunction, inflammation, neuronal loss and finally to dementia (De Strooper and Karran, 2016). Recently, evidence has been reported that Aβ protein acts by increasing tau pathology through the formation of tau species capable of producing new aggregates (Bennett et al., 2017).

After acute inflammatory damage, the brain glial cells respond to repair the tissue. If the stimulus persists, it produces an inflammatory chronic state that leads to neuronal dysfunction, injury, and loss (Streit et al., 2004; Calsolaro and Edison, 2016). As mentioned before, inflammation is one of the possible causes in the development of AD (Wyss-Coray, 2006). The increase in Aβ deposition induces the activation of astrocytes as well as microglia (Cagnin et al., 2001). These activated cells can release both pro- and anti-inflammatory mediators, leading to a state of chronic inflammation in the tissue. This inflammation not only occurs in response to Aβ deposition, but is also capable of generating, via feedback mechanisms, more Aβ while weakening the mechanisms responsible for its elimination (Parpura et al., 2012).

The Soluble Aβ oligomers and Aβ fibrils can react to various receptors expressed by microglia, including CD14, CD36, CD47, α6β1 integrin, class A scavenger receptor, receptor for advanced glycosylation end products (RAGE) and TLRs (Stewart et al., 2010). The RAGE is an important cell-surface receptor for Aβ in the endothelial cells, neurons, and microglia, and increased expression in these cell types has been demonstrated in AD (Yan et al., 1996). The interaction of Aβ with RAGE causes oxidative stress in neurons, enhances inflammatory responses in microglia, and is involved in reversed transport of Aβ across the BBB in endothelial cells (Deane et al., 2012). The binding of Aβ to CD36 (cell surface microglial co-receptor) promotes the TLR4 and/or TLR6 phosphorylation and activation, resulting in the production of inflammatory cytokines and chemokines (Stewart et al., 2010).

Recently, an alternative pathway has been described for intracellular signaling produced by the binding of Aβ to microglial cells, activating NLRP3 inflammasome (Heneka et al., 2013; Sheedy et al., 2013). NLRP3 inflammasome is an intracellular protein complex. Their assembly and activation regulates activation of caspase-1, which catalyzes the cleavage and activation of proinflammatory cytokines of the IL-1β family, promoting the secretion of these, now biologically active, cytokines. These cytokines could induce neuronal degeneration (Gold and El Khoury, 2015). In addition, NLRP3 inflammasome activation reduces phagocytosis of Aβ by microglial cells, thus increasing the Aβ depositions and contributing to the pathogenesis of AD (Garlanda et al., 2013; Gold and El Khoury, 2015).

Microglial cells are important for the normal functioning of neurons in the CNS. They provide trophic support to neurons and regulate synapses. The altered microglial behavior could induce neuronal degeneration in AD (Southam et al., 2016). During development, microglia are involved in synapse elimination and these mechanisms may be aberrantly reactivated in the aged brain, contributing to the synapse loss in AD. The synapse loss in the hippocampus and association cortices is an early hallmark of AD and strongly correlates with cognitive impairment (Hong et al., 2016). In the healthy development of the brain, the proteins of complement participate in synapse pruning. Synapses to be cleared express C3 and binding to CR3 on microglia, resulting in microglial phagocytosis of the synapse (Schafer et al., 2012; Southam et al., 2016). In the healthy adult brain, these complement components are downregulated. However, in aging brains, C1q and C3 are highly upregulated and are deposited on synapses, particularly in the hippocampus, the most vulnerable region in the synapse loss in AD (Bialas and Stevens, 2013). These findings highlight the importance of complement regulation for normal synaptic maintenance (Southam et al., 2016). In addition, it has been shown that Aβ can bind and regulate the expression and localization of complement proteins in the AD brain. An upregulation has been observed in the complement proteins (C1q, C3, and C4) localized in senile plaques also known as neuritic plaques (Hong et al., 2016).

Microglial cells can use additional mechanisms for synapsis regulation. The release of brain-derived neurotrophic factor (BDNF) by microglial cells induces synaptic pruning. However, the depletion of this factor in the microglia results in learning and memory impairment (Parkhurst et al., 2013). The activation of the fractalkine receptor (CX3CR1) in microglial cells, increases synaptic strength. However, deficiency in this receptor results in a reduced hippocampal synaptic plasticity (Rogers et al., 2011; Clark et al., 2015).

It has been reported that in the later stages of AD, there is destruction of axons, dendrites, and synapses, in which microglia has a relevant role (Parpura et al., 2012). In AD brains reactive microglia has been found colocalized with amyloid plaques. In addition, the reactive astrocytes accumulate around senile plaques next to the activated microglia (Heneka et al., 2015). In brain, astrocytes as well as microglia are capable of capturing Aβ for degradation (Pihlaja et al., 2011). In AD patients, astrocytes in the entorhinal cortex accumulate Aβ, this accumulation being positively correlated with the extent of AD (Nagele et al., 2003). Moreover, astrocytes can also induce microglia to perform Aβ phagocytosis by regulating the release of the apo E and the ATP-binding cassette (ABCA) protein. Studies *in vitro* have demonstrated that microglial phagocytosis of Aβ is more effective in the presence of supernatants derived from astrocytes (Terwel et al., 2011). In AD, mutations in ABCA7 can cause a loss of receptor activity, resulting in reduced microglia phagocytic function (Southam et al., 2016).

Microglial senescence can enhance the sensitivity of microglia to inflammatory stimuli; this phenomenon is called "priming" (Heneka et al., 2015). In addition, aged microglia show reduced phagocytic capacity. This process could be due partly to a reduction in the ability of microglia to recognize phagocytic targets (Udeochu et al., 2016). Both inflammation and reduced microglial phagocytic capacity in AD can contribute to the decline in synaptic plasticity observed in this pathology (Ritzel et al., 2015; Udeochu et al., 2016).

In AD, protein aggregation is caused by declining of protein homeostasis (proteostasis) (Mosher and Wyss-Coray, 2014). As mentioned above, Aβ deposits can attract and activate microglia. Presumably, microglial proliferation around plaques could serve as a line of defense to limit the deposition of amyloid. Nonetheless, it seems that microglial cells clustered around Aβ− deposits have become incapable of removing the amyloid (Calsolaro and Edison, 2016). The sustained exposure to cytokines, chemokines and Aβ, could be responsible for the functional impairment of microglial cells located around Aβ− deposits (Heneka et al., 2015). In addition, microglial-specific genetic alterations may be related to this microglial dysfunction. The expression of beclin 1, a protein associated with autophagy pathway, is reduced in the brain of patients with AD, leading to disruption in phagocytosis and retromer-mediated recycling of the phagocytic receptors CD36 and TREM2 in microglia (Mosher and Wyss-Coray, 2014).

Similarly, mutations in TREM2 can trigger the loss of phagocytic capacity in microglial cells. TREM2 inhibits pro-inflammatory cytokine production, facilitates phagocytosis and promotes cell survival. Thus, TREM2 dysfunction could induce the loss of the homeostasis in the tissue (Painter et al., 2015). Missense mutations in TREM2 lead to a significant risk of developing AD (Jonsson et al., 2013; Meyer-Luehmann and Prinz, 2015).

As mentioned above, in AD the Aβ peptide that is aggregated extracellularly in the neuritic plaques produces an inflammatory environment and a chronic activation of microglial and astroglial cells (D'Andrea, 2005). Activated microglia can shed MVs in response to several signals, including cytokines. These MVs contain bioactive molecules (i.e., IL-1β, proteases, and MHC-II) which modulate the activity of neuronal and non-neuronal cells (Antonucci et al., 2012). In AD patients, the production of MVs is very high, reflecting microgliosis. These extracellular vesicles can be isolated form cerebrospinal fluid (Guerriero et al., 2016).

In patients with AD, an upregulation of iNOS has been found. In the course of AD, cytokines stimulate iNOS in microglia and astrocytes, generating high NO levels (Vodovotz et al., 1996). NO can interact with signaling cascades and regulate gene transcription, impair mitochondrial respiration or directly induce neuron death by apoptosis or necrosis (Parpura et al., 2012). In addition, the NO can promote the nitration of Aβ, increasing their propensity to aggregate (Kummer et al., 2011; Heneka et al., 2015).

In late-onset Alzheimer's disease (LOAD), accumulating Aβ and NO harm the cells of the cerebral vessel, causing the onset of cerebral amyloid angiopathy (Nelson et al., 2016). The neurovascular unit, constituted by cerebral blood vessels, perivascular glia and neurons, are associated with distinct inflammatory, functional, and morphological alterations in AD (Heneka et al., 2015). In LOAD, damaged blood vessels can hinder neurogenesis from neural stem cells in the subventricular zone and hippocampus, preventing the processing and storage of new memories (Licht and Keshet, 2015; Chiarini et al., 2016).

Recently, it has been suggested that the involvement of glial cells in AD is related with the transient receptor potential melastatin member 2 (TRPM2). This receptor, besides regulating synaptic plasticity and glial cell activation, also modulates oxidative stress and inflammation (Yuruker et al., 2015). TRPM2 channel can be activated by Aβ. The activation of these channels in microglia and astrocytes leads to Ca^{2+} overload and subsequent inflammation and oxidative stress. All of this causes mitochondrial dysfunction, $[Ca^{2+}]_I$ increase, Aβ accumulation, glutamate-receptor dysfunction, and finally plasticity alterations and dementia (Yuruker et al., 2015; Wang et al., 2016).

PARKINSON AND MICROGLIA

PD is characterized by α-synuclein (α-syn) accumulation, dopaminergic neuron loss and inflammation (Beach et al., 2014; Wang et al., 2015). The pathological hallmark of this disorder is the presence of Lewy bodies. The Braak hypothesis has suggested that PD begins in the olfactory bulb or the gastrointestinal tract. These areas are constantly exposed to the environment, and in them, the Lewy bodies accumulate (Kannarkat et al., 2013). Lewy bodies are constituted mainly by misfolded α-syn and other intraneuronal protein aggregates such as tau and ubiquitin proteins (Campello et al., 2013; George and Brundin, 2015). The nitration, phosphorylation, and ubiquitination of α-syn can promote their pathological accumulation, inducing neurodegeneration (Giasson et al., 2000; Tofaris et al., 2003; Anderson et al., 2006). In addition, missense mutations in α-syn can produce the protein aggregation in familial PD (Conway et al., 1998).

Reportedly, α-syn can induce microglial activation, which in turn can promote α-syn phagocytosis (Cao et al., 2012) and neuroinflammation. The neuroinflammation leads to the loss of dopaminergic neurons and drives the chronic progression of neurodegeneration in PD (Schapansky et al., 2015). Accumulations of activated microglia have been found around dopaminergic neurons in postmortem human brains (Hamza et al., 2010). Microglial cells can be activated by α-syn, via TLRs, initiating an immune response (Fellner et al., 2013). Specifically, the stimulation of TRL2 and TRL4 in the microglia induces signaling cascades involved in the inflammatory response. It has been shown in PD patients that TLR2 colocalized with CD68+ amoeboid microglia indicates microglial activation at the sites of neuronal loss (Doorn et al., 2014). Also, TRL4 can induce microglial phagocytosis of α-syn. Deficiencies in this receptor can prompt poor α-syn clearance and neurodegeneration (Fellner et al., 2013).

The clearance of α-syn also can be promoted by the leucine-rich repeat kinase 2 (LRRK2) gene. This gene has been proposed as a regulator of the microglial response (Schapansky et al., 2015). LRRK2 is the most commonly mutated gene in both idiopathic and familial PD. Pathogenic mutations in LRRK2 influence the ability of microglia to internalize and degrade α-syn, exacerbating α-syn-induced microglial pathology, and neuroinflammation (Schapansky et al., 2015). In addition, other genes whose mutations are responsible for rare familial forms of PD have been identified, including, SNCA, PARKIN, DJ-1, and PINK1 (Chao et al., 2014).

Persistent microglial activation is known to exert harmful effects that result in dopaminergic neuron death. One of the most important signaling pathways associated with the microglial activation in PD involves nuclear factor-kappa B (NF-kB) (Zhang et al., 2017). The activation of this factor could increase the release of proinflammatory cytokines such TNF-α and interleukin 1β by microglial cells (Mogi et al., 1996; McLaughlin et al., 2006). In addition, proinflammatory mediators such as TNF-α, IL-1β, and IFN-γ have been found at higher levels in the midbrain of PD patients (Wang et al., 2015). Immunomodulators, including the CX3CL1, CD200, CD22, CD47, CD95, and neural cell adhesion molecule, sustain the rest state of microglia under normal conditions (Chang et al., 2000; Sheridan and Murphy, 2013). In rat PD models, both deficiency CX3CL1 or CX3CR1 as well as the dysfunction of CD200-CD200R signaling have been shown to increase microglial activation and the degeneration of DA neurons (Wang et al., 2011; Zhang et al., 2011).

The cytokines released by activated microglia can attract peripheral immune cells (e.g., CD4 T-cell) to the brain. *In vivo* and *in vitro* studies have demonstrated that overexpression of α-syn can induce the MHC-II expression by microglia. The MHC-II expression in microglia cells can play an important role in the immune responses (innate and adaptive) in PD (Michelucci et al., 2009; Harms et al., 2013; Gonzalez et al., 2015).

In addition, dopaminergic neurons seem to be especially sensitive to several factors that can induce cell damage and eventually cell death. It has been suggested that mitochondrial malfunction leads to reduced energy metabolism and induces neuroinflammation via NO and ROS production, which ultimately entails neurodegeneration (Vivekanantham et al., 2015). The production of NO and superoxide exerted by activated microglia in PD can cause the degeneration of dopaminergic neurons (Appel et al., 2010). The high cytosolic concentrations of free DA can produce oxidative stress and can interact with α-syn, promoting the neurodegenerative process (Mosharov et al., 2006). In addition, the neuromelanin (dark, complex endogenous polymer derived from DA) can activate microglial cells, inducing neuroinflammation and neurodegeneration of dopaminergic neurons in PD (Zecca et al., 2008; Herrera et al., 2015).

Neuroinflammation is produced by the set of integrated responses of all the CNS immune cells including microglia, astrocytes and infiltrating T-lymphocytes (Le et al., 2016). Gliosis in the PD is an atypical activation where astrogliosis is largely absent while the microglia is highly activated by the disease. The low astroglial response may be caused by degeneration due to an increase of α-syn in the astrocyte (Stefanova et al., 2001; Orr et al., 2002; Sofroniew and Vinters, 2010). Astrocytes are responsible for secreting glutathione and transporting to neurons in response to neural excitatory stimuli. A lower level of glutathione has been detected in the CNS of PD patients, and thus the antioxidant capacity in the tissue could be impaired, probably secondary to the astroglial defect (Olanow and Tatton, 1999).

Recently, the kinurenic pathway (KP) has been implicated in the inflammatory and neurotoxic processes in PD. Astrocytes produce a neuroactive component of KP, kynurenic acid, considered to be neuroprotective. By contrast, quinolinic acid, released by microglia, can activate the NMDA receptor-signaling pathway, leading to excitotoxicity and increasing the inflammatory response. Based on this, KP may represent an important target to prevent the progression of the underlying neurodegeneration observed in PD (Lim C. K. et al., 2017).

Nowdays, it has been reported that prothrombin kringle-2 (pKr-2), which is a domain of prothrombin (which is produced by active thrombin), could be involved in PD. Also, pKr-2 induced DA neuronal death in an experimental PD model (Kim et al., 2010). In addition, in PD patient's pKr-2 expression is significantly increased and co-localized in activated microglial in the substantia nigra, leading to disruption of the nigrostriatal DA projection. This disruption could be mediated through the neurotoxic inflammatory events brought about by the pKr-2 upregulation, wich trigger microglial activation via TLR4. On the basic of these results, limiting pKr-2-induced microglial activation may be an effective therapeutic strategy for protecting DA neurons (Leem et al., 2016).

NEURODEGENERATIVE DISEASES AND THE EYE

Alzheimer's Disease

Classically, the damage in AD was thought to be restricted mainly to the brain. However, in the last few decades it has been demonstrated that patients with AD often develop visual anomalies, which are correlated with abnormalities in the eye. Among them, there is a reduction in the number of optic nerve head axons and a decrease in the thickness of the peripapillary and macular retinal nerve fiber layer (RNFL) (Tsai et al., 1991; Hedges et al., 1996; Danesh-Meyer et al., 2006; Iseri et al., 2006; Paquet et al., 2007; Garcia-Martin et al., 2014; Salobrar-Garcia et al., 2015; Salobrar-García et al., 2016c) (**Table 1**). One of the earliest symptoms of AD could be the thinning of the RGC layer and visual spatial impairment (Kesler et al., 2011). Postmortem studies in AD retinas, have demonstrated that, in addition to RGC loss, melanopsin retinal ganglion cells (mRGC) are lost. There is evidence that mRGCs may be affected primarily by Aβ pathology in AD (La Morgia et al., 2011). This mRGC deficiency could be correlated with a circadian dysfunction (La Morgia et al., 2011) in which AD patients tend to be more active during the night in comparison with the day (Hatfield et al., 2004; Hooghiemstra et al., 2015). In addition, in the retina of AD patients as well as AD human postmortem specimens the presence of Aβ plaques has been demonstrated. Aβ deposition was observed from the outer nuclear layer (ONL) to nerve fiber layer (NFL), being more abundant in the superior region of the retina where greater neuronal degeneration has been detected (Hardy and Selkoe, 2002; Selkoe, 2004, 2008; Alexandrov et al., 2011; Ratnayaka et al., 2015; Hart et al., 2016; **Table 1**). In AD patients, the alloform Aβ42 is increased (Alexandrov et al., 2011). This alloform presents higher cellular toxicity, more aggregation capacity, and a more direct relation with AD pathology (Qiu et al., 2015). Aβ42 peptide accumulation in the retina may contribute to retinal degeneration and visual impairment in AD (Hardy and Selkoe, 2002; Selkoe, 2004, 2008; Alexandrov et al., 2011; Ratnayaka et al., 2015; Hart et al., 2016; **Figure 1A**, **Table 1**). However, recently Williams et al. in AD patients found no evidence of deposits or accumulations of Tau, Aβ, TDP-43, ubiquitin or α-syn in any part of the eyeball (Williams E. A. et al., 2017).

Aβ plaques have also been detected in the retina of transgenic mouse models of AD (APP_{swe} / $PS1_{\Delta E9}$, Tg2576AD, 3xTg-AD, PSAPP, 5xFAD; Hsiao et al., 1996; Holcomb et al., 1998; Takeuchi et al., 2000; Lukiw et al., 2001; Oddo et al., 2003; Kumar-Singh et al., 2005; Oakley et al., 2006; Philipson et al., 2010; Koronyo-Hamaoui et al., 2011). Overall, in these mice, Aβ plaques were found principally in the NFL, ganglion cell layer (GCL), inner plexiform layer (IPL), inner nuclear layer (INL) and outer plexiform layer (OPL) (**Table 1**). In APP_{swe} / $PS1_{\Delta E9}$ transgenic mice, Aβ plaques appeared in the retina of young transgenic AD mice at presymptomatic stages, as early as 2.5 months, preceding their detection in the brain. This situation points out a correlation between retinal and brain pathology in AD. The detection of retinal Aβ might potentially provide an alternative noninvasive approach to assess the progression of AD. In relation to this last point, it has been demonstrated that the systemic administration of curcumin to AD mice resulted in specific *in vivo* labeling of retinal Aβ plaques. This finding provides the basis for the development of a high-resolution noninvasive optical-imaging technique for detecting Aβ plaques in the retina, allowing the early diagnosis and follow up of AD (Koronyo-Hamaoui et al., 2011; Kayabasi et al., 2014). In addition, curcumin has been revealed to be a novel agent for treating AD through different neuroprotective mechanisms, such as inhibition of Aβ aggregation and decrease in neuroinflammation (Maiti and Dunbar, 2016; Lakey-Beitia et al., 2017).

In addition to Aβ plaques, pTau was observed from OPL to GCL in the retina of AD patients. Also, pTau has been found from the ONL to GCL in the transgenic mouse (Liu et al., 2009). It has been postulated that pTau could be potentially a marker for the AD disease (Lim J. K. et al., 2016). In a model of transgenic mice P301S tau, early accumulation of pTau and βIII-tubulin in the NFL of the retina was demonstrated. This accumulation was accompanied by somatodendritic redistribution of pTau and the subsequent development of tau inclusions in a group of RGCs. In the optic nerve of this transgenic model, at 5 months of age, damaged axons were detected presenting phospho-tau, neurofilaments, amyloid precursor protein and ubiquitin accumulations, as well as disordered filaments and degenerating mitochondria and organelles (Gasparini et al., 2011). These observations suggest that tau may alter axonal transport. This alteration is an early event in tau-induced neuronal dysfunction and corroborates previous findings in mouse models of tautopathy and glaucoma, showing that axonal degeneration precedes neuronal loss (Schlamp et al., 2006; Leroy et al., 2007; **Figure 1A**, **Table 1**).

A significant upregulation of inflammation (evidenced by astroglial and microglial activation) has been found in the retinas of AD mouse models in relation to Aβ plaques (Parnell et al., 2012). Ning et al. (2008) observed an age-dependent increment in Aβ in the retina of the double transgenic mice model APP_{swe} / $PS1_{\Delta E9}$. This increment was accompanied by increases in the inflammatory cytokine MCP-1, the microglial marker F4/80, and the TUNNEL-positive cells in the RGC layer. Thus, the authors suggested that Aβ played a major role in the inflammation and neurodegeneration in AD. In the same transgenic model, Perez et al. (2009) observed significantly greater microglial activity. Microglial activation could occur early in the retina and could be involved in the elimination or turnover of Aβ deposition. In addition, activated microglia could trigger a neuroinflammatory response, which may contribute to a disorganization of the retina, as demonstrated by electroretinogram functional alterations (Krasodomska et al., 2010; **Table 1**). This neuroinflammatory response associated with Aβ plaques and pTau, has also been observed in Tg2576AD mice. In these animals, there was a significant increase in Iba1 cells (a microglial marker) and an increase in the glial fibrillary acidic protein (GFAP) immunoreactivity (a marker of astrocytes) (**Figure 1A**). The vaccination with Aβ oligomer antigen reduced Aβ retinal deposits in these transgenic mice. However, the microvascular Aβ deposition as well as the microglial infiltration and astrogliosis were increased and were associated with the disruption of retinal architecture (Liu et al., 2009). Other studies support the involvement of the neuroinflammation in the AD progression. These studies analyzed the role of the complement in this disease (Parnell et al., 2012). Deficits have been found in the expression of the innate immune-repressor complement factor H (CFH) associated with significant increases of Aβ42 peptides in brains and retinas of transgenic models of AD (Veerhuis, 2011). CFH functions as a cofactor in the inactivation of C3b in the alternative complement pathway, and thus low CFH levels result in complement activation, triggering inflammation in the retina and brain (Alexandrov et al., 2011). In the transgenic rat model (TgF344-AD) also has been observed, along with Aβ deposition, microglial recruitment, and complement activation in association with a decline in visual function (Tsai et al., 2014; **Table 1**).

Parkinson's Disease

As mentioned above, PD is a motor disorder associated with degeneration of dopaminergic neurons in the substantia nigra (Inzelberg et al., 2004). In this disease, high levels of α-syn

TABLE 1 | Retinal changes associated with AD, PD, and glaucoma.

		AD	PD	Glaucoma
			References	
Retinal thickness decrease		Tsai et al., 1991; Hedges et al., 1996; Danesh-Meyer et al., 2006; Iseri et al., 2006; Paquet et al., 2007; Kesler et al., 2011; Garcia-Martin et al., 2014; Maldonado et al., 2015; Salobrar-Garcia et al., 2015, 2016a,b; Salobrar-García et al., 2016c	Inzelberg et al., 2004; Yu et al., 2014; Stemplewitz et al., 2015; Boeke et al., 2016; Satue et al., 2017	Leung, 2016; Fallon et al., 2017
Inner retinal involvement		La Morgia et al., 2011	Bodis-Wollner, 1990; Tatton et al., 1990; Surguchov et al., 2001; Cuenca et al., 2005; Hajee et al., 2009; Bodis-Wollner et al., 2014	Rojas et al., 2014
Outer retinal involvement		Hardy and Selkoe, 2002; Selkoe, 2004, 2008; Ratnayaka et al., 2015; Hart et al., 2016	Maurage et al., 2003; Esteve-Rudd et al., 2011	
Protein deposits in retina	Aβ	Hsiao et al., 1996; Holcomb et al., 1998; Takeuchi et al., 2000; Lukiw et al., 2001; Hardy and Selkoe, 2002; Oddo et al., 2003; Selkoe, 2004, 2008; Kumar-Singh et al., 2005; Oakley et al., 2006; Philipson et al., 2010; Alexandrov et al., 2011; Koronyo-Hamaoui et al., 2011; Kayabasi et al., 2014; Qiu et al., 2015; Ratnayaka et al., 2015; Hart et al., 2016		McKinnon et al., 2002; McKinnon, 2003; Goldblum et al., 2007
	pTau	Liu et al., 2009; Gasparini et al., 2011; Lim J. K. et al., 2016		Gupta et al., 2008; Ning et al., 2008; Bolos et al., 2017
	α-syn		Surguchov et al., 2001; Maurage et al., 2003; Bodis-Wollner et al., 2014	
	γ-syn			Surgucheva et al., 2002
Microglial activation		Ning et al., 2008; Perez et al., 2009; Parnell et al., 2012	Chen et al., 2003; Nagel et al., 2009; Cho et al., 2012	Kreutzberg, 1995; Neufeld et al., 1997; Giulian and Ingeman, 1988; Wax et al., 1998; Neufeld, 1999; Shareef et al., 1999; Tezel et al., 2001; Yang et al., 2001b; Yuan and Neufeld, 2001; Naskar et al., 2002; Steele et al., 2005; Taylor et al., 2005; Nakazawa et al., 2006; Stasi et al., 2006; Vidal et al., 2006; Farina et al., 2007; Inman and Horner, 2007; Johnson et al., 2007; Hammam et al., 2008; Tezel, 2009; Ebneter et al., 2010; Graeber and Streit, 2010; Luo et al., 2010; Bosco et al., 2011, 2012; Kettenmann et al., 2011; London et al., 2011; Bosco et al., 2012; Gallego et al., 2012; Varnum and Ikezu, 2012; de Hoz et al., 2013; Gramlich et al., 2013; Pinazo-Duran et al., 2013; Astafurov et al., 2014; Cherry et al., 2014; Gonzalez et al., 2014; Jones and Bouvier, 2014; Lee et al., 2014; Rojas et al., 2014; Karlstetter et al., 2015; Madeira et al., 2015; Ransohoff and El Khoury, 2015; Chidlow et al., 2016; Bolos et al., 2017; Williams E. A. et al., 2017

(Continued)

TABLE 1 | Continued

	AD	PD	Glaucoma
		References	
Neurodegeneration	Hatfield et al., 2004; Schlamp et al., 2006; Leroy et al., 2007; Liu et al., 2009; La Morgia et al., 2011; Veerhuis, 2011; Parnell et al., 2012; Tsai et al., 2014; Hooghiemstra et al., 2015	Bodis-Wollner, 1990; Tatton et al., 1990; Cuenca et al., 2005	Neufeld, 1999; Yuan and Neufeld, 2001; Steele et al., 2005; Garden and Möller, 2006; Quigley and Broman, 2006; Stasi et al., 2006; Koizumi et al., 2007; Langmann, 2007; Ohsawa et al., 2007; Wu et al., 2007; Tezel, 2009; Karlstetter et al., 2010, 2015; Taylor et al., 2011; Rojas et al., 2014; Wang et al., 2014; Bosco et al., 2016; Chidlow et al., 2016
Blood-retinal barrier breakdown			Farina et al., 2007; Tezel, 2009; London et al., 2011; Howell et al., 2012; Gonzalez et al., 2014; Karlstetter et al., 2015; Breen et al., 2016
Visual impairment	Krasodomska et al., 2010; Tsai et al., 2014	Djamgoz et al., 1997	

AD, Alzheimer's Disease; PD, Parkinson's Disease; Aβ, beta-amyloid; pTau, hyperphosphorylated tau protein; α-syn, α-synuclein; γ-syn, γ-synuclein.

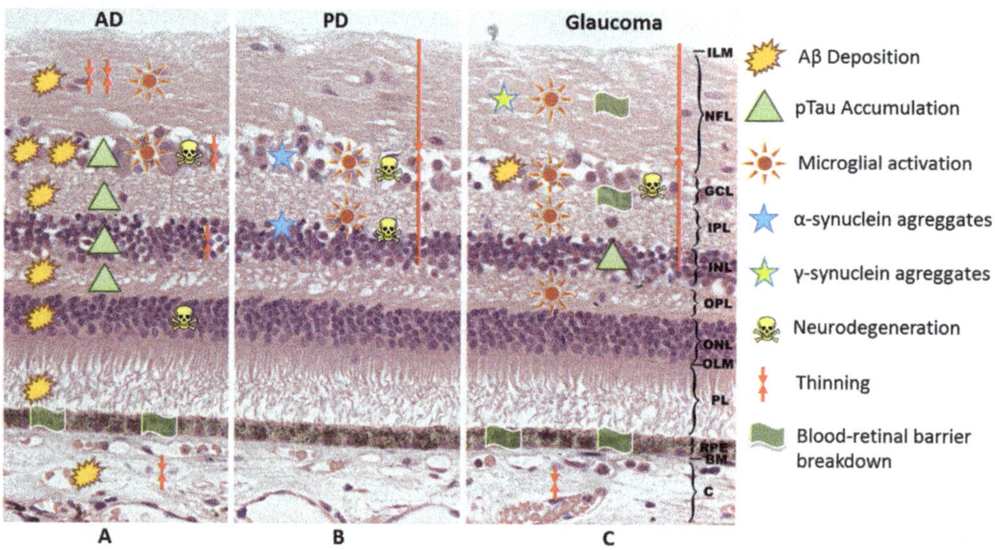

FIGURE 1 | Schematic representation of the hypothetical events associated with the neuroinflammation in AD **(A)**, PD **(B)**, and glaucoma **(C)**. AD, Alzheimer's Disease; PD, Parkinson's Disease; ILM, inner limitant membrane; NFL, nerve fiber layer; GCL, ganglion cell layer; IPL, inner plexiform layer; INL, inner nuclear layer; OPL, outer plexiform layer; ONL, outer nuclear layer; OLM, outer limitant membrane; PL, photoreceptor layer; RPE, retinal pigment epithelium; BM, Bruch membrane; C, choroid; Aβ, beta-amyloid; pTau, phosphorylated tau.

are found in midbrain dopaminergic neurons (Neystat et al., 1999; Solano et al., 2000; Braak et al., 2003; Kingsbury et al., 2004; Alafuzoff and Parkkinen, 2014). Moreover, abnormalities in visual function have been reported (Bodis-Wollner, 1990; Nowacka et al., 2014) in PD patients and correlated with changes in retinal tissue (La Morgia et al., 2013; Yu et al., 2014) (**Table 1**).

In the normal retina of vertebrates, α-syn is expressed at photoreceptor axon terminals of vertebrates, as well as in several subtypes of bipolar and amacrine retinal cells. This protein is present in presynaptic, but not postsynaptic, terminals of retinal neurons in both IPL and OPL, where it could be associated with synaptic vesicles to modulate neurotransmission (Martinez-Navarrete et al., 2007). However, α-syn aggregates are related to neurodegenerative disorders, including PD. In postmortem PD eyes, α-syn aggregates have been observed inside the neurons of different retinal layers, including the border of the INL, the IPL, and the GCL. These locations suggest a substrate for the visual impairment in PD (Bodis-Wollner et al., 2014). Maurage et al. also reported the presence of α-syn inclusions in the OPL and a lower cone density in a patient suffering dementia with Lewy bodies (Maurage et al., 2003). Additionally, in transgenic mice overexpressing α-syn, an accumulation of this protein has been found in the INL, GCL, and NFL (Surguchov et al., 2001; **Figure 1B**, **Table 1**).

In PD, in addition to substantia nigra dopaminergic neuron degeneration, the DA content in the retina diminishes. This deficiency could alter visual processing by altering the ganglion cells receptive fields (Djamgoz et al., 1997). Retinas having a dopaminergic deficiency associated with the loss of amacrine cells, which provide input to the ganglion cells, can lose RGCs. This fact is has been observed both in human PD and in PD model in monkeys treated with 1-methyl-4-phenyl-1,2,3,6-tetrahydropyridine (MPTP) (selective neurotoxin which destroys DA neurons) (Bodis-Wollner, 1990; Tatton et al., 1990; Cuenca et al., 2005). This loss can be mediated by the impoverished dopaminergic input, which contributes to an alteration in the glutamate production and the atrophy of inferotemporal circumpapillary RNFL in PD patients (Inzelberg et al., 2004). These data agree with the observations in PD patients, in which a thinning of inner retinal layer (15–20%) has been demonstrated in the macular region. This percentage of thinning does not necessarily cause a vision loss (Hajee et al., 2009; **Figure 1B**, **Table 1**). Also in the retina of mice treated with rotenone (pesticide that elicits DA neuron degenerations), an experimental model of PD, a correlation between functional and structural alterations were located in the retina, specifically in the photoreceptors and their synaptic connections with second-order neurons (Esteve-Rudd et al., 2011).

Very few studies analyze retinal glial cells in PD. In a transgenic mouse model overexpressing α-syn, an accumulation of α-syn has been found in glial cells of the INL (Surguchov et al., 2001). In a PD model with the administration of MPTP increased GFAP immunostaining, glutamine synthetase (Müller cell marker), and CD11b (microglial marker) were detected, indicating an activation of retinal glial cells (Chen et al., 2003). In the same experimental model, Nagel et al. also observed astrogliosis in retinal tissue, without changes in the number of tyrosine hydroxylase (TH)+ amacrine cells, postulating that other retinal neurons can be affected, even non-neuronal cells (Nagel et al., 2009). In addition, a non-proliferative gliosis of GFAP+ Müller cells was found in the MPTP model of PD. This gliosis was accompanied of milder declines in TH+ amacrine cells, followed by stronger recoveries without neurogenesis (Cho et al., 2012). Müller cells constitute the main glial cell type in the retina where it interacts with virtually all cells displaying functions relevant to retinal physiology. Müller cells are able to synthesize and release DA to the extracellular medium. Thus, the dopaminergic Müller cells can be used as a source of DA in cell-therapy procedures (Stutz et al., 2014; **Table 1**).

Glaucoma

Glaucoma, the second leading cause of blindness in the world, is characterized by the irreversible RGC loss, leading to a vision loss (Quigley and Broman, 2006). In the early stages of the disease, the reactivation of the glial cells leads to the progression of glaucomatous damage (Tezel, 2009). As mentioned above, when neurons are damaged, microglial cells respond by adopting an activated phenotype (Kreutzberg, 1995; Graeber and Streit, 2010). In glaucoma, activated microglia can exhibit morphological changes, proliferate, migrate, or can change the expression of different enzymes, receptors, growth factors, and cytokines (Rojas et al., 2014). An overexpression of these latter inflammatory mediators can contribute to retinal degeneration (Langmann, 2007; Karlstetter et al., 2010). Also, microglia can act as antigen-presenting cells and even transform into phagocytes (Luo et al., 2010; Kettenmann et al., 2011; Karlstetter et al., 2015; Ransohoff and El Khoury, 2015). Unfortunately the role of the microglia in the pathophysiology of glaucoma is poorly understood, and thus better knowledge of the function of microglial cells in this disease is necessary.

As mentioned above, microglial activation is one of the first events in glaucomatous neurodegeneration (Williams P. A. et al., 2017), but even this activation is prior to the RGC loss (Ebneter et al., 2010; Bosco et al., 2011). In experimental glaucoma models, it has been observed that after treatment with minocycline (Bosco et al., 2008) or with a high dose of irradiation (Bosco et al., 2012), there was a reduction of microglial activation and thus lower RGC death. In addition, in DBA-2J mice a significant quantitative correlation has been established between the microgliosis and the axon loss in the optic nerve (Bosco et al., 2016; **Figure 1C**, **Table 1**).

Neurons can induce an inflammatory response in microglial cells after an injury. Nucleotides released by damaged neurons can up-regulate the purinergic receptors of the microglia, activating their phagocytic ability, motility, and migration (Koizumi et al., 2007; Ohsawa et al., 2007; Wu et al., 2007). It has been demonstrated, in an experimental mouse glaucoma model, that deficiencies in the activation of CX3R1 increase microglial activity, neurotoxicity, and the RGC death (Wang et al., 2014). In addition, in the experimental model of glaucoma, there is an early change in the CD200R/CD200 expression which regulates the microglial activity and precedes RGC death (Taylor et al., 2011). The damaged neurons can release head-shock proteins (HSP), triggering the oxidative response in the microglial cells. These proteins can activate the innate immune system via TRLs in the glaucoma (Tezel, 2009; Karlstetter et al., 2015). In the human glaucoma, high levels of HSP27, HSP60, HSP7, and antibodies against HSPs (Cagnin et al., 2001; Streit et al., 2004; Wyss-Coray, 2006; Stewart et al., 2010; Parpura et al., 2012; Calsolaro and Edison, 2016; De Strooper and Karran, 2016; Bennett et al., 2017) have been found. Furthermore, the dying neurons release the protein HMGB1, which binds to the CD11b receptor of the microglia to induce the production of inflammatory and neurotoxic factors. In experimental glaucoma the elimination of the CD11b receptor has a neuroprotective role since it prevents the microglial activation (Nakazawa et al., 2006).

In glaucoma patients, an overexpression of γ–synuclein has been demonstrated in ganglion cell axons as well as in glial cells of the lamina and postlamina cribosa of the optic nerve. Synuclein has an important role in neurodegenerative diseases, and these findings suggest possible synuclein involvement in glaucomatous alterations in the optic nerve (Surgucheva et al., 2002).

In experimental glaucoma and in the DBA/2j spontaneous mouse glaucoma model, amyloid precursor protein and Aβ were found in the RGCs (**Figure 1C**) in relation to increased IOP (McKinnon et al., 2002; McKinnon, 2003; Goldblum et al., 2007). In addition, abnormal tau (AT8) and phosphorylated tau were found to be present in human ocular tissues of uncontolled IOP and in donor eyes with glaucoma (Gupta et al., 2008; Ning et al., 2008). This implies that Aβ accumulation in the retina is involved in the pathogenesis of glaucoma, this Aβ deposition being related to microglial activation and neuroinflammation (Bolos et al., 2017; **Figure 1C**, **Table 1**).

When microglia are activated, they can adopt different morphologies. In experimental models of glaucoma, activated microglia acquire several morphological phenotypes: stellate cells with thick processes, hyper-ramified cells, rounded cells, amoeboid cells (which act as macrophages, phagocytizing cellular debris) and rod-like microglia. The rod-like microglia are related to neurodegeneration, in the experimental glaucoma model, and the presence of this cell type is restricted to eyes with neuronal damage. It seems that the rod-like microglia might be involved in the active removal or "stripping" of the synaptic contacts (Gallego et al., 2012; de Hoz et al., 2013; Rojas et al., 2014).

In addition to the different morphologies, activated microglia can adopt different functional phenotypes in response to neuronal damage. After injury, the cytokines released by the damaged cells (e.g., IFN-γ) give rise to the microglial activation, acquiring a M1-like phenotype. This phenotype is characterized by production of proteolytic enzymes and pro-inflammatory cytokines (TNF-α, IL-1β, IL-6, IL-12, and NO) promoting tissue inflammation (Varnum and Ikezu, 2012; Gonzalez et al., 2014; Jones and Bouvier, 2014). In human glaucoma and in the experimental models of glaucoma, high levels of these pro-inflammatory cytokines have been found (Neufeld et al., 1997; Shareef et al., 1999; Tezel et al., 2001; Nakazawa et al., 2006; Vidal et al., 2006; Lee et al., 2014; Madeira et al., 2015).

In experimental glaucoma, it has been observed that the activated microglia can migrate to remove the damaged or dead cells (Bosco et al., 2012; Rojas et al., 2014). In the human glaucoma the amoeboid microglia are located in the lamina cribrosa phagocyting the damaged axons (Neufeld, 1999). The morphology change of the microglia from the ramified shape to the amoeboid phagocytic shape is associated with the expression of different surface markers such as: MHC-II (OX6), CD68, Griffonia simplicifolia isolectin B4, complement receptor 3 (CD11b/CD18, OX42), and F4/80 (Kreutzberg, 1996; Streit et al., 1999). In a unilateral experimental glaucoma model, CD68 expression (a member of the scavenger-receptor family) was observed in the retinal microglia (Rojas et al., 2014). The migration and the proliferation of the microglial cells are regulated by soluble factors or by the extracellular matrix changes of damaged CNS tissues. It has been found that microglia of the optic-nerve head express different matrix metalloproteinases and their inhibitors, indicating their participation in the remodeling of the extracellular matrix (Yuan and Neufeld, 2001; Garden and Möller, 2006).

The activation of the microglia also involves higher numbers of microglial cells. This fact it has been observed in human glaucoma and in glaucoma animal models (Giulian and Ingeman, 1988; Yuan and Neufeld, 2001; Naskar et al., 2002; Inman and Horner, 2007; Johnson et al., 2007; Gallego et al., 2012; de Hoz et al., 2013; Rojas et al., 2014). The microglia mitosis can be stimulated by neurotrophic factors (BDNF, NT-3) and several cytokines (macrophage colony-stimulating factors, granulocyte macrophage CSF, IL-1β, IL-4, and IFN-γ) (Garden and Möller, 2006).

In the classical M1 activation, the MHC II, CD86, and Fcγ receptors are up-regulated, because this phenotype is oriented to antigen presentation and the killing of intracellular pathogens (Taylor et al., 2005; Cherry et al., 2014). Under physiological conditions, some microglial cells express very low levels of MHC-II, although certain pro-inflammatory cytokines (e.g., TNF-α or IFN-γ) can upregulate MHC-II expression by microglial cells. In this context, both for glaucoma patients (Yang et al., 2001b; Tezel, 2009; Ebneter et al., 2010) and in animal models of glaucoma (Ebneter et al., 2010; Gallego et al., 2012; de Hoz et al., 2013; Rojas et al., 2014) there is evidence for increased expression of MHC-II molecules in glial cells. In a glaucoma model, after 15 days of ocular hypertension (OHT), most of microglial cells were MHC-II + while the CD86 expression was observed only in some amoeboid and rounded Iba-1+cells in the NFL and the GCL (Rojas et al., 2014). The fact that most of microglial cells were CD86- could prevent T-cell activation by their omission of co-stimulation, leading to a downregulation of the immune response (Broderick et al., 2000). In addition, in an experimental glaucoma model the MHC-II upregulation by the activated microglia in the optic nerve could be associated with more severe RGC degeneration (Chidlow et al., 2016). It has been observed in an experimental glaucoma model that caffeine administration decreases the microglia MHC-II upregulation reducing microglial activation and increasing RGC survival (Madeira et al., 2016).

After M1 activation, the microglial cells can return to a state of rest, adopting a transitory state of M2 activation. In this state, the microglia can upregulate CD68, CD206, and Ym1 (Menzies et al., 2010; Komori et al., 2011; Varnum and Ikezu, 2012; Jones and Bouvier, 2014; Zhou et al., 2014). In an experimental model of unilateral glaucoma, it was observed that the only cells expressing Ym1 were amoeboid Iba-1 + cells in the NFL and GCL of the OHT retinas. The authors postulated that most of the microglial cells in this OHT model were serving functions not related with the M2 microglial phenotype (Rojas et al., 2014).

In glaucomatous eyes, the chronic stress in the tissue can induce the rupture of the blood-retinal barrier, allowing the contact of nervous tissue of the retina and the optic nerve with systemic immune cells (Tezel, 2009). In addition, chemokines (CCL2, CCL5, CCL20, CXCL10, CXCL12, CXCL1, CXCL2, and CX3CL1) released by reactive astrocytes can recruit dendritic cells, microglia, monocytes/macrophages, and T-cells into the inflamed tissue (Farina et al., 2007; Gonzalez et al., 2014). In a chronic glaucoma model DBA/2J, the loss of CX3CL1 signaling increased the infiltration of peripheral macrophages (Breen et al., 2016). The role of monocytes in the survival of RGCs is controversial. In an experimental model of OHT it was observed that an increased number of monocytes could be protective (London et al., 2011). However, in a genetic model of glaucoma (DBA/2J) the irradiation that lowered the number of monocytes boosted RGC survival (Howell et al., 2012).

In addition, the blood retinal barrier breakdown (**Figure 1C**, **Table 1**) can allow the entry of complement proteins, thus activating the complement in the retinal tissue (Karlstetter et al.,

2015). For retinal homeostasis, the level of complement proteins should be low. However, the complement constituents can be activated by inflammatory cytokines (e.g., TNF-α, INF-γ, and IL-6) produced under inflammatory conditions such as glaucoma (Karlstetter et al., 2015). In the retina of the glaucomatous eyes an upregulation of the component complement C1q has been observed (Steele et al., 2005; Stasi et al., 2006). Microglial cells respond to C1q upregulation by eliminating the targeted synapses (Steele et al., 2005; Stasi et al., 2006). Thus, the involvement of the immune system in glaucomatous pathology has been postulated. Recently, it has been suggested that oral microbiome could be related to glaucoma pathophysiology, through microglial activation mediated through TLR4 signaling and complement upregulation (Astafurov et al., 2014). Apart from the chronic activation of resident immunoregulatory glial cells, the presence of plasma cells in the retina, and the complement activation (Tezel, 2009), high levels of autoantibodies and deposition of immunoglobulins have been found in the glaucomatous neurodegeneration (Wax et al., 1998; Hammam et al., 2008; Gramlich et al., 2013; Pinazo-Duran et al., 2013). It has even been speculated that the glaucoma would be mediated by an autoimmune mechanism and that both innate and adaptive responses accompany this pathology (Tezel, 2009, 2013). The serum of glaucoma patients has been found to contain high levels of antibodies (e.g., against HSPs; Maruyama et al., 2000; Wax et al., 2001; Tezel et al., 2004; Grus et al., 2008). Moreover, serum alteration of the populations of T-cell repertoires and of interleukin-2 receptors has been detected (Yang et al., 2001a). In view of the evidence mentioned above, the immune response could be involved in the pathogenesis of the glaucoma.

CONCLUSION

AD, PD, and glaucoma are neurodegenerative diseases that share a common pathogenic mechanism, in which the neuroinflammation, in the form of microglial activation, plays an important part. The differential activation of microglia (M1 or M2 phenotypes) can produce a neurotoxic or neuroprotective environment, and could constitute a key in neuroinflammation regulation. In the search for a new strategy to control neuroinflammation, it might be more effective to change the M1 phenotype to the M2 phenotype than to block microglial activation completely. In the regulation of microglial activation, several cell types including, neurons, astrocytes, and T-cells are involved. When the neuroinflammatory process is triggered by protein aggregates (Aß, α-syn, pTau etc.), peripheral immune cells infiltrate CNS and prompt more activation on resident microglia, favoring neuroinflammatory processes.

Neuroinflammatory processes occur not only in the brain but also in the retina, because the retina is a projection of the CNS. Thus AD, PD, and glaucoma share neuroinflammatory changes in the retinal tissue. The follow up of neuroinflammatory processes in the retinal tissue may be useful for the early diagnosis and monitoring of neurodegenerative diseases. Future research could therefore address these issues to provide fuller knowledge of neuroinflammatory events that occur in AD, PD, and glaucoma, especially the contribution of microglia. This might help in the development of new therapeutic strategies to control neuroinflammation and thereby spur progress in treating these neurodegenerative diseases.

AUTHOR CONTRIBUTIONS

Conception of the work: Rd, JS, AR, ES, BR, AT, and JR. Acquisition, analysis and interpretation of data for the work: Rd, JS, AR, ES, and JR. Bibliographic research: Rd, JS, AR, ES, DA, PR, IL, and JR. Drafting the work: Rd, JS, AR, ES, DA, IL, and JR. Revising critically for important intellectual content: Rd, JS, AR, ES, DA, IL, PR, BR, AT, and JR. Final approval of the version to be published Rd, JS, AR, ES, IL, DA, PR, BR, AT, and JR. Agreement to be accountable for all aspects of the work in ensuring that questions related to the accuracy or integrity of any part of the work are appropriately investigated and resolved: Rd, JS, AR, ES, DA, IL, PR, BR, AT, and JR.

FUNDING

This work was supported by the Ophthalmological Network OFTARED (RD16/0008/0005: Enfermedades oculares: "Prevención, detección precoz, tratamiento y rehabilitación de las patologías oculares."), of the Institute of Health of Carlos III of the Spanish Ministry of Economy. This work has been funded by the PN I+D+i 2008–2011, by the ISCIII-Subdirección General de Redes y Centros de Investigación Cooperativa, and by the European programme FEDER. SAF-2014-53779-R: Neuroinflamación en glaucoma: Secuenciación de la alteración glial y de la barrera hematorretiniana. AINES encapsulados en microparticulas de PLGA como terapia neuroprotectora" from the Spanish Ministry of Economy and Competitiveness. Grants to Elena Salobrar-Garcia are currently supported by a Predoctoral Fellowship (FPU) from the Spanish Ministry of Education, Culture and Sport.

ACKNOWLEDGMENTS

David Nesbitt corrected the English version of this work.

REFERENCES

Alafuzoff, I., and Parkkinen, L. (2014). Staged pathology in Parkinson's disease. *Parkinsonism Relat. Disord.* 20 (Suppl. 1), S57–S61. doi: 10.1016/S1353-8020(13)70016-6

Alexandrov, P. N., Pogue, A., Bhattacharjee, S., and Lukiw, W. J. (2011). Retinal amyloid peptides and complement factor H in transgenic models of Alzheimer's disease. *Neuroreport* 22, 623–627. doi: 10.1097/WNR.0b013e3283497334

Anderson, J. P., Walker, D. E., Goldstein, J. M., de Laat, R., Banducci, K., Caccavello, R. J., et al. (2006). Phosphorylation of Ser-129 is the dominant pathological modification of alpha-synuclein in familial and sporadic Lewy body disease. *J. Biol. Chem.* 281, 29739–29752. doi: 10.1074/jbc.M600933200

Andreasson, K. I., Bachstetter, A. D., Colonna, M., Ginhoux, F., Holmes, C., Lamb, B., et al. (2016). Targeting innate immunity for neurodegenerative disorders of the central nervous system. *J. Neurochem.* 138, 653–693. doi: 10.1111/jnc.13667

Antonucci, F., Turola, E., Riganti, L., Caleo, M., Gabrielli, M., Perrotta, C., et al. (2012). Microvesicles released from microglia stimulate synaptic activity via enhanced sphingolipid metabolism. *EMBO J.* 31, 1231–1240. doi: 10.1038/emboj.2011.489

Appel, S. H., Beers, D. R., and Henkel, J. S. (2010). T cell-microglial dialogue in Parkinson's disease and amyotrophic lateral sclerosis: are we listening? *Trends Immunol.* 31, 7–17. doi: 10.1016/j.it.2009.09.003

Astafurov, K., Elhawy, E., Ren, L., Dong, C. Q., Igboin, C., Hyman, L., et al. (2014). Oral microbiome link to neurodegeneration in glaucoma. *PLoS ONE* 9:e104416. doi: 10.1371/journal.pone.0104416

Beach, T. G., Carew, J., Serrano, G., Adler, C. H., Shill, H. A., Sue, L. I., et al. (2014). Phosphorylated alpha-synuclein-immunoreactive retinal neuronal elements in Parkinson's disease subjects. *Neurosci. Lett.* 571, 34–38. doi: 10.1016/j.neulet.2014.04.027

Bennett, R. E., DeVos, S. L., Dujardin, S., Corjuc, B., Gor, R., Gonzalez, J., et al. (2017). Enhanced tau aggregation in the presence of Amyloid β. *Am. J. Pathol.* 187, 1601–1612. doi: 10.1016/j.ajpath.2017.03.011

Bialas, A. R., and Stevens, B. (2013). TGF-beta signaling regulates neuronal C1q expression and developmental synaptic refinement. *Nat. Neurosci.* 16, 1773–1782. doi: 10.1038/nn.3560

Block, M. L., Zecca, L., and Hong, J. S. (2007). Microglia-mediated neurotoxicity: uncovering the molecular mechanisms. *Nat. Rev. Neurosci.* 8, 57–69. doi: 10.1038/nrn2038

Bodis-Wollner, I. (1990). Visual deficits related to dopamine deficiency in experimental animals and Parkinson's disease patients. *Trends Neurosci.* 13, 296–302. doi: 10.1016/0166-2236(90)90113-O

Bodis-Wollner, I., Kozlowski, P. B., Glazman, S., and Miri, S. (2014). Alpha-Synuclein in the inner retina in Parkinson disease. *Ann. Neurol.* 75, 964–966. doi: 10.1002/ana.24182

Boeke, A., Rosen, D., Mastrianni, J., Xie, T., and Bernard, J. (2016). Optical coherence tomography as potential biomarker in Parkinson's disease and Alzheimer's disease (P5. 177). *Neurology* 86(16 Suppl.), P5. 177.

Bolos, M., Perea, J. R., and Avila, J. (2017). Alzheimer's disease as an inflammatory disease. *Biomol. Concepts* 8, 37–43. doi: 10.1515/bmc-2016-0029

Bosco, A., Breen, K. T., Anderson, S. R., Steele, M. R., Calkins, D. J., and Vetter, M. L. (2016). Glial coverage in the optic nerve expands in proportion to optic axon loss in chronic mouse glaucoma. *Exp. Eye Res.* 150, 34–43. doi: 10.1016/j.exer.2016.01.014

Bosco, A., Crish, S. D., Steele, M. R., Romero, C. O., Inman, D. M., Horner, P. J., et al. (2012). Early reduction of microglia activation by irradiation in a model of chronic glaucoma. *PLoS ONE* 7:e43602. doi: 10.1371/journal.pone.0043602

Bosco, A., Inman, D. M., Steele, M. R., Wu, G., Soto, I., Marsh-Armstrong, N., et al. (2008). Reduced retina microglial activation and improved optic nerve integrity with minocycline treatment in the DBA/2J mouse model of glaucoma. *Invest. Ophthalmol. Vis. Sci.* 49, 1437–1446. doi: 10.1167/iovs.07-1337

Bosco, A., Steele, M. R., and Vetter, M. L. (2011). Early microglia activation in a mouse model of chronic glaucoma. *J. Comp. Neurol.* 519, 599–620. doi: 10.1002/cne.22516

Braak, H., Del Tredici, K., Rub, U., de Vos, R. A., Jansen Steur, E. N., and Braak, E. (2003). Staging of brain pathology related to sporadic Parkinson's disease. *Neurobiol. Aging* 24, 197–211. doi: 10.1016/S0197-4580(02)00065-9

Breen, K. T., Anderson, S. R., Steele, M. R., Calkins, D. J., Bosco, A., and Vetter, M. L. (2016). Loss of fractalkine signaling exacerbates axon transport dysfunction in a chronic model of glaucoma. *Front. Neurosci.* 10:526. doi: 10.3389/fnins.2016.00526

Broderick, C., Duncan, L., Taylor, N., and Dick, A. D. (2000). IFN-gamma and LPS-mediated IL-10-dependent suppression of retinal microglial activation. *Invest. Ophthalmol. Vis. Sci.* 41, 2613–2622.

Brown, G. C., and Neher, J. J. (2014). Microglial phagocytosis of live neurons. *Nat. Rev. Neurosci.* 15, 209–216. doi: 10.1038/nrn3710

Brown, G. C., and Vilalta, A. (2015). How microglia kill neurons. *Brain Res.* 1628(Pt B), 288–297. doi: 10.1016/j.brainres.2015.08.031

Burguillos, M. A., Deierborg, T., Kavanagh, E., Persson, A., Hajji, N., Garcia-Quintanilla, A., et al. (2011). Caspase signalling controls microglia activation and neurotoxicity. *Nature* 472, 319–324. doi: 10.1038/nature09788

Cagnin, A., Brooks, D. J., Kennedy, A. M., Gunn, R. N., Myers, R., Turkheimer, F. E., et al. (2001). *In-vivo* measurement of activated microglia in dementia. *Lancet* 358, 461–467. doi: 10.1016/S0140-6736(01)05625-2

Calabrese, V., Scapagnini, G., Giuffrida Stella, A. M., Bates, T. E., and Clark, J. B. (2001). Mitochondrial involvement in brain function and dysfunction: relevance to aging, neurodegenerative disorders and longevity. *Neurochem. Res.* 26, 739–764. doi: 10.1023/A:1010955807739

Calsolaro, V., and Edison, P. (2016). Neuroinflammation in Alzheimer's disease: current evidence and future directions. *Alzheimers Dement.* 12, 719–732. doi: 10.1016/j.jalz.2016.02.010

Campello, L., Esteve-Rudd, J., Cuenca, N., and Martin-Nieto, J. (2013). The ubiquitin-proteasome system in retinal health and disease. *Mol. Neurobiol.* 47, 790–810. doi: 10.1007/s12035-012-8391-5

Cao, S., Standaert, D. G., and Harms, A. S. (2012). The gamma chain subunit of Fc receptors is required for alpha-synuclein-induced pro-inflammatory signaling in microglia. *J. Neuroinflammat.* 9, 259-2094-9-259. doi: 10.1186/1742-2094-9-259

Chang, R. C., Hudson, P., Wilson, B., Haddon, L., and Hong, J. S. (2000). Influence of neurons on lipopolysaccharide-stimulated production of nitric oxide and tumor necrosis factor-alpha by cultured glia. *Brain Res.* 853, 236–244. doi: 10.1016/S0006-8993(99)02255-6

Chao, Y., Wong, S. C., and Tan, E. K. (2014). Evidence of inflammatory system involvement in Parkinson's disease. *Biomed Res. Int.* 2014:308654. doi: 10.1155/2014/308654

Chen, S. T., Hsu, J. R., Hsu, P. C., and Chuang, J. I. (2003). The retina as a novel *in vivo* model for studying the role of molecules of the Bcl-2 family in relation to MPTP neurotoxicity. *Neurochem. Res.* 28, 805–814. doi: 10.1023/A:1023298604347

Cherry, J. D., Olschowka, J. A., and O'Banion, M. K. (2014). Neuroinflammation and M2 microglia: the good, the bad, and the inflamed. *J. Neuroinflammat.* 11:98. doi: 10.1186/1742-2094-11-98

Chiarini, A., Armato, U., Liu, D., and Dal Pra, I. (2016). Calcium-sensing receptors of human neural cells play crucial roles in Alzheimer's disease. *Front. Physiol.* 7:134. doi: 10.3389/fphys.2016.00134

Chidlow, G., Ebneter, A., Wood, J. P., and Casson, R. J. (2016). Evidence supporting an association between expression of major histocompatibility complex II by microglia and optic nerve degeneration during experimental glaucoma. *J. Glaucoma* 25, 681–691. doi: 10.1097/IJG.0000000000000447

Cho, K. I., Searle, K., Webb, M., Yi, H., and Ferreira, P. A. (2012). Ranbp2 haploinsufficiency mediates distinct cellular and biochemical phenotypes in brain and retinal dopaminergic and glia cells elicited by the Parkinsonian neurotoxin, 1-methyl-4-phenyl-1,2,3,6-tetrahydropyridine (MPTP). *Cell. Mol. Life Sci.* 69, 3511–3527. doi: 10.1007/s00018-012-1071-9

Chrysostomou, V., Rezania, F., Trounce, I. A., and Crowston, J. G. (2013). Oxidative stress and mitochondrial dysfunction in glaucoma. *Curr. Opin. Pharmacol.* 13, 12–15. doi: 10.1016/j.coph.2012.09.008

Clark, A. K., Gruber-Schoffnegger, D., Drdla-Schutting, R., Gerhold, K. J., Malcangio, M., and Sandkuhler, J. (2015). Selective activation of microglia facilitates synaptic strength. *J. Neurosci.* 35, 4552–4570. doi: 10.1523/JNEUROSCI.2061-14.2015

Conway, K. A., Harper, J. D., and Lansbury, P. T. (1998). Accelerated *in vitro* fibril formation by a mutant alpha-synuclein linked to early-onset Parkinson disease. *Nat. Med.* 4, 1318–1320. doi: 10.1038/3311

Cosenza-Nashat, M., Zhao, M. L., Suh, H. S., Morgan, J., Natividad, R., Morgello, S., et al. (2009). Expression of the translocator protein of 18 kDa by microglia, macrophages and astrocytes based on immunohistochemical localization in abnormal human brain. *Neuropathol. Appl. Neurobiol.* 35, 306–328. doi: 10.1111/j.1365-2990.2008.01006.x

Cuenca, N., Fernández-Sánchez, L., Campello, L., Maneu, V., De la Villa, P., Lax, P., et al. (2014). Cellular responses following retinal injuries and therapeutic approaches for neurodegenerative diseases. *Prog. Retin. Eye Res.* 43, 17–75. doi: 10.1016/j.preteyeres.2014.07.001

Cuenca, N., Herrero, M. T., Angulo, A., de Juan, E., Martinez-Navarrete, G. C., Lopez, S., et al. (2005). Morphological impairments in retinal neurons of the scotopic visual pathway in a monkey model of Parkinson's disease. *J. Comp. Neurol.* 493, 261–273. doi: 10.1002/cne.20761

da Fonseca, A. C., Matias, D., Garcia, C., Amaral, R., Geraldo, L. H., Freitas, C., et al. (2014). The impact of microglial activation on blood-brain barrier in brain diseases. *Front. Cell Neurosci.* 8:362. doi: 10.3389/fncel.2014.00362

D'Andrea, M. R. (2005). Add Alzheimer's disease to the list of autoimmune diseases. *Med. Hypotheses* 64, 458–463. doi: 10.1016/j.mehy.2004.08.024

Danesh-Meyer, H. V., Birch, H., Ku, J. Y., Carroll, S., and Gamble, G. (2006). Reduction of optic nerve fibers in patients with Alzheimer disease identified by laser imaging. *Neurology* 67, 1852–1854. doi: 10.1212/01.wnl.0000244490.07925.8b

Dauer, W., and Przedborski, S. (2003). Parkinson's disease: mechanisms and models. *Neuron* 39, 889–909. doi: 10.1016/s0896-6273(03)00568-3

de Hoz, R., Gallego, B. I., Ramírez, A. I., Rojas, B., Salazar, J. J., Valiente-Soriano, F. J., et al. (2013). Rod-like microglia are restricted to eyes with laser-induced ocular hypertension but absent from the microglial changes in the contralateral untreated eye. *PLoS ONE* 8:e83733. doi: 10.1371/journal.pone.0083733

de Hoz, R., Rojas, B., Ramirez, A. I., Salazar, J. J., Gallego, B. I., Trivino, A., et al. (2016). Retinal Macroglial Responses in Health and Disease. *Biomed. Res. Int.* 2016:2954721. doi: 10.1155/2016/2954721

de Lau, L. M., and Breteler, M. M. (2006). Epidemiology of Parkinson's disease. *Lancet Neurol* 5, 525–535. doi: 10.1016/S1474-4422(06)70471-9

De Strooper, B., and Karran, E. (2016). The cellular phase of Alzheimer's disease. *Cell* 164, 603–615. doi: 10.1016/j.cell.2015.12.056

Deane, R., Singh, I., Sagare, A. P., Bell, R. D., Ross, N. T., LaRue, B., et al. (2012). A multimodal RAGE-specific inhibitor reduces amyloid beta-mediated brain disorder in a mouse model of Alzheimer disease. *J. Clin. Invest.* 122, 1377–1392. doi: 10.1172/JCI58642

Ding, Y. M., Jaumotte, J. D., Signore, A. P., and Zigmond, M. J. (2004). Effects of 6-hydroxydopamine on primary cultures of substantia nigra: specific damage to dopamine neurons and the impact of glial cell line-derived neurotrophic factor. *J. Neurochem.* 89, 776–787. doi: 10.1111/j.1471-4159.2004.02415.x

Djamgoz, M. B., Hankins, M. W., Hirano, J., and Archer, S. N. (1997). Neurobiology of retinal dopamine in relation to degenerative states of the tissue. *Vision Res.* 37, 3509–3529. doi: 10.1016/S0042-6989(97)00129-6

Doorn, K. J., Moors, T., Drukarch, B., van de Berg, W. D., Lucassen, P. J., and van Dam, A. M. (2014). Microglial phenotypes and toll-like receptor 2 in the substantia nigra and hippocampus of incidental Lewy body disease cases and Parkinson's disease patients. *Acta Neuropathol. Commun.* 2:90-014-0090-1. doi: 10.1186/s40478-014-0090-1

Dudvarski Stankovic, N., Teodorczyk, M., Ploen, R., Zipp, F., and Schmidt, M. H. (2016). Microglia-blood vessel interactions: a double-edged sword in brain pathologies. *Acta Neuropathol.* 131, 347–363. doi: 10.1007/s00401-015-1524-y

Ebneter, A., Casson, R. J., Wood, J. P., and Chidlow, G. (2010). Microglial activation in the visual pathway in experimental glaucoma: spatiotemporal characterization and correlation with axonal injury. *Invest. Ophthalmol. Vis. Sci.* 51, 6448–6460. doi: 10.1167/iovs.10-5284

Esteve-Rudd, J., Fernandez-Sanchez, L., Lax, P., De Juan, E., Martin-Nieto, J., and Cuenca, N. (2011). Rotenone induces degeneration of photoreceptors and impairs the dopaminergic system in the rat retina. *Neurobiol. Dis.* 44, 102–115. doi: 10.1016/j.nbd.2011.06.009

Fakhoury, M. (2016). Immune-mediated processes in neurodegeneration: where do we stand? *J. Neurol.* 263, 1683–1701. doi: 10.1007/s00415-016-8052-0

Fallon, M., Valero, O., Pazos, M., and Antón, A. (2017). Diagnostic accuracy of imaging devices in glaucoma: a meta-analysis. *Surv. Ophthalmol.* 62, 446–461. doi: 10.1016/j.survophthal.2017.01.001

Farina, C., Aloisi, F., and Meinl, E. (2007). Astrocytes are active players in cerebral innate immunity. *Trends Immunol.* 28, 138–145. doi: 10.1016/j.it.2007.01.005

Fellner, L., Irschick, R., Schanda, K., Reindl, M., Klimaschewski, L., Poewe, W., et al. (2013). Toll-like receptor 4 is required for α-synuclein dependent activation of microglia and astroglia. *Glia* 61, 349–360. doi: 10.1002/glia.22437

Fu, R., Shen, Q., Xu, P., Luo, J. J., and Tang, Y. (2014). Phagocytosis of microglia in the central nervous system diseases. *Mol. Neurobiol.* 49, 1422–1434. doi: 10.1007/s12035-013-8620-6

Gallego, B. I., Salazar, J. J., de Hoz, R., Rojas, B., Ramírez, A. I., Salinas-Navarro, M., et al. (2012). IOP induces upregulation of GFAP and MHC-II and microglia reactivity in mice retina contralateral to experimental glaucoma. *J. Neuroinflammat.* 9:92. doi: 10.1186/1742-2094-9-92

Garcia-Martin, E. S., Rojas, B., Ramirez, A. I., de Hoz, R., Salazar, J. J., Yubero, R., et al. (2014). Macular thickness as a potential biomarker of mild Alzheimer's disease. *Ophthalmology* 121, 1149–1151.e3. doi: 10.1016/j.ophtha.2013.12.023

Garcia-Ospina, G. P., Jimenez-Del Rio, M., Lopera, F., and Velez-Pardo, C. (2003). Neuronal DNA damage correlates with a positive detection of c-Jun, nuclear factor kB, p53 and Par-4 transcription factors in Alzheimer's disease. *Rev. Neurol* 36, 1004–1010.

Garden, G. A., and Möller, T. (2006). Microglia biology in health and disease. *J. Neuroimmune Pharmacol.* 1, 127–137. doi: 10.1007/s11481-006-9015-5

Garlanda, C., Dinarello, C. A., and Mantovani, A. (2013). The interleukin-1 family: back to the future. *Immunity* 39, 1003–1018. doi: 10.1016/j.immuni.2013.11.010

Gasparini, L., Crowther, R. A., Martin, K. R., Berg, N., Coleman, M., Goedert, M., et al. (2011). Tau inclusions in retinal ganglion cells of human P301S tau transgenic mice: effects on axonal viability. *Neurobiol. Aging* 32, 419–433. doi: 10.1016/j.neurobiolaging.2009.03.002

Gazulla, J., and Cavero-Nagore, M. (2006). Glutamate and Alzheimer's disease. *Rev. Neurol* 42, 427–432.

George, S., and Brundin, P. (2015). Immunotherapy in Parkinson's disease: micromanaging Alpha-Synuclein aggregation. *J. Parkinsons Dis.* 5, 413–424. doi: 10.3233/JPD-150630

Ghiso, J. A., Doudevski, I., Ritch, R., and Rostagno, A. A. (2013). Alzheimer's disease and glaucoma: mechanistic similarities and differences. *J. Glaucoma* 22(Suppl. 5), S36–S38. doi: 10.1097/IJG.0b013e3182934af6

Giasson, B. I., Duda, J. E., Murray, I. V., Chen, Q., Souza, J. M., Hurtig, H. I., et al. (2000). Oxidative damage linked to neurodegeneration by selective alpha-synuclein nitration in synucleinopathy lesions. *Science* 290, 985–989. doi: 10.1126/science.290.5493.985

Giulian, D., and Ingeman, J. E. (1988). Colony-stimulating factors as promoters of ameboid microglia. *J. Neurosci.* 8, 4707–4717.

Glass, C. K., Saijo, K., Winner, B., Marchetto, M. C., and Gage, F. H. (2010). Mechanisms underlying inflammation in neurodegeneration. *Cell* 140, 918–934. doi: 10.1016/j.cell.2010.02.016

Glezer, I., Simard, A. R., and Rivest, S. (2007). Neuroprotective role of the innate immune system by microglia. *Neuroscience* 147, 867–883. doi: 10.1016/j.neuroscience.2007.02.055

Gold, M., and El Khoury, J. (2015). beta-amyloid, microglia, and the inflammasome in Alzheimer's disease. *Semin. Immunopathol.* 37, 607–611. doi: 10.1007/s00281-015-0518-0

Goldblum, D., Kipfer-Kauer, A., Sarra, G. M., Wolf, S., and Frueh, B. E. (2007). Distribution of amyloid precursor protein and amyloid-beta immunoreactivity in DBA/2J glaucomatous mouse retinas. *Invest. Ophthalmol. Vis. Sci.* 48, 5085–5090. doi: 10.1167/iovs.06-1249

Gonzalez, H., Contreras, F., and Pacheco, R. (2015). Regulation of the neurodegenerative process associated to Parkinson's disease by CD4+ T-cells. *J. Neuroimmune Pharmacol.* 10, 561–575. doi: 10.1007/s11481-015-9618-9

Gonzalez, H., Elgueta, D., Montoya, A., and Pacheco, R. (2014). Neuroimmune regulation of microglial activity involved in neuroinflammation and neurodegenerative diseases. *J. Neuroimmunol.* 274, 1–13. doi: 10.1016/j.jneuroim.2014.07.012

Gordon, R., Anantharam, V., Kanthasamy, A. G., and Kanthasamy, A. (2012). Proteolytic activation of proapoptotic kinase protein kinase Cdelta by tumor necrosis factor alpha death receptor signaling in dopaminergic neurons during neuroinflammation. *J. Neuroinflammat.* 9, 1–18. doi: 10.1186/1742-2094-9-82

Graeber, M. B., and Streit, W. J. (2010). Microglia: biology and pathology. *Acta Neuropathol.* 119, 89–105. doi: 10.1007/s00401-009-0622-0

Gramlich, O. W., Beck, S., von Hohenstein-Blaul, N., Boehm, N., Ziegler, A., Vetter, J. M., et al. (2013). Enhanced insight into the autoimmune component of glaucoma: IgG autoantibody accumulation and pro-inflammatory conditions in human glaucomatous retina. *PLoS ONE* 8:e57557. doi: 10.1371/journal.pone.0057557

Grus, F. H., Joachim, S. C., Wuenschig, D., Rieck, J., and Pfeiffer, N. (2008). Autoimmunity and glaucoma. *J. Glaucoma* 17, 79–84. doi: 10.1097/IJG.0b013e318156a592

Guerriero, F., Sgarlata, C., Francis, M., Maurizi, N., Faragli, A., Perna, S., et al. (2016). Neuroinflammation, immune system and Alzheimer disease: searching for the missing link. *Aging Clin. Exp. Res.* doi: 10.1007/s40520-016-0637-z. [Epub ahead of print].

Guimaraes, J. S., Freire, M. A., Lima, R. R., Souza-Rodrigues, R. D., Costa, A. M., dos Santos, C. D., et al. (2009). Mechanisms of secondary degeneration in the central nervous system during acute neural disorders and white matter damage. *Rev. Neurol.* 48, 304–310.

Gupta, N., Ang, L. C., Noel de Tilly, L., Bidaisee, L., and Yucel, Y. H. (2006). Human glaucoma and neural degeneration in intracranial optic nerve, lateral geniculate nucleus, and visual cortex. *Br. J. Ophthalmol.* 90, 674–678. doi: 10.1136/bjo.2005.086769

Gupta, N., Fong, J., Ang, L. C., and Yucel, Y. H. (2008). Retinal tau pathology in human glaucomas. *Can. J. Ophthalmol.* 43, 53–60. doi: 10.3129/i07-185

Gupta, N., Ly, T., Zhang, Q., Kaufman, P. L., Weinreb, R. N., and Yucel, Y. H. (2007). Chronic ocular hypertension induces dendrite pathology in the lateral geniculate nucleus of the brain. *Exp. Eye Res.* 84, 176–184. doi: 10.1016/j.exer.2006.09.013

Hajee, M. E., March, W. F., Lazzaro, D. R., Wolintz, A. H., Shrier, E. M., Glazman, S., et al. (2009). Inner retinal layer thinning in Parkinson disease. *Arch. Ophthalmol.* 127, 737–741. doi: 10.1001/archophthalmol.2009.106

Hammam, T., Montgomery, D., Morris, D., and Imrie, F. (2008). Prevalence of serum autoantibodies and paraproteins in patients with glaucoma. *Eye (Lond).* 22, 349–353. doi: 10.1038/sj.eye.6702613

Hamza, T. H., Zabetian, C. P., Tenesa, A., Laederach, A., Montimurro, J., Yearout, D., et al. (2010). Common genetic variation in the HLA region is associated with late-onset sporadic Parkinson's disease. *Nat. Genet.* 42, 781–785. doi: 10.1038/ng.642

Han, J., Wang, M., Ren, M., and Lou, H. (2017). Contributions of triggering-receptor-expressed-on-myeloid-cells-2 to neurological diseases. *Int. J. Neurosci.* 127, 368–375. doi: 10.1080/00207454.2016.1264072

Hanisch, U. K., and Kettenmann, H. (2007). Microglia: active sensor and versatile effector cells in the normal and pathologic brain. *Nat. Neurosci.* 10, 1387–1394. doi: 10.1038/nn1997

Hardy, J., and Selkoe, D. J. (2002). The amyloid hypothesis of Alzheimer's disease: progress and problems on the road to therapeutics. *Science* 297, 353–356. doi: 10.1126/science.1072994

Harms, A. S., Cao, S., Rowse, A. L., Thome, A. D., Li, X., Mangieri, L. R., et al. (2013). MHCII is required for alpha-synuclein-induced activation of microglia, CD4 T cell proliferation, and dopaminergic neurodegeneration. *J. Neurosci.* 33, 9592–9600. doi: 10.1523/JNEUROSCI.5610-12.2013

Hart, N. J., Koronyo, Y., Black, K. L., and Koronyo-Hamaoui, M. (2016). Ocular indicators of Alzheimer's: exploring disease in the retina. *Acta Neuropathol.* 132, 767–787. doi: 10.1007/s00401-016-1613-6

Hatfield, C. F., Herbert, J., van Someren, E. J., Hodges, J. R., and Hastings, M. H. (2004). Disrupted daily activity/rest cycles in relation to daily cortisol rhythms of home-dwelling patients with early Alzheimer's dementia. *Brain* 127(Pt 5), 1061–1074. doi: 10.1093/brain/awh129

Hedges, T. R., III, Perez Galves, R., Speigelman, D., Barbas, N. R., Peli, E., et al. (1996). Retinal nerve fiber layer abnormalities in Alzheimer's disease. *Acta Ophthalmol. Scand.* 74, 271–275. doi: 10.1111/j.1600-0420.1996.tb00090.x

Heneka, M. T., Carson, M. J., El Khoury, J., Landreth, G. E., Brosseron, F., Feinstein, D. L., et al. (2015). Neuroinflammation in Alzheimer's disease. *Lancet Neurol.* 14, 388–405. doi: 10.1016/S1474-4422(15)70016-5

Heneka, M. T., Kummer, M. P., Stutz, A., Delekate, A., Schwartz, S., Vieira-Saecker, A., et al. (2013). NLRP3 is activated in Alzheimer's disease and contributes to pathology in APP/PS1 mice. *Nature* 493, 674–678. doi: 10.1038/nature11729

Hernández-Montiel, H. L. (2006). Aspectos moleculares y prospectos de terapias en la enfermedad de Parkinson. *Bioquimia* 31, 146–158.

Herrera, A. J., Espinosa-Oliva, A. M., Carrillo-Jimenez, A., Oliva-Martin, M. J., Garcia-Revilla, J., Garcia-Quintanilla, A., et al. (2015). Relevance of chronic stress and the two faces of microglia in Parkinson's disease. *Front. Cell Neurosci.* 9:312. doi: 10.3389/fncel.2015.00312

Holcomb, L., Gordon, M. N., McGowan, E., Yu, X., Benkovic, S., Jantzen, P., et al. (1998). Accelerated Alzheimer-type phenotype in transgenic mice carrying both mutant amyloid precursor protein and presenilin 1 transgenes. *Nat. Med.* 4, 97–100. doi: 10.1038/nm0198-097

Hong, S., Dissing-Olesen, L., and Stevens, B. (2016). New insights on the role of microglia in synaptic pruning in health and disease. *Curr. Opin. Neurobiol.* 36, 128–134. doi: 10.1016/j.conb.2015.12.004

Hooghiemstra, A. M., Eggermont, L. H., Scheltens, P., van der Flier, W. M., and Scherder, E. J. (2015). The rest-activity rhythm and physical activity in early-onset dementia. *Alzheimer Dis. Assoc. Disord* 29, 45–49. doi: 10.1097/WAD.0000000000000037

Howell, G. R., Soto, I., Zhu, X., Ryan, M., Macalinao, D. G., Sousa, G. L., et al. (2012). Radiation treatment inhibits monocyte entry into the optic nerve head and prevents neuronal damage in a mouse model of glaucoma. *J. Clin. Invest.* 122, 1246–1261. doi: 10.1172/JCI61135

Hsiao, K., Chapman, P., Nilsen, S., Eckman, C., Harigaya, Y., Younkin, S., et al. (1996). Correlative memory deficits, Abeta elevation, and amyloid plaques in transgenic mice. *Science* 274, 99–102.

Hsieh, C. L., Koike, M., Spusta, S. C., Niemi, E. C., Yenari, M., Nakamura, M. C., et al. (2009). A role for TREM2 ligands in the phagocytosis of apoptotic neuronal cells by microglia. *J. Neurochem.* 109, 1144–1156. doi: 10.1111/j.1471-4159.2009.06042.x

Inman, D. M., and Horner, P. J. (2007). Reactive nonproliferative gliosis predominates in a chronic mouse model of glaucoma. *Glia* 55, 942–953. doi: 10.1002/glia.20516

Inzelberg, R., Ramirez, J. A., Nisipeanu, P., and Ophir, A. (2004). Retinal nerve fiber layer thinning in Parkinson disease. *Vision Res.* 44, 2793–2797. doi: 10.1016/j.visres.2004.06.009

Iseri, P. K., Altinas, O., Tokay, T., and Yuksel, N. (2006). Relationship between cognitive impairment and retinal morphological and visual functional abnormalities in Alzheimer disease. *J. Neuroophthalmol.* 26, 18–24. doi: 10.1097/01.wno.0000204645.56873.26

Jack, C. S., Arbour, N., Manusow, J., Montgrain, V., Blain, M., McCrea, E., et al. (2005). TLR signaling tailors innate immune responses in human microglia and astrocytes. *J. Immunol.* 175, 4320–4330. doi: 10.4049/jimmunol.175.7.4320

Johnson, E. C., Jia, L., Cepurna, W. O., Doser, T. A., and Morrison, J. C. (2007). Global changes in optic nerve head gene expression after exposure to elevated intraocular pressure in a rat glaucoma model. *Invest. Ophthalmol. Vis. Sci.* 48, 3161–3177. doi: 10.1167/iovs.06-1282

Jones, E. V., and Bouvier, D. S. (2014). Astrocyte-secreted matricellular proteins in CNS remodelling during development and disease. *Neural Plast.* 2014:321209. doi: 10.1155/2014/321209

Jonsson, T., Stefansson, H., Steinberg, S., Jonsdottir, I., Jonsson, P. V., Snaedal, J., et al. (2013). Variant of TREM2 associated with the risk of Alzheimer's disease. *N. Engl. J. Med.* 368, 107–116. doi: 10.1056/NEJMoa1211103

Kaarniranta, K., Salminen, A., Haapasalo, A., Soininen, H., and Hiltunen, M. (2011). Age-related macular degeneration (AMD): Alzheimer's disease in the eye? *J. Alzheimer's Dis.* 24, 615–631. doi: 10.3233/JAD-2011-101908

Kannarkat, G. T., Boss, J. M., and Tansey, M. G. (2013). The role of innate and adaptive immunity in Parkinson's disease. *J. Parkinsons Dis.* 3, 493–514. doi: 10.3233/JPD-130250

Karlstetter, M., Ebert, S., and Langmann, T. (2010). Microglia in the healthy and degenerating retina: Insights from novel mouse models. *Immunobiology* 215, 685–691. doi: 10.1016/j.imbio.2010.05.010

Karlstetter, M., Scholz, R., Rutar, M., Wong, W. T., Provis, J. M., and Langmann, T. (2015). Retinal microglia: just bystander or target for therapy? *Prog. Retin. Eye Res.* 45, 30–57. doi: 10.1016/j.preteyeres.2014.11.004

Kayabasi, U., Sergott, R. C., and Rispoli, M. (2014). Retinal examination for the diagnosis of Alzheimer's disease. *Int. J. Ophthal. Pathol.* 3:4. doi: 10.4172/2324-8599.1000145

Kesler, A., Vakhapova, V., Korczyn, A. D., Naftaliev, E., and Neudorfer, M. (2011). Retinal thickness in patients with mild cognitive impairment and Alzheimer's disease. *Clin. Neurol Neurosurg.* 113, 523–526. doi: 10.1016/j.clineuro.2011.02.014

Kettenmann, H., Hanisch, U., Noda, M., and Verkhratsky, A. (2011). Physiology of Microglia. *Physiol. Rev.* 91, 461–553. doi: 10.1152/physrev.00011.2010

Kim, S. R., Chung, E. S., Bok, E., Baik, H. H., Chung, Y. C., Won, S. Y., et al. (2010). Prothrombin kringle-2 induces death of mesencephalic dopaminergic neurons *in vivo* and *in vitro* via microglial activation. *J. Neurosci. Res.* 88, 1537–1548. doi: 10.1002/jnr.22318

Kingsbury, A. E., Daniel, S. E., Sangha, H., Eisen, S., Lees, A. J., and Foster, O. J. (2004). Alteration in alpha-synuclein mRNA expression in Parkinson's disease. *Mov. Disord.* 19, 162–170. doi: 10.1002/mds.10683

Koizumi, S., Shigemoto-Mogami, Y., Nasu-Tada, K., Shinozaki, Y., Ohsawa, K., Tsuda, M., et al. (2007). UDP acting at P2Y6 receptors is a mediator of microglial phagocytosis. *Nature* 446, 1091–1095. doi: 10.1038/nature05704

Komori, T., Morikawa, Y., Inada, T., Hisaoka, T., and Senba, E. (2011). Site-specific subtypes of macrophages recruited after peripheral nerve injury. *Neuroreport* 22, 911–917. doi: 10.1097/WNR.0b013e32834cd76a

Koronyo-Hamaoui, M., Koronyo, Y., Ljubimov, A. V., Miller, C. A., Ko, M. K., Black, K. L., et al. (2011). Identification of amyloid plaques in retinas from Alzheimer's patients and noninvasive *in vivo* optical imaging of retinal plaques in a mouse model. *Neuroimage* 54(Suppl. 1), S204–S217. doi: 10.1016/j.neuroimage.2010.06.020

Krasodomska, K., Lubinski, W., Potemkowski, A., and Honczarenko, K. (2010). Pattern electroretinogram (PERG) and pattern visual evoked potential (PVEP) in the early stages of Alzheimer's disease. *Doc. Ophthalmol.* 121, 111–121. doi: 10.1007/s10633-010-9238-x

Kreutzberg, G. (1995). Microglia, the first line of defence in brain pathologies. *Arzneimittelforschung* 45, 357–360.

Kreutzberg, G. W. (1996). Microglia: a sensor for pathological events in the CNS. *Trends Neurosci.* 19, 312–318. doi: 10.1016/0166-2236(96)10049-7

Kumar-Singh, S., Pirici, D., McGowan, E., Serneels, S., Ceuterick, C., Hardy, J., et al. (2005). Dense-core plaques in Tg2576 and PSAPP mouse models of Alzheimer's disease are centered on vessel walls. *Am. J. Pathol.* 167, 527–543. doi: 10.1016/S0002-9440(10)62995-1

Kummer, M. P., Hermes, M., Delekarte, A., Hammerschmidt, T., Kumar, S., Terwel, D., et al. (2011). Nitration of tyrosine 10 critically enhances amyloid beta aggregation and plaque formation. *Neuron* 71, 833–844. doi: 10.1016/j.neuron.2011.07.001

La Morgia, C., Barboni, P., Rizzo, G., Carbonelli, M., Savini, G., Scaglione, C., et al. (2013). Loss of temporal retinal nerve fibers in Parkinson disease: a mitochondrial pattern? *Eur. J. Neurol.* 20, 198–201. doi: 10.1111/j.1468-1331.2012.03701.x

La Morgia, C., Ross-Cisneros, F. N., Hannibal, J., Montagna, P., Sadun, A. A., and Carelli, V. (2011). Melanopsin-expressing retinal ganglion cells: implications for human diseases. *Vision Res.* 51, 296–302. doi: 10.1016/j.visres.2010.07.023

Lakey-Beitia, J., González, Y., Doens, D., Stephens, D. E., Santamaría, R., Murillo, E., et al. (2017). Assessment of novel curcumin derivatives as potent inhibitors of inflammation and Amyloid-β aggregation in Alzheimer's disease. *J. Alzheimer's Dis.* doi: 10.3233/JAD-170071. [Epub ahead of print].

Langmann, T. (2007). Microglia activation in retinal degeneration. *J. Leukoc. Biol.* 81, 1345–1351. doi: 10.1189/jlb.0207114

Lascaratos, G., Garway-Heath, D. F., Willoughby, C. E., Chau, K., and Schapira, A. H. V. (2012). Mitochondrial dysfunction in glaucoma: understanding genetic influences. *Mitochondrion* 12, 202–212. doi: 10.1016/j.mito.2011.11.004

Lauro, C., Cipriani, R., Catalano, M., Trettel, F., Chece, G., Brusadin, V., et al. (2010). Adenosine A1 receptors and microglial cells mediate CX3CL1-induced protection of hippocampal neurons against Glu-induced death. *Neuropsychopharmacology* 35, 1550–1559. doi: 10.1038/npp.2010.26

Lauro, C., Di Angelantonio, S., Cipriani, R., Sobrero, F., Antonilli, L., Brusadin, V., et al. (2008). Activity of adenosine receptors type 1 Is required for CX3CL1-mediated neuroprotection and neuromodulation in hippocampal neurons. *J. Immunol.* 180, 7590–7596. doi: 10.4049/jimmunol.180.11.7590

Le, W., Wu, J., and Tang, Y. (2016). Protective microglia and their regulation in Parkinson's disease. *Front. Mol. Neurosci.* 9:89. doi: 10.3389/fnmol.2016.00089

Lee, J., Shin, J., Chun, M., and Oh, S. (2014). Morphological analyses on retinal glial responses to glaucomatous injury evoked by venous cauterization. *Appl. Microsc.* 44, 21–29. doi: 10.9729/AM.2014.44.1.21

Lee, S., Van Bergen, N. J., Kong, G. Y., Chrysostomou, V., Waugh, H. S., O'Neill, E. C., et al. (2011). Mitochondrial dysfunction in glaucoma and emerging bioenergetic therapies. *Exp. Eye Res.* 93, 204–212. doi: 10.1016/j.exer.2010.07.015

Leem, E., Jeong, K. H., Won, S. Y., Shin, W. H., and Kim, S. R. (2016). Prothrombin Kringle-2: a potential inflammatory pathogen in the parkinsonian dopaminergic system. *Exp. Neurobiol.* 25, 147–155. doi: 10.5607/en.2016.25.4.147

Leroy, K., Bretteville, A., Schindowski, K., Gilissen, E., Authelet, M., De Decker, R., et al. (2007). Early axonopathy preceding neurofibrillary tangles in mutant tau transgenic mice. *Am. J. Pathol.* 171, 976–992. doi: 10.2353/ajpath.2007.070345

Leung, C. K. (2016). Optical coherence tomography imaging for glaucoma - today and tomorrow. *Asia Pac. J. Ophthalmol. (Phila)* 5, 11–16. doi: 10.1097/APO.0000000000000179

Licht, T., and Keshet, E. (2015). The vascular niche in adult neurogenesis. *Mech. Dev.* 138(Pt 1), 56–62. doi: 10.1016/j.mod.2015.06.001

Liddelow, S. A., Guttenplan, K. A., Clarke, L. E., Bennett, F. C., Bohlen, C. J., Schirmer, L., et al. (2017). Neurotoxic reactive astrocytes are induced by activated microglia. *Nature* 541, 481–487. doi: 10.1038/nature21029

Lim, C. K., Fernández-Gomez, F. J., Braidy, N., Estrada, C., Costa, C., Costa, S., et al. (2017). Involvement of the kynurenine pathway in the pathogenesis of Parkinson's disease. *Prog. Neurobiol.* 155, 76–95. doi: 10.1016/j.pneurobio.2015.12.009

Lim, J. K., Li, Q. X., He, Z., Vingrys, A. J., Wong, V. H., Currier, N., et al. (2016). The eye as a biomarker for Alzheimer's disease. *Front. Neurosci.* 10:536. doi: 10.3389/fnins.2016.00536

Linnartz, B., Kopatz, J., Tenner, A. J., and Neumann, H. (2012). Sialic acid on the neuronal glycocalyx prevents complement C1 binding and complement receptor-3-mediated removal by microglia. *J. Neurosci.* 32, 946–952. doi: 10.1523/JNEUROSCI.3830-11.2012

Liu, B., Rasool, S., Yang, Z., Glabe, C. G., Schreiber, S. S., Ge, J., et al. (2009). Amyloid-peptide vaccinations reduce {beta}-amyloid plaques but exacerbate vascular deposition and inflammation in the retina of Alzheimer's transgenic mice. *Am. J. Pathol.* 175, 2099–2110. doi: 10.2353/ajpath.2009.090159

London, A., Itskovich, E., Benhar, I., Kalchenko, V., Mack, M., Jung, S., et al. (2011). Neuroprotection and progenitor cell renewal in the injured adult murine retina requires healing monocyte-derived macrophages. *J. Exp. Med.* 208, 23–39. doi: 10.1084/jem.20101202

Lukiw, W. J., Gordon, W. C., Rogaev, E. I., Thompson, H., and Bazan, N. G. (2001). Presenilin-2 (PS2) expression up-regulation in a model of retinopathy of prematurity and pathoangiogenesis. *Neuroreport* 12, 53–57. doi: 10.1097/00001756-200101220-00019

Lull, M. E., and Block, M. L. (2010). Microglial Activation and Chronic Neurodegeneration. *Neurotherapeutics* 7, 354–365. doi: 10.1016/j.nurt.2010.05.014

Luo, C., Chen, M., and Xu, H. (2011). Complement gene expression and regulation in mouse retina and retinal pigment epithelium/choroid. *Mol. Vis.* 17, 1588–1597.

Luo, X., Ding, J., and Chen, S. (2010). Microglia in the aging brain: relevance to neurodegeneration. *Mol. Neurodegen.* 5:12. doi: 10.1186/1750-1326-5-12

MacCormick, I. J., Czanner, G., and Faragher, B. (2015). Developing retinal biomarkers of neurological disease: an analytical perspective. *Biomark Med.* 9, 691–701. doi: 10.2217/bmm.15.17

Madeira, M. H., Boia, R., Santos, P. F., Ambrosio, A. F., and Santiago, A. R. (2015). Contribution of microglia-mediated neuroinflammation to retinal degenerative diseases. *Mediat. Inflamm.* 2015:673090. doi: 10.1155/2015/673090

Madeira, M. H., Ortin-Martinez, A., Nadal-Nicolas, F., Ambrosio, A. F., Vidal-Sanz, M., Agudo-Barriuso, M., et al. (2016). Caffeine administration prevents retinal neuroinflammation and loss of retinal ganglion cells in an animal model of glaucoma. *Sci. Rep.* 6:27532. doi: 10.1038/srep27532

Magni, P., Ruscica, M., Dozio, E., Rizzi, E., Beretta, G., and Maffei Facino, R. (2012). Parthenolide inhibits the LPS-induced secretion of IL-6 and TNF-alpha and NF-kappaB nuclear translocation in BV-2 microglia. *Phytother Res.* 26, 1405–1409. doi: 10.1002/ptr.3732

Maiti, P., and Dunbar, G. L. (2016). Rationale for curcumin therapy in Alzheimer's disease. *ARC J. Neurosci.* 1, 10–16. doi: 10.20431/2456-057X.0103002

Maldonado, R. S., Mettu, P., El-Dairi, M., and Bhatti, M. T. (2015). The application of optical coherence tomography in neurologic diseases. *Neurol. Clin. Pract.* 5, 460–469. doi: 10.1212/cpj.0000000000000187

Martínez-Lazcano, J. C., Boll-Woehrlen, M. C., Hernández-Melesio, M., Rubio-Osornio, M., Sánchez-Mendoza, M., and Ríos, C. (2010). Radicales libres y estrés oxidativo en las enfermedades neurodegenerativas. *Mensaje Bioquim* 34, 43–59.

Martinez-Navarrete, G. C., Martin-Nieto, J., Esteve-Rudd, J., Angulo, A., and Cuenca, N. (2007). Alpha synuclein gene expression profile in the retina of vertebrates. *Mol. Vis.* 13, 949–961.

Maruyama, I., Ohguro, H., and Ikeda, Y. (2000). Retinal ganglion cells recognized by serum autoantibody against γ-enolase found in glaucoma patients. *Invest. Ophthalmol. Vis. Sci.* 41, 1657–1665.

Mattson, M. P. (2000). Apoptosis in neurodegenerative disorders. *Nat. Rev. Mol. Cell Biol.* 1, 120–129. doi: 10.1038/35040009

Maurage, C. A., Ruchoux, M. M., de Vos, R., Surguchov, A., and Destee, A. (2003). Retinal involvement in dementia with Lewy bodies: a clue to hallucinations? *Ann. Neurol.* 54, 542–547. doi: 10.1002/ana.10730

McKinnon, S. J. (2003). Glaucoma: ocular Alzheimer's disease. *Front. Biosci* 8, s1140–s1156. doi: 10.2741/1172

McKinnon, S. J., Lehman, D. M., Kerrigan-Baumrind, L. A., Merges, C. A., Pease, M. E., Kerrigan, D. F., et al. (2002). Caspase activation and amyloid precursor protein cleavage in rat ocular hypertension. *Invest. Ophthalmol. Vis. Sci.* 43, 1077–1087.

McLaughlin, P., Zhou, Y., Ma, T., Liu, J., Zhang, W., Hong, J. S., et al. (2006). Proteomic analysis of microglial contribution to mouse strain-dependent dopaminergic neurotoxicity. *Glia* 53, 567–582. doi: 10.1002/glia.20294

Menzies, F. M., Henriquez, F. L., Alexander, J., and Roberts, C. W. (2010). Sequential expression of macrophage anti-microbial/inflammatory and wound healing markers following innate, alternative and classical activation. *Clin. Exp. Immunol.* 160, 369–379. doi: 10.1111/j.1365-2249.2009.04086.x

Meyer-Luehmann, M., and Prinz, M. (2015). Myeloid cells in Alzheimer's disease: culprits, victims or innocent bystanders? *Trends Neurosci.* 38, 659–668. doi: 10.1016/j.tins.2015.08.011

Michelucci, A., Heurtaux, T., Grandbarbe, L., Morga, E., and Heuschling, P. (2009). Characterization of the microglial phenotype under specific pro-inflammatory and anti-inflammatory conditions: effects of oligomeric and fibrillar amyloid-beta. *J. Neuroimmunol.* 210, 3–12. doi: 10.1016/j.jneuroim.2009.02.003

Mirzaei, N., Tang, S. P., Ashworth, S., Coello, C., Plisson, C., Passchier, J., et al. (2016). *In vivo* imaging of microglial activation by positron emission tomography with [(11)C]PBR28 in the 5XFAD model of Alzheimer's disease. *Glia* 64, 993–1006. doi: 10.1002/glia.22978

Mogi, M., Harada, M., Narabayashi, H., Inagaki, H., Minami, M., and Nagatsu, T. (1996). Interleukin (IL)-1 beta, IL-2, IL-4, IL-6 and transforming growth factor-alpha levels are elevated in ventricular cerebrospinal fluid in juvenile parkinsonism and Parkinson's disease. *Neurosci. Lett.* 211, 13–16. doi: 10.1016/0304-3940(96)12706-3

Mosharov, E. V., Staal, R. G., Bove, J., Prou, D., Hananiya, A., Markov, D., et al. (2006). Alpha-synuclein overexpression increases cytosolic catecholamine concentration. *J. Neurosci.* 26, 9304–9311. doi: 10.1523/JNEUROSCI.0519-06.2006

Mosher, K. I., and Wyss-Coray, T. (2014). Microglial dysfunction in brain aging and Alzheimer's disease. *Biochem. Pharmacol.* 88, 594–604. doi: 10.1016/j.bcp.2014.01.008

Nagel, F., Bahr, M., and Dietz, G. P. (2009). Tyrosine hydroxylase-positive amacrine interneurons in the mouse retina are resistant against the application of various parkinsonian toxins. *Brain Res. Bull.* 79, 303–309. doi: 10.1016/j.brainresbull.2009.04.010

Nagele, R. G., D'Andrea, M. R., Lee, H., Venkataraman, V., and Wang, H.-Y. (2003). Astrocytes accumulate Aβ42 and give rise to astrocytic amyloid plaques in Alzheimer disease brains. *Brain Res.* 971, 197–209. doi: 10.1016/S0006-8993(03)02361-8

Nakazawa, T., Nakazawa, C., Matsubara, A., Noda, K., Hisatomi, T., She, H., et al. (2006). Tumor necrosis factor-alpha mediates oligodendrocyte death and delayed retinal ganglion cell loss in a mouse model of glaucoma. *J. Neurosci.* 26, 12633–12641. doi: 10.1523/JNEUROSCI.2801-06.2006

Naskar, R., Wissing, M., and Thanos, S. (2002). Detection of early neuron degeneration and accompanying microglial responses in the retina of a rat model of glaucoma. *Invest. Ophthalmol. Vis. Sci.* 43, 2962–2968.

Nelson, A. R., Sweeney, M. D., Sagare, A. P., and Zlokovic, B. V. (2016). Neurovascular dysfunction and neurodegeneration in dementia and Alzheimer's disease. *Biochim. Biophys. Acta* 1862, 887–900. doi: 10.1016/j.bbadis.2015.12.016

Neufeld, A. H. (1999). Microglia in the optic nerve head and the region of parapapillary chorioretinal atrophy in glaucoma. *Arch. Ophthalmol.* 117, 1050–1056. doi: 10.1001/archopht.117.8.1050

Neufeld, A. H., Hernandez, M. R., and Gonzalez, M. (1997). Nitric oxide synthase in the human glaucomatous optic nerve head. *Arch. Ophthalmol.* 115, 497–503. doi: 10.1001/archopht.1997.01100150499009

Neystat, M., Lynch, T., Przedborski, S., Kholodilov, N., Rzhetskaya, M., and Burke, R. E. (1999). Alpha-synuclein expression in substantia nigra and cortex in Parkinson's disease. *Mov. Disord.* 14, 417–422. doi: 10.1002/1531-8257(199905)14:3<417::AID-MDS1005>3.0.CO;2-X

Nickells, R. W. (1999). Apoptosis of retinal ganglion cells in glaucoma: an update of the molecular pathways involved in cell death. *Surv. Ophthalmol.* 43(Suppl. 1), S151–S161. doi: 10.1016/S0039-6257(99)00029-6

Nigro, A., Colombo, F., Casella, G., Finardi, A., Verderio, C., and Furlan, R. (2016). Myeloid extracellular vesicles: messengers from the demented brain. *Front. Immunol.* 7:17. doi: 10.3389/fimmu.2016.00017

Ning, A., Cui, J., To, E., Ashe, K. H., and Matsubara, J. (2008). Amyloid-beta deposits lead to retinal degeneration in a mouse model of Alzheimer disease. *Invest. Ophthalmol. Vis. Sci.* 49, 5136–5143. doi: 10.1167/iovs.08-1849

Nowacka, B., Lubinski, W., Honczarenko, K., Potemkowski, A., and Safranow, K. (2014). Ophthalmological features of Parkinson disease. *Med. Sci. Monit.* 20, 2243–2249. doi: 10.12659/MSM.890861

Oakley, H., Cole, S. L., Logan, S., Maus, E., Shao, P., Craft, J., et al. (2006). Intraneuronal beta-amyloid aggregates, neurodegeneration, and neuron loss in transgenic mice with five familial Alzheimer's disease mutations: potential factors in amyloid plaque formation. *J. Neurosci.* 26, 10129–10140. doi: 10.1523/JNEUROSCI.1202-06.2006

Oddo, S., Caccamo, A., Shepherd, J. D., Murphy, M. P., Golde, T. E., Kayed, R., et al. (2003). Triple-transgenic model of Alzheimer's disease with plaques and tangles: intracellular Abeta and synaptic dysfunction. *Neuron* 39, 409–421. doi: 10.1016/s0896-6273(03)00434-3

Ohsawa, K., Irino, Y., Nakamura, Y., Akazawa, C., Inoue, K., and Kohsaka, S. (2007). Involvement of P2X4 and P2Y12 receptors in ATP-induced microglial chemotaxis. *Glia* 55, 604–616. doi: 10.1002/glia.20489

Olanow, C. W., and Tatton, W. G. (1999). Etiology and pathogenesis of Parkinson's disease. *Annu. Rev. Neurosci.* 22, 123–144. doi: 10.1146/annurev.neuro.22.1.123

Orr, C. F., Rowe, D. B., and Halliday, G. M. (2002). An inflammatory review of Parkinson's disease. *Prog. Neurobiol.* 68, 325–340. doi: 10.1016/S0301-0082(02)00127-2

Owen, D. R., and Matthews, P. M. (2011). Imaging brain microglial activation using positron emission tomography and translocator protein-specific radioligands. *Int. Rev. Neurobiol.* 101, 19–39. doi: 10.1016/B978-0-12-387718-5.00002-X

Painter, M. M., Atagi, Y., Liu, C. C., Rademakers, R., Xu, H., Fryer, J. D., et al. (2015). TREM2 in CNS homeostasis and neurodegenerative disease. *Mol. Neurodegener.* 10:43-015-0040-9. doi: 10.1186/s13024-015-0040-9

Paolicelli, R. C., Bolasco, G., Pagani, F., Maggi, L., Scianni, M., Panzanelli, P., et al. (2011). Synaptic pruning by microglia is necessary for normal brain development. *Science* 333, 1456–1458. doi: 10.1126/science.1202529

Paquet, C., Boissonnot, M., Roger, F., Dighiero, P., Gil, R., and Hugon, J. (2007). Abnormal retinal thickness in patients with mild cognitive impairment and Alzheimer's disease. *Neurosci. Lett.* 420, 97–99. doi: 10.1016/j.neulet.2007.02.090

Park, S., and Ou, Y. (2013). "Neurodegeneration in Glaucoma and Alzheimer's disease," in *Recent Advances in Ophthalmology Research*, ed G. Dimitrova (New York, NY: Nova Science Publishers), 59.

Parkhurst, C. N., Yang, G., Ninan, I., Savas, J. N., Yates, J. R. III, Lafaille, J. J., et al. (2013). Microglia promote learning-dependent synapse formation through brain-derived neurotrophic factor. *Cell* 155, 1596–1609. doi: 10.1016/j.cell.2013.11.030

Parnell, M., Guo, L., Abdi, M., and Cordeiro, M. F. (2012). Ocular manifestations of Alzheimer's disease in animal models. *Int. J. Alzheimers Dis.* 2012:786494. doi: 10.1155/2012/786494

Parpura, V., Heneka, M. T., Montana, V., Oliet, S. H., Schousboe, A., Haydon, P. G., et al. (2012). Glial cells in (patho)physiology. *J. Neurochem.* 121, 4–27. doi: 10.1111/j.1471-4159.2012.07664.x

Pasqualetti, G., Brooks, D. J., and Edison, P. (2015). The role of neuroinflammation in dementias. *Curr. Neurol Neurosci. Rep.* 15:17-015-0531-7. doi: 10.1007/s11910-015-0531-7

Pérez, M. A., and Arancibia, S. R. (2007). Estrés oxidativo y neurodegeneración:¿ causa o consecuencia. *Arch. Neurocienc.* 12, 45–54.

Perez, S. E., Lumayag, S., Kovacs, B., Mufson, E. J., and Xu, S. (2009). Beta-amyloid deposition and functional impairment in the retina of the APPswe/PS1DeltaE9 transgenic mouse model of Alzheimer's disease. *Invest. Ophthalmol. Vis. Sci.* 50, 793–800. doi: 10.1167/iovs.08-2384

Philipson, O., Lord, A., Gumucio, A., O'Callaghan, P., Lannfelt, L., and Nilsson, L. N. (2010). Animal models of amyloid-beta-related pathologies in Alzheimer's disease. *FEBS J.* 277, 1389–1409. doi: 10.1111/j.1742-4658.2010.07564.x

Pihlaja, R., Koistinaho, J., Kauppinen, R., Sandholm, J., Tanila, H., and Koistinaho, M. (2011). Multiple cellular and molecular mechanisms are involved in human Abeta clearance by transplanted adult astrocytes. *Glia* 59, 1643–1657. doi: 10.1002/glia.21212

Pinazo-Duran, M. D., Zanon-Moreno, V., Garcia-Medina, J. J., and Gallego-Pinazo, R. (2013). Evaluation of presumptive biomarkers of oxidative stress, immune response and apoptosis in primary open-angle glaucoma. *Curr. Opin. Pharmacol.* 13, 98–107. doi: 10.1016/j.coph.2012.10.007

Qiu, T., Liu, Q., Chen, Y. X., Zhao, Y. F., and Li, Y. M. (2015). Aβ42 and Aβ40: similarities and differences. *J. Pept. Sci.* 21, 522–529. doi: 10.1002/psc.2789

Quigley, H. A., and Broman, A. T. (2006). The number of people with glaucoma worldwide in 2010 and 2020. *Br. J. Ophthalmol.* 90, 262–267. doi: 10.1136/bjo.2005.081224

Quigley, H. A., Dunkelberger, G. R., and Green, W. R. (1988). Chronic human glaucoma causing selectively greater loss of large optic nerve fibers. *Ophthalmology* 95, 357–363. doi: 10.1016/S0161-6420(88)33176-3

Ransohoff, R. M., and Cardona, A. E. (2010). The myeloid cells of the central nervous system parenchyma. *Nature* 468, 253–262. doi: 10.1038/nature09615

Ransohoff, R. M., and El Khoury, J. (2015). Microglia in health and disease. *Cold Spring Harb. Perspect. Biol.* 8:a020560. doi: 10.1101/cshperspect.a020560

Ratnayaka, J. A., Serpell, L. C., and Lotery, A. J. (2015). Dementia of the eye: the role of amyloid beta in retinal degeneration. *Eye (Lond).* 29, 1013–1026. doi: 10.1038/eye.2015.100

Ritzel, R. M., Patel, A. R., Pan, S., Crapser, J., Hammond, M., Jellison, E., et al. (2015). Age- and location-related changes in microglial function. *Neurobiol. Aging* 36, 2153–2163. doi: 10.1016/j.neurobiolaging.2015.02.016

Rogers, J. T., Morganti, J. M., Bachstetter, A. D., Hudson, C. E., Peters, M. M., Grimmig, B. A., et al. (2011). CX3CR1 deficiency leads to impairment of hippocampal cognitive function and synaptic plasticity. *J. Neurosci.* 31, 16241–16250. doi: 10.1523/JNEUROSCI.3667-11.2011

Rojas, B., Gallego, B. I., Ramírez, A. I., Salazar, J. J., de Hoz, R., Valiente-Soriano, F. J., et al. (2014). Microglia in mouse retina contralateral to experimental glaucoma exhibit multiple signs of activation in all retinal layers. *J. Neuroinflammat.* 11:133. doi: 10.1186/1742-2094-11-133

Salobrar-Garcia, E., Garcia, Y., Lostao, C., Jañez, L., de Hoz, R., Rojas, B., et al. (2016a). Maculopapillary analysis in the posterior pole in patients with mild Alzheimer's disease. *Acta Ophthalmol.* doi: 10.1111/j.1755-3768.2016.0372

Salobrar-Garcia, E., Hoyas, I., Leal, M., de Hoz, R., Rojas, B., Ramirez, A. I., et al. (2015). Analysis of retinal peripapillary segmentation in early Alzheimer's disease patients. *Biomed. Res. Int.* 2015:636548. doi: 10.1155/2015/636548

Salobrar-Garcia, E., Leal, M., Hoyas, I., Salazar, J. J., Ramirez, A. I., de Hoz, R., et al. (2016b). Early changes in mild Alzheimer's disease in the neuroretinal rim segmentation. *Acta Ophthalmol.* doi: 10.1111/j.1755-3768.2016.0449

Salobrar-García, E., Ramírez, A. I., de Hoz, R., Rojas, P., Salazar, J. J., Rojas, B., et al. (2016c). "Ocular manifestations of dementia: the eye and its role in the diagnosis and monitoring, Chapter 15" in *Update on Dementia*, ed D. Moretti (InTech). doi: 10.5772/64490

Satue, M., Rodrigo, M. J., Obis, J., Vilades, E., Gracia, H., Otin, S., et al. (2017). Evaluation of progressive visual dysfunction and retinal degeneration in patients with Parkinson's disease. *Invest. Ophthalmol. Vis. Sci.* 58, 1151–1157. doi: 10.1167/iovs.16-20460

Schafer, D. P., Lehrman, E. K., Kautzman, A. G., Koyama, R., Mardinly, A. R., Yamasaki, R., et al. (2012). Microglia sculpt postnatal neural circuits in an activity and complement-dependent manner. *Neuron* 74, 691–705. doi: 10.1016/j.neuron.2012.03.026

Schapansky, J., Nardozzi, J. D., and LaVoie, M. J. (2015). The complex relationships between microglia, alpha-synuclein, and LRRK2 in Parkinson's disease. *Neuroscience* 302, 74–88. doi: 10.1016/j.neuroscience.2014.09.049

Schlamp, C. L., Li, Y., Dietz, J. A., Janssen, K. T., and Nickells, R. W. (2006). Progressive ganglion cell loss and optic nerve degeneration in DBA/2J mice is variable and asymmetric. *BMC Neurosci.* 7:66. doi: 10.1186/1471-2202-7-66

Selkoe, D. J. (2004). Cell biology of protein misfolding: the examples of Alzheimer's and Parkinson's diseases. *Nat. Cell Biol.* 6, 1054–1061. doi: 10.1038/ncb1104-1054

Selkoe, D. J. (2008). Soluble oligomers of the amyloid beta-protein impair synaptic plasticity and behavior. *Behav. Brain Res.* 192, 106–113. doi: 10.1016/j.bbr.2008.02.016

Shareef, S., Sawada, A., and Neufeld, A. H. (1999). Isoforms of nitric oxide synthase in the optic nerves of rat eyes with chronic moderately elevated intraocular pressure. *Invest. Ophthalmol. Vis. Sci.* 40, 2884–2891.

Sharma, S., and Lipincott, W. (2017). Biomarkers in Alzheimer's disease-recent update. *Curr. Alzheimer Res.* doi: 10.2174/1567205014666170220141822. [Epub ahead of print].

Sheedy, F. J., Grebe, A., Rayner, K. J., Kalantari, P., Ramkhelawon, B., Carpenter, S. B., et al. (2013). CD36 coordinates NLRP3 inflammasome activation by facilitating intracellular nucleation of soluble ligands into particulate ligands in sterile inflammation. *Nat. Immunol.* 14, 812–820. doi: 10.1038/ni.2639

Sheridan, G. K., and Murphy, K. J. (2013). Neuron-glia crosstalk in health and disease: fractalkine and CX3CR1 take centre stage. *Open Biol.* 3:130181. doi: 10.1098/rsob.130181

Simard, A. R., Soulet, D., Gowing, G., Julien, J. P., and Rivest, S. (2006). Bone marrow-derived microglia play a critical role in restricting senile plaque formation in Alzheimer's disease. *Neuron* 49, 489–502. doi: 10.1016/j.neuron.2006.01.022

Sofroniew, M., and Vinters, H. (2010). Astrocytes: biology and pathology. *Acta Neuropathol.* 119, 7–35. doi: 10.1007/s00401-009-0619-8

Solano, S. M., Miller, D. W., Augood, S. J., Young, A. B., and Penney, J. B. Jr. (2000). Expression of α-synuclein, parkin, and ubiquitin carboxy-terminal hydrolase L1 mRNA in human brain: genes associated with familial Parkinson's disease. *Ann. Neurol.* 47, 201–210. doi: 10.1002/1531-8249(200002)47:2<201::AID-ANA10>3.0.CO;2-F

Southam, K. A., Vincent, A. J., and Small, D. H. (2016). Do Microglia default on network maintenance in Alzheimer's disease? *J. Alzheimers Dis.* 51, 657–669. doi: 10.3233/JAD-151075

Stasi, K., Nagel, D., Yang, X., Wang, R. F., Ren, L., Podos, S. M., et al. (2006). Complement component 1Q (C1Q) upregulation in retina of murine, primate, and human glaucomatous eyes. *Invest. Ophthalmol. Vis. Sci.* 47, 1024–1029. doi: 10.1167/iovs.05-0830

Steele, M. R., Inman, D. M., Sappington, R. R., Golestaneh, N., Marsh–Armstrong, N., Calkins, D., et al. (2005). Whole retinal microarray analysis of DBA/2J mice: a model for glaucoma. *Invest. Ophthalmol. Vis. Sci.* 46, 48. doi: 10.1167/iovs.05-0865

Stefanova, N., Klimaschewski, L., Poewe, W., Wenning, G. K., and Reindl, M. (2001). Glial cell death induced by overexpression of alpha-synuclein. *J. Neurosci. Res.* 65, 432–438. doi: 10.1002/jnr.1171

Stemplewitz, B., Keseru, M., Bittersohl, D., Buhmann, C., Skevas, C., Richard, G., et al. (2015). Scanning laser polarimetry and spectral domain optical coherence tomography for the detection of retinal changes in Parkinson's disease. *Acta Ophthalmol.* 93, e672–e677. doi: 10.1111/aos.12764

Stewart, C. R., Stuart, L. M., Wilkinson, K., van Gils, J. M., Deng, J., Halle, A., et al. (2010). CD36 ligands promote sterile inflammation through assembly of a Toll-like receptor 4 and 6 heterodimer. *Nat. Immunol.* 11, 155–161. doi: 10.1038/ni.1836

Streit, W. J., Conde, J. R., Fendrick, S. E., Flanary, B. E., and Mariani, C. L. (2005). Role of microglia in the central nervous system's immune response. *Neurol. Res.* 27, 685–691. doi: 10.1179/016164105X49463

Streit, W. J., Mrak, R. E., and Griffin, W. S. (2004). Microglia and neuroinflammation: a pathological perspective. *J. Neuroinflammat.* 1:14. doi: 10.1186/1742-2094-1-14

Streit, W. J., Walter, S. A., and Pennell, N. A. (1999). Reactive microgliosis. *Progr. Neurobiol.* 57, 563–581. doi: 10.1016/S0301-0082(98)00069-0

Stutz, B., da Conceicao, F. S., Santos, L. E., Cadilhe, D. V., Fleming, R. L., Acquarone, M., et al. (2014). Murine dopaminergic Muller cells restore motor function in a model of Parkinson's disease. *J. Neurochem.* 128, 829–840. doi: 10.1111/jnc.12475

Suh, H.-S., Zhao, M.-L., Derico, L., Choi, N., and Lee, S. C. (2013). Insulin-like growth factor 1 and 2 (IGF1, IGF2) expression in human microglia: differential regulation by inflammatory mediators. *J. Neuroinflammat.* 10:805. doi: 10.1186/1742-2094-10-37

Surgucheva, I., McMahan, B., Ahmed, F., Tomarev, S., Wax, M. B., and Surguchov, A. (2002). Synucleins in glaucoma: implication of gamma-synuclein in glaucomatous alterations in the optic nerve. *J. Neurosci. Res.* 68, 97–106. doi: 10.1002/jnr.10198

Surguchov, A., McMahan, B., Masliah, E., and Surgucheva, I. (2001). Synucleins in ocular tissues. *J. Neurosci. Res.* 65, 68–77. doi: 10.1002/jnr.1129

Takeuchi, A., Irizarry, M. C., Duff, K., Saido, T. C., Hsiao Ashe, K., Hasegawa, M., et al. (2000). Age-related amyloid beta deposition in transgenic mice overexpressing both Alzheimer mutant presenilin 1 and amyloid beta precursor protein Swedish mutant is not associated with global neuronal loss. *Am. J. Pathol.* 157, 331–339. doi: 10.1016/S0002-9440(10)64544-0

Tang, Y., and Le, W. (2016). Differential roles of M1 and M2 microglia in neurodegenerative diseases. *Mol. Neurobiol.* 53, 1181–1194. doi: 10.1007/s12035-014-9070-5

Tatton, W. G., Kwan, M. M., Verrier, M. C., Seniuk, N. A., and Theriault, E. (1990). MPTP produces reversible disappearance of tyrosine hydroxylase-containing retinal amacrine cells. *Brain Res.* 527, 21–31. doi: 10.1016/0006-8993(90)91056-M

Taylor, P. R., Martinez-Pomares, L., Stacey, M., Lin, H., Brown, G. D., and Gordon, S. (2005). Macrophage receptors and immune recognition. *Annu. Rev. Immunol.* 23, 901–944. doi: 10.1146/annurev.immunol.23.021704.115816

Taylor, S., Calder, C. J., Albon, J., Erichsen, J. T., Boulton, M. E., and Morgan, J. E. (2011). Involvement of the CD200 receptor complex in microglia activation in experimental glaucoma. *Exp. Eye Res.* 92, 338–343. doi: 10.1016/j.exer.2011.01.012

Terwel, D., Steffensen, K. R., Verghese, P. B., Kummer, M. P., Gustafsson, J. A., Holtzman, D. M., et al. (2011). Critical role of astroglial apolipoprotein E and liver X receptor-alpha expression for microglial Abeta phagocytosis. *J. Neurosci.* 31, 7049–7059. doi: 10.1523/JNEUROSCI.6546-10.2011

Tezel, G. (2009). the Fourth ARVO/Pfizer Ophthalmics Research Institute Conference,Working Group. The role of glia, mitochondria, and the immune system in glaucoma. *Invest. Ophthalmol. Vis. Sci.* 50, 1001–1012. doi: 10.1167/iovs.08-2717

Tezel, G. (2013). Immune regulation toward immunomodulation for neuroprotection in glaucoma. *Curr. Opin. Pharmacol.* 13, 23–31. doi: 10.1016/j.coph.2012.09.013

Tezel, G., Li, L. Y., Patil, R. V., and Wax, M. B. (2001). TNF-α and TNF-α receptor-1 in the retina of normal and glaucomatous eyes. *Invest. Ophthalmol. Vis. Sci.* 42, 1787–1794.

Tezel, G., Yang, J., and Wax, M. B. (2004). Heat shock proteins, immunity and glaucoma. *Brain Res. Bull.* 62, 473–480. doi: 10.1016/S0361-9230(03)00074-1

Tofaris, G. K., Razzaq, A., Ghetti, B., Lilley, K. S., and Spillantini, M. G. (2003). Ubiquitination of alpha-synuclein in Lewy bodies is a pathological event not associated with impairment of proteasome function. *J. Biol. Chem.* 278, 44405–44411. doi: 10.1074/jbc.M308041200

Tsai, C. S., Ritch, R., Schwartz, B., Lee, S. S., Miller, N. R., Chi, T., et al. (1991). Optic nerve head and nerve fiber layer in Alzheimer's disease. *Arch. Ophthalmol.* 109, 199–204. doi: 10.1001/archopht.1991.01080020045040

Tsai, Y., Lu, B., Ljubimov, A. V., Girman, S., Ross-Cisneros, F. N., Sadun, A. A., et al. (2014). Ocular changes in TgF344-AD rat model of Alzheimer's disease. *Invest. Ophthalmol. Vis. Sci.* 55, 523–534. doi: 10.1167/iovs.13-12888

Udeochu, J. C., Shea, J. M., and Villeda, S. A. (2016). Microglia communication: parallels between aging and Alzheimer's disease. *Clin. Exp. Neuroimmunol.* 7, 114–125. doi: 10.1111/cen3.12307

Uttara, B., Singh, A. V., Zamboni, P., and Mahajan, R. T. (2009). Oxidative stress and neurodegenerative diseases: a review of upstream and downstream antioxidant therapeutic options. *Curr. Neuropharmacol.* 7, 65–74. doi: 10.2174/157015909787602823

van Boxel-Dezaire, A. H., Rani, M. R., and Stark, G. R. (2006). Complex modulation of cell type-specific signaling in response to type I interferons. *Immunity* 25, 361–372. doi: 10.1016/j.immuni.2006.08.014

Varnum, M. M., and Ikezu, T. (2012). The classification of microglial activation phenotypes on neurodegeneration and regeneration in Alzheimer's disease brain. *Arch. Immunol. Ther. Exp.* 60, 251–266. doi: 10.1007/s00005-012-0181-2

Veerhuis, R. (2011). Histological and direct evidence for the role of complement in the neuroinflammation of AD. *Curr. Alzheimer Res.* 8, 34–58. doi: 10.2174/156720511794604589

Verkhratsky, A., and Butt, A. M. (2013). *Glial Physiology and Pathophysiology.* Oxford: Wiley-Blackwell-John Wiley & Sons.

Verkhratsky, A., Parpura, V., Pekna, M., Pekny, M., and Sofroniew, M. (2014). Glia in the pathogenesis of neurodegenerative diseases. *Biochem. Soc. Trans.* 42, 1291–1301. doi: 10.1042/BST20140107

Vidal, L., Díaz, F., Villena, A., Moreno, M., Campos, J. G., and de Vargas, I. P. (2006). Nitric oxide synthase in retina and optic nerve head of rat with increased intraocular pressure and effect of timolol. *Brain Res. Bull.* 70, 406–413. doi: 10.1016/j.brainresbull.2006.07.009

Vivekanantham, S., Shah, S., Dewji, R., Dewji, A., Khatri, C., and Ologunde, R. (2015). Neuroinflammation in Parkinson's disease: role in neurodegeneration and tissue repair. *Int. J. Neurosci.* 125, 717–725. doi: 10.3109/00207454.2014.982795

Vodovotz, Y., Lucia, M. S., Flanders, K. C., Chesler, L., Xie, Q. W., Smith, T. W., et al. (1996). Inducible nitric oxide synthase in tangle-bearing neurons of patients with Alzheimer's disease. *J. Exp. Med.* 184, 1425–1433. doi: 10.1084/jem.184.4.1425

Wang, K., Peng, B., and Lin, B. (2014). Fractalkine receptor regulates microglial neurotoxicity in an experimental mouse glaucoma model. *Glia* 62, 1943–1954 doi: 10 1002/glia 22715

Wang, J., Jackson, M. F., and Xie, Y. F. (2016). Glia and TRPM2 channels in plasticity of central nervous system and Alzheimer's diseases. *Neural Plast.* 2016:1680905. doi: 10.1155/2016/1680905

Wang, Q., Liu, Y., and Zhou, J. (2015). Neuroinflammation in Parkinson's disease and its potential as therapeutic target. *Transl. Neurodegener.* 4:19-015-0042-0. eCollection 2015. doi: 10.1186/s40035-015-0042-0

Wang, X. J., Zhang, S., Yan, Z. Q., Zhao, Y. X., Zhou, H. Y., Wang, Y., et al. (2011). Impaired CD200-CD200R-mediated microglia silencing enhances midbrain dopaminergic neurodegeneration: roles of aging, superoxide, NADPH oxidase, and p38 MAPK. *Free Radic. Biol. Med.* 50, 1094–1106. doi: 10.1016/j.freeradbiomed.2011.01.032

Wax, M. B., Tezel, G., and Edward, P. D. (1998). Clinical and ocular histopathological findings in a patient with normal-pressure glaucoma. *Arch. Ophthalmol.* 116, 993–1001. doi: 10.1001/archopht.116.8.993

Wax, M. B., Tezel, G., Kawase, K., and Kitazawa, Y. (2001). Serum autoantibodies to heat shock proteins in glaucoma patients from Japan and the United States. *Ophthalmology* 108, 296–302. doi: 10.1016/S0161-6420(00)00525-X

Williams, E. A., McGuone, D., Frosch, M. P., Hyman, B. T., Laver, N., and Stemmer-Rachamimov, A. (2017). Absence of Alzheimer disease neuropathologic changes in eyes of subjects with Alzheimer disease. *J. Neuropathol. Exp. Neurol.* 76, 376–383. doi: 10.1093/jnen/nlx020

Williams, P. A., Marsh-Armstrong, N., Howell, G. R. (2017). Lasker/IRRF initiative on astrocytes and glaucomatous neurodegeneration participants. Neuroinflammation in glaucoma: a new opportunity. *Exp. Eye Res.* 157, 20–27. doi: 10.1016/j.exer.2017.02.014

Wostyn, P., Audenaert, K., and De Deyn, P. P. (2010). Alzheimer's disease: cerebral glaucoma? *Med. Hypotheses* 74, 973–977. doi: 10.1016/j.mehy.2009.12.019

Wu, L., Vadakkan, K. I., and Zhuo, M. (2007). ATP-induced chemotaxis of microglial processes requires P2Y receptor-activated initiation of outward potassium currents. *Glia* 55, 810–821. doi: 10.1002/glia.20500

Wyss-Coray, T. (2006). Inflammation in Alzheimer disease: driving force, bystander or beneficial response? *Nat. Med.* 12, 1005–1015. doi: 10.1038/nm1484

Xu, L., He, D., and Bai, Y. (2016). Microglia-mediated inflammation and neurodegenerative disease. *Mol. Neurobiol.* 53, 6709–6715. doi: 10.1007/s12035-015-9593-4

Yan, S. D., Chen, X., Fu, J., Chen, M., Zhu, H., Roher, A., et al. (1996). RAGE and amyloid-beta peptide neurotoxicity in Alzheimer's disease. *Nature* 382, 685–691.

Yan, Z., Gibson, S. A., Buckley, J. A., Qin, H., and Benveniste, E. N. (2016). Role of the JAK/STAT signaling pathway in regulation of innate immunity in neuroinflammatory diseases. *Clin. Immunol.* doi: 10.1016/j.clim.2016.09.014. [Epub ahead of print].

Yang, J., Patil, R. V., Yu, H., Gordon, M., and Wax, M. B. (2001a). T cell subsets and sIL-2R/IL-2 levels in patients with glaucoma. *Am. J. Ophthalmol.* 131, 421–426. doi: 10.1016/S0002-9394(00)00862-X

Yang, J., Yang, P., Tezel, G., Patil, R. V., Hernandez, M. R., and Wax, M. B. (2001b). Induction of HLA-DR expression in human lamina cribrosa astrocytes by cytokines and simulated ischemia. *Invest. Ophthalmol. Vis. Sci.* 42, 365–371.

Yu, J. G., Feng, Y. F., Xiang, Y., Huang, J. H., Savini, G., Parisi, V., et al. (2014). Retinal nerve fiber layer thickness changes in Parkinson disease: a meta-analysis. *PLoS ONE* 9:e85718. doi: 10.1371/journal.pone.0085718

Yuan, L., and Neufeld, A. H. (2001). Activated microglia in the human glaucomatous optic nerve head. *J. Neurosci. Res.* 64, 523–532. doi: 10.1002/jnr.1104

Yucel, Y. H., Zhang, Q., Weinreb, R. N., Kaufman, P. L., and Gupta, N. (2003). Effects of retinal ganglion cell loss on magno-, parvo-, koniocellular pathways in the lateral geniculate nucleus and visual cortex in glaucoma. *Prog. Retin. Eye Res.* 22, 465–481. doi: 10.1016/S1350-9462(03)00026-0

Yuruker, V., Naziroglu, M., and Senol, N. (2015). Reduction in traumatic brain injury-induced oxidative stress, apoptosis, and calcium entry in rat hippocampus by melatonin: possible involvement of TRPM2 channels. *Metab. Brain Dis.* 30, 223–231. doi: 10.1007/s11011-014-9623-3

Zecca, L., Wilms, H., Geick, S., Claasen, J. H., Brandenburg, L. O., Holzknecht, C., et al. (2008). Human neuromelanin induces neuroinflammation and neurodegeneration in the rat substantia nigra: implications for Parkinson's disease. *Acta Neuropathol.* 116, 47–55. doi: 10.1007/s00401-008-0361-7

Zhang, Q. S., Heng, Y., Yuan, Y. H., and Chen, N. H. (2017). Pathological alpha-synuclein exacerbates the progression of Parkinson's disease through microglial activation. *Toxicol Lett* 265, 30–37. doi: 10.1016/j.toxlet.2016.11.002

Zhang, S., Wang, X.-J., Tian, L.-P., Pan, J., Lu, G.-Q., Zhang, Y.-J., et al. (2011). CD200-CD200R dysfunction exacerbates microglial activation and dopaminergic neurodegeneration in a rat model of Parkinson's disease. *J. Neuroinflammat.* 8:154. doi: 10.1186/1742-2094-8-154

Zhou, X., He, X., and Ren, Y. (2014). Function of microglia and macrophages in secondary damage after spinal cord injury. *Neural Regen. Res* 9, 1787–1795. doi: 10.4103/1673-5374.143423

16

Modulation of Microglial Activity by Rho-Kinase (ROCK) Inhibition as Therapeutic Strategy in Parkinson's Disease and Amyotrophic Lateral Sclerosis

*Anna-Elisa Roser[1,2], Lars Tönges[3] and Paul Lingor[1,2]**

[1]Department of Neurology, University Medicine Göttingen, Göttingen, Germany, [2]DFG Cluster of Excellence Nanoscale Microscopy and Molecular Physiology of the Brain (CNMPB), University Medicine Göttingen, Göttingen, Germany, [3]Department of Neurology, Ruhr-Universität Bochum, Bochum, Germany

***Correspondence:**
Paul Lingor
plingor@gwdg.de

Neurodegenerative diseases are characterized by the progressive degeneration of neurons in the central and peripheral nervous system (CNS, PNS), resulting in a reduced innervation of target structures and a loss of function. A shared characteristic of many neurodegenerative diseases is the infiltration of microglial cells into affected brain regions. During early disease stages microglial cells often display a rather neuroprotective phenotype, but switch to a more pro-inflammatory neurotoxic phenotype in later stages of the disease, contributing to the neurodegeneration. Activation of the Rho kinase (ROCK) pathway appears to be instrumental for the modulation of the microglial phenotype: increased ROCK activity in microglia mediates mechanisms of the inflammatory response and is associated with improved motility, increased production of reactive oxygen species (ROS) and release of inflammatory cytokines. Recently, several studies suggested inhibition of ROCK signaling as a promising treatment option for neurodegenerative diseases. In this review article, we discuss the contribution of microglial activity and phenotype switch to the pathophysiology of Parkinson's disease (PD) and Amyotrophic lateral sclerosis (ALS), two devastating neurodegenerative diseases without disease-modifying treatment options. Furthermore, we describe how ROCK inhibition can influence the microglial phenotype in disease models and explore ROCK inhibition as a future treatment option for PD and ALS.

Keywords: microglial polarization, Parkinson's disease, amyotrophic lateral sclerosis, ROCK, ROCK inhibition, neuroinflammation

INTRODUCTION

The idea that neurodegenerative disorders (NDD) are primarily caused by a particular susceptibility of neuronal subpopulations to damaging insults is challenged by the observation that a pronounced infiltration of microglia into affected brain regions is a common hallmark of NDD. The discovery of a microglial phenotype switch from an immune-suppressive neuroprotective to a pro-inflammatory neurotoxic phenotype emphasizes the importance of a microglial contribution to the formation and course of NDD. One major regulator of microglial activity is the Rho-kinase (ROCK) signaling pathway. ROCK is a serine/threonine kinase that is expressed as two homologs, ROCK1 and

ROCK2. The two isoforms share similar structure and function, but show differences in their abundance. ROCK1 is the dominant form in liver, lung, testes, blood and the immune system, whereas ROCK2 is dominant in the brain and muscles (Nakagawa et al., 1996; Hashimoto et al., 1999). ROCK activity is regulated by its upstream regulators, the Rho-GTPases RhoA and RhoC, which belong to the Ras-superfamily (Leung et al., 1996; Hashimoto et al., 1999). Active ROCK phosphorylates numerous downstream targets which are involved in regulation of cell shape and motility as well as apoptosis and cell survival. In microglial cells the ROCK pathway is involved in regulation of migration, phagocytosis and release of inflammatory cytokines and thus mediates the microglial phenotype (Yan et al., 2012; Borrajo et al., 2014a). Additionally, there is accumulating evidence that ROCK is increased in microglial cells in Parkinson's disease (PD) and Amyotrophic lateral sclerosis (ALS; Conti et al., 2014; Saal et al., 2017). Thus, inhibition of the ROCK pathway could be a promising treatment option for NDD. In this review article, we show how ROCK inhibition can influence the microglial phenotype, discuss the microglial contribution to the pathophysiology of PD and ALS and explore ROCK inhibition as a treatment option for PD and ALS.

MICROGLIAL POLARIZATION AND PHENOTYPES

Microglia are the resident innate immune cells with a macrophage-like capacity in the otherwise immune-privileged central nervous system (CNS; Kettenmann et al., 2011). Microglial cells fulfill a broad variety of functions and can commit to different reactive phenotypes (Schwartz et al., 2006; Hanisch and Kettenmann, 2007). In the healthy brain microglia occur in a so-called "resting" state with a ramified phenotype, which presents highly motile processes that continuously scan their environment. The processes can detect even slight aberrations in neural signal propagation and in occurrence and quantity of extracellular molecules. Thus, "resting" microglia serve mainly in the surveillance and maintenance of the CNS homeostasis (Kettenmann et al., 2011; Wolf et al., 2017). Under pathological conditions microglia can be "activated", e.g., by infectious agents, tissue damage or functional modifications of neighboring neurons. This is accompanied by a drastic morphological change towards an ameboid phenotype and an altered expression of surface molecules and releasable factors (Kettenmann et al., 2011; Hu et al., 2015) that is strongly dependent on the brain region and the nature of the activating agent. It was shown that microglia isolated from different brain regions and the spinal cord differ in the severity of a pro-inflammatory response (Baskar Jesudasan et al., 2014). Activated microglia can be classified according to the peripheral macrophage classification system in "M1" and "M2" microglia, even though this oversimplified model only represents two extreme activation states and it has become clear that microglial activation is a highly dynamic process with more than the two polarities (Franco and Fernández-Suárez, 2015; Tang and Le, 2016; Wolf et al., 2017). The "M1" phenotype is associated with the release of proinflammatory cytokines (e.g., TNF-α, IL-1β), nitric oxide (NO) and reactive oxygen species (ROS) and bears the risk of harming neuronal cells with prolonged activation (Hanisch and Kettenmann, 2007; Tang and Le, 2016). The "M2" phenotype provides a rather neuroprotective environment by the release of anti-inflammatory cytokines (e.g., IL-4, IL-10, IL-13) or growth factors such as TGF-β and promotes tissue repair and regeneration. A growing body of evidence suggests different "M2" subpopulations with distinct biological functions (Hu et al., 2015; Tang and Le, 2016).

THE ROLE OF ROCK ACTIVITY FOR THE INFLAMMATORY RESPONSE OF MICROGLIA

ROCK activity plays a crucial role in microglial activation. It has been shown that it is involved in the regulation of key features of microglial activitiy like migration, phagocytosis and release of cytokines and chemokines (Barcia et al., 2012; Yan et al., 2012; Borrajo et al., 2014a). Microglia are migratory cells that can travel along chemokine gradients towards a site of infection or injury. Motility is a process that mainly reflects the dynamic organization of the actin cytoskeleton and that is critically controlled by the Rho family of small GTPases (Welch and Mullins, 2002). ROCK maintains stress fibers and focal adhesions, whereas Rac organizes the formation of filopodia, both necessary structures for migration (Nobes and Hall, 1995). For phagocytotic cells like microglia, the remodeling of the actin cytoskeleton is not only important for migration, but also enables them to engulf particles and cellular debris. Even though phagocytosis is initiated by different receptors, downstream they all lead to activation of Rho GTPases for remodeling of the actin cytoskeleton (Chimini and Chavrier, 2000). As migration and phagocytosis are strongly dependent on the actin cytoskeleton the involvement of ROCK activity in these processes is not surprising. Interestingly, however, ROCK signaling plays also a role in microglial release of cytokines and chemokines, a process that is initiated by binding of ligands to specific surface receptors, e.g., purinergic receptors, toll-like receptors (TLRs) or angiotensin type receptors (Olson and Miller, 2004; Inoue, 2006; Rodriguez-Perez et al., 2015). Activation of purinergic receptors for extracellular nucleotides leads to microglial motility, chemotaxis and release of cytokines, NO and superoxides. Downstream of purinergic receptors different effector molecules are activated, among them JNK and MAPK signaling pathways and ROCK (Erb et al., 2006; Färber and Kettenmann, 2006). Another important family of receptors for the activation of microglia are TLRs. They have a variety of downstream targets including the RhoA-ROCK signaling pathway (Oda and Kitano, 2006). Microglial release of cytokines and chemokines is also mediated by angiotensin type receptors by activation of the nicotinamide adenine dinucleotide phosphate (NADPH)-oxidase complex and the ROCK signaling pathway (Rodriguez-Perez et al., 2015). There are several studies employing inhibition of ROCK that emphasize the significant role of this pathway for the microglial activation process. In a rat model of neuropathic pain, ROCK inhibition prevented morphological changes in microglia as well as microglia-neuron interactions (Tatsumi et al., 2015). In a mouse model for hypoxia and reoxygenation it was shown that ROCK inhibition by Fasudil led to a reduced expression of microglial inducible nitric oxide synthase (iNOS). Furthermore, treatment with the isoquinoline-type ROCK-inhibitor Fasudil reduced the microglial release of the pro-inflammatory factors NO, IL-1β, IL-6 and TNF-α (Ding et al., 2010). Similar findings were made in the rat retina (Tura et al., 2009). Additionally, there is strong evidence that the ROCK pathway is involved in modulation of the microglial phenotype. Even though there are no studies showing that ROCK activity is increased in a certain microglial phenotype, there are reports from different models showing that inhibition of ROCK leads to a phenotypic shift from "M1" towards "M2" microglia, suggesting that ROCK activation is necessary for maintenance of the pro-inflammatory "M1" phenotype. These phenotypic shifts were associated with a decrease in the release of the pro-inflammatory factors NO, IL-1β, IL-6 and TNF-α and increased the release of the anti-inflammatory factor IL-10 in cultured microglia (Ding et al., 2010). A similar suppression of the pro-inflammatory cytokines was observed in a mouse model after Fasudil-treatment (Tönges et al., 2014). Taken together, there is robust evidence that ROCK activity plays an important role in activation of microglia and the determination of its reactive phenotype.

MICROGLIAL ACTIVITY IN PD

PD is the second most common neurodegenerative disorder worldwide with a prevalence of about 0.3% in industrialized countries (Dexter and Jenner, 2013). One of its characteristics is a progressive degeneration of the dopaminergic nigrostriatal projections and their cell bodies in the substantia nigra. This leads to a lack of striatal dopamine and imbalanced basal ganglia signaling, causing severe motor deficits (Jankovic, 2008). Approximately 5% of all PD cases are inherited and caused by mutations in different genes or duplications/triplications of the α-synuclein locus. However, the majority of the PD cases occurs sporadically without identifiable cause (Dexter and Jenner, 2013).

There are numerous *in vitro* and animal studies suggesting a link between the loss of dopaminergic neurons and activation of microglia in the substantia nigra in PD. In animals treated with the neurotoxins 6-hydroxydopamine (6-OHDA) or 1-Methyl-4-phenyl-1,2,3,6-tetrahydropyridin (MPTP) an increased microglial infiltration and activation has been described (Akiyama and McGeer, 1989; Członkowska et al., 1996; Cicchetti et al., 2002; Gao et al., 2002; Noelker et al., 2013). Similar observations could be made in monkeys treated with MPTP. Here, a prolonged activation of microglia was observed even 1 year after MPTP treatment (Barcia et al., 2004). Interestingly, the postmortem tissues of human MPTP users showed also a prolonged activation of reactive microglia, even years after the acute intoxication (Langston et al., 1999). Furthermore, aggregated α-synuclein, one of the main hallmarks of PD, released from dying neurons leads to a microglial activation towards the pro-inflammatory "M1" phenotype (Zhang et al., 2005; Reynolds et al., 2008; Lee et al., 2010). It is possible to visualize reactive microglia *in vivo* by positron emission topography (PET) employing radiotracers that bind to surface structures of activated microglia, such as the isoquinoline-derivative and translocator protein (TSPO)-ligand [^{11}C]-PK11195 (Bartels and Leenders, 2007). Different PET studies could confirm an increased microglial activation in the midbrain of PD patients that was correlated to disease progression (Ouchi et al., 2005; Gerhard et al., 2006; Koshimori et al., 2015). This goes in line with a study reporting that the pro-inflammatory cytokines TNFα, IL-6 and IL-1β were elevated in the cerebrospinal fluid (CSF) of PD patients (Qin et al., 2016). So far, all evidence on hand points towards an increased microglial activation with a pro-inflammatory "M1" phenotype that might contribute to PD progression. Little is known about the "M2" phenotype in PD.

Abnormal activity of ROCK associated with an increased inflammatory response was demonstrated in the substantia nigra of the MPTP mouse model for PD (Villar-Cheda et al., 2012). Additionally, our group could show that in postmortem tissue of PD patients compared to age-matched controls ROCK expression is increased in glial cells (Saal et al., 2017). It has been shown that, as the two phenotypes can transit into each other, treatment with a ROCK inhibitor skews "M1" toward "M2" microglia in experimental PD models and thus, is a promising therapeutic option for the treatment of PD (Zhao et al., 2015; He et al., 2016; summarized in **Figure 1**).

MICROGLIAL ACTIVATION IN ALS

ALS is a chronic progressive NDD with a fatal disease course. Because of the involvement of upper and lower motoneurons with subsequent impairment of the CNS corticopyramidal tract and peripheral motor axons patients suffer from progressive muscle weakness and paralysis, which ultimately leads to death within 3–5 years. The large majority of ALS is sporadic but there are also familial cases which have a genetic predisposition (e.g., mutations in the SOD1 gene or DNA repeat expansions in C9orf72; Paez-Colasante et al., 2015).

The immune system and neuroinflammation are strongly implicated in ALS progression and comprise microglial activation, T-cell-independent macrophage activation, monocyte recruitment to diseased tissue and dysregulation of immune-related genes in human ALS patients (Henkel et al., 2013; Philips and Rothstein, 2014). This neuroinflammatory response accompanies neuronal cell death with microglial cells being the first cell type to be activated (Evans et al., 2013). In human postmortem studies, reactive microglia were detected in regions which play an important role in motor function (motor cortex, motor nuclei of the brainstem, corticospinal tract, spinal cord; Kawamata et al., 1992; Moisse and Strong, 2006). Recently, microglia were also visualized in ALS patients using integrated MR/PET and the radioligand [^{11}C]-PBR28 that also binds to TSPO (Alshikho et al., 2016).

While a functional analysis of microglia in living human subjects remains difficult, there are various experimental approaches. In ALS mouse models, microgliosis occurs as well in

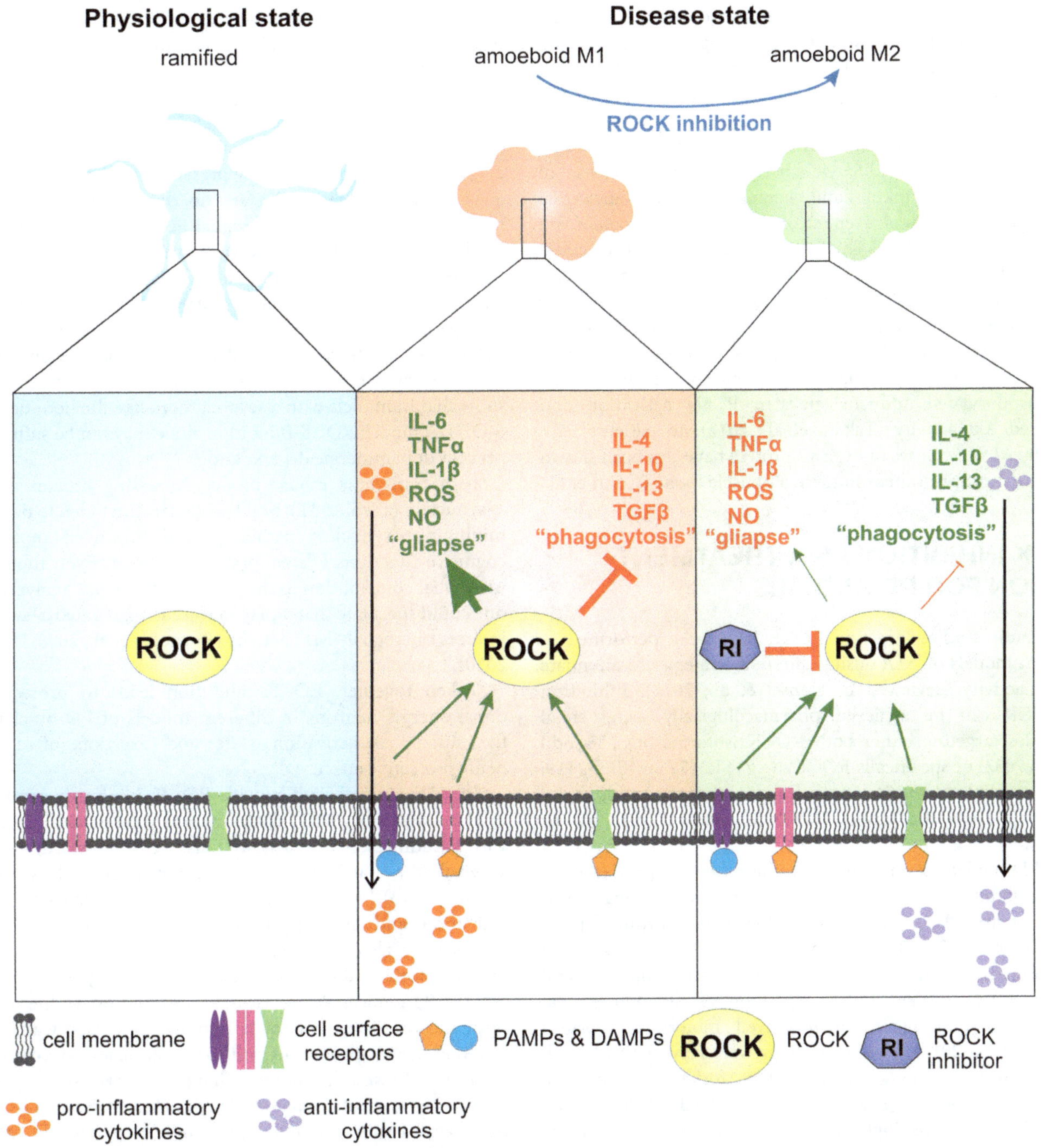

FIGURE 1 | The role of Rho-kinase (ROCK) activity and ROCK inhibition in microglia in Parkinson's disease (PD) and amyotrophic lateral sclerosis (ALS). In their physiological "ramified" stage microglia are continuously scanning their environment. For simplification, constitutive ROCK activity is disregarded in this illustration. Upon binding of pathogen- or danger associated molecular patterns (PAMPs or DAMPs; e.g., α-synuclein) to cell surface receptors microglia are activated, showing a "M1" phenotype that is associated with increased ROCK activity. This leads to a drastic change in morphology towards an ameboid shape, release of pro-inflammatory cytokines and chemokines and increased formation of microglia-neuron contacts ("gliapses"). Upon ROCK inhibition by a ROCK inhibitor the microglial phenotype changes towards a more "M2"-like phenotype, leading to the release of anti-inflammatory cytokines and growth factors and less "gliapse" formation.

pre-symptomatic as in symptomatic SOD1.G93A mice (Gerber et al., 2012; Tönges et al., 2014) and in SOD1.G37R mice (Boillée et al., 2006). Here, *in vivo* imaging could demonstrate that microglial cells were highly reactive in pre-symptomatic stages but lost this ability with disease progression (Dibaj et al., 2011). Phenotyping of mSOD1.G93A microglia suggests a predominant M2-type in early onset SOD1.G93A mice and a rather classically activated M1-type at end stage (Liao et al., 2012) indicating that the function of microglia changes during disease progression and both protective or harmful effects may be exerted depending on the particular situation (summarized in **Figure 1**).

When both, wildtype and mSOD1(G93A) primary microglia were stimulated with LPS, we observed a strong release of pro-inflammatory cytokines and chemokines in both microglial cells types, which was even stronger in the wildtype form (Tönges et al., 2014). This inflammatory response could be effectively attenuated when cells were co-treated with ROCK inhibitor Fasudil. This underlines that ROCK is considerably involved in the modulation of microglial cell function. In line with this, SOD1.G93A mice were shown to exhibit enhanced ROCK activity leading to increased levels of phosphorylated adducin, elevated PTEN activation and decreased Akt activity (Takata et al., 2013). In patients with sporadic ALS, increases of ROCK2 protein have also been shown and were most prominent in skeletal muscle tissue (Conti et al., 2014).

ROCK INHIBITION AS A TREATMENT OPTION FOR PD AND ALS

Therapeutic studies targeting ROCK have been performed in different models of NDD using different strategies to attenuate ROCK activity (reviewed in Hensel et al., 2015). Inhibition of ROCK can be achieved pharmacologically using small molecules targeting either both ROCK isoforms (e.g., Fasudil and Y-27632) or specifically ROCK2 (e.g., SR3677 and SLx-2119; Defert and Boland, 2017). Another approach is the employment of genetic tools that target ROCK expression (e.g., sh- or siRNA).

In PD models, several studies using different approaches of ROCK inhibition have been published (reviewed in Labandeira-Garcia et al., 2015). In a medium severe subchronic MPTP mouse model of PD (30 mg/kg body weight for five consecutive days) oral treatment with Fasudil led to protection of nigral dopaminergic neurons and preservation of the nigrostriatal projections, resulting in an improved motor performance (Tönges et al., 2012). Similar findings were reported in MPTP treated mice (30 mg/kg body weight for five consecutive days) that received the ROCK inhibitor Y-27632 (Villar-Cheda et al., 2012). Interestingly, the effects were attributed both, to a direct neuroprotective effect, which was also present in a microglia-free neuronal culture (Tönges et al., 2012), and to an inhibition of the microglial response (Villar-Cheda et al., 2012). Another study could show that inhibition of the microglial response is essential for the neuroprotective effects of ROCK inhibition in the MPP^+-mediated dopaminergic degeneration (Borrajo et al., 2014b). Additionally, it was shown that MPTP treatment leads to microglial activation and increased formation of microglia-neuron contacts, so called "gliapses". Treatment with Fasudil prevented microglial activation and led to increased dopaminergic neuron survival (Barcia et al., 2012).

In another toxin-induced PD model that shows a more severe lesion, the high dose (4 μg/2 μl) striatal 6-OHDA model, oral treatment with Fasudil could not reduce dopaminergic degeneration in mice (Tatenhorst et al., 2014). Using shRNAs that diminished ROCK2 in nigral neurons in the same model, we could show decreased dopaminergic cell death in the substantia nigra. However, striatal fiber density and dopamine contents were not significantly preserved in these animals (Saal et al., 2015). So far, there are no descriptions of the effect of ROCK inhibition on microglial activation in the 6-OHDA model, even though it is known that microglial activation and ROS production contribute to 6-OHDA induced dopaminergic neurodegeneration (Rodriguez-Pallares et al., 2007). The extent of dopaminergic neuron loss in the two described toxin-induced PD models is strongly dependent on the dosage and, in the 6-OHDA model, site of administration. The described studies show that in models with a severe lesion, like the here-described 6-OHDA model, ROCK inhibition alone may not be sufficient to prevent dopaminergic degeneration.

In a transgenic mouse model expressing human mutated α-synuclein (aSyn.A53T), oral Fasudil treatment led to decreased midbrain α-synuclein pathology and improved motor and cognitive functions (Tatenhorst et al., 2016). Even though the microglial contribution to the phenotype was not analyzed here, one could speculate that it plays a role, as aggregated α-synuclein induces microglial "M1" activity (Reynolds et al., 2008; Lee et al., 2010).

Taken together, ROCK inhibition leads to protection of dopaminergic neurons in different models of PD by changing the microglial activation state and exertion of a direct neuroprotective effect.

In ALS, animal studies with ROCK inhibitors are limited to the transgenic SOD1.G93A mouse model. Oral treatment with Fasudil resulted in a slowed disease progression, increased survival time and attenuated motor neuron loss (Takata et al., 2013), which was mediated by decreased PTEN activation and an increase in PI3K-Akt signaling. Similar effects were also observed in our own analysis. Additionally, pre-symptomatically applied Fasudil modified glial responses in SOD1.G93A mice. While astroglial infiltration in the anterior horn was decreased, microglia numbers increased with Fasudil treatment. Furthermore, an *in vitro* activation analysis of primary microglia showed that Fasudil changes the release of cytokines towards an anti-inflammatory profile. Thus, it can be postulated that Fasudil shifts the microglial phenotype towards "M2" in SOD1 mice (Tönges et al., 2014). In animals, where the treatment started with disease onset and thus pathology was already advanced, survival, basic neurological scoring, motoneuron pathology and microglial infiltration could not be significantly improved by Fasudil. However, even in this paradigm the treated animals showed a better motor performance compared to non-treated animals (Günther et al., 2017). In another study, treatment with the 4-aminopyridine ROCK-inhibitor Y-27632 improved motor function in male SOD1.G93A mice (Günther et al., 2014). Since both Fasudil and Y-27632 are not completely selective for ROCK, inhibition of other kinases may also contribute to their effects. Nevertheless, the biological efficacy of these two molecules with chemically distinct back bones strongly argues for ROCK as their main pharmacologically relevant target.

PHARMACOLOGICAL ROCK INHIBITORS

In recent years a large number of pharmacological ROCK inhibitors have been developed, most of them belonging either to the chemical group of isoquinoline derivates (e.g., Fasudil; Ripasudil) or aminopyridines (e.g., Y-27632; Feng et al., 2016; Defert and Boland, 2017). The majority of ROCK inhibitors are Type 1 ATP competitive kinase inhibitors that block the transfer of the terminal phosphate from ATP to the respective substrate (Liu and Gray, 2006). In biomedical research Fasudil and Y-27632 are the most extensively used ROCK inhibitors, even though they are less selective against different other kinases and show a limited potency (Feng et al., 2016). Thus, off-target effects that might have contributed to the results have to be considered in studies that used these drugs. Consequently, to date there is only limited data demonstrating the effect of selective or isoform-selective pharmacological ROCK inhibition (reviewed in Defert and Boland, 2017). Development of selective ROCK2 inhibitors would be especially important for the treatment of NDD as ROCK2 is the dominating isoform in the CNS. Furthermore, selective ROCK2 inhibition would minimize the risk of hypotension, a major side effect of long-term treatment with non-selective ROCK inhibitors. So far, two ROCK inhibitors have been licensed for clinical use, both in Japan; Fasudil for the treatment of cerebral vasospasms (Mueller et al., 2005) and Ripasudil for glaucoma treatment (Garnock-Jones, 2014). Possible adverse events under systemic Fasudil treatment are abnormal elevation of liver enzymes (<2%), renal dysfunction (<2%) and hypotension (<5%) that occurred in a small number of treated patients, thus indicating excellent tolerability (Suzuki et al., 2007). In addition, several new compounds are tested in preclinical and clinical trials, exploring the potential of pharmacological ROCK inhibition a promising therapeutic strategy for the treatment of NDD.

CONCLUDING REMARKS AND PROSPECTS FOR CLINICAL APPLICATION

Taken together, there is an obvious microglial contribution to the pathogenesis of PD and ALS and ROCK plays an important role in mediating the microglial inflammatory response. Different studies showed that inhibition of ROCK changes the microglial phenotype from the pro-inflammatory "M1" towards the beneficial "M2" and that it enhances clinically relevant outcomes in models of different NDDs making it an auspicious treatment strategy. Fasudil is already licensed in Japan for the treatment of vasospasms following subarachnoidal hemorrhage and its safety for short-term treatment was proven in several preclinical and clinical trials (Fukumoto et al., 2013; Takata et al., 2013). As NDDs are chronic diseases, long-term effects of systemic ROCK inhibition will have to be evaluated, even though first preclinical long-term studies show excellent tolerability and safety (Tatenhorst et al., 2016). Translational trials in human patients are now needed to evaluate the tolerability, safety and efficacy of ROCK inhibition as a treatment strategy for NDDs.

AUTHOR CONTRIBUTIONS

A-ER developed the idea under the lead of PL, performed literature research, wrote and finalized the manuscript and prepared the figure. LT was involved in literature research, writing and revision of the manuscript. PL developed the idea for this review and revised the manuscript. All authors have seen and approved the final version.

REFERENCES

Akiyama, H., and McGeer, P. L. (1989). Microglial response to 6-hydroxydopamine-induced substantia nigra lesions. *Brain Res.* 489, 247–253. doi: 10.1016/0006-8993(89)90857-3

Alshikho, M. J., Zürcher, N. R., Loggia, M. L., Cernasov, P., Chonde, D. B., Izquierdo Garcia, D., et al. (2016). Glial activation colocalizes with structural abnormalities in amyotrophic lateral sclerosis. *Neurology* 87, 2554–2561. doi: 10.1212/WNL.0000000000003427

Barcia, C., Sánchez Bahillo, A. S., Fernández-Villalba, E., Bautista, V., Poza Y Poza, M., Fernández-Barreiro, A., et al. (2004). Evidence of active microglia in substantia nigra pars compacta of parkinsonian monkeys 1 year after MPTP exposure. *Glia* 46, 402–409. doi: 10.1002/glia.20015

Barcia, C., Ros, C. M., Annese, V., Carrillo-de Sauvage, M. A., Ros-Bernal, F., Gómez, A., et al. (2012). ROCK/Cdc42-mediated microglial motility and gliapse formation lead to phagocytosis of degenerating dopaminergic neurons *in vivo*. *Sci. Rep.* 2:809. doi: 10.1038/srep00809

Bartels, A. L., and Leenders, K. L. (2007). Neuroinflammation in the pathophysiology of Parkinson's disease: evidence from animal models to human *in vivo* studies with [^{11}C]-PK11195 PET. *Mov. Disord.* 22, 1852–1856. doi: 10.1002/mds.21552

Baskar Jesudasan, S. J., Todd, K. G., and Winship, I. R. (2014). Reduced inflammatory phenotype in microglia derived from neonatal rat spinal cord versus brain. *PLoS One* 9:e99443. doi: 10.1371/journal.pone.0099443

Boillée, S., Yamanaka, K., Lobsiger, C. S., Copeland, N. G., Jenkins, N. A., Kassiotis, G., et al. (2006). Onset and progression in inherited ALS determined by motor neurons and microglia. *Science* 312, 1389–1392. doi: 10.1126/science.1123511

Borrajo, A., Rodriguez-Perez, A. I., Diaz-Ruiz, C., Guerra, M. J., and Labandeira-Garcia, J. L. (2014a). Microglial TNF-α mediates enhancement of dopaminergic degeneration by brain angiotensin. *Glia* 62, 145–157. doi: 10.1002/glia.22595

Borrajo, A., Rodriguez-Perez, A. I., Villar-Cheda, B., Guerra, M. J., and Labandeira-Garcia, J. L. (2014b). Inhibition of the microglial response is essential for the neuroprotective effects of Rho-kinase inhibitors on MPTP-induced dopaminergic cell death. *Neuropharmacology* 85, 1–8. doi: 10.1016/j.neuropharm.2014.05.021

Chimini, G., and Chavrier, P. (2000). Function of Rho family proteins in actin dynamics during phagocytosis and engulfment. *Nat. Cell Biol.* 2, E191–E196. doi: 10.1038/35036454

Cicchetti, F., Brownell, A. L., Williams, K., Chen, Y. I., Livni, E., and Isacson, O. (2002). Neuroinflammation of the nigrostriatal pathway during progressive 6-OHDA dopamine degeneration in rats monitored by immunohistochemistry and PET imaging. *Eur. J. Neurosci.* 15, 991–998. doi: 10.1046/j.1460-9568.2002.01938.x

Conti, A., Riva, N., Pesca, M., Iannaccone, S., Cannistraci, C. V., Corbo, M., et al. (2014). Increased expression of Myosin binding protein H in the skeletal muscle of amyotrophic lateral sclerosis patients. *Biochim. Biophys. Acta* 1842, 99–106. doi: 10.1016/j.bbadis.2013.10.013

Członkowska, A., Kohutnicka, M., Kurkowska-Jastrzębska, I., and Członkowski, A. (1996). Microglial reaction in MPTP (1-methyl-4-phenyl-1,2,3,6-tetrahydropyridine) induced Parkinson's disease mice model. *Neurodegeneration* 5, 137–143. doi: 10.1006/neur.1996.0020

Defert, O., and Boland, S. (2017). Rho kinase inhibitors: a patent review (2014–2016). *Expert Opin. Ther. Pat.* 27, 507–515. doi: 10.1080/13543776.2017.1272579

Dexter, D. T., and Jenner, P. (2013). Parkinson disease: from pathology to molecular disease mechanisms. *Free Radic. Biol. Med.* 62, 132–144. doi: 10.1016/j.freeradbiomed.2013.01.018

Dibaj, P., Steffens, H., Zschüntzsch, J., Nadrigny, F., Schomburg, E. D., Kirchhoff, F., et al. (2011). *In vivo* imaging reveals distinct inflammatory activity of CNS microglia versus PNS macrophages in a mouse model for ALS. *PLoS One* 6:e17910. doi: 10.1371/journal.pone.0017910

Ding, J., Li, Q. Y., Wang, X., Sun, C. H., Lu, C. Z., and Xiao, B. G. (2010). Fasudil protects hippocampal neurons against hypoxia-reoxygenation injury by suppressing microglial inflammatory responses in mice. *J. Neurochem.* 114, 1619–1629. doi: 10.1111/j.1471-4159.2010.06876.x

Erb, L., Liao, Z., Seye, C. I., and Weisman, G. A. (2006). P2 receptors: intracellular signaling. *Pflugers Arch.* 452, 552–562. doi: 10.1007/s00424-006-0069-2

Evans, M. C., Couch, Y., Sibson, N., and Turner, M. R. (2013). Inflammation and neurovascular changes in amyotrophic lateral sclerosis. *Mol. Cell. Neurosci.* 53, 34–41. doi: 10.1016/j.mcn.2012.10.008

Färber, K., and Kettenmann, H. (2006). Purinergic signaling and microglia. *Pflugers Arch.* 452, 615–621. doi: 10.1007/s00424-006-0064-7

Feng, Y., LoGrasso, P. V., Defert, O., and Li, R. (2016). Rho kinase (ROCK) inhibitors and their therapeutic potential. *J. Med. Chem.* 59, 2269–2300. doi: 10.1021/acs.jmedchem.5b00683

Franco, R., and Fernández-Suárez, D. (2015). Alternatively activated microglia and macrophages in the central nervous system. *Prog. Neurobiol.* 131, 65–86. doi: 10.1016/j.pneurobio.2015.05.003

Fukumoto, Y., Yamada, N., Matsubara, H., Mizoguchi, M., Uchino, K., Yao, A., et al. (2013). Double-blind, placebo-controlled clinical trial with a rho-kinase inhibitor in pulmonary arterial hypertension. *Circ. J.* 77, 2619–2625. doi: 10.1253/circj.cj-13-0443

Gao, H.-M., Jiang, J., Wilson, B., Zhang, W., Hong, J.-S., and Liu, B. (2002). Microglial activation-mediated delayed and progressive degeneration of rat nigral dopaminergic neurons: relevance to Parkinson's disease. *J. Neurochem.* 81, 1285–1297. doi: 10.1046/j.1471-4159.2002.00928.x

Garnock-Jones, K. P. (2014). Ripasudil: first global approval. *Drugs* 74, 2211–2215. doi: 10.1007/s40265-014-0333-2

Gerber, Y. N., Sabourin, J.-C., Rabano, M., Vivanco, M. D. M., and Perrin, F. E. (2012). Early functional deficit and microglial disturbances in a mouse model of amyotrophic lateral sclerosis. *PLoS One* 7:e36000. doi: 10.1371/journal.pone.0036000

Gerhard, A., Pavese, N., Hotton, G., Turkheimer, F., Es, M., Hammers, A., et al. (2006). *In vivo* imaging of microglial activation with $[^{11}C](R)$-PK11195 PET in idiopathic Parkinson's disease. *Neurobiol. Dis.* 21, 404–412. doi: 10.1016/j.nbd.2005.08.002

Günther, R., Balck, A., Koch, J. C., Nientiedt, T., Sereda, M., Bähr, M., et al. (2017). Rho kinase inhibition with fasudil in the SOD1G93A mouse model of amyotrophic lateral sclerosis—symptomatic treatment potential after disease onset. *Front. Pharmacol.* 8:17. doi: 10.3389/fphar.2017.00017

Günther, R., Saal, K.-A., Suhr, M., Scheer, D., Koch, J. C., Bähr, M., et al. (2014). The Rho kinase inhibitor Y-27632 improves motor performance in male SOD1G93A mice. *Front. Neurosci.* 8:304. doi: 10.3389/fnins.2014.00304

Hanisch, U.-K., and Kettenmann, H. (2007). Microglia: active sensor and versatile effector cells in the normal and pathologic brain. *Nat. Neurosci.* 10, 1387–1394. doi: 10.1038/nn1997

Hashimoto, R., Nakamura, Y., Kosako, H., Amano, M., Kaibuchi, K., Inagaki, M., et al. (1999). Distribution of Rho-kinase in the bovine brain. *Biochem. Biophys. Res. Commun.* 263, 575–579. doi: 10.1006/bbrc.1999.1409

He, Q., Li, Y., Guo, S., Wang, Y., Lin, W., Zhang, Q., et al. (2016). Inhibition of Rho-kinase by Fasudil protects dopamine neurons and attenuates inflammatory response in an intranasal lipopolysaccharide-mediated Parkinson's model. *Eur. J. Neurosci.* 43, 41–52. doi: 10.1111/ejn.13132

Henkel, J. S., Beers, D. R., Wen, S., Rivera, A. L., Toennis, K. M., Appel, J. E., et al. (2013). Regulatory T-lymphocytes mediate amyotrophic lateral sclerosis progression and survival. *EMBO Mol. Med.* 5, 64–79. doi: 10.1002/emmm.201201544

Hensel, N., Rademacher, S., and Claus, P. (2015). Chatting with the neighbors: crosstalk between Rho-kinase (ROCK) and other signaling pathways for treatment of neurological disorders. *Front. Neurosci.* 9:198. doi: 10.3389/fnins.2015.00198

Hu, X., Leak, R. K., Shi, Y., Suenaga, J., Gao, Y., Zheng, P., et al. (2015). Microglial and macrophage polarization—new prospects for brain repair. *Nat. Rev. Neurol.* 11, 56–64. doi: 10.14800/macrophage.679

Inoue, K. (2006). The function of microglia through purinergic receptors: neuropathic pain and cytokine release. *Pharmacol. Ther.* 109, 210–226. doi: 10.1016/j.pharmthera.2005.07.001

Jankovic, J. (2008). Parkinson's disease: clinical features and diagnosis. *J. Neurol. Neurosurg. Psychiatry* 79, 368–376. doi: 10.1136/jnnp.2007.131045

Kawamata, T., Akiyama, H., Yamada, T., and McGeer, P. L. (1992). Immunologic reactions in amyotrophic lateral sclerosis brain and spinal cord tissue. *Am. J. Pathol.* 140, 691–707.

Kettenmann, H., Hanisch, U., Noda, M., and Verkhratsky, A. (2011). Physiology of microglia. *Physiol. Rev.* 91, 461–553. doi: 10.1152/physrev.00011.2010

Koshimori, Y., Ko, J.-H., Mizrahi, R., Rusjan, P., Mabrouk, R., Jacobs, M. F., et al. (2015). Imaging striatal microglial activation in patients with Parkinson's disease. *PLoS One* 10:e0138721. doi: 10.1371/journal.pone.0138721

Labandeira-Garcia, J. L., Rodríguez-Perez, A. I., Villar-Cheda, B., Borrajo, A., Dominguez-Meijide, A., and Guerra, M. J. (2015). Rho kinase and dopaminergic degeneration: a promising therapeutic target for Parkinson's disease. *Neuroscientist* 21, 616–629. doi: 10.1177/1073858414554954

Langston, J. W., Forno, L. S., Tetrud, J., Reeves, A. G., Kaplan, J. A., and Karluk, D. (1999). Evidence of active nerve cell degeneration in the substantia nigra of humans years after 1-methyl-4-phenyl-1,2,3,6-tetrahydrophyridine exposure. *Ann. Neurol.* 46, 598–605. doi: 10.1002/1531-8249(199910)46:4<598::AID-ANA7>3.0.CO;2-F

Lee, E.-J., Woo, M.-S., Moon, P.-G., Baek, M.-C., Choi, I.-Y., Kim, W.-K., et al. (2010). α-synuclein activates microglia by inducing the expressions of matrix metalloproteinases and the subsequent activation of protease-activated receptor-1. *J. Immunol.* 185, 615–623. doi: 10.4049/jimmunol.0903480

Leung, T., Chen, X. Q., Manser, E., and Lim, L. (1996). The p160 RhoA-binding kinase ROK α is a member of a kinase family and is involved in the reorganization of the cytoskeleton. *Mol. Cell. Biol.* 16, 5313–5327. doi: 10.1128/mcb.16.10.5313

Liao, B., Zhao, W., Beers, D. R., Henkel, J. S., and Appel, S. H. (2012). Transformation from a neuroprotective to a neurotoxic microglial phenotype in a mouse model of ALS. *Exp. Neurol.* 237, 147–152. doi: 10.1016/j.expneurol.2012.06.011

Liu, Y., and Gray, N. S. (2006). Rational design of inhibitors that bind to inactive kinase conformations. *Nat. Chem. Biol.* 2, 358–364. doi: 10.1038/nchembio799

Moisse, K., and Strong, M. J. (2006). Innate immunity in amyotrophic lateral sclerosis. *Biochim. Biophys. Acta* 1762, 1083–1093. doi: 10.1016/j.bbadis.2006.03.001

Mueller, B. K., Mack, H., and Teusch, N. (2005). Rho kinase, a promising drug target for neurological disorders. *Nat. Rev. Drug Discov.* 4, 387–398. doi: 10.1038/nrd1719

Nakagawa, O., Fujisawa, K., Ishizaki, T., Saito, Y., Nakao, K., and Narumiya, S. (1996). ROCK-I and ROCK-II, two isoforms of Rho-associated coiled-coil forming protein serine/threonine kinase in mice. *FEBS Lett.* 392, 189–193. doi: 10.1016/0014-5793(96)00811-3

Nobes, C. D., and Hall, A. (1995). Rho, Rac and Cdc42 GTPases regulate the assembly of multimolecular focal complexes associated with actin stress fibers, lamellipodia and filopodia. *Cell* 81, 53–62. doi: 10.1016/0092-8674(95)90370-4

Noelker, C., Morel, L., Lescot, T., Osterloh, A., Alvarez-Fischer, D., Breloer, M., et al. (2013). Toll like receptor 4 mediates cell death in a mouse MPTP model of Parkinson disease. *Sci. Rep.* 3:1393. doi: 10.1038/srep01393

Oda, K., and Kitano, H. (2006). A comprehensive map of the toll-like receptor signaling network. *Mol. Syst. Biol.* 2:2006.0015. doi: 10.1038/msb4100057

Olson, J. K., and Miller, S. D. (2004). Microglia initiate central nervous system innate and adaptive immune responses through multiple TLRs. *J. Immunol.* 173, 3916–3924. doi: 10.4049/jimmunol.173.6.3916

Ouchi, Y., Yoshikawa, E., Sekine, Y., Futatsubashi, M., Kanno, T., Ogusu, T., et al. (2005). Microglial activation and dopamine terminal loss in early Parkinson's disease. *Ann. Neurol.* 57, 168–175. doi: 10.1002/ana.20338

Paez-Colasante, X., Figueroa-Romero, C., Sakowski, S. A., Goutman, S. A., and Feldman, E. L. (2015). Amyotrophic lateral sclerosis: mechanisms and therapeutics in the epigenomic era. *Nat. Rev. Neurol.* 11, 266–279. doi: 10.1038/nrneurol.2015.57

Philips, T., and Rothstein, J. D. (2014). Glial cells in amyotrophic lateral sclerosis. *Exp. Neurol.* 262, 111–120. doi: 10.1016/j.expneurol.2014.05.015

Qin, X.-Y., Zhang, S.-P., Cao, C., Loh, Y. P., and Cheng, Y. (2016). Aberrations in peripheral inflammatory cytokine levels in Parkinson disease. *JAMA Neurol.* 73, 1316–1324. doi: 10.1001/jamaneurol.2016.2742

Reynolds, A. D., Kadiu, I., Garg, S. K., Glanzer, J. G., Nordgren, T., Ciborowski, P., et al. (2008). Nitrated α-synuclein and microglial neuroregulatory activities. *J. Neuroimmune Pharmacol.* 3, 59–74. doi: 10.1007/s11481-008-9100-z

Rodriguez-Pallares, J., Parga, J. A., Muñoz, A., Rey, P., Guerra, M. J., and Labandeira-Garcia, J. L. (2007). Mechanism of 6-hydroxydopamine neurotoxicity: the role of NADPH oxidase and microglial activation in 6-hydroxydopamine-induced degeneration of dopaminergic neurons. *J. Neurochem.* 103, 145–156. doi: 10.1111/j.1471-4159.2007.04699.x

Rodriguez-Perez, A. I., Borrajo, A., Rodriguez-Pallares, J., Guerra, M. J., and Labandeira-Garcia, J. L. (2015). Interaction between NADPH-oxidase and Rho-kinase in angiotensin II-induced microglial activation. *Glia* 63, 466–482. doi: 10.1002/glia.22765

Saal, K.-A., Galter, D., Roeber, S., Bähr, M., Tönges, L., and Lingor, P. (2017). Altered expression of growth associated protein-43 and Rho kinase in human patients with Parkinson's disease. *Brain Pathol.* 27, 13–25. doi: 10.1111/bpa.12346

Saal, K.-A., Koch, J. C., Tatenhorst, L., Szegö, E. M., Ribas, V. T., Michel, U., et al. (2015). AAV.shRNA-mediated downregulation of ROCK2 attenuates degeneration of dopaminergic neurons in toxin-induced models of Parkinson's disease *in vitro* and *in vivo*. *Neurobiol. Dis.* 73, 150–162. doi: 10.1016/j.nbd.2014.09.013

Schwartz, M., Butovsky, O., Brück, W., and Hanisch, U.-K. (2006). Microglial phenotype: is the commitment reversible? *Trends Neurosci.* 29, 68–74. doi: 10.1016/j.tins.2005.12.005

Suzuki, Y., Shibuya, M., Satoh, S., Sugimoto, Y., and Takakura, K. (2007). A postmarketing surveillance study of fasudil treatment after aneurysmal subarachnoid hemorrhage. *Surg. Neurol.* 68, 126–131; discussion 131–132. doi: 10.1016/j.surneu.2006.10.037

Takata, M., Tanaka, H., Kimura, M., Nagahara, Y., Tanaka, K., Kawasaki, K., et al. (2013). Fasudil, a rho kinase inhibitor, limits motor neuron loss in experimental models of amyotrophic lateral sclerosis. *Br. J. Pharmacol.* 170, 341–351. doi: 10.1111/bph.12277

Tang, Y., and Le, W. (2016). Differential roles of M1 and M2 microglia in neurodegenerative diseases. *Mol. Neurobiol.* 53, 1181–1194. doi: 10.1007/s12035-014-9070-5

Tatenhorst, L., Eckermann, K., Dambeck, V., Fonseca-Ornelas, L., Walle, H., Lopes da Fonseca, T., et al. (2016). Fasudil attenuates aggregation of α-synuclein in models of Parkinson's disease. *Acta Neuropathol. Commun.* 4:39. doi: 10.1186/s40478-016-0310-y

Tatenhorst, L., Tönges, L., Saal, K.-A., Koch, J. C., Szegö, É. M., Bähr, M., et al. (2014). Rho kinase inhibition by fasudil in the striatal 6-hydroxydopamine lesion mouse model of Parkinson disease. *J. Neuropathol. Exp. Neurol.* 73, 770–779. doi: 10.1097/NEN.0000000000000095

Tatsumi, E., Yamanaka, H., Kobayashi, K., Yagi, H., Sakagami, M., and Noguchi, K. (2015). RhoA/ROCK pathway mediates p38 MAPK activation and morphological changes downstream of P2Y12/13 receptors in spinal microglia in neuropathic pain. *Glia* 63, 216–228. doi: 10.1002/glia.22745

Tönges, L., Frank, T., Tatenhorst, L., Saal, K. A., Koch, J. C., Szego, É. M., et al. (2012). Inhibition of rho kinase enhances survival of dopaminergic neurons and attenuates axonal loss in a mouse model of Parkinson's disease. *Brain* 135, 3355–3370. doi: 10.1093/brain/aws254

Tönges, L., Günther, R., Suhr, M., Jansen, J., Balck, A., Saal, K.-A., et al. (2014). Rho kinase inhibition modulates microglia activation and improves survival in a model of amyotrophic lateral sclerosis. *Glia* 62, 217–232. doi: 10.1002/glia.22601

Tura, A., Schuettauf, F., Monnier, P. P., Bartz-Schmidt, K. U., and Henke-Fahle, S. (2009). Efficacy of Rho-kinase inhibition in promoting cell survival and reducing reactive gliosis in the rodent retina. *Investig. Ophthalmol. Vis. Sci.* 50, 452–461. doi: 10.1167/iovs.08-1973

Villar-Cheda, B., Dominguez-Meijide, A., Joglar, B., Rodriguez-Perez, A. I., Guerra, M. J., and Labandeira-Garcia, J. L. (2012). Involvement of microglial RhoA/Rho-Kinase pathway activation in the dopaminergic neuron death. Role of angiotensin via angiotensin type 1 receptors. *Neurobiol. Dis.* 47, 268–279. doi: 10.1016/j.nbd.2012.04.010

Welch, M. D., and Mullins, R. D. (2002). Cellular control of actin nucleation. *Annu. Rev. Cell Dev. Biol.* 18, 247–288. doi: 10.1146/annurev.cellbio.18.040202.112133

Wolf, S. A., Boddeke, H. W. G. M., and Kettenmann, H. (2017). Microglia in physiology and disease. *Annu. Rev. Physiol.* 79, 619–643. doi: 10.1146/annurev-physiol-022516-034406

Yan, J., Zhou, X., Guo, J. J., Mao, L., Wang, Y. J., Sun, J., et al. (2012). Nogo-66 inhibits adhesion and migration of microglia via GTPase Rho pathway *in vitro*. *J. Neurochem.* 120, 721–731. doi: 10.1111/j.1471-4159.2011.07619.x

Zhang, W., Wang, T., Pei, Z., Miller, D. S., Wu, X., Block, M. L., et al. (2005). Aggregated α-synuclein activates microglia: a process leading to disease progression in Parkinson's disease. *FASEB J.* 19, 533–542. doi: 10.1096/fj.04-2751com

Zhao, Y., Zhang, Q., Xi, J., Li, Y., Ma, C., and Xiao, B. (2015). Multitarget intervention of Fasudil in the neuroprotection of dopaminergic neurons in MPTP-mouse model of Parkinson's disease. *J. Neurol. Sci.* 353, 28–37. doi: 10.1016/j.jns.2015.03.022

17

Mild Inflammatory Profile without Gliosis in the c-Rel Deficient Mouse Modeling a Late-Onset Parkinsonism

Vanessa Porrini [1†], Mariana Mota [1†], Edoardo Parrella [1], Arianna Bellucci [1], Marina Benarese [1], Lara Faggi [1], Paolo Tonin [2], Pier F. Spano [1,2] and Marina Pizzi [1,2]*

[1]*Laboratory of Pharmacology, Department of Molecular and Translational Medicine, University of Brescia, Brescia, Italy,* [2]*IRCCS, San Camillo Hospital, Venice, Italy*

Correspondence:
Marina Pizzi
marina.pizzi@unibs.it

†These authors have contributed equally to this work.

The impact of neuroinflammation and microglial activation to Parkinson's disease (PD) progression is still debated. Post-mortem analysis of PD brains has shown that neuroinflammation and microgliosis are key features of end-stage disease. However, microglia neuroimaging studies and evaluation of cerebrospinal fluid (CSF) cytokines in PD patients at earlier stages do not support the occurrence of a pronounced neuroinflammatory process. PD animal models recapitulating the motor and non-motor features of the disease, and the slow and progressive neuropathology, can be of great advantage in understanding whether and how neuroinflammation associates with the onset of symptoms and neuronal loss. We recently described that 18-month-old NF-κB/c-Rel deficient mice (c-rel$^{-/-}$) develop a spontaneous late-onset PD-like phenotype encompassing L-DOPA-responsive motor impairment, nigrostriatal neuron degeneration, α-synuclein and iron accumulation. To assess whether inflammation and microglial activation accompany the onset and the progression of PD-like pathology, we investigated the expression of cytokines (*interleukin 1 beta (Il1b), interleukin 6 (Il6)*) and microglial/macrophage activation markers (*Fc gamma receptor III (Fcgr3), mannose receptor 1 (Mrc1), chitinase-like 3 (Ym1), arginase 1 (Arg 1), triggering receptor expressed on myeloid cells 2 (Trem2)*), together with microglial ionized calcium binding adapter molecule 1 (Iba1) and astrocyte glial fibrillary acidic protein (GFAP) immunolabeling, in the substantia nigra (SN) of c-rel$^{-/-}$ mice, at premotor (4- and 13-month-old) and motor phases (18-month-old). By quantitative real-time RT-PCR we found increased M2c microglial/macrophage markers expression (*Mrc1* and *Arg1*) in 4-month-old c-rel$^{-/-}$ mice. M2-type transcription dropped down in 13-month-old c-rel$^{-/-}$ mice. At this age, the pro-inflammatory *Il1b*, but not *Il6* or the microglia-macrophage M1-polarization marker *Fcgr3*/CD16, increased when compared to wild-type (wt). Furthermore, no significant variation in the transcription of inflammatory and microglial/macrophage activation genes was present in 18-month-old c-rel$^{-/-}$ mice, that display motor dysfunctions and dopaminergic neuronal loss. Immunofluorescence analysis of Iba1-positive cells in the

Abbreviations: Arg1, arginase 1; CNS, central nervous system; CSF, cerebrospinal fluid; DAT, dopamine transporter; Fcgr3, Fc gamma receptor III, also known as CD16; GFAP, glial fibrillary acidic protein; Iba1, ionized calcium binding adapter molecule 1; Il6, interleukin 6; Il1b, interleukin 1 beta; Mrc1, mannose receptor 1; PD, Parkinson's disease; qRT-PCR, real-time quantitative reverse transcription-polymerase chain reaction; SN, substantia nigra; Trem2, triggering receptor expressed on myeloid cells 2; Ym1, chitinase-like 3.

SN revealed no sign of overt microglial activation in c-rel$^{-/-}$ mice at all the time-points. MRC1-Iba1-positive cells were identified as non-parenchymal macrophages in 4-month-old c-rel$^{-/-}$ mice. Finally, no sign of astrogliosis was detected in the SN of the diverse animal groups. In conclusion, this study supports the presence of a mild inflammatory profile without evident signs of gliosis in c-rel$^{-/-}$ mice up to 18 months of age. It suggests that symptomatic PD-like phenotype can develop in the absence of concomitant severe inflammatory process.

Keywords: c-Rel, neuroinflammation, microglia, Parkinson's disease, astrocytes, substantia nigra

INTRODUCTION

Parkinson's disease (PD) is the major neurodegenerative motor disorder worldwide, characterized by motor symptoms such as bradykinesia, resting tremor and rigidity. Key hallmarks of the brains of affected patients are the loss of dopaminergic neurons of substantia nigra (SN) pars compacta and Lewy bodies, intracellular inclusions mainly composed by aggregated α-synuclein (Poewe et al., 2017). Although the neuropathological features of the disease have been well described, the biological basis of neuronal death still needs to be clarified. Nonetheless, processes such as neuroinflammation and microglial activation have been proposed to contribute to the onset of PD (Poewe et al., 2017).

Microglia, the resident immune cells of the brain (Aguzzi et al., 2013), are essential for brain homeostasis in physiological conditions (Nimmerjahn et al., 2005; Neumann et al., 2009; Miyamoto et al., 2013). During brain injury, microglia become activated, which can be either detrimental or protective for neuronal cells in the central nervous system (CNS; Hayakawa et al., 2008; Brites and Vaz, 2014; Hu et al., 2015). The opposite role of microglia in brain diseases has been hypothesized to arise from the fact that these cells can adopt diverse activation states (Tang and Le, 2016). In particular, the classification of monocyte-derived macrophages into classically (M1) and alternatively activated (M2) was later applied to microglia (Gordon, 2003). While the M1 state has been associated with pro-inflammatory responses (Hu et al., 2015), the alternatively activated state M2 has been found to be related to healing and scavenging. In addition, three different M2 sub-classes have been described: M2a, M2b and M2c, that have been associated with tissue repair, regulation of inflammation and tissue remodeling, and debris and iron scavenging, respectively (David and Kroner, 2011).

The first evidence of increased microglial activation in post-mortem brains of PD patients was published by McGeer and collaborators almost 30 years ago (McGeer et al., 1988). Since then, microgliosis and inflammation have been thought to play a role in PD pathogenesis and/or progression (Long-Smith et al., 2009). On the other hand, the relevance of astrogliosis in PD pathology remains debated (Hirsch and Hunot, 2009), due to contrasting results of studies in PD patients (Knott et al., 1999; Mirza et al., 2000; Thannickal et al., 2007; Song et al., 2009; Tong et al., 2015). Indeed, post-mortem analysis of PD brains showed increased reactive microglia in the SN around the surviving dopaminergic neurons, as well as an augmented level of cytokines (McGeer et al., 1988; Mogi et al., 1994a; Banati et al., 1998; Imamura et al., 2003), indicating a clear involvement of microglia and inflammation at the end stage of the disease. In order to evaluate neuroinflammation during different stages of the disease, several studies have analyzed the content of cytokines in the cerebrospinal fluid (CSF) of patients affected by PD, which is considered a representative indicator of pathological brain states. Earlier studies found an increase in the levels of cytokines, such as interleukin 6 (IL-6), interleukin 1 beta (IL-1β), TNFα and TGF-β, in CSF from relatively small cohorts of PD patients (Mogi et al., 1994b, 1995, 1996; Blum-Degen et al., 1995; Vawter et al., 1996; Müller et al., 1998). On the other hand, more recent studies on larger patients' cohorts showed no differences in the CSF levels of IL-6 and TNFα (Lindqvist et al., 2013), and fractalkine (Shi et al., 2011), in PD subjects compared to controls. Thus, while clear neuroinflammatory pathology has been established in the post-mortem brain of late-stage PD, it remains arguable the participation of inflammatory processes with microglial activation in the earlier and progressive stages of PD.

Animal models of PD could be valuable tools to investigate whether inflammation with microglial activation, and its diverse activation states, occurs along with SN degeneration and the onset of motor dysfunction. However, none of the available models fully recapitulates the pathological hallmarks and the slow progression of PD (Cebrián et al., 2015). Thus, the importance of these pathological features to the onset and worsening of the disease is still an open question.

We have previously shown that mice deficient for the NF-κB c-Rel nuclear factor (c-rel$^{-/-}$ mice) develop a late-onset parkinsonism (Baiguera et al., 2012) characterized by significant impairment in spontaneous motor activity. They displayed an L-DOPA-reversible hypo-motility and gait-related deficits at 18 months, but not at younger ages (Baiguera et al., 2012). The motor deficits observed in aged c-rel$^{-/-}$ mice were accompanied by a significant loss of dopaminergic neurons and accumulation of α-synuclein aggregates in the SN, marked reduction of dopaminergic terminals and dopamine content in the striatum, as well as increased expression of divalent metal transporter 1 and iron staining in SN and striatum (Baiguera et al., 2012). Furthermore, we described that the SN and striatum of 18-month-old c-rel$^{-/-}$ mice displayed a significant increase in the area of CD11b-positive microglia (Baiguera et al., 2012). More recently, we found that c-rel$^{-/-}$ mice displayed progressive accumulation of pathological α-synuclein in SN, as well as striatal loss of dopamine transporter (DAT) as early as 12 months of age, when they did not show either motor impairment or loss of dopaminergic neurons in the SN yet (Lanzillotta et al., 2015; Parrella et al., submitted). In this premotor phase (2–13 months of age), c-rel$^{-/-}$ showed non-motor symptoms typical of PD, such as hyposmia and gastrointestinal dysfunctions (Lanzillotta et al., 2015; Parrella et al., submitted).

In this study, we investigated whether there is a temporal correlation between inflammatory transcription and microglial/astrocyte activation with the development of the spontaneous PD-like pathology in c-rel$^{-/-}$ mice. We evaluated markers of inflammation and microglial/macrophage activation, as well as signs of gliosis, in the premotor and motor stages of c-rel$^{-/-}$ mice at 4, 13 and 18 months of age.

MATERIALS AND METHODS

Experimental Animals

C57BL/6 mice carrying the c-Rel gene null mutation (c-rel$^{-/-}$) were originally generated by inserting the neomycin cassette into the fifth exon of the *c-Rel* gene (Liou et al., 1999). The genotypes were confirmed by PCR analysis (Baiguera et al., 2012) and western blot, and both lines were continued by homozygous breeding. The c-rel$^{-/-}$ and c-rel$^{+/+}$ wild-type (wt) mice were housed in the animal facility of the Department of Molecular and Translational Medicine of the University of Brescia. Animals were maintained in standard cages under 12/12 h light/dark cycles with *ad libitum* access to food and water. Humidity and room temperature were maintained constant. This study was carried out in accordance with the recommendations of the Directive 2010/63/EU of the European Parliament and of the Council of 22 September 2010 on the protection of animals used for scientific purposes. The protocol was approved by the animal-welfare body of the University of Brescia. Male 4-, 13- and 18-month-old mice were used for this study.

Real-Time Quantitative Reverse Transcription-Polymerase Chain Reaction (qRT-PCR)

Total RNA was purified from SN using the RNeasy Mini Kit for total RNA extractions (Qiagen). Total RNA (1 μg) was reverse transcribed using the Quantitect® Reverse Transcription Kit (Qiagen) according to manufacture instructions. Retrotranscribed cDNA (1–5 μL) was amplified using iQ™ SYBR Green Supermix (Bio-Rad) and 10 μM optimized forward and reverse primers. PCR reaction was performed using the standard program in ViiA7™ Real-Time PCR System (Applied Biosystems). Each reaction was performed at least in triplicate. For standardization of quantification, beta-Actin *(Actb)* was used as housekeeping gene. Data were analyzed following the comparative Ct method. The following primers were used for real-time quantitative reverse transcription-polymerase chain reaction (qRT-PCR):

- *arginase 1 (Arg1)*: For GTGTACATTGGCTTGCGAGA; Rev AATCGGCCTTTTCTTCCTTC
- *Actb*: For GGCTCTTTTCCAGCCTTCCT; Rev ATGCCT GGGTACATGGTGGT
- *Fc gamma receptor III (Fcgr3)*: For TATCGGTG TCAAATGGAGCA; Rev GCACCT TAGCGTGATGGTTT
- *Il6*: For CCTACCCCAATTTCCAATGCT; Rev TATTTT CTGACCACAGTGAGGAAT
- *Il1b*: For GGCTTCAGGCAGGCAGTATC; Rev TAATGG GAACGTCACACACC
- *mannose receptor 1 (Mrc1)*: For AAGGTTCGGGATTGTG GAG; Rev AATCGGCCTTTTCTTCCTTC
- *triggering receptor expressed on myeloid cells 2 (Trem2)*: For CACTCTGAAGAACCTCCAAGC; Rev ATTCCTGGAG GTGCTGTGTT
- *chitinase-like 3 (Ym1)*: For GCCCACCAGGAAAGTACACA; Rev CACGGCACCTCCTAAATTGT

Immunofluorescence

Mice were anesthetized with chloral hydrate (400 mg/kg intraperitoneally) and transcardially perfused with PBS (Sigma-Aldrich) and 4% (w/v) ice-cold paraformaldehyde (PFA). Brains were postfixed in 4% PFA at 4°C for 2 h, followed by cryoprotection in 30% sucrose in PBS until cut. Coronal slices (15 μm-thick) were cut to obtain serial sections of the SN (anterior–posterior 2.54–3.40 mm), using bregma-based coordinates (Paxinos and Franklin, 2012).

Immunofluorescence for the ionized calcium binding adapter molecule 1 (Iba1) and glial fibrillary acidic protein (GFAP) antibodies was initiated by performing antigen retrieval (Tris-EDTA Buffer pH 9, 90°C, 10 min), followed by permeabilization and blocking. Then, sections were incubated overnight at 4°C with the primary antibodies rabbit anti-Iba1 (1:500, Wako #019-19741) or mouse anti-GFAP (1:100, Sigma #G3893). The following day, slices were incubated for 1 h at room temperature with the secondary antibodies goat anti-rabbit Alexa Fluor 488 (1:1000, Jackson ImmunoResearch #111-545-144), for Iba1, and goat anti-mouse Alexa Fluor 488 (1:800, Jackson ImmunoResearch #115-546-071), for GFAP. Lastly, sections were incubated with Hoechst 33342 (1 mg/mL, Sigma-Aldrich) to stain cellular nuclei.

Double immunofluorescence staining for MRC1 and Iba1 was initiated by performing antigen retrieval, permeabilization and blocking, followed by an overnight incubation at 4°C with rat anti-mouse MRC1 (1:50, Bio-Rad #MCA2235). Sections were then incubated for 1 h at room temperature in biotinylated goat anti-rat (1:400, Vector laboratories #BA-9401) followed by streptavidin-Alexa Fluor 488 (1:1000, ThermoFisher Scientific #S11227). Then, the sections were incubated 2 h at 37°C in the second primary antibody rabbit anti-Iba1, goat anti-rabbit Alexa Fluor 488, and Hoechst 33342.

Double immunofluorescence staining for IL-1β and Iba1 was performed by incubating sections in goat anti-Iba1 (1:100, Novus Biologicals #NB 300-270) overnight at 4°C followed by donkey anti-goat Alexa Fluor 488 (1:500, Jackson ImmunoResearch #705-545-147). Slices were then incubated in the second primary antibody rabbit anti-IL-1β (1:50, Abcam #ab9722) overnight at 4°C, followed by biotinylated goat anti-rabbit (1:400, Vector laboratories #BA-1000), streptavidin-Alexa Fluor 488, and lastly Hoechst 33342. In order to check antibody specificity, control (blank) reactions with no primary antibodies were run in parallel.

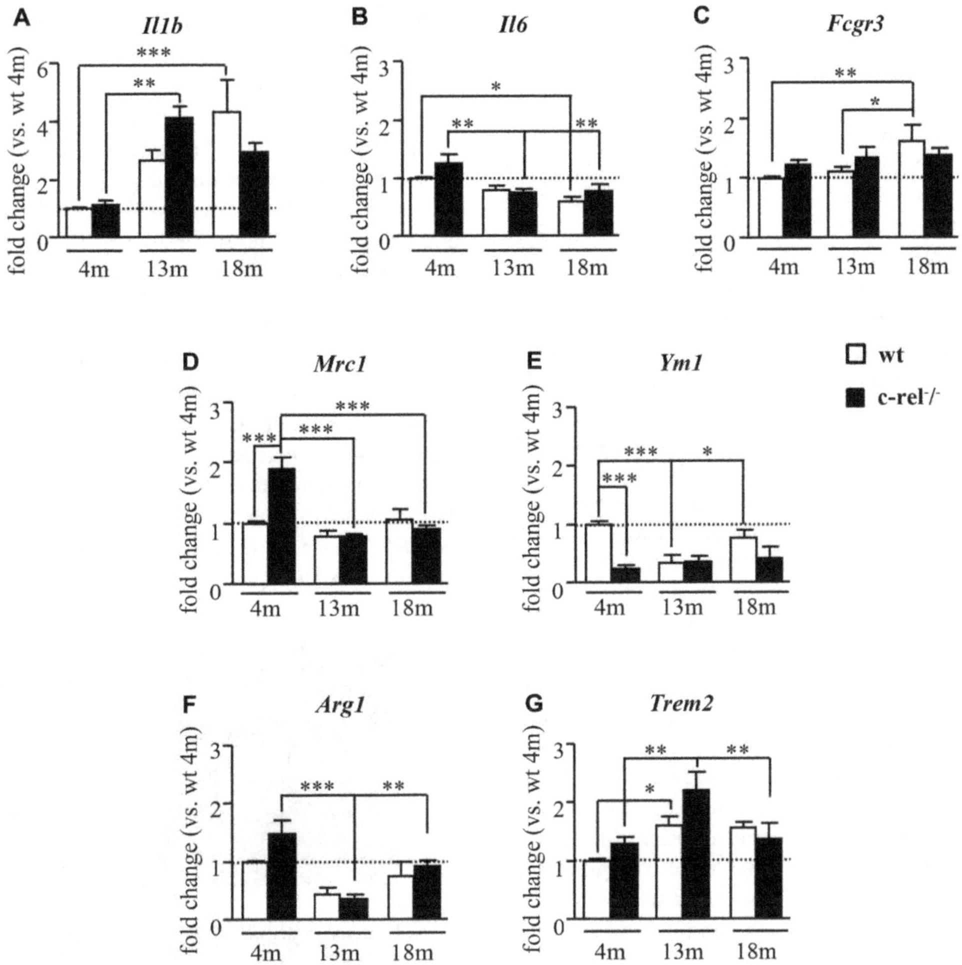

FIGURE 1 | Inflammatory and microglial/macrophage mRNA expression profile in c-rel$^{-/-}$ and wild-type (wt) mice. Real-time quantitative reverse transcription-polymerase chain reaction (qRT-PCR) analysis of pro-inflammatory cytokines, interleukin 1 beta (*Il1b*) and *interleukin 6* (*Il6*; **A,B**), and microglial/macrophage activation markers, *Fc gamma receptor III* (*Fcgr3*; **C**), for M1 phenotype; *mannose receptor 1* (*Mrc1*; **D**), *chitinase-like 3* (*Ym1*; **E**), *arginase 1* (*Arg1*); **(F)**, and *triggering receptor expressed on myeloid cells 2* (*Trem2*); **(G)**, for M2 state in substantia nigra (SN) of 4, 13 and 18 months of age mice (n = 4–6 animals per group). Four-month-old c-rel$^{-/-}$ mice showed increased expression of M2c microglial marker *Mrc1* and *Arg1*, associated with marked decrease of *Ym1* transcription. At 13 months of age, c-Rel deficient mice displayed an upregulation in *Il1b* transcription compared to younger c-rel$^{-/-}$ mice, while no differences in microglial M2 markers were found in c-rel$^{-/-}$ mice compared to wt group. No biologically relevant variations in all the analyzed markers were evident in 18-month-old c-rel$^{-/-}$ mice compared to wt. Data are presented as mean ± SEM. *$P < 0.05$, **$p < 0.01$, ***$p < 0.001$; two-way analysis of variance (ANOVA) followed by Bonferroni test for comparison vs. 4-month-old wt mice.

Microscopy

Immunofluorescence stainings were analyzed by an inverted light/epifluorescence microscope (Olympus IX50; Olympus), and pictures were captured with a digital camera (Olympus XC 30) and cellSens Software (Olympus) and analyzed in a blinded manner. Images were adjusted for brightness and contrast with Adobe Photoshop (Adobe system) software.

Statistical Analysis

Statistical analysis was performed with the GraphPad Prism program (GraphPad Software). qRT-PCR data was analyzed by two-way analysis of variance (ANOVA) followed by Bonferroni *post hoc* test. Data are presented as mean ± SEM. $P < 0.05$ was considered as significant.

RESULTS

Age-Related Alterations in the Expression of Inflammatory and Microglial/Macrophage Activation Markers in the Substantia Nigra of c-Rel Deficient Mice

We first evaluated the expression of general markers of inflammation and specific markers for the diverse microglial/macrophage activation states, M1 (pro-inflammatory) and M2 (anti-inflammatory, phagocytic) by qRT-PCR on SN RNA extracts of wt and c-rel$^{-/-}$ mice at 4, 13 and 18 months. In particular, we analyzed the pro-inflammatory markers *Il1b* and *Il6*, that are widely expressed in the CNS, and *Fcgr3*/CD16, that is specifically expressed by M1-polarized microglia/macrophages. Moreover, we determined the expression of *Mrc1*, *Ym1*, *Arg1* and *Trem2*, specific markers for the M2 activation state of microglia/macrophages.

At 4 months of age, no differences were found in the mRNA expression of the pro-inflammatory markers *Il1b* and *Il6*, and M1 microglia/macrophage marker *Fcgr3* in the SN of c-rel$^{-/-}$ mice when compared to wt (**Figures 1A–C**). At 13 months of age, a statistically significant increase of *Il1b* expression was detected only in c-rel$^{-/-}$ mice (**Figure 1A**). This age-dependent increase in *Il1b* transcription was also detected in the wt mice at 18 months of age (**Figure 1A**). Interestingly, the levels of *Il1b* in 18-month-old c-rel$^{-/-}$ mice were not significantly different from those observed at 4 months (**Figure 1A**). However, no biologically relevant, albeit statistically significant, differences in the expression of *Il6* or *Fcgr3* were observed between c-rel$^{-/-}$ and wt mice at all the time points analyzed (**Figures 1B,C**). These analyses only showed an age-related decrease of *Il6*, occurring in both mouse lines, and a statistically significant increase of *Fcgr3* in 18-month-old wt mice (**Figure 1C**). On the other hand, the analysis of the expression of M2 markers in 4-month-old mice showed a significant increase of *Mrc1* and a trend to increase for *Arg1* transcription in c-rel$^{-/-}$ mice when compared to wt, while *Ym1* resulted significantly downregulated (**Figures 1D–F**). No significant difference in *Trem2* was detected between c-rel$^{-/-}$ and wt mice at this age (**Figure 1G**). This expression pattern seems to indicate a polarization of microglia/macrophages towards a particular M2 state named M2c, that is associated with tissue repair, as well as to debris and iron scavenging (David and Kroner, 2011), in 4-month-old c-rel$^{-/-}$ mice. However, the M2c activation state was no longer detectable in 13-month-old c-rel$^{-/-}$ mice. Indeed, at this age, *Mrc1* and *Arg1* transcripts resulted downregulated in c-rel$^{-/-}$ mice when compared to 4-month-old mice, while *Ym1* expression remained unchanged (**Figures 1D–F**). On the other hand, we observed a significant increase in *Trem2* transcription in 13-month-old c-Rel deficient mice when compared to younger animals (**Figure 1G**). Though similar changes were found in wt mice (**Figure 1G**). Finally, we did not observe biologically relevant changes in the expression of all M2 markers between c-rel$^{-/-}$ and wt mice at either 13 or 18 months of age, thus suggesting a limited involvement of the M2 polarization of microglia/macrophages in the SN of older c-rel$^{-/-}$ mice.

These data support the occurrence of M2c-like pattern of expression in the SN of c-rel$^{-/-}$ mice at 4 months of age, when they do not display any sign of degeneration in this area yet. It is followed by a mild inflammatory state characterized by *Ilb* expression in 13-month-old c-rel$^{-/-}$ mice, when they develop a loss of DAT immunostaining in the striatum (Lanzillotta et al., 2015).

Immunohistochemical Characterization of Mild Inflammatory Profile in the Substantia Nigra of c-Rel Deficient Mice

To assess microglial activation in the premotor and motor phases of PD-like pathology, we analyzed the immunoreactivity for Iba1, a constitutive marker of microglia and macrophages, in the SN of 4-, 13- and 18-month-old c-rel$^{-/-}$ mice and age-matched wt animals. Iba1 was expressed similarly, both in distribution and morphology, in c-rel$^{-/-}$ and wt mice, at all the considered ages (**Figure 2**). These data appeared contrasting to our previous findings showing an increased immunoreactivity for CD11b in the SN of 18-month-old c-rel$^{-/-}$ mice (Baiguera et al., 2012).

To identify the origin of the increased *Mrc1* transcription in the SN of 4-month-old c-rel$^{-/-}$ mice, double immunofluorescence staining with MRC1 and Iba1 was performed in brain sections of these animals. MRC1 immunoreactivity was not detected in Iba1-positive parenchymal microglia, but instead in Iba1-positive cells located at CNS interfaces (**Figure 3**). These non-ramified cells were identified as non-parenchymal or CNS macrophages, namely

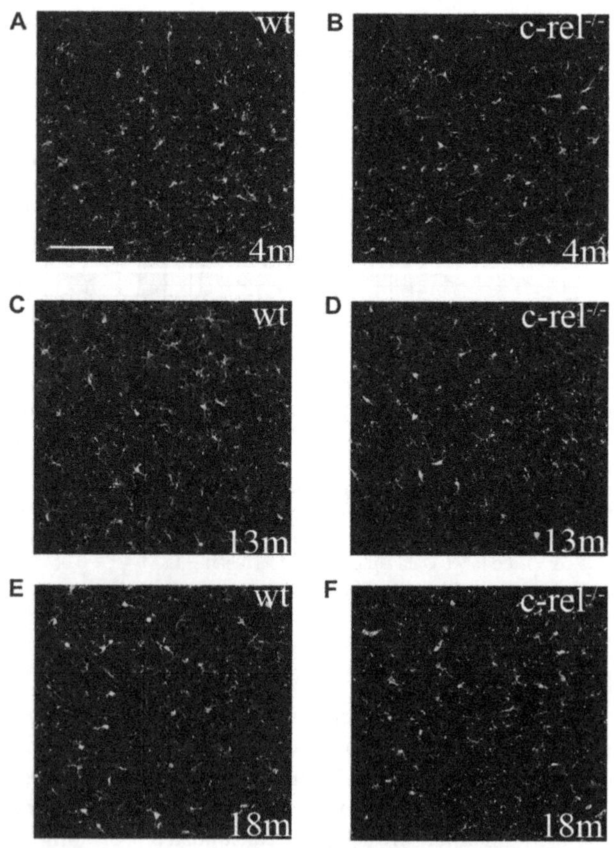

FIGURE 2 | Ionized calcium binding adapter molecule 1 (Iba1) immunoreactivity in c-rel$^{-/-}$ and wt mice. Pictures of SN sections from 4- **(A,B)**, 13- **(C,D)** and 18-month-old animals **(E,F)** illustrating Iba1 immunostaining. No evident changes in microglial activation were found in c-rel$^{-/-}$ mice **(B,D,F)** compared to age-matched wt **(A,C,E)**. Immunofluorescence images are representative of five sections from each animal (n = 3 animals per group). Abbreviations: SN, substantia nigra. Scale bar: in **(A)** = 100 μm for **(A–F)**.

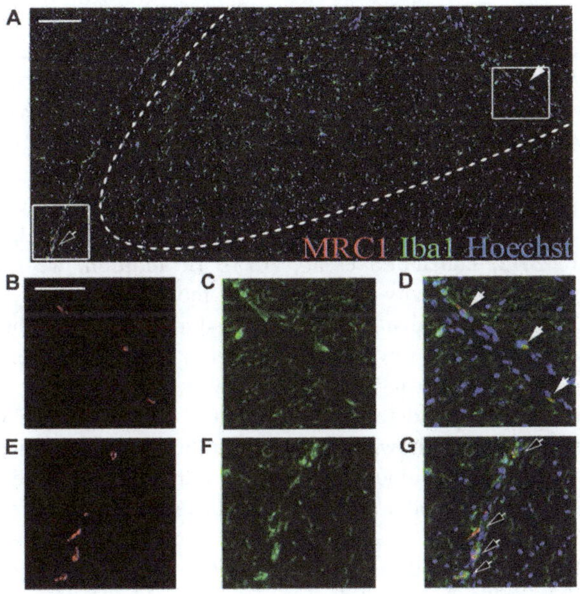

FIGURE 3 | Non-parenchymal macrophages are immunoreactive to MRC1. **(A)** MRC1 (red) and Iba1 (green) double-labeled cells are localized at CNS interfaces (closed and open arrows) and not in the SN parenchyma (delimited by the dashed line) in 4-month-old c-rel$^{-/-}$ mice. **(B–D)** Higher magnification of MRC1-Iba1 double-labeled perivascular macrophages (closed arrow) and Iba1-positive microglia in the SN. **(E,F)** Higher magnification of MRC1-Iba1 double-labeled meningeal macrophages (open arrows), and Iba1-positive microglia, outside the SN. Upper image **(A)** is representative of five sections from each animal (n = 3). Abbreviations: CNS, central nervous system; SN, substantia nigra. Scale bars: in **(A)** = 100 μm; in **(B)** = 50 μm for **(B–G)**.

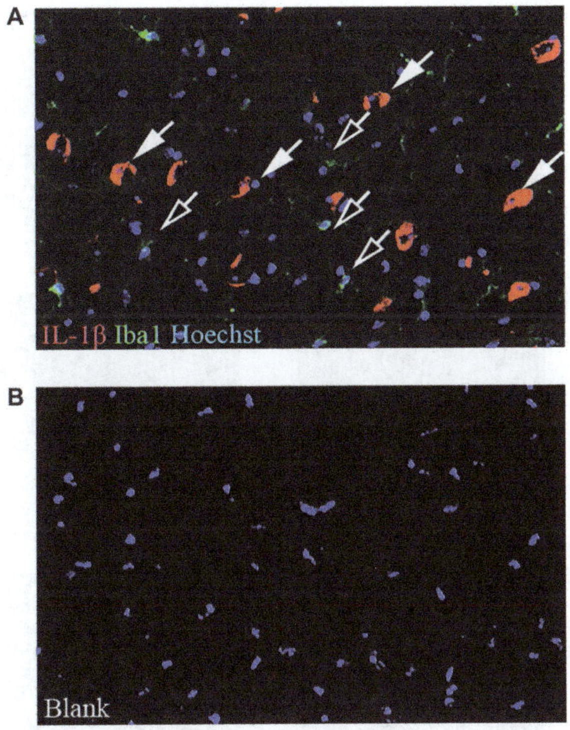

FIGURE 4 | IL-1β localization in the SN. **(A)** Representative image of IL-1β (red) and Iba1 (green) immunofluorescence with Hoechst (blue) staining in the SN of 13-month-old c-rel$^{-/-}$ mice. Closed arrows highlight IL-1β-positive cells. Open arrows highlight Iba1-positive cells. The image is representative of five sections from each animal (n = 3). **(B)** Blank control. Abbreviations: SN, substantia nigra. Scale bar: in **(A)** = 100 μm for **(A,B)**.

perivascular or meningeal, depending on their localization and morphology (Goldmann et al., 2016). Considering that the aim of the present work was to study parenchymal microglia in the SN, we chose not to proceed with the analysis of these few macrophages limited to CNS borders, though it would definitely be interesting to focus our attention on these cells in a future study.

To establish the source of the increased *Il1b* mRNA in the SN of c-rel$^{-/-}$ mice at 13 months of age, SN sections from these mice were immunolabeled for IL-1β and Iba1. IL-1β expression was mostly found in cells negative for Iba1 in 13-month-old c-rel$^{-/-}$ mice (**Figure 4**). Considering their morphology, we speculate these IL-1β-positive Iba1-negative cells are neurons.

The immunoreactivity for GFAP, an astrocyte marker, was performed to analyze astrocyte activation in the SN of c-rel$^{-/-}$ mice. In line with our earlier results (Baiguera et al., 2012), no signs of astrogliosis were detected in SN sections of 18-month-old c-rel$^{-/-}$ mice. Likewise, no increased reactivity to GFAP was identified in 4- or 13-month-old c-rel$^{-/-}$ mice, when compared to wt animals (**Figure 5**).

DISCUSSION

The present study shows that merely a mild inflammatory process, lacking a pronounced activation of microglia and astrocytes, anticipates SN degeneration in c-rel$^{-/-}$ mouse, a novel animal model of late-onset parkinsonism (Baiguera et al., 2012).

Although several animal models of PD have been established in the last decades, none of them showed to develop both the parkinsonian motor and non-motor symptoms (Cebrián et al., 2015). Furthermore, most models display rapid dopaminergic neuron degeneration, not replicating the slow, aging-dependent neuronal loss characteristic of the sporadic human disease (Tieu, 2011). Recently, we have observed that, between 2 and 13 months of age, c-rel$^{-/-}$ mice manifest olfactory deficits and gut dysfunctions, which are accompanied by progressive α-synuclein accumulation in the SN and reduction of DAT immunoreactivity in the striatum (Parrella et al., submitted). These alterations, that are reminiscent of prodromal PD, anticipate the onset of the motor disturbances and dopaminergic neuronal loss in the SN that become evident at 18 months (Baiguera et al., 2012). The aim of the present study was to investigate whether inflammation and glial activation may be associated with or anticipate the onset of PD-like neuropathological alterations reported in the brain of c-rel$^{-/-}$ mice.

The analysis of inflammation-related transcripts in the SN of 4-month-old c-rel$^{-/-}$ mice revealed increased expression of *Mrc1* and *Arg1* with respect to wt mice. The transcription of these factors was associated with a decreased *Ym1* expression, supporting the presence of the M2c-type

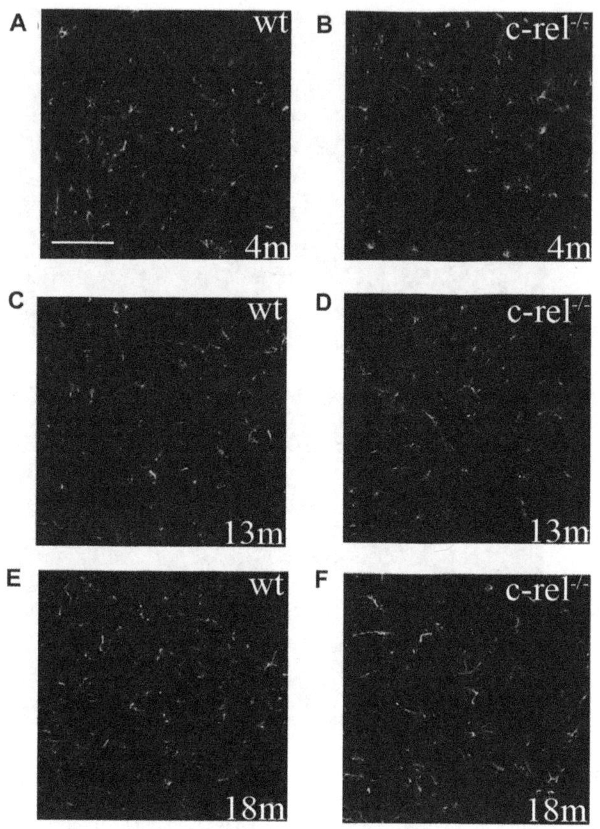

FIGURE 5 | GFAP immunoreactivity in c-rel$^{-/-}$ and wt mice. Pictures of SN sections from 4- **(A,B)**, 13- **(C,D)** and 18-month-old **(E,F)** animals illustrating GFAP astroglial immunostaining. No evident changes in astroglial activation were found in c-rel$^{-/-}$ mice **(B,D,F)** compared to age-matched wt **(A,C,E)**. Immunofluorescence images are representative of five sections from each animal (n = 3 animals per group). Abbreviations: GFAP, glial fibrillary acidic protein; SN, substantia nigra. Scale bar: in **(A)** = 100 μm for **(A–F)**.

microglial/macrophages associated with iron scavenging (David and Kroner, 2011) in the SN of c-rel$^{-/-}$ mice. The M2c microglial/macrophage polarization appeared to be transient as it dropped down at 13 and 18 months of age. Although a role for M2c-type microglia/macrophages in the onset and progression of the PD-like disease has yet to be established, our findings suggest that M2c "sentinel cells" in the SN of c-rel$^{-/-}$ mice are indeed reacting to harmful signals already present in brain milieu of young animals. On the contrary the loss of this M2c-phenotype might contribute to the accumulation of iron and likely α-synuclein in the SN of older c-rel$^{-/-}$ mice (Baiguera et al., 2012).

The double labeling of MRC1 and Iba1 in the SN of these mice allowed us to identify the MRC1-Iba1-positive cells as non-parenchymal or CNS macrophages, rather than microglia. This is in agreement with recently published data demonstrating that the marker MRC1 is specific for CNS macrophages, but not microglia, in mice (Goldmann et al., 2016) and humans (Melief et al., 2012). It suggests that the observed changes in the expression of *Mrc1* might reflect macrophage rather than microglial alterations.

Notably, at 13 months of age, the reduction in the expression of M2c-specific markers was accompanied by a significant increase of *Il1b*, but not *Il6* or *Fcgr3* transcription, which is suggestive of a mild inflammatory profile in the c-rel$^{-/-}$ brain. In wt mice, a similar increase of *Il1b* expression became evident only at 18 months of age. As an augment of IL-1β is recognized to be a feature of brain aging (Maher et al., 2004), the anticipation of *Il1b* expression in c-rel$^{-/-}$ mice supports that c-Rel deficiency accelerates the aging and neurodegeneration of the SN (Baiguera et al., 2012; Lanzillotta et al., 2015). In addition, we found that immunoreactivity for IL-1β was mostly localized within Iba1-negative cells displaying a neuronal morphology in the SN of c-rel$^{-/-}$ mice. However, we cannot exclude that other cell types, such as microglia, might contribute to the higher level of *Il1b* transcripts detected by qRT-PCR. This is in line with previous findings showing transcription but no transduction of IL-1β in peripheral blood mononuclear cells, as well as in the SN of a PD mouse model (Schindler et al., 1990a,b; Depino et al., 2003).

Anyhow, we could not detect differences in the morphology of Iba1-positive microglia/macrophages in the SN of c-rel$^{-/-}$ mice, at all the considered ages, though we previously described the presence of activated CD11b-positive cells in the SN of 18-month-old c-rel$^{-/-}$ mice (Baiguera et al., 2012). This discrepancy may be ascribed to the use of different microglial/macrophage markers in the two studies. Indeed, several authors reported that CD11b and Iba1 can lead to different staining patterns (Korzhevskii and Kirik, 2016; Lee et al., 2016; Scholtzova et al., 2017), which depends on the microglial/macrophage activation state (Ji et al., 2007). In particular, CD11b, although being an unspecific marker for microglia and macrophages, as it is also expressed in monocytes and granulocytes (Korzhevskii and Kirik, 2016), detects preferentially the activated microglial/macrophage state. This is related to the fact that resting microglia display low expression for membrane receptors, including CD11b, which become upregulated upon activation (Kreutzberg, 1996). On the other hand, Iba1 is a specific microglial/macrophage marker, but not especially sensitive to the activated form (Liaury et al., 2012; Korzhevskii and Kirik, 2016). Previous evidence by Liaury et al. showed increases in immunoreactivity for CD11b without significant difference in Iba1 in the hippocampal dentate gyrus of Gunn rats, an animal model of schizophrenia (Liaury et al., 2012). We can assume that microglia may adopt a minor "intermediate" state of activation detectable only by immunolabeling CD11b in c-rel$^{-/-}$ mice. The Iba1-labeled microglia, by depicting microglial morphology at all the activation states, is a realistic representation of the mild inflammatory condition present in c-rel$^{-/-}$ mice. The blunt inflammatory response is also supported by the GFAP staining for astrocytes in SN of c-rel$^{-/-}$ mice. As previously reported (Baiguera et al., 2012), c-rel$^{-/-}$ mice showed no signs of astrogliosis, accordingly to findings in PD patients (Mirza et al., 2000; Song et al., 2009; Tong et al., 2015). The role of astrocytes in PD pathology remains controversial (Hirsch and Hunot, 2009). Moreover, microglial activation does not necessarily lead to the release of proinflammatory cytokines (Depino et al., 2003). As mentioned above, it has been found that peripheral blood mononuclear cells, that are able to transcribe but not translate *Il1b*, upon receiving a secondary inflammatory stimulus, respond excessively by releasing disproportionate quantities of inflammatory cytokines, a phenomenon that is known as cell priming (Schindler et al., 1990a,b). Therefore, we hypothesize that this "intermediate" microglial activation state in 18-month-old c-rel$^{-/-}$ mice could belong to "primed" microglia. Interestingly, neurodegenerative diseases and normal aging are responsible for microglial priming or sensitization (Norden and Godbout, 2013). In a model of accelerated aging, primed microglia showed an exaggerated response to peripheral lipopolysaccharide injection (Raj et al., 2014). Since PD patients frequently suffer from infections, being even one of the main causes of death (Beyer et al., 2001), it cannot be excluded that peripheral infections trigger an excessive brain inflammatory response at the symptomatic motor stage of the disease. Diverse factors, such as nutrition (Seidl et al., 2014; Agim and Cannon, 2015) and physical exercise (LaHue et al., 2016), that have been assumed to influence the progression of PD, could very well contribute to modulate the neuroinflammatory process (Spencer et al., 2012; Orr et al., 2013). If we consider that c-rel$^{-/-}$ mice exhibit increased susceptibility to brain aging, it would be remarkable confirming the presence and role of primed microglia in this animal model, by evaluating its reactivity upon a peripheral inflammatory stimulus in further investigations. Moreover, our findings do not clarify the origin of a putative microglial "priming" and whether c-rel$^{-/-}$ mice display an impaired neuronal resilience at 12 months of age, as suggested by the increased *Il1b* expression in SN and loss of DAT in the striatum (Lanzillotta et al., 2015).

Definitely, whether and how inflammation contributes to PD pathology is still debated. Post-mortem analysis of PD brains has shown reactive microglia in the SN of patients at the end stage of the disease (McGeer et al., 1988; Imamura et al., 2003). The assessment of microglial activation *in vivo* at earlier stages of PD can be achieved by positron emission tomography (PET) imaging of radioligand binding to mitochondrial translocator protein 18 kDa (TSPO), a molecule expressed during microglial activation (Banati et al., 1997). However, genetic polymorphisms in TSPO cause an elevated variability in binding affinity, which is the main limitation of this technique (Owen et al., 2012; Yoder et al., 2013). In two studies that have controlled for TSPO rs6791 polymorphism, no differences were seen in [18F]-FEPPA binding in PD patients compared to controls (Koshimori et al., 2015; Ghadery et al., 2017). Thus, whilst microglial activation seems to be a pathological hallmark of end-stage PD, small-scale studies on the activation of microglia in patients at initial phases of the disease suggest there is no association of microgliosis with early disease progression. These findings are also supported by recent investigations showing no difference in CSF cytokine content in patients with mild PD (Shi et al., 2011; Lindqvist et al., 2013). By rising some concerns about the role of inflammation as a trigger of the disease, this scenario deserves confirmation in large-scale studies.

In conclusion, our findings hint that severe inflammation, and particularly microglial pro-inflammatory activation, is not a key hallmark of PD-like phenotype in c-Rel deficient mice. So far, we have analyzed microglial activation in mice up to 18 months of age, when dopaminergic neuronal loss in the SN is about 40% (Baiguera et al., 2012). The moderate amount of neuronal degeneration leads us to speculate that, at this age, c-rel$^{-/-}$ mice are modeling a mild PD. Thus, we cannot exclude that c-rel$^{-/-}$ mice may develop strong microgliosis at older ages, similar to what is found in post mortem brains of late-stage PD subjects (McGeer et al., 1988; Imamura et al., 2003). These findings own potentially relevant implications for understanding the role of neuroinflammation in PD.

AUTHOR CONTRIBUTIONS

VP, MM and MP conceived and designed the experiments; VP, MM, EP and MB performed the experiments; VP, MM and LF analyzed the data; PT and PFS contributed to results interpretation; VP, MM, AB and MP wrote the article.

FUNDING

This work was funded by Seventh Framework Programme (FP7 Project No. 607962), by Fondazione Cariplo (2014-0769) and by University of Brescia ("BIOMANE"-Health and Wealth project).

REFERENCES

Agim, Z. S., and Cannon, J. R. (2015). Dietary factors in the etiology of Parkinson's disease. *Biomed Res. Int.* 2015:672838. doi: 10.1155/2015/672838

Aguzzi, A., Barres, B. A., and Bennett, M. L. (2013). Microglia: scapegoat, saboteur, or something else? *Science* 339, 156–161. doi: 10.1126/science.1227901

Baiguera, C., Alghisi, M., Pinna, A., Bellucci, A., De Luca, M. A., Frau, L., et al. (2012). Late-onset Parkinsonism in NFκB/c-Rel-deficient mice. *Brain* 135, 2750–2765. doi: 10.1093/brain/aws193

Banati, R. B., Daniel, S. E., and Blunt, S. B. (1998). Glial pathology but absence of apoptotic nigral neurons in long-standing Parkinson's disease. *Mov. Disord.* 13, 221–227. doi: 10.1002/mds.870130205

Banati, R. B., Myers, R., and Kreutzberg, G. W. (1997). PK ('peripheral benzodiazepine')—binding sites in the CNS indicate early and discrete brain lesions: microautoradiographic detection of [3H]PK11195 binding to activated microglia. *J. Neurocytol.* 26, 77–82. doi: 10.1023/A:1018567510105

Beyer, M. K., Herlofson, K., Arsland, D., and Larsen, J. P. (2001). Causes of death in a community-based study of Parkinson's disease. *Acta Neurol. Scand.* 103, 7–11. doi: 10.1034/j.1600-0404.2001.00191.x

Blum-Degen, D., Müller, T., Kuhn, W., Gerlach, M., Przuntek, H., and Riederer, P. (1995). Interleukin-1 β and interleukin-6 are elevated in the cerebrospinal fluid of Alzheimer's and de novo Parkinson's disease patients. *Neurosci. Lett.* 202, 17–20. doi: 10.1016/0304-3940(95)12192-7

Brites, D., and Vaz, A. R. (2014). Microglia centered pathogenesis in ALS: insights in cell interconnectivity. *Front. Cell. Neurosci.* 8:117. doi: 10.3389/fncel.2014.00117

Cebrián, C., Loike, J. D., and Sulzer, D. (2015). Neuroinflammation in Parkinson's disease animal models: a cell stress response or a step in neurodegeneration? *Curr. Top. Behav. Neurosci.* 22, 237–270. doi: 10.1007/7854_2014_356

David, S., and Kroner, A. (2011). Repertoire of microglial and macrophage responses after spinal cord injury. *Nat. Rev. Neurosci.* 12, 388–399. doi: 10.1038/nrn3053

Depino, A. M., Earl, C., Kaczmarczyk, E., Ferrari, C., Besedovsky, H., del Rey, A., et al. (2003). Microglial activation with atypical proinflammatory cytokine expression in a rat model of Parkinson's disease. *Eur. J. Neurosci.* 18, 2731–2742. doi: 10.1111/j.1460-9568.2003.03014.x

Ghadery, C., Koshimori, Y., Coakeley, S., Harris, M., Rusjan, P., Kim, J., et al. (2017). Microglial activation in Parkinson's disease using $[^{18}F]$-FEPPA. *J. Neuroinflammation* 14:8. doi: 10.1186/s12974-016-0778-1

Goldmann, T., Wieghofer, P., Jordão, M. J., Prutek, F., Hagemeyer, N., Frenzel, K., et al. (2016). Origin, fate and dynamics of macrophages at central nervous system interfaces. *Nat. Immunol.* 17, 797–805. doi: 10.1038/ni.3423

Gordon, S. (2003). Alternative activation of macrophages. *Nat. Rev. Immunol.* 3, 23–35. doi: 10.1038/nri978

Hayakawa, K., Mishima, K., Nozako, M., Hazekawa, M., Mishima, S., Fujioka, M., et al. (2008). Delayed treatment with minocycline ameliorates neurologic impairment through activated microglia expressing a high-mobility group box1-inhibiting mechanism. *Stroke* 39, 951–958. doi: 10.1161/STROKEAHA.107.495820

Hirsch, E. C., and Hunot, S. (2009). Neuroinflammation in Parkinson's disease: a target for neuroprotection? *Lancet Neurol.* 8, 382–397. doi: 10.1016/S1474-4422(09)70062-6

Hu, X., Leak, R. K., Shi, Y., Suenaga, J., Gao, Y., Zheng, P., et al. (2015). Microglial and macrophage polarization—new prospects for brain repair. *Nat. Rev. Neurol.* 11, 56–64. doi: 10.1038/nrneurol.2014.207

Imamura, K., Hishikawa, N., Sawada, M., Nagatsu, T., Yoshida, M., and Hashizume, Y. (2003). Distribution of major histocompatibility complex class II-positive microglia and cytokine profile of Parkinson's disease brains. *Acta Neuropathol.* 106, 518–526. doi: 10.1007/s00401-003-0766-2

Ji, K. A., Yang, M. S., Jeong, H. K., Min, K. J., Kang, S. H., Jou, I., et al. (2007). Resident microglia die and infiltrated neutrophils and monocytes become major inflammatory cells in lipopolysaccharide-injected brain. *Glia* 55, 1577–1588. doi: 10.1002/glia.20571

Knott, C., Wilkin, G. P., and Stern, G. (1999). Astrocytes and microglia in the substantia nigra and caudate-putamen in Parkinson's disease. *Parkinsonism Relat Disord.* 5, 115–122. doi: 10.1016/s1353-8020(99)00022-x

Korzhevskii, D. E., and Kirik, O. V. (2016). Brain microglia and microglial markers. *Neurosci. Behav. Physiol.* 46, 284–290. doi: 10.1007/s11055-016-0231-z

Koshimori, Y., Ko, J. H., Mizrahi, R., Rusjan, P., Mabrouk, R., Jacobs, M. F., et al. (2015). Imaging striatal microglial activation in patients with Parkinson's disease. *PLoS One* 10:e0138721. doi: 10.1371/journal.pone.0138721

Kreutzberg, G. W. (1996). Microglia: a sensor for pathological events in the CNS. *Trends Neurosci.* 19, 312–318. doi: 10.1016/0166-2236(96)10049-7

LaHue, S. C., Comella, C. L., and Tanner, C. M. (2016). The best medicine? The influence of physical activity and inactivity on Parkinson's disease. *Mov. Disord.* 31, 1444–1454. doi: 10.1002/mds.26728

Lanzillotta, A., Porrini, V., Bellucci, A., Benarese, M., Branca, C., Parrella, E., et al. (2015). NF-κB in innate neuroprotection and age-related neurodegenerative diseases. *Front. Neurol.* 6:98. doi: 10.3389/fneur.2015.00098

Lee, A., O'Halloran, C., DenBleyker, M., Bisulco, S., Möller, T., and Adams, K. (2016). "Microglia identification methods," in *Reference Module in Biomedical Sciences*, ed. M. Caplan (Amsterdam: Elsevier).

Liaury, K., Miyaoka, T., Tsumori, T., Furuya, M., Wake, R., Ieda, M., et al. (2012). Morphological features of microglial cells in the hippocampal dentate gyrus of Gunn rat: a possible schizophrenia animal model. *J. Neuroinflammation* 9:56. doi: 10.1186/1742-2094-9-56

Lindqvist, D., Hall, S., Surova, Y., Nielsen, H. M., Janelidze, S., Brundin, L., et al. (2013). Cerebrospinal fluid inflammatory markers in Parkinson's disease—associations with depression, fatigue, and cognitive impairment. *Brain Behav. Immun.* 33, 183–189. doi: 10.1016/j.bbi.2013.07.007

Liou, H. C., Jin, Z., Tumang, J., Andjelic, S., Smith, K. A., and Liou, M. L. (1999). c-Rel is crucial for lymphocyte proliferation but dispensable for T cell effector function. *Int. Immunol.* 11, 361–371. doi: 10.1093/intimm/11.3.361

Long-Smith, C. M., Sullivan, A. M., and Nolan, Y. M. (2009). The influence of microglia on the pathogenesis of Parkinson's disease. *Prog. Neurobiol.* 89, 277–287. doi: 10.1016/j.pneurobio.2009.08.001

Maher, F. O., Martin, D. S., and Lynch, M. A. (2004). Increased IL-1β in cortex of aged rats is accompanied by downregulation of ERK and PI-3 kinase. *Neurobiol. Aging* 25, 795–806. doi: 10.1016/s0197-4580(03)00181-7

McGeer, P. L., Itagaki, S., Boyes, B. E., and McGeer, E. G. (1988). Reactive microglia are positive for HLA-DR in the substantia nigra of Parkinson's and Alzheimer's disease brains. *Neurology* 38, 1285–1291. doi: 10.1212/WNL.38.8.1285

Melief, J., Koning, N., Schuurman, K. G., Van De Garde, M. D., Smolders, J., Hoek, R. M., et al. (2012). Phenotyping primary human microglia: tight regulation of LPS responsiveness. *Glia* 60, 1506–1517. doi: 10.1002/glia.22370

Mirza, B., Hadberg, H., Thomsen, P., and Moos, T. (2000). The absence of reactive astrocytosis is indicative of a unique inflammatory process in Parkinson's disease. *Neuroscience* 95, 425–432. doi: 10.1016/s0306-4522(99)00455-8

Miyamoto, A., Wake, H., Moorhouse, A. J., and Nabekura, J. (2013). Microglia and synapse interactions: fine tuning neural circuits and candidate molecules. *Front. Cell. Neurosci.* 7:70. doi: 10.3389/fncel.2013.00070

Mogi, M., Harada, M., Kondo, T., Narabayashi, H., Riederer, P., and Nagatsu, T. (1995). Transforming growth factor-β1 levels are elevated in the striatum and in ventricular cerebrospinal fluid in Parkinson's disease. *Neurosci. Lett.* 193, 129–132. doi: 10.1016/0304-3940(95)11686-q

Mogi, M., Harada, M., Kondo, T., Riederer, P., Inagaki, H., Minami, M., et al. (1994a). Interleukin-1 β, interleukin-6, epidermal growth factor and transforming growth factor-α are elevated in the brain from parkinsonian patients. *Neurosci. Lett.* 180, 147–150. doi: 10.1016/0304-3940(94)90508-8

Mogi, M., Harada, M., Riederer, P., Narabayashi, H., Fujita, K., and Nagatsu, T. (1994b). Tumor necrosis factor-α (TNF-α) increases both in the brain and in the cerebrospinal fluid from parkinsonian patients. *Neurosci. Lett.* 165, 208–210. doi: 10.1016/0304-3940(94)90746-3

Mogi, M., Harada, M., Narabayashi, H., Inagaki, H., Minami, M., and Nagatsu, T. (1996). Interleukin (IL)-1 β, IL-2, IL-4, IL-6 and transforming growth factor-α levels are elevated in ventricular cerebrospinal fluid in juvenile parkinsonism and Parkinson's disease. *Neurosci. Lett.* 211, 13–16. doi: 10.1016/0304-3940(96)12706-3

Müller, T., Blum-Degen, D., Przuntek, H., and Kuhn, W. (1998). Interleukin-6 levels in cerebrospinal fluid inversely correlate to severity of Parkinson's disease. *Acta Neurol. Scand.* 98, 142–144. doi: 10.1111/j.1600-0404.1998.tb01736.x

Neumann, H., Kotter, M. R., and Franklin, R. J. (2009). Debris clearance by microglia: an essential link between degeneration and regeneration. *Brain* 132, 288–295. doi: 10.1093/brain/awn109

Nimmerjahn, A., Kirchhoff, F., and Helmchen, F. (2005). Resting microglial cells are highly dynamic surveillants of brain parenchyma *in vivo*. *Science* 308, 1314–1318. doi: 10.1515/nf-2005-0304

Norden, D. M., and Godbout, J. P. (2013). Review: microglia of the aged brain: primed to be activated and resistant to regulation. *Neuropathol. Appl. Neurobiol.* 39, 19–34. doi: 10.1111/j.1365-2990.2012.01306.x

Orr, S. K., Trépanier, M. O., and Bazinet, R. P. (2013). n-3 Polyunsaturated fatty acids in animal models with neuroinflammation. *Prostaglandins Leukot. Essent. Fatty Acids* 88, 97–103. doi: 10.1016/j.plefa.2012.05.008

Owen, D. R., Yeo, A. J., Gunn, R. N., Song, K., Wadsworth, G., Lewis, A., et al. (2012). An 18-kDa translocator protein (TSPO) polymorphism explains differences in binding affinity of the PET radioligand PBR28. *J. Cereb. Blood Flow Metab.* 32, 1–5. doi: 10.1038/jcbfm.2011.147

Paxinos, G., and Franklin, K. B. J. (2012). *Paxinos and Franklin's the Mouse Brain in Stereotaxic Coordinates.* 4th Edn. San Diego, CA: Academic Press.

Poewe, W., Seppi, K., Tanner, C. M., Halliday, G. M., Brundin, P., Volkmann, J., et al. (2017). Parkinson disease. *Nat. Rev. Dis. Primers* 3:17013. doi: 10.1038/nrdp.2017.13

Raj, D. D., Jaarsma, D., Holtman, I. R., Olah, M., Ferreira, F. M., Schaafsma, W., et al. (2014). Priming of microglia in a DNA-repair deficient model of accelerated aging. *Neurobiol. Aging* 35, 2147–2160. doi: 10.1016/j.neurobiolaging.2014.03.025

Schindler, R., Clark, B. D., and Dinarello, C. A. (1990a). Dissociation between interleukin-1 β mRNA and protein synthesis in human peripheral blood mononuclear cells. *J. Biol. Chem.* 265, 10232–10237.

Schindler, R., Gelfand, J. A., and Dinarello, C. A. (1990b). Recombinant C5a stimulates transcription rather than translation of interleukin-1 (IL-1) and tumor necrosis factor: translational signal provided by lipopolysaccharide or IL-1 itself. *Blood* 76, 1631–1638.

Scholtzova, H., Do, E., Dhakal, S., Sun, Y., Liu, S., Mehta, P. D., et al. (2017). Innate immunity stimulation via toll-like receptor 9 ameliorates vascular amyloid pathology in Tg-SwDI mice with associated cognitive benefits. *J. Neurosci.* 37, 936–959. doi: 10.1523/JNEUROSCI.1967-16.2016

Seidl, S. E., Santiago, J. A., Bilyk, H., and Potashkin, J. A. (2014). The emerging role of nutrition in Parkinson's disease. *Front. Aging Neurosci.* 6:36. doi: 10.3389/fnagi.2014.00036

Shi, M., Bradner, J., Hancock, A. M., Chung, K. A., Quinn, J. F., Peskind, E. R., et al. (2011). Cerebrospinal fluid biomarkers for Parkinson disease diagnosis and progression. *Ann. Neurol.* 69, 570–580. doi: 10.1002/ana.22311

Song, Y. J., Halliday, G. M., Holton, J. L., Lashley, T., O'Sullivan, S. S., McCann, H., et al. (2009). Degeneration in different parkinsonian syndromes relates to astrocyte type and astrocyte protein expression. *J. Neuropathol. Exp. Neurol.* 68, 1073–1083. doi: 10.1097/NEN.0b013e3181b66f1b

Spencer, J. P., Vafeiadou, K., Williams, R. J., and Vauzour, D. (2012). Neuroinflammation: modulation by flavonoids and mechanisms of action. *Mol. Aspects Med.* 33, 83–97. doi: 10.1016/j.mam.2011.10.016

Tang, Y., and Le, W. (2016). Differential roles of M1 and M2 microglia in neurodegenerative diseases. *Mol. Neurobiol.* 53, 1181–1194. doi: 10.1007/s12035-014-9070-5

Thannickal, T. C., Lai, Y. Y., and Siegel, J. M. (2007). Hypocretin (orexin) cell loss in Parkinson's disease. *Brain* 130, 1586–1595. doi: 10.1093/brain/awm097

Tieu, K. (2011). A guide to neurotoxic animal models of Parkinson's disease. *Cold Spring Harb. Perspect. Med.* 1:a009316. doi: 10.1101/cshperspect.a009316

Tong, J., Ang, L. C., Williams, B., Furukawa, Y., Fitzmaurice, P., Guttman, M., et al. (2015). Low levels of astroglial markers in Parkinson's disease: relationship to α-synuclein accumulation. *Neurobiol. Dis.* 82, 243–253. doi: 10.1016/j.nbd.2015.06.010

Vawter, M. P., Dillon-Carter, O., Tourtellotte, W. W., Carvey, P., and Freed, W. J. (1996). TGFβ1 and TGFβ2 concentrations are elevated in Parkinson's disease in ventricular cerebrospinal fluid. *Exp. Neurol.* 142, 313–322. doi: 10.1006/exnr.1996.0200

Yoder, K. K., Nho, K., Risacher, S. L., Kim, S., Shen, L., and Saykin, A. J. (2013). Influence of TSPO genotype on 11C-PBR28 standardized uptake values. *J. Nucl. Med.* 54, 1320–1322. doi: 10.2967/jnumed.112.118885

18

Brain Renin-Angiotensin System and Microglial Polarization: Implications for Aging and Neurodegeneration

Jose L. Labandeira-Garcia[1,2], Ana I. Rodríguez-Perez[1,2], Pablo Garrido-Gil[1,2], Jannette Rodriguez-Pallares[1,2], Jose L. Lanciego[2,3] and Maria J. Guerra[1,2]*

[1]Laboratory of Neuroanatomy and Experimental Neurology, Department of Morphological Sciences, Center for Research in Molecular Medicine and Chronic Diseases (CIMUS), University of Santiago de Compostela, Santiago de Compostela, Spain, [2]Networking Research Center on Neurodegenerative Diseases (CIBERNED), Madrid, Spain, [3]Neurosciences Division, Center for Applied Medical Research (CIMA), University of Navarra, Pamplona, Spain

***Correspondence:**
Jose L. Labandeira-Garcia
joseluis.labandeira@usc.es

Microglia can transform into proinflammatory/classically activated (M1) or anti-inflammatory/alternatively activated (M2) phenotypes following environmental signals related to physiological conditions or brain lesions. An adequate transition from the M1 (proinflammatory) to M2 (immunoregulatory) phenotype is necessary to counteract brain damage. Several factors involved in microglial polarization have already been identified. However, the effects of the brain renin-angiotensin system (RAS) on microglial polarization are less known. It is well known that there is a "classical" circulating RAS; however, a second RAS (local or tissue RAS) has been observed in many tissues, including brain. The locally formed angiotensin is involved in local pathological changes of these tissues and modulates immune cells, which are equipped with all the components of the RAS. There are also recent data showing that brain RAS plays a major role in microglial polarization. Level of microglial NADPH-oxidase (Nox) activation is a major regulator of the shift between M1/proinflammatory and M2/immunoregulatory microglial phenotypes so that Nox activation promotes the proinflammatory and inhibits the immunoregulatory phenotype. Angiotensin II (Ang II), via its type 1 receptor (AT1), is a major activator of the NADPH-oxidase complex, leading to pro-oxidative and pro-inflammatory effects. However, these effects are counteracted by a RAS opposite arm constituted by Angiotensin II/AT2 receptor signaling and Angiotensin 1–7/Mas receptor (MasR) signaling. In addition, activation of prorenin-renin receptors may contribute to activation of the proinflammatory phenotype. Aged brains showed upregulation of AT1 and downregulation of AT2 receptor expression, which may contribute to a pro-oxidative pro-inflammatory state and the increase in neuron vulnerability. Several recent studies have shown interactions between the brain RAS and different factors involved in microglial polarization, such as estrogens, Rho kinase (ROCK), insulin-like growth factor-1 (IGF-1), tumor necrosis factor α (TNF)-α, iron, peroxisome proliferator-activated receptor gamma, and toll-like receptors (TLRs). Metabolic reprogramming has recently been involved in the regulation of the neuroinflammatory response. Interestingly, we have recently observed a mitochondrial RAS, which is altered in aged brains. In conclusion, dysregulation of brain RAS plays a major role in aging-related changes and neurodegeneration by exacerbation of oxidative stress (OS) and neuroinflammation, which may be attenuated by pharmacological manipulation of RAS components.

Keywords: angiotensin, microglia, NADPH-oxidase, neuroinflammation, neuroprotection, Nox, oxidative stress, Parkinson

INTRODUCTION

In the late 19th century, Franz Nissl first described microglia as staebchenzellen (rod cells) for their rod-shaped nuclei. In 1913, Santiago Ramón y Cajal described these cells as a "third element", and in 1919 microglial cells were characterized by his disciple Pío del Río Hortega as a phagocytic and distinct non-neural and non-astrocytic population. During embryonic development, primitive yolk sac myeloid progenitors enter the brain and differentiate into microglial cells (Alliot et al., 1999; Ginhoux et al., 2010). It is usually estimated that around 10% of the adult brain cells are microglial cells (Carson et al., 2006; Kettenmann et al., 2011). In the adult mouse brain, microglia constitute 5%–12% of all glial cells, although these cells are not evenly distributed throughout the brain, ranging from 5% in the cerebral cortex to 12% in the substantia nigra (Lawson et al., 1990; Mittelbronn et al., 2001; Harry and Kraft, 2012). There are tissue-specific macrophages in practically all tissues of the body (Gautier et al., 2012), and microglial cells have been considered as the resident macrophages in the brain. Consistent with this, the resident microglia mediate the brain immune and inflammatory responses (Hu et al., 2014; Prinz and Priller, 2014). Although microglia and brain macrophages express several common protein markers, microglial cells have a particular molecular signature, which is different to other circulating and tissue-resident macrophagic cells (Hickman et al., 2013; Butovsky et al., 2014).

Microglial cells have been classically described to exist in two states, resting and activated state. In the healthy brain, neurons produce several immunosuppressive proteins, which keep microglia in a classical inactivated state (Harrison et al., 1998; Hoek et al., 2000). However, the initial concept of resting microglia has been modified, and recent studies have shown that the classical "resting" microglia are highly active by scanning of the surrounding region for disturbances in physiological conditions (Davalos et al., 2005; Nimmerjahn et al., 2005). Furthermore, it is now generally admitted that the term activation includes a set of several "activated" states. The classical concept of either "good" or "bad" activation states of microglia has to be reconsidered, and substituted by a range of different types of functional activation. Microglia can develop a number of different phenotypes and functions to preserve brain homeostasis depending on their environment.

MICROGLIAL POLARIZATION

The dual role of microglia is associated with different polarization of microglia under different context, particularly after brain injury (Hu et al., 2014; Franco and Fernández-Suárez, 2015; Kim et al., 2015). Microglia can develop into proinflammatory/classically activated (M1) or anti-inflammatory/alternatively activated (M2) phenotypes depending on the signals present at different stages after brain lesions. M1/proinflammatory microglia produces proinflammatory mediators and free radicals that exacerbate neuronal death. Alternatively, M2/immunoregulatory microglia induce brain repair and regeneration, produce growth factors and anti-inflammatory cytokines to protect neurons and resolve inflammation. In addition, as primarily described in the periphery, several subclasses of M2/immunoregulatory activation have been identified. The M2a activation state has a main function of suppression of inflammation. A second state of alternative activation is classified as "M2c", which has been suggested to restore the tissue after the inflammatory process has been attenuated (Gordon, 2003; Colton, 2009; Sica and Mantovani, 2012). The class termed "M2b" is least understood; M2b has been involved in both pro- or anti-inflammatory responses and related to memory immune responses (Mantovani et al., 2004; Edwards et al., 2006). The functional polarization of microglia is modulated by several receptors, transcription factors, acute phase proteins, and metabolic states. Toll-like receptors (TLRs), nucleotide-binding oligomerization domains (NODs) and NOD-like receptors are known to play a major role in microglia-mediated inflammation (Ransohoff and Perry, 2009; Ransohoff and Brown, 2012). Upregulation and release of reactive oxygen species (ROS) and activation of inducible nitric oxide synthase (iNOS), followed by the release of reactive nitrogen species (RNS), are hallmarks of M1 macrophages/microglia (MacMicking et al., 1997). Upregulation of the enzyme arginase 1 (Arg1) is considered as an specific marker of M2 macrophages/microglia (Sica and Bronte, 2007; Chhor et al., 2013).

An adequate progression from the proinflammatory/M1 to immunoregulatory/M2 phenotype is necessary to efficiently counteract brain lesions. However, when this process is dysregulated, the persistent release of inflammatory cytokines and ROS induces neuron death and enhances brain damage (Kigerl et al., 2009). Interestingly, microglial activation and enhanced neuroinflammatory responses have been observed in major neurodegenerative diseases (Frank-Cannon et al., 2009). Persistently proinflammatory polarized microglia and release of proinflammatory cytokines leads to a pro-oxidative and proinflammatory milieu and enhances neurodegeneration (Heneka et al., 2015; Tang and Le, 2016). New therapeutical strategies are necessary to modulate microglial activation and drive microglia polarization to a protective phenotype (Koenigsknecht-Talboo and Landreth, 2005; Porrini et al., 2015).

Proinflammatory phenotype polarization can be induced by stimulation with compounds such as the TLR-4 agonist lipopolysaccharide (LPS), interferon (IFN)-γ, Interleukin (IL)-17A and tumor necrosis factor-α (TNF)-α. Alternatively, stimuli such as IL-4, IL-10, or transforming growth factor β (TGF)-β induce the M2/immunoregulatory phenotype. However, the effects of the brain renin-angiotensin system (RAS) on microglial polarization are less known. It has been shown that angiotensin modulates immune cells in peripheral tissues, and that inflammatory cells have all RAS components, including angiotensin II (Ang II). Ang II receptor antagonists are modulators of macrophagic polarization in different tissues such adipose tissue, lung, kidney, or tumors (Fujisaka et al., 2011; Ma et al., 2011; Liu et al., 2012; Shrestha et al., 2016). There are also recent data showing that brain RAS plays a major role in microglial polarization.

THE RENIN-ANGIOTENSIN SYSTEM

The RAS was initially considered as a circulating humoral system, with functions in regulating blood pressure and in sodium and water homeostasis. Ang II, which is the most important effector peptide of the RAS, is formed by the sequential action of two enzymes (renin and angiotensin converting enzyme, ACE) on angiotensinogen. Ang II acts via type 1 and 2 (AT1 and AT2) receptors (Unger et al., 1996; Oro et al., 2007; Jones et al., 2008). AT1 and AT2 receptors have usually opposite effects on several cell functions (Chabrashvili et al., 2003; Jones et al., 2008). A number of data suggest, however, that interactions between AT1 and AT2 receptors may be more complex, and additional studies are necessary. Furthermore, new RAS components have emerged, which appear to contribute to further regulate the system (see below; **Figure 1**).

In addition to the "classical" circulating RAS, a second RAS (local or tissue RAS) has been observed in several tissues. A local independent RAS has also been observed in the brain (Ganong, 1994; Re, 2004). The local systems have all components

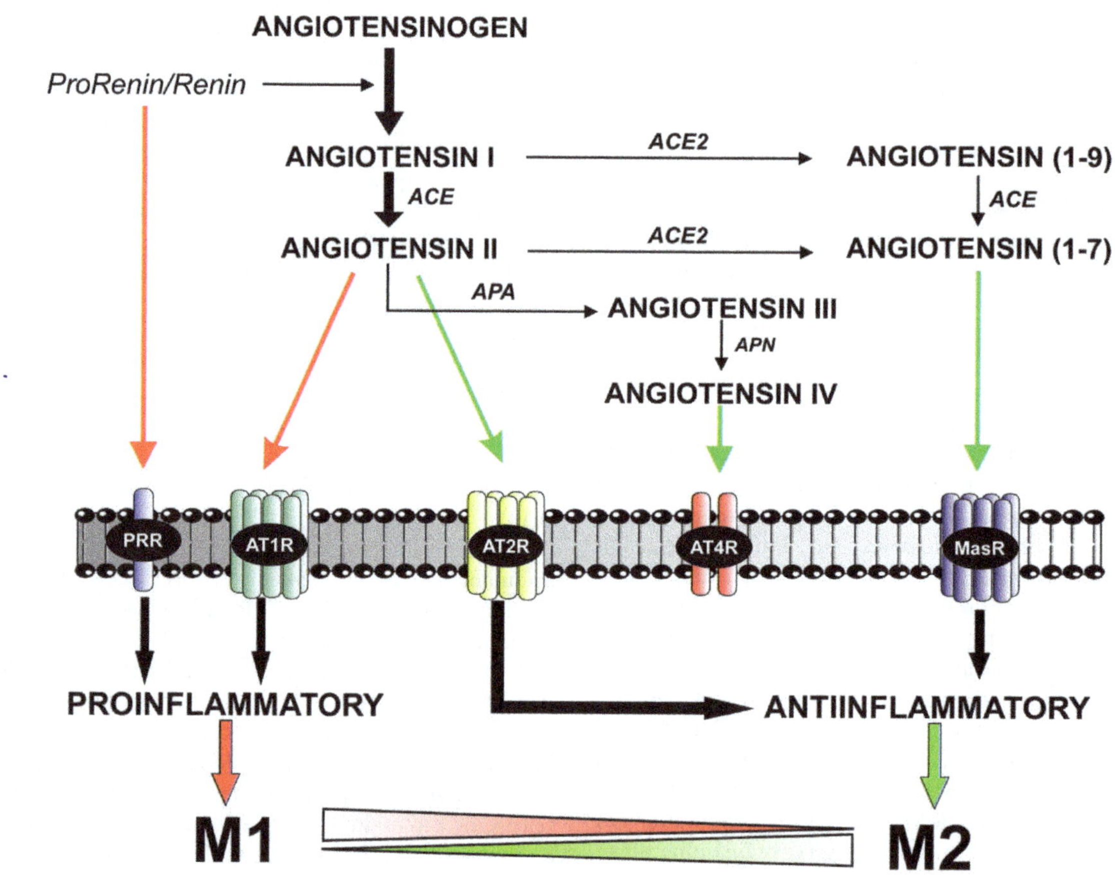

FIGURE 1 | The brain renin–angiotensin system (RAS). Angiotensin II is formed by the sequential action of two enzymes prorenin-renin (that forms angiotensin I) and ACE on the precursor protein angiotensinogen. Renin and its precursor prorenin also act on specific PRR receptors. In addition to angiotensin II, several angiotensin peptides such as Angiotensin (1–7), angiotensin III and angiotensin IV are formed from angiotensin I and II by the action of ACE2, APA and APN. Angiotensin II, via AT1 receptors, induces pro-inflammatory effects and M1 phenotype. However, these effects are counteracted by a RAS opposite arm constituted by angiotensin II/AT2 receptor signaling and Angiotensin 1–7/MasR signaling. In addition, activation of prorenin-renin receptors may contribute to activation of the proinflammatory phenotype. Abbreviations: ACE, angiotensin converting enzyme; ACE2, angiotensin converting enzyme 2; APA, aminopeptidase A; APN, aminopeptidase N; AT1R, angiotensin type 1 receptor; AT2R, angiotensin type 2 receptor; AT4R, angiotensin type 4 receptor; MasR, Mas receptor; PRR, prorenin/renin receptor.

observed in the circulating RAS. The local Ang II plays a relevant function in pathological changes of the corresponding tissues (Ruiz-Ortega et al., 2001; Suzuki et al., 2003). Tissue Ang II, via AT1 receptors, induces oxidative stress (OS) damage by activation of the NADPH-oxidase complex (Nox; Touyz, 2004; Garrido and Griendling, 2009). In different types of cells, PKC mediates initiation of AT1-induced Nox activation (Plumb et al., 2005; Herrera et al., 2010), which was also confirmed in microglial cells (Joglar et al., 2009). However, this initial generation of superoxide/H_2O_2 activates multiple downstream signals and transcription factors that may further amplify Nox oxidase activity in a multistep process that remains to be totally clarified (Seshiah et al., 2002; Balakumar and Jagadeesh, 2014). Consistent with this, we have recently shown that Nox-derived superoxide activates NFκB and the RhoA/Rho kinase pathway in microglial cells, which further increased Nox activation via p38 MAPK (Borrajo et al., 2014a; Rodriguez-Perez et al., 2015a).

More recent studies on local RAS have identified new components and mechanisms controlling RAS effects (**Figure 1**). New ACE homologs such as ACE2 and Chymase have been observed in different cells and tissues (Bacani and Frishman, 2006; Hamming et al., 2007). In addition to Ang II, several angiotensin peptides such as Ang (1–7), Ang III and Ang IV have been shown to have functional effects. Ang IV may act via specific AT4 receptors (Albiston et al., 2001). Ang (1–7), via a G-protein coupled receptor Mas (Santos et al., 2003), may counteract the effects of activation of AT1 by Ang II (Clark et al., 2001; Kostenis et al., 2005). A specific receptor for renin and its precursor prorenin (prorenin/renin receptor, PRR) may be of particular interest for the brain RAS (Nguyen et al., 2002). High levels of PRR were found in heart, brain, placenta and adipocytes, and lower level of expression in other tissues (Nguyen, 2011). PRR play a dual function (Nguyen and Contrepas, 2008; Shan et al., 2008): (i) Ang II-mediated effects; after binding to PRR, the catalytic activity of renin to hydrolyze angiotensinogen into angiotensin increases by about 4–5 times, and the precursor prorenin acquires catalytic properties similar to those of renin and (ii) Ang II-independent actions; PRR trigger their own signaling pathway that leads to pro-oxidative effects similar to those induced by activation of AT1 receptors.

THE BRAIN RAS

Initially, it was considered that the effects of RAS in the CNS were a consequence of the activity of the circulating RAS, acting through the circumventricular organs, on neurons regulating blood pressure and sodium and water homeostasis (Phillips and de Oliveira, 2008), because active components of the RAS, particularly Ang II, do not cross the blood-brain barrier (Harding et al., 1988). However, a local and independent RAS has now been identified in the brain. Astrocytes are the major source of brain angiotensinogen (Stornetta et al., 1988; Milsted et al., 1990), with only a small contribution from neurons (Kumar et al., 1988; Thomas et al., 1992).

Different RAS components were observed in several brain regions. In the basal ganglia, particularly in the nigrostriatal dopaminergic system, we have shown a local RAS using laser confocal microscopy and other methods such as *in situ* hybridization, laser microdissection and PCR or western blotting. In the substantia nigra, both AT1 and AT2 receptors were observed in dopaminergic neurons, astrocytes and microglia of rats (Rodriguez-Pallares et al., 2008), mice (Joglar et al., 2009), non-human primates (Valenzuela et al., 2010; Garrido-Gil et al., 2013b, 2017) and human brains (Garrido-Gil et al., 2013b). In addition, AT1 and AT2 receptors were observed in dopaminergic neurons and glial cells in primary cell cultures of the nigral region and several neuronal and glial cell lines (Rodriguez-Pallares et al., 2004, 2008; Joglar et al., 2009; Rodriguez-Perez et al., 2015a). In some studies, expression of AT1 receptors was not detected in microglial cells (Benicky et al., 2009). However, it is known that the level of microglial AT1 receptor expression is low in control (classically non-activated) microglia and is highly upregulated as part of the pro-inflammatory microglial response (Miyoshi et al., 2008; Rodriguez-Perez et al., 2015a; Dominguez-Meijide et al., 2017). Detection of AT1 expression may depend on the sensitivity threshold of the methodology used, and the level of pro-inflammatory activation of the microglial cells that are being analyzed. In addition, cytoplasmatic and membrane Nox subunits were located in dopaminergic neurons, astrocytes and microglia (Rodriguez-Pallares et al., 2007, 2008; Joglar et al., 2009).

A MAJOR ROLE FOR THE NADPH-OXIDASE COMPLEX ACTIVATION IN POLARIZATION TO PROINFLAMMATORY/M1 PHENOTYPE

The complex NADPH-oxidase is a multi-component enzyme constituted by three cytosolic subunits (p40, p47 and p67) and at least two membrane subunits (gp91 and p22). The complex is inactive when the different subunits are spatially isolated. After stimulation, the complex is assembled and activated. In cells, mitochondria and the membrane NADPH-oxidase complex are the major sources of ROS (Babior, 2004). In addition, NADPH oxidase-derived ROS enhance production of ROS by mitochondria, intracellular iron uptake and other intracellular ROS sources (Cai, 2005). It is known that there is a ROS-mediated cross-talk signaling between the membrane Nox and mitochondria (Sheh et al., 2007; Alberici et al., 2009). This feed-forward mechanism enhances and sustains ROS production. Most cells appear to have Nox. However, Nox produces high levels of oxidants in phagocytes and low levels of ROS, particularly for signaling function, in other cell types (including neurons and glial cells). Initially, Nox-derived ROS may have been developed in cells as a signaling system, and then specialized as a defense system in macrophages (Babior, 2004). In phagocytes-neutrophiles and monocytes, Nox produces high levels of extracellular superoxide/ROS to eliminate invading microorganisms or unwanted cells (Babior, 2004; West et al., 2011). Superoxide induces tissue damage after being transformed into toxic species such as hydrogen peroxide and peroxynitrite, formed after reaction with NO. Furthermore, in the presence of Nox, iNOS oxidation of L-arginine (L-ARG) produces NO (MacMicking et al., 1997). ROS derived from Nox may also act indirectly by enhancing the production of proteases (Reeves et al., 2002). In macrophages and microglial cells, Nox-derived ROS also act on intracellular signaling pathways involved in microglial or macrophage activation and the release of proinflammatory signals (Qin et al., 2004).

Ang II, VIA AT1 RECEPTORS, IS A MAJOR ACTIVATOR OF THE NADPH-OXIDASE COMPLEX. ROLE IN BRAIN DISEASES AND NEURODEGENERATION

Abnormal upregulation of local Ang II induces OS and exacerbates inflammation. As indicated above, Ang II, via its AT1 receptor, is a major activator of the NADPH-oxidase complex (Zalba et al., 2001; Hoogwerf, 2010), and NADPH-dependent oxidases mediate several key aspects of OS and inflammatory processes that are involved in major degenerative diseases in peripheral tissues (Griendling et al., 2000; Münzel and Keaney, 2001). In the brain, the RAS has been involved in several disorders such as anxiety and stress (Peng et al., 2002), depressive illness (Saab et al., 2007), and alcohol intake (Maul et al., 2005). Inhibition of AT1 receptors has been reported to improve aging-related deficits in learning, spatial working memory and motor performance (Hellner et al., 2005; Kerr et al., 2005). AT1 receptor blockers and ACE inhibitors (ACEIs) have been shown to inhibit inflammation in the central nervous system (Platten et al., 2009; Stegbauer et al., 2009). Indeed, AT1 receptor antagonists exerted positive effects in several processes mediated by microglial activation and neuroinflammation, such as experimental models of multiple sclerosis (Platten et al., 2009; Stegbauer et al., 2009), Alzheimer's disease (AD; Kehoe and Wilcock, 2007; Mogi and Horiuchi, 2009; Torika et al., 2016) and brain ischemia (Iwanami et al., 2010). Consistent with this, several clinical and genetic studies suggest a relationship between AD and RAS (reviewed in Savaskan, 2005; Kehoe and Wilcock, 2007; Mogi and Horiuchi, 2009). In a series of recent studies in animal models of PD, we have also observed that the brain RAS plays a major role in progression of dopaminergic degeneration.

A number of experimental and clinical data suggest that neuroinflammation is a factor for the progression of dopaminergic neuron degeneration. Both PD patients (Ouchi et al., 2005; Ghadery et al., 2017) and PD animal models (Cicchetti et al., 2002; Rodriguez-Pallares et al., 2007) show enhanced microglial reaction in the substantia nigra and striatum (**Figure 2**). It was initially considered that the increase in the microglial response was a consequence of the neuronal death to remove dead cells and debris, although this inflammatory process may also lead to additional damage of the surrounding neurons and progression of neurodegeneration, as reported for several autoimmune diseases (Vowinckel et al., 1997). However, it has been shown that microglial response and Nox

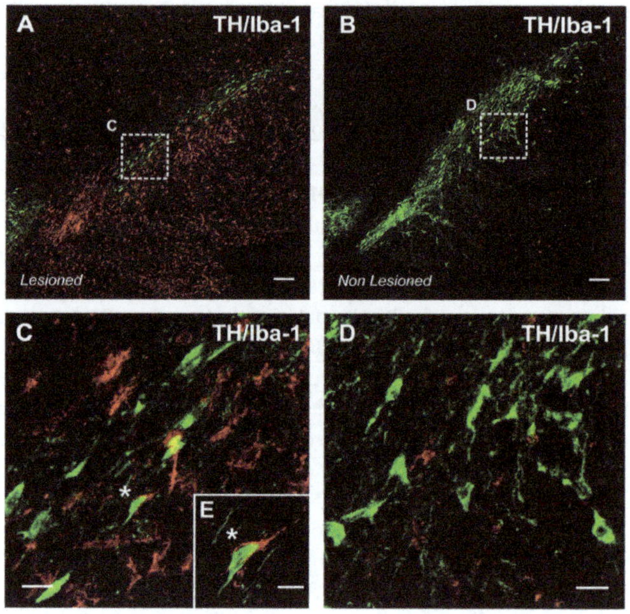

FIGURE 2 | Intense microglial activation in a degenerating rat substantia nigra (A), iba-1 positive red immunofluorescence. A high density of activated microglial cells is observed in the nigral region surrounding the dopaminergic cells. The degeneration of dopaminergic neurons (green; tyrosine hydroxylase, TH immunolabeled cells) was triggered by over expression of alpha-synuclein (not shown) after unilateral injection of adeno-associated viral vectors encoding alpha-synuclein. The contralateral non-lesioned substantia nigra of the same tissue section **(B)** shows scattered microglial cells in an apparent classical "non-activated" state. The areas squared in **(A,B)** are magnified in **(C–E)**, and a close interaction between a dopaminergic neuron and a microglial cell (asterisks) is shown in **(E)**. Scale bar: 100 μm **(A,B)**, 20 μm **(C,D)** and 10 μm **(E)**.

activation are major factors for triggering neuronal degeneration, acting synergistically with different pathogenic factors to induce neurodegeneration at early stages of the disease (Gao et al., 2003; Wu et al., 2003). In different PD models, we observed that Ang II increased the neurotoxic effect of low doses of dopaminergic neurotoxins, and that administration of ACE inhibitors (Lopez-Real et al., 2005; Muñoz et al., 2006) or AT1 receptor antagonists (Rey et al., 2007; Rodriguez-Pallares et al., 2008; Joglar et al., 2009) induced significant protection of dopaminergic neurons and reduction in neurotoxin-induced levels of protein oxidation and lipid peroxidation (Sánchez-Iglesias et al., 2007). Nox inhibitors also blocked the enhancing effect of Ang II on dopaminergic neurodegeneration, which confirmed that Nox activation and Nox-induced ROS play a major role in the Ang II-induced increase in neuronal loss (Rey et al., 2007; Rodriguez-Pallares et al., 2008; Joglar et al., 2009). In summary (Labandeira-Garcia et al., 2013; Labandeira-García et al., 2014), we suggest that Ang II acts by a double mechanism; in dopaminergic neurons (i.e., CNS resident cells), Ang II acts on AT1 receptors to produce low levels of intraneuronal ROS by activation of neuronal Nox. In addition, Ang II acts on microglia (i.e., inflammatory cells), and activation of the microglial AT1/ Nox axis induces the generation of high levels of superoxide and superoxide-derived ROS that, after being released to the extracellular medium, may lead to neuronal damage. In addition, a small amount of microglial ROS is used as a microglial second messenger in intracellular pathways that regulate the inflammatory response (Babior, 2004; Qin et al., 2004). Consistent with this, overactivation of the Ang II/AT1/Nox axis enhances vulnerability of dopaminergic neurons and synergistically contributes to initiation and progression of the disease. The role of brain RAS in dopaminergic neuron death and possibly in PD has also been shown by a number of studies from different research groups (Grammatopoulos et al., 2007; Zawada et al., 2011; Sonsalla et al., 2013).

OVERACTIVATION OF THE Ang II/AT1/NADPH-OXIDASE AXIS IN AGING

Aging is the major risk factor for neurodegenerative diseases, and particularly for PD and AD (McCormack et al., 2004; Collier et al., 2007). Aged tissues, including brain tissue, are characterized by a proinflammatory, pro-oxidant state that leads to exacerbated responses to lesions and enhanced vulnerability to neurodegeneration (Csiszar et al., 2003; Choi et al., 2010). Consistent with this, age-related diseases such as hypertension, diabetes and atherosclerosis show increased NADPH-oxidase activity (Griendling et al., 2000; Mehta and Griendling, 2007). It is known that tissue Ang II, acting on AT1 receptors, plays a major role in inflammatory processes that induce age-related degenerative changes (Heymes et al., 1998; Basso et al., 2005). In normal non-pathological states, there is a tight regulation of Ang II-induced ROS (de Cavanagh et al., 2004; Garrido and Griendling, 2009). However, a marked hyperactivity of the Ang/AT1/Nox axis has been observed in aged tissues (Min et al., 2009; Cassis et al., 2010). Consistent with this, mice null for AT1 receptors showed longevity, which was related to a decrease in OS together with an increase in expression of the prosurvival gene sirtuin 3 and mitochondrial protection (Benigni et al., 2009; de Cavanagh et al., 2011; Valenzuela et al., 2016). Furthermore, AT1 receptor deletion decreased age-related progression of atherosclerosis (Umemoto, 2008).

We observed that the increase in AT1/Nox activity in the substantia nigra of aged rats plays a major role in the increase in vulnerability of dopaminergic neurons with aging (**Figure 3**). In aged animals, neurotoxins induced higher levels of dopaminergic neuron loss than in young animals (Sugama et al., 2003; McCormack et al., 2004), and nigral RAS was involved in this effect (Villar-Cheda et al., 2012b). A significant increase in Nox activity and levels of the pro-inflammatory cytokines IL-1β and TNF-α was observed in aged rats, which revealed a pro-oxidative and pro-inflammatory state in the aged substantia nigra. Aged rats also showed upregulation of AT1 receptor expression and down-regulation of AT2 receptor expression, which was inhibited by administration of the AT1 receptor blocker candesartan. The aging-related increase in AT1 receptors may lead to the increase in the Nox-derived OS and dopaminergic cell vulnerability to degeneration. In aged rats, Nox activation is further increased by the lack of the compensatory upregulation of AT2 receptors (see below), which was observed in young rats after upregulation of AT1 receptor signaling (Villar-Cheda et al., 2010). Aging-related loss of striatal D2 and D1 receptors (Wang et al., 1998; Ishibashi et al., 2009) and alteration of the dopaminergic system (Kubis et al., 2000; Collier et al., 2007; Cruz-Muros et al., 2009) have been observed in experimental models and human brains. It is also known that Ang II, via AT1 receptors, increases the release of dopamine (Mendelsohn et al., 1993; Brown et al., 1996; Dominguez-Meijide et al., 2014). Therefore, the upregulation of the Ang II/AT1/Nox axis that we observed in aged rats may be a compensatory change to counteract the decreased levels of dopamine or dopamine receptors (Villar-Cheda et al., 2012b, 2014). However, in addition to the dopaminergic down-regulation, other factors are probably involved in the aging-related upregulation of AT1/Nox activity, as aging has been shown to be associated with overactivation of the AngII/AT1/Nox axis in different tissues (Thompson et al., 2000; Min et al., 2009; Cassis et al., 2010).

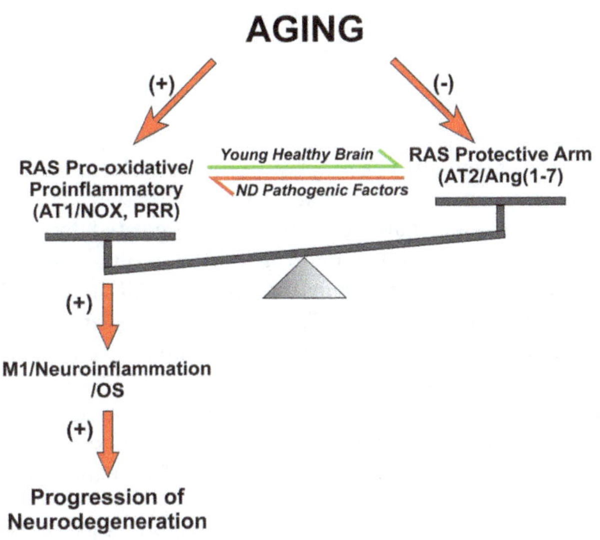

FIGURE 3 | Dysregulation of brain RAS with aging and other pathogenic factors. In young and healthy brains the balance between the RAS pro-oxidative/proinflammatory and protective arms are tight regulated for physiological functions. Aging is associated with overactivation of the Ras pro-oxidative/proinflammatory arm and lack of compensatory upregulation of the protective arm, which leads to a pro-oxidative pro-inflammatory state and increased vulnerability to neurodegeneration. Other pathogenic factors involved in triggering neurodegeneration may also increase the activity of the RAS pro-inflammatory axis. Abbreviations: Ang, angiotensin; AT1, angiotensin type 1 receptor; AT2, angiotensin type 2 receptor; ND, neurodegenerative; Nox, NADPH-oxidase; OS, oxidative stress; PRR, prorenin/renin receptor.

THE ROLE OF OTHER ANGIOTENSIN RECEPTORS IN REGULATION OF MICROGLIAL POLARIZATION

Level of Nox activation has been suggested to be a major factor for regulation of the shift between proinflammatory/M1 and M2/immunoregulatory microglial phenotypes, so that Nox activation promotes proinflammatory and suppress the immunoregulatory phenotype (Choi et al., 2012). Consistent with this, AT1 receptor antagonists reduce proinflammatory microglia activation and promote immunoregulatory microglia polarization (Saavedra, 2012; Rodriguez-Perez et al., 2016; Torika et al., 2016). The classical Ang II/AT1/Nox pro-oxidative and pro-inflammatory axis plays a major role in the RAS effects both in the brain and peripheral tissues. However, it is now known that these effects are regulated by a RAS opposite arm constituted by Ang II/AT2 receptor signaling and Ang1-7/MasR signaling. A number of recent data suggest that activation of AT2 and/or MasRs plays an anti-oxidative/anti-inflammatory role. In addition, activation of PRR appears to contribute to activation of proinflammatory phenotype. However, the mechanisms involved in the interaction between different RAS receptors signaling to regulate microglial polarization and neuroinflammation are still unclear (**Figure 4**).

AT2 receptors counteract the effects of AT1 receptor activation and promote the M2/immunoregulatory phenotype. Reciprocal interaction between AT1 and AT2 receptors may regulate the effect of Ang II on cells (Sohn et al., 2000). Several studies in different types of cells have shown that AT2 activation decreases AT1 expression and NADPH-oxidase activation, leading to decrease in inflammatory responses (Jin et al., 2012; Yang et al., 2012; Lu et al., 2015). However, the intracellular pathways responsible for the interactions have not been clarified, and several mechanisms may be involved (Wu et al., 2004; Rompe et al., 2010; Yang et al., 2012; Dhande et al., 2013). Consistent with this, treatment with AT2 agonists led to reduction in the inflammatory responses, which were increased in AT2 receptor KO mice (Dhande et al., 2013; Iwanami et al., 2015). In the nigrostriatal system of young animals, we observed that upregulation of AT1 receptors was accompanied by a simultaneous and apparently compensatory upregulation of AT2 receptors (Villar-Cheda et al., 2010). In the nigra and striatum of aged rats, there was an increase in the expression of AT1 receptors and Nox activation; however, there was a lack of compensatory increase in AT2 expression (Villar-Cheda et al., 2010, 2012b). In aged animals, a decrease in AT2 receptor expression may lead to further increase in the pro-oxidative, pro-inflammatory effects and neuron vulnerability induced by activation of upregulated AT1 receptors.

MasRs, together with AT2 receptors, are considered major components of the RAS protective arm, which mediates actions opposing to AT1 (Bader, 2013; Villela et al., 2015). The ACE2 transforms Ang II into the heptapeptide Ang (1–7), which activates MasRs. It was observed that Mas-protooncogene is primarily expressed in the brain (Bunnemann et al., 1990; Von Bohlen und Halbach et al., 2000), and MasRs were identified in neurons, astrocytes and glial cells (Gallagher et al., 2006; Liu et al., 2016). Several recent studies suggest that activation of the Ang (1–7)/Mas axis inhibits the M1 inflammatory response in microglial cells and peripheral macrophages (Hammer et al., 2016; Liu et al., 2016; Tao et al., 2016). However, the cellular mechanisms involved in these effects remain to be clarified.

PRRs have been identified in neurons, astrocytes and microglial cells in rodents and primates, including humans (Valenzuela et al., 2010; Garrido-Gil et al., 2013b). PRR, together with AT1 receptors, promote the inflammatory response and the M1/proinflammatory phenotype (Shi et al., 2014; Zhu et al., 2015). The mechanisms involved in interactions of PRR and other RAS receptors to regulate microglial polarization remain to be investigated. The peptide Ang IV and its receptor have been involved in a number of functions in the CNS (Wright et al., 2015). There are a few data on possible involvement of Ang IV in inflammatory responses in peripheral tissues (Esteban et al., 2005; Kong et al., 2015). However, there are no data on the involvement of Ang IV in the neuroinflammatory response.

INTERACTIONS BETWEEN RAS AND OTHER MICROGLIAL POLARIZATION REGULATORS

A number of studies have shown interactions or mutual regulation between RAS and different compounds involved in neuroinflammation and microglial polarization, such as estrogens, Rho kinase (ROCK), insulin-like growth factor-1 (IGF-1), TNF-α, iron, peroxisome proliferator-activated receptor gamma (PPARγ), and TLRs.

Estrogens protect neurons by mechanisms that are still unclear. However, modulation of the glial neuroinflammatory response plays a major role in the estrogen-induced neuroprotection (Morale et al., 2006; Suzuki et al., 2007; Vegeto et al., 2008). In several recent studies using PD models, we observed that estrogens modulate brain RAS and neuroinflammation acting both on astrocytes and microglia (Rodriguez-Perez et al., 2010, 2012, 2015b; Labandeira-Garcia et al., 2016). We observed that activation of microglial estrogen receptor (ER) β with the agonist 2,3-Bis-4-hydroxyphenyl-propionitrile (DPN)) inhibited the Ang II-induced increase in levels of several major mediators of the microglial inflammatory response such as IL-1β and ROCK (Villar-Cheda et al., 2012a; Rodriguez-Perez et al., 2013, 2015a).

RhoA/ROCK is a major modulator of the actin cytoskeleton, which regulates migration of microglia and other inflammatory cells (Yan et al., 2012; Labandeira-Garcia et al., 2015) into lesioned areas (Greenwood et al., 2003; Honing et al., 2004). RhoA/ROCK induces changes in the actin cytoskeleton necessary for cell motility, process retraction and cell spreading, which characterize activation of inflammatory cells, including microglia (Bernhart et al., 2010). Activation of the microglial RhoA/ROCK pathway plays a major role in the effect of Ang II/AT1/Nox axis on microglial polarization and neurodegeneration. This was shown in rodents (Barcia et al., 2012; Villar-Cheda et al., 2012a), and confirmed using mesencephalic cultures lacking microglial cells (Villar-Cheda et al., 2012a; Borrajo et al., 2014b). During Ang II-induced microglial activation, a crosstalk signaling between Nox and ROCK has been observed: Ang II-induced Nox activation led to superoxide production, NF-κB translocation and Rho-kinase activation. In addition, Rho-kinase activation

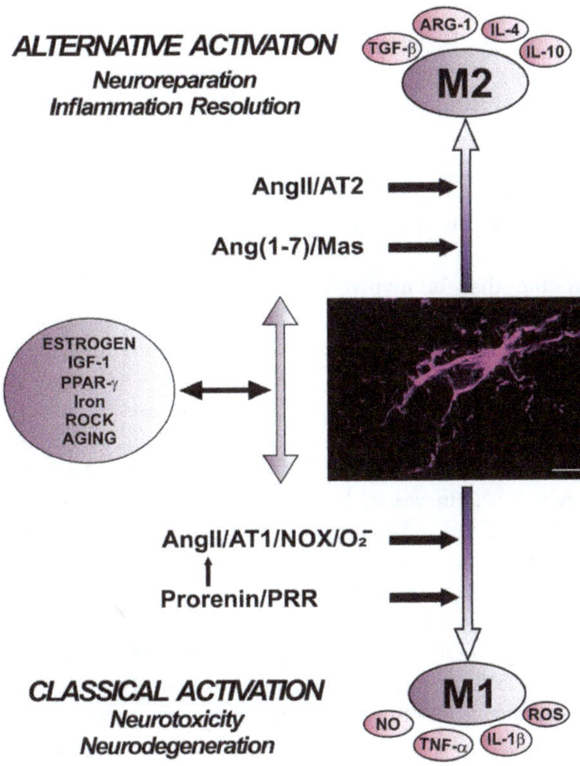

FIGURE 4 | Role of different angiotensin receptors in regulation of microglial polarization, and interactions with other microglial polarization regulators. Angiotensin II, via AT1 receptor and Nox activation, and prorenin/renin, via PRR, induce pro-inflammatory effects and M1 phenotype, which is associated to increased levels of ROS, NO, TNF-α and IL-1β. These effects are counteracted by a RAS opposite arm constituted by angiotensin II/AT2 receptor signaling and Angiotensin 1–7/MasR signaling, which promote anti-inflammatory effects and M2 phenotype, which is also associated to TGF-β, IL-4, IL-10, and Arg-1 overexpression. In addition, there are interactions between RAS and different compounds involved in neuroinflammation and microglial polarization, such as estrogens, ROCK, IGF1, TNF-α, iron, PPARγ, and toll-like receptors. Abbreviations: Ang, angiotensin; ARG-1, arginase 1; AT1, angiotensin type 1 receptor; AT2, angiotensin type 2 receptor; IGF1, insulin-like growth factor-1; IL, interleukin; MasR, Mas receptor; NO, nitric oxide; Nox, NADPH-oxidase; O_2^-, superoxide; PPARγ, peroxisome proliferator-activated receptor gamma; PRR, prorenin/renin receptor; ROCK, Rho kinase; ROS, reactive oxygen species; TGF-β, transforming growth factor β; TNF-α tumor necrosis factor α. Scale bar: 7.5 μm.

was involved in regulation of NADPH-oxidase activation via p38 mitogen-activated protein kinase. Moreover, Rho-kinase activation, via NF-κB, upregulated angiotensin type-1 receptor expression in microglial cells through a feed-forward mechanism (Rodriguez-Perez et al., 2015a).

For many years, IGF-1 was considered a cytoprotective factor. However, it has also been suggested that IGF-1 may be detrimental to health, and that reduced IGF-1 levels lead to prolonged life (Tao et al., 2007; Suh et al., 2008). Local brain IGF-1 is produced by neurons and glial cells (Quesada et al., 2007; Suh et al., 2013), but the effects of IGF-1 in the brain and particularly in the aged brain are unclear (Bartke et al., 2003; Brown-Borg, 2007). Inhibitory effects on the neuroinflammatory response (Nadjar et al., 2009), improvement in mitochondrial function (Puche et al., 2008), inhibition of OS and Sirtuin-1 activation (Vinciguerra et al., 2009; Tran et al., 2014) have been suggested as possible mechanisms. Interestingly, the brain RAS has been shown to be involved in neuroinflammation (Borrajo et al., 2014a; Rodriguez-Perez et al., 2015a), mitochondrial function (Zawada et al., 2011; Rodriguez-Pallares et al., 2012) and Sirtuin-1 activity (Diaz-Ruiz et al., 2015). Recently, we observed a reciprocal regulation between IGF-1 and RAS (Rodriguez-Perez et al., 2016): IGF-1 inhibited AT1/Nox activity in neurons and glial cells (i.e., it decreased AT1, increased AT2 and decreased angiotensinogen expression); conversely, Ang II—via AT1 receptors—increased the levels of IGF-1 in microglial cells, while activation of AT2 receptors decreased IGF-1 levels. We observed that Ang II, via AT1 receptors, induced an increase in markers of the proinflammatory phenotype, which was blocked by treatment with IGF-1, suggesting that induction of microglial IGF-1 by Ang II and other OS and pro-inflammatory inducers may play a major role in repressing the M1-neurotoxic phenotype and transition to an M2-repair/regenerative phenotype. Our study showed that IGF-1 and the local RAS interact to inhibit or activate neuroinflammation (i.e., transition from the M1/proinflammatory to the M2/immunoregulatory phenotype). However, in brains from aged rats, particularly in the substantia nigra, we observed increased Ang II/AT1/Nox activity, while IGF-I levels remained decreased. The loss of the mechanism that upregulates IGF-1 to inhibit the AT1/Nox axis (Rodriguez-Perez et al., 2016) may lead to the loss of capacity of microglia to undergo M2/immunoregulatory activation and the pro-oxidative and pro-inflammatory state that characterizes the aged brain, and particularly the aged substantia nigra (Rey et al., 2007; Villar-Cheda et al., 2012b). IGF-1 and the local RAS may interact to inhibit or activate neuroinflammation and this important mechanism may be impaired in aged animals.

TNF-α is a pro-inflammatory cytokine that is involved in the pathogenesis of several neurodegenerative diseases (Hofman et al., 1989; Fillit et al., 1991; Mogi et al., 1994). In particular, dopaminergic neurons are highly vulnerable to TNF-α (McGuire et al., 2001; Qin et al., 2007; Harms et al., 2012). In primary mesencephalic cultures, we have recently observed that administration of low doses of the neurotoxin MPP^+ led to significant dopaminergic cell death, which was increased by co-treatment with Ang II and decreased by administration of TNF-α blockers (Borrajo et al., 2014a). Furthermore, treatment with Ang II induced a marked increase in levels of TNF-α in primary mesencephalic cultures, which was blocked by administration of AT1 receptor antagonists, NADPH-oxidase inhibitors and NFK-β blockers. In cultures lacking microglial cells, however, levels of TNF-α were not significantly affected by administration of Ang II. We also observed that AT1 receptors, NADPH-oxidase, Rho-kinase and NFK-β were involved in the release of TNF-α by microglia (Borrajo et al., 2014a). These results revealed an important functional interaction between Ang II and TNF-α, and also that microglial TNF-α is a major mediator of Ang II-induced neuroinflammation and dopaminergic neurodegeneration.

Microglia play a major role in iron storage and homeostasis, and Ang II modulates microglial ferritin/iron storage levels and the neuroinflammatory response (Garrido-Gil et al., 2013a). Microglial ferritin levels (i.e., iron storage by ferritin) change in response to OS and microglial activation, and the release of iron from ferritin in activated microglia may enhance the oxidative damage derived from the proinflammatory microglial response (Mehlhase et al., 2006). Consistent with this, we observed in PD models that intense RAS overactivity and OS induced an increase in microglial labile iron and a decrease in ferritin levels. Although some data are controversial (Zecca et al., 2001), it is usually accepted that iron and ferritin increase in the substantia nigra with aging (Dusek et al., 2012). Aging-related increase in microglial ferritin has been associated to a less efficient control of iron homeostasis by senescent microglia (Lopes et al., 2008). In several studies in aged rats, we observed hyperactivity of the AT1/Nox axis in the substantia nigra, together with an increase in the levels of iron and ferritin, which were inhibited by AT1 receptor blockers such as candesartan. This suggests that overactivity of the Ang II/AT1/Nox axis plays a key role in aging-related iron and ferritin increase in the substantia nigra (Garrido-Gil et al., 2013a). The aging-associated upregulation of Ang II/AT1/Nox activity may lead to upregulation of iron storage by microglia and induce a pro-oxidative pro-inflammatory state and higher vulnerability of dopaminergic cells to degeneration with aging (Collier et al., 2007; Villar-Cheda et al., 2009, 2012b).

PPAR-γ is a member of a group of nuclear receptors (PPARs), which have been related to regulation of macrophage and adipocyte differentiation, as well as glucose and lipid metabolism and energy homeostasis. PPAR-γ receptors are also involved in inhibition of expression of different inflammatory cytokines and downregulation of the inflammatory process (Jiang et al., 1998; Ricote et al., 1998). PPAR-γ receptors are also involved in regulation of microglial activation and suppression of the proinflammatory phenotype (Bernardo et al., 2000; Mrak and Landreth, 2004). It was also shown that activation of the PPAR-γ induces the microglial immunoregulatory/M2 phenotype (Benoit et al., 2008; Rajaram et al., 2010). PPARγ agonists have been suggested as promising therapy for neurodegenerative diseases enhanced by neuroinflammation such as AD and PD (Schintu et al., 2009; Mandrekar-Colucci et al., 2012). Several studies have shown that AT1 receptor antagonists activate PPARγ. This has been related to pharmacological properties of some AT1 blockers such as telmisartan (Xu et al., 2015). However, studies using AT1 null mice revealed that blockage of AT1 receptors, independently of the pharmacological properties of the antagonists, also inhibits neuroinflammation and neurodegeneration (Garrido-Gil et al., 2012). Inhibition of AT1 with antagonists (ARBs), in addition to inhibition of proinflammatory polarization (see above), leads to activation of PPAR-γ and promotes the immunoregulatory phenotype by a double mechanism: by a pharmacological AT1-independent PPARγ agonistic effect (with more or less activation potency depending on the type of ARB), and by a direct effect of the blockage of the AT1 itself, which also induces PPARγ activation (Garrido-Gil et al., 2012). Among ARBS, the role of PPARγ activation in anti-inflammatory effects is particularly important for telmisartan, both at peripheral and CNS levels (Garrido-Gil et al., 2012; Pang et al., 2012; Wang et al., 2014; Villapol and Saavedra, 2015).

TLRs such as TLR2 and TLR4 are known to mediate classical microglial activation and neuroinflammation (Rietdijk et al., 2016). An increasing number of studies suggest a functional interaction or crosstalk between AT1 receptors and TLR4 and/or TLR2 (Biancardi et al., 2016). AT1 receptor antagonists inhibit TLRs in different immune effector cells both in peripheral tissues (Dasu et al., 2009; Cheng et al., 2011) and in brain microglia (Daniele et al., 2015; Biancardi et al., 2016). Ang II, via AT1, has been shown to increase TLR4 expression and Ang II-mediated ROS production and Ang II-induced microglial activation was blunted in TLR4 deficient mice (Rietdijk et al., 2016). The mechanisms involved in Ang II/AT1/TLRs interactions remain unknown.

Several recent studies suggest a pivotal role of metabolic reprogramming in the regulation of the innate inflammatory response (Galván-Peña and O'Neill, 2014; Tannahill et al., 2015). In the context of the peripheral immune cells, a shift in the cellular metabolism from oxidative phosphorylation to a erobic glycolysis for energy production favors the polarization toward a proinflammatory phenotype. More recently, the link between polarization and mitochondrial energy metabolism has been considered in microglia (see for review Orihuela et al., 2016). Interestingly, we have recently shown that an intracellular RAS, including AT1 and AT2 receptors, exists in brain mitochondria (Valenzuela et al., 2016). Activation of mitochondrial AT1 receptors regulates (by activation of mitochondrial Nox4) levels of superoxide and increases mitochondrial respiration. Mitochondrial AT2 receptors are much more abundant and downregulate mitochondrial respiration via NO production. Interestingly, altered expression of mitochondrial angiotensin receptors was observed in aged rats. Altered expression of AT1 and AT2 receptors with aging may contribute to mitochondrial dysfunction, neuroinflammation and neurodegeneration.

CONCLUSION

Dysregulation of brain RAS plays a major role in aging-related changes and neurodegeneration by exacerbation of OS and neuroinflammation, which may be attenuated by pharmacological manipulation of RAS components. Angiotensin II (via AT1 receptor and Nox activation) and prorenin/renin (via PRR) induce pro-inflammatory effects and M1 microglial phenotype. These effects are counteracted by a RAS opposite arm constituted by angiotensin II/AT2 receptor signaling and Angiotensin 1-7/MasR signaling, which promote anti-inflammatory effects and M2 microglial phenotype. In addition, there are interactions between RAS and different compounds involved in neuroinflammation and microglial polarization, such as estrogens, ROCK, IGF1, TNF-α, iron, PPARγ and TLRs. Pharmacological manipulation of brain RAS components may be an interesting therapeutical approach for neurodegenerative diseases and aging-related processes in which OS and neuroinflammation play a major role.

AUTHOR CONTRIBUTIONS

All authors have contributed to this work and approved its final version for submission. JLL-G developed the idea for this review article and wrote the manuscript. AIR-P prepared the figures and was involved in literature review, and revision of the manuscript. JLL prepared the viral vectors used for activation of microglia in Figure 2, and revised the manuscript. PG-G, JR-P and MJG were involved in literature review, and preparation of the manuscript.

ACKNOWLEDGMENTS

The work reported here was supported by Spanish Ministry of Science and Innovation (BFU2015-70523), Spanish Ministry of Health (RD12/0019/0020, RD16/0011/0016 and CIBERNED), Galician Government (XUGA GRC2014/002) and European Regional Development Fund (FEDER).

REFERENCES

Alberici, L. C., Oliveira, H. C., Paim, B. A., Mantello, C. C., Augusto, A. C., Zecchin, K. G., et al. (2009). Mitochondrial ATP-sensitive K^+ channels as redox signals to liver mitochondria in response to hypertriglyceridemia. *Free Radic. Biol. Med.* 47, 1432–1439. doi: 10.1016/j.freeradbiomed.2009.08.013

Albiston, A. L., McDowall, S. G., Matsacos, D., Sim, P., Clune, E., Mustafa, T., et al. (2001). Evidence that the angiotensin IV (AT_4) receptor is the enzyme insulin-regulated aminopeptidase. *J. Biol. Chem.* 276, 48623–48626. doi: 10.1074/jbc.c100512200

Alliot, F., Godin, I., and Pessac, B. (1999). Microglia derive from progenitors, originating from the yolk sac, and which proliferate in the brain. *Dev. Brain Res.* 117, 145–152. doi: 10.1016/s0165-3806(99)00113-3

Babior, B. M. (2004). NADPH oxidase. *Curr. Opin. Immunol.* 16, 42–47. doi: 10.1016/j.coi.2003.12.001

Bacani, C., and Frishman, W. H. (2006). Chymase: a new pharmacologic target in cardiovascular disease. *Cardiol. Rev.* 14, 187–193. doi: 10.1097/01.crd.0000195220.62533.c5

Bader, M. (2013). ACE2, angiotensin-(1–7), and Mas: the other side of the coin. *Pflugers Arch.* 465, 79–85. doi: 10.1007/s00424-012-1120-0

Balakumar, P., and Jagadeesh, G. (2014). A century old renin-angiotensin system still grows with endless possibilities: AT1 receptor signaling cascades in cardiovascular physiopathology. *Cell. Signal.* 26, 2147–2160. doi: 10.1016/j.cellsig.2014.06.011

Barcia, C., Ros, C. M., Annese, V., Carrillo-de Sauvage, M. A., Ros-Bernal, F., Gómez, A., et al. (2012). ROCK/Cdc42-mediated microglial motility and gliapse formation lead to phagocytosis of degenerating dopaminergic neurons *in vivo*. *Sci. Rep.* 2:809. doi: 10.1038/srep00809

Bartke, A., Chandrashekar, V., Dominici, F., Turyn, D., Kinney, B., Steger, R., et al. (2003). Insulin-like growth factor 1 (IGF-1) and aging: controversies and new insights. *Biogerontology* 4, 1–8. doi: 10.1023/A:1022448532248

Basso, N., Paglia, N., Stella, I., de Cavanagh, E. M., Ferder, L., del Rosario Lores Arnaiz, M., et al. (2005). Protective effect of the inhibition of the renin-angiotensin system on aging. *Regul. Pept.* 128, 247–252. doi: 10.1016/j.regpep.2004.12.027

Benicky, J., Sánchez-Lemus, E., Pavel, J., and Saavedra, J. M. (2009). Anti-inflammatory effects of angiotensin receptor blockers in the brain and the periphery. *Cell. Mol. Neurobiol.* 29, 781–792. doi: 10.1007/s10571-009-9368-4

Benigni, A., Corna, D., Zoja, C., Sonzogni, A., Latini, R., Salio, M., et al. (2009). Disruption of the Ang II type 1 receptor promotes longevity in mice. *J. Clin. Invest.* 119, 524–530. doi: 10.1172/JCI36703

Benoit, M., Desnues, B., and Mege, J. L. (2008). Macrophage polarization in bacterial infections. *J. Immunol.* 181, 3733–3739. doi: 10.4049/jimmunol.181.6.3733

Bernardo, A., Levi, G., and Minghetti, L. (2000). Role of the peroxisome proliferator-activated receptor-γ (PPAR-γ) and its natural ligand 15-deoxy-$\Delta^{12,14}$-prostaglandin J_2 in the regulation of microglial functions. *Eur. J. Neurosci.* 12, 2215–2223. doi: 10.1046/j.1460-9568.2000.00110.x

Bernhart, E., Kollroser, M., Rechberger, G., Reicher, H., Heinemann, A., Schratl, P., et al. (2010). Lysophosphatidic acid receptor activation affects the C13NJ microglia cell line proteome leading to alterations in glycolysis, motility, and cytoskeletal architecture. *Proteomics* 10, 141–158. doi: 10.1002/pmic.200900195

Biancardi, V. C., Stranahan, A. M., Krause, E. G., de Kloet, A. D., and Stern, J. E. (2016). Cross talk between AT1 receptors and Toll-like receptor 4 in microglia contributes to angiotensin II-derived ROS production in the hypothalamic paraventricular nucleus. *Am. J. Physiol. Heart Circ. Physiol.* 310, H404–H415. doi: 10.1152/ajpheart.00247.2015

Borrajo, A., Rodriguez-Perez, A. I., Diaz-Ruiz, C., Guerra, M. J., and Labandeira-Garcia, J. L. (2014a). Microglial TNF-α mediates enhancement of dopaminergic degeneration by brain angiotensin. *Glia* 62, 145–157. doi: 10.1002/glia.22595

Borrajo, A., Rodriguez-Perez, A. I., Villar-Cheda, B., Guerra, M. J., and Labandeira-Garcia, J. L. (2014b). Inhibition of the microglial response is essential for the neuroprotective effects of Rho-kinase inhibitors on MPTP-induced dopaminergic cell death. *Neuropharmacology* 85, 1–8. doi: 10.1016/j.neuropharm.2014.05.021

Brown, D. C., Steward, L. J., Ge, J., and Barnes, N. M. (1996). Ability of angiotensin II to modulate striatal dopamine release via the AT1 receptor *in vitro* and *in vivo*. *Br. J. Pharmacol.* 118, 414–420. doi: 10.1111/j.1476-5381.1996.tb15418.x

Brown-Borg, H. M. (2007). Hormonal regulation of longevity in mammals. *Ageing Res. Rev.* 6, 28–45. doi: 10.1016/j.arr.2007.02.005

Bunnemann, B., Fuxe, K., Metzger, R., Mullins, J., Jackson, T. R., Hanley, M. R., et al. (1990). Autoradiographic localization of mas proto-oncogene mRNA in adult rat brain using *in situ* hybridization. *Neurosci. Lett.* 114, 147–153. doi: 10.1016/0304-3940(90)90063-f

Butovsky, O., Jedrychowski, M. P., Moore, C. S., Cialic, R., Lanser, A. J., Gabriely, G., et al. (2014). Identification of a unique TGF-β-dependent molecular and functional signature in microglia. *Nat. Neurosci.* 17, 131–143. doi: 10.1038/nn.3599

Cai, H. (2005). NAD(P)H oxidase-dependent self-propagation of hydrogen peroxide and vascular disease. *Circ. Res.* 96, 818–822. doi: 10.1161/01.res.0000163631.07205.fb

Carson, M. J., Doose, J. M., Melchior, B., Schmid, C. D., and Ploix, C. C. (2006). CNS immune privilege: hiding in plain sight. *Immunol. Rev.* 213, 48–65. doi: 10.1111/j.1600-065x.2006.00441.x

Cassis, P., Conti, S., Remuzzi, G., and Benigni, A. (2010). Angiotensin receptors as determinants of life span. *Pflugers Arch.* 459, 325–332. doi: 10.1007/s00424-009-0725-4

Chabrashvili, T., Kitiyakara, C., Blau, J., Karber, A., Aslam, S., Welch, W. J., et al. (2003). Effects of ANG II type 1 and 2 receptors on oxidative stress, renal NADPH oxidase and SOD expression. *Am. J. Physiol. Regul. Integr. Comp. Physiol.* 285, R117–R124. doi: 10.1152/ajpregu.00476.2002

Cheng, X. W., Song, H., Sasaki, T., Hu, L., Inoue, A., Bando, Y. K., et al. (2011). Angiotensin type 1 receptor blocker reduces intimal neovascularization and plaque growth in apolipoprotein E-deficient mice. *Hypertension* 57, 981–989. doi: 10.1161/HYPERTENSIONAHA.110.168385

Chhor, V., Le Charpentier, T., Lebon, S., Oré, M. V., Celador, I. L., Josserand, J., et al. (2013). Characterization of phenotype markers and neuronotoxic potential of polarised primary microglia *in vitro*. *Brain Behav. Immun.* 32, 70–85. doi: 10.1016/j.bbi.2013.02.005

Choi, S.-H., Aid, S., Kim, H.-W., Jackson, S. H., and Bosetti, F. (2012). Inhibition of NADPH oxidase promotes alternative and anti-inflammatory microglial activation during neuroinflammation. *J. Neurochem.* 120, 292–301. doi: 10.1111/j.1471-4159.2011.07572.x

Choi, D.-Y., Zhang, J., and Bing, G. (2010). Aging enhances the neuroinflammatory response and α-synuclein nitration in rats. *Neurobiol. Aging* 31, 1649–1653. doi: 10.1016/j.neurobiolaging.2008.09.010

Cicchetti, F., Brownell, A. L., Williams, K., Chen, Y. I., Livni, E., and Isacson, O. (2002). Neuroinflammation of the nigrostriatal pathway during progressive 6-OHDA dopamine degeneration in rats monitored by immunohistochemistry and PET imaging. *Eur. J. Neurosci.* 15, 991–998. doi: 10.1046/j.1460-9568.2002.01938.x

Clark, M. A., Diz, D. I., and Tallant, E. A. (2001). Angiotensin-(1–7) downregulates the angiotensin II type 1 receptor in vascular smooth muscle cells. *Hypertension* 37, 1141–1146. doi: 10.1161/01.hyp.37.4.1141

Collier, T. J., Lipton, J., Daley, B. F., Palfi, S., Chu, Y., Sortwell, C., et al. (2007). Aging-related changes in the nigrostriatal dopamine system and the response to MPTP in nonhuman primates: diminished compensatory mechanisms as a prelude to parkinsonism. *Neurobiol. Dis.* 26, 56–65. doi: 10.1016/j.nbd.2006.11.013

Colton, C. A. (2009). Heterogeneity of microglial activation in the innate immune response in the brain. *J. Neuroimmune Pharmacol.* 4, 399–418. doi: 10.1007/s11481-009-9164-4

Cruz-Muros, I., Afonso-Oramas, D., Abreu, P., Pérez-Delgado, M. M., Rodriguez, M., and González-Hernández, T. (2009). Aging effects on the dopamine transporter expression and compensatory mechanisms. *Neurobiol. Aging* 30, 973–986. doi: 10.1016/j.neurobiolaging.2007.09.009

Csiszar, A., Ungvari, Z., Koller, A., Edwards, J. G., and Kaley, G. (2003). Aging-induced proinflammatory shift in cytokine expression profile in coronary arteries. *FASEB J.* 17, 1183–1185. doi: 10.1096/fj.02-1049fje

Daniele, S. G., Béraud, D., Davenport, C., Cheng, K., Yin, H., and Maguire-Zeiss, K. A. (2015). Activation of MyD88-dependent TLR1/2 signaling by misfolded α-synuclein, a protein linked to neurodegenerative disorders. *Sci. Signal.* 8:ra45. doi: 10.1126/scisignal.2005965

Dasu, M. R., Riosvelasco, A. C., and Jialal, I. (2009). Candesartan inhibits Toll-like receptor expression and activity both *in vitro* and *in vivo*. *Atherosclerosis* 202, 76–83. doi: 10.1016/j.atherosclerosis.2008.04.010

Davalos, D., Grutzendler, J., Yang, G., Kim, J. V., Zuo, Y., Jung, S., et al. (2005). ATP mediates rapid microglial response to local brain injury *in vivo*. *Nat. Neurosci.* 8, 752–758. doi: 10.1038/nn1472

de Cavanagh, E. M., Inserra, F., and Ferder, L. (2011). Angiotensin II blockade: a strategy to slow ageing by protecting mitochondria? *Cardiovasc. Res.* 89, 31–40. doi: 10.1093/cvr/cvq285

de Cavanagh, E. M., Piotrkowski, B., and Fraga, C. G. (2004). Concerted action of the renin-angiotensin system, mitochondria, and antioxidant defenses in aging. *Mol. Aspects Med.* 25, 27–36. doi: 10.1016/j.mam.2004.02.006

Dhande, I., Ali, Q., and Hussain, T. (2013). Proximal tubule angiotensin AT2 receptors mediate an anti-inflammatory response via interleukin-10: role in renoprotection in obese rats. *Hypertension* 61, 1218–1226. doi: 10.1161/HYPERTENSIONAHA.111.00422

Diaz-Ruiz, C., Rodriguez-Perez, A. I., Beiroa, D., Rodriguez-Pallares, J., and Labandeira-Garcia, J. L. (2015). Reciprocal regulation between sirtuin-1 and angiotensin-II in the substantia nigra: implications for aging and neurodegeneration. *Oncotarget* 6, 26675–26689. doi: 10.18632/oncotarget.5596

Dominguez-Meijide, A., Rodriguez-Perez, A. I., Diaz-Ruiz, C., Guerra, M. J., and Labandeira-Garcia, J. L. (2017). Dopamine modulates astroglial and microglial activity via glial renin-angiotensin system in cultures. *Brain Behav. Immun.* 62, 277–290. doi: 10.1016/j.bbi.2017.02.013

Dominguez-Meijide, A., Villar-Cheda, B., Garrido-Gil, P., Sierrra-Paredes, G., Guerra, M. J., and Labandeira-Garcia, J. L. (2014). Effect of chronic treatment with angiotensin type 1 receptor antagonists on striatal dopamine levels in normal rats and in a rat model of Parkinson's disease treated with L-DOPA. *Neuropharmacology* 76, 156–168. doi: 10.1016/j.neuropharm.2013.07.016

Dusek, P., Jankovic, J., and Le, W. (2012). Iron dysregulation in movement disorders. *Neurobiol. Dis.* 46, 1–18. doi: 10.1016/j.nbd.2011.12.054

Edwards, J. P., Zhang, X., Frauwirth, K. A., and Mosser, D. M. (2006). Biochemical and functional characterization of three activated macrophage populations. *J. Leukoc. Biol.* 80, 1298–1307. doi: 10.1189/jlb.0406249

Esteban, V., Ruperez, M., Sánchez-López, E., Rodriguez-Vita, J., Lorenzo, O., Demaegdt, H., et al. (2005). Angiotensin IV activates the nuclear transcription factor-κB and related proinflammatory genes in vascular smooth muscle cells. *Circ. Res.* 96, 965–973. doi: 10.1161/01.res.0000166326.91395.74

Fillit, H., Ding, W. H., Buee, L., Kalman, J., Altstiel, L., Lawlor, B., et al. (1991). Elevated circulating tumor necrosis factor levels in Alzheimer's disease. *Neurosci. Lett.* 129, 318–320. doi: 10.1016/0304-3940(91)90490-k

Franco, R., and Fernández-Suárez, D. (2015). Alternatively activated microglia and macrophages in the central nervous system. *Prog. Neurobiol.* 131, 65–86. doi: 10.1016/j.pneurobio.2015.05.003

Frank-Cannon, T. C., Alto, L. T., McAlpine, F. E., and Tansey, M. G. (2009). Does neuroinflammation fan the flame in neurodegenerative diseases? *Mol. Neurodegener.* 4:47. doi: 10.1186/1750-1326-4-47

Fujisaka, S., Usui, I., Kanatani, Y., Ikutani, M., Takasaki, I., Tsuneyama, K., et al. (2011). Telmisartan improves insulin resistance and modulates adipose tissue macrophage polarization in high-fat-fed mice. *Endocrinology* 152, 1789–1799. doi: 10.1210/en.2010-1312

Gallagher, P. E., Chappell, M. C., Ferrario, C. M., and Tallant, E. A. (2006). Distinct roles for ANG II and ANG-(1–7) in the regulation of angiotensin-converting enzyme 2 in rat astrocytes. *Am. J. Physiol. Cell Physiol.* 290, C420–C426. doi: 10.1152/ajpcell.00409.2004

Galván-Peña, S. A., and O'Neill, L. A. (2014). Metabolic reprograming in macrophage polarization. *Front. Immunol.* 5:420. doi: 10.3389/fimmu.2014.00420

Ganong, W. F. (1994). Origin of the angiotensin II secreted by cells. *Proc. Soc. Exp. Biol. Med.* 205, 213–219. doi: 10.3181/00379727-205-43699a

Gao, H. M., Liu, B., Zhang, W., and Hong, J. S. (2003). Critical role of microglial NADPH oxidase-derived free radicals in the *in vitro* MPTP model of Parkinson's disease. *FASEB J.* 17, 1954–1956. doi: 10.1096/fj.03-0109fje

Garrido, A. M., and Griendling, K. K. (2009). NADPH oxidases and angiotensin II receptor signaling. *Mol. Cell. Endocrinol.* 302, 148–158. doi: 10.1016/j.mce.2008.11.003

Garrido-Gil, P., Joglar, B., Rodriguez-Perez, A. I., Guerra, M. J., and Labandeira-Garcia, J. L. (2012). Involvement of PPAR-γ in the neuroprotective and anti-inflammatory effects of angiotensin type 1 receptor inhibition: effects of the receptor antagonist telmisartan and receptor deletion in a mouse MPTP model of Parkinson's disease. *J. Neuroinflammation* 9:38. doi: 10.1186/1742-2094-9-38

Garrido-Gil, P., Rodriguez-Pallares, J., Dominguez-Meijide, A., Guerra, M. J., and Labandeira-Garcia, J. L. (2013a). Brain angiotensin regulates iron homeostasis in dopaminergic neurons and microglial cells. *Exp. Neurol.* 250, 384–396. doi: 10.1016/j.expneurol.2013.10.013

Garrido-Gil, P., Valenzuela, R., Villar-Cheda, B., Lanciego, J. L., and Labandeira-Garcia, J. L. (2013b). Expression of angiotensinogen and receptors for angiotensin and prorenin in the monkey and human substantia nigra: an intracellular renin-angiotensin system in the nigra. *Brain Struct. Funct.* 218, 373–388. doi: 10.1007/s00429-012-0402-9

Garrido-Gil, P., Rodriguez-Perez, A. I., Fernandez-Rodriguez, P., Lanciego, J. L., and Labandeira-Garcia, J. L. (2017). Expression of angiotensinogen and receptors for angiotensin and prorenin in the rat and monkey striatal neurons and glial cells. *Brain Struct. Funct.* doi: 10.1007/s00429-016-1357-z [Epub ahead of print].

Gautier, E. L., Shay, T., Miller, J., Greter, M., Jakubzick, C., Ivanov, S., et al. (2012). Gene-expression profiles and transcriptional regulatory pathways that underlie the identity and diversity of mouse tissue macrophages. *Nat. Immunol.* 13, 1118–1128. doi: 10.1038/ni.2419

Ghadery, C., Koshimori, Y., Coakeley, S., Harris, M., Rusjan, P., Kim, J., et al. (2017). Microglial activation in Parkinson's disease using [^{18}F]-FEPPA. *J. Neuroinflammation* 14:8. doi: 10.1186/s12974-016-0778-1

Ginhoux, F., Greter, M., Leboeuf, M., Nandi, S., See, P., Gokhan, S., et al. (2010). Fate mapping analysis reveals that adult microglia derive from primitive macrophages. *Science* 330, 841–845. doi: 10.1126/science.1194637

Gordon, S. (2003). Alternative activation of macrophages. *Nat. Rev. Immunol.* 3, 23–35. doi: 10.1038/nri978

Grammatopoulos, T. N., Jones, S. M., Ahmadi, F. A., Hoover, B. R., Snell, L. D., Skoch, J., et al. (2007). Angiotensin type 1 receptor antagonist losartan, reduces MPTP-induced degeneration of dopaminergic neurons in substantia nigra. *Mol. Neurodegener.* 2:1. doi: 10.1186/1750-1326-2-1

Greenwood, J., Walters, C. E., Pryce, G., Kanuga, N., Beraud, E., Baker, D., et al. (2003). Lovastatin inhibits brain endothelial cell Rho-mediated lymphocyte migration and attenuates experimental autoimmune encephalomyelitis. *FASEB J.* 17, 905–907. doi: 10.1096/fj.02-1014fje

Griendling, K. K., Sorescu, D., and Ushio-Fukai, M. (2000). NAD(P)H oxidase: role in cardiovascular biology and disease. *Circ. Res.* 86, 494–501. doi: 10.1161/01.res.86.5.494

Hammer, A., Yang, G., Friedrich, J., Kovacs, A., Lee, D. H., Grave, K., et al. (2016). Role of the receptor Mas in macrophage-mediated inflammation *in vivo*. *Proc. Natl. Acad. Sci. U S A* 113, 14109–14114. doi: 10.1073/pnas.1612668113

Hamming, I., Cooper, M. E., Haagmans, B. L., Hooper, N. M., Korstanje, R., Osterhaus, A. D., et al. (2007). The emerging role of ACE2 in physiology and disease. *J. Pathol.* 212, 1–11. doi: 10.1002/path.2162

Harding, J. W., Sullivan, M. J., Hanesworth, J. M., Cushing, L. L., and Wright, J. W. (1988). Inability of [125I]Sar1, Ile8-angiotensin II to move between the blood and cerebrospinal fluid compartments. *J. Neurochem.* 50, 554–557. doi: 10.1111/j.1471-4159.1988.tb02946.x

Harms, A. S., Lee, J. K., Nguyen, T. A., Chang, J., Ruhn, K. M., Treviño, I., et al. (2012). Regulation of microglia effector functions by tumor necrosis factor signaling. *Glia* 60, 189–202. doi: 10.1002/glia.21254

Harrison, J. K., Jiang, Y., Chen, S., Xia, Y., Maciejewski, D., McNamara, R. K., et al. (1998). Role for neuronally derived fractalkine in mediating interactions between neurons and CX3CR1-expressing microglia. *Proc. Natl. Acad. Sci. U S A* 95, 10896–10901. doi: 10.1073/pnas.95.18.10896

Harry, G. J., and Kraft, A. D. (2012). Microglia in the developing brain: a potential target with lifetime effects. *Neurotoxicology* 33, 191–206. doi: 10.1016/j.neuro.2012.01.012

Hellner, K., Walther, T., Schubert, M., and Albrecht, D. (2005). Angiotensin-(1–7) enhances LTP in the hippocampus through the G-protein-coupled receptor Mas. *Mol. Cell. Neurosci.* 29, 427–435. doi: 10.1016/j.mcn.2005.03.012

Heneka, M. T., Carson, M. J., El Khoury, J., Landreth, G. E., Brosseron, F., Feinstein, D. L., et al. (2015). Neuroinflammation in Alzheimer's disease. *Lancet Neurol.* 14, 388–405. doi: 10.1016/S1474-4422(15)70016-5

Herrera, M., Silva, G. B., and Garvin, J. L. (2010). Angiotensin II stimulates thick ascending limb superoxide production via protein kinase C^{α}-dependent NADPH oxidase activation. *J. Biol. Chem.* 285, 21323–21328. doi: 10.1074/jbc.M110.109157

Heymes, C., Silvestre, J. S., Llorens-Cortes, C., Chevalier, B., Marotte, F., Levy, B. I., et al. (1998). Cardiac senescence is associated with enhanced expression of angiotensin II receptor subtypes. *Endocrinology* 139, 2579–2587. doi: 10.1210/en.139.5.2579

Hickman, S. E., Kingery, N. D., Ohsumi, T. K., Borowsky, M. L., Wang, L. C., Means, T. K., et al. (2013). The microglial sensome revealed by direct RNA sequencing. *Nat. Neurosci.* 16, 1896–1905. doi: 10.1038/nn.3554

Hoek, R. M., Ruuls, S. R., Murphy, C. A., Wright, G. J., Goddard, R., Zurawski, S. M., et al. (2000). Down-regulation of the macrophage lineage through interaction with OX2 (CD200). *Science* 290, 1768–1771. doi: 10.1126/science.290.5497.1768

Hofman, F. M., Hinton, D. R., Johnson, K., and Merrill, J. E. (1989). Tumor necrosis factor identified in multiple sclerosis brain. *J. Exp. Med.* 170, 607–612. doi: 10.1084/jem.170.2.607

Honing, H., van den Berg, T. K., van der Pol, S. M., Dijkstra, C. D., van der Kammen, R. A., Collard, J. G., et al. (2004). RhoA activation promotes transendothelial migration of monocytes via ROCK. *J. Leukoc. Biol.* 75, 523–528. doi: 10.1189/jlb.0203054

Hoogwerf, B. J. (2010). Renin-angiotensin system blockade and cardiovascular and renal protection. *Am. J. Cardiol.* 105, 30A–35A. doi: 10.1016/j.amjcard.2009.10.009

Hu, X., Liou, A. K., Leak, R. K., Xu, M., An, C., Suenaga, J., et al. (2014). Neurobiology of microglial action in CNS injuries: receptor-mediated signaling mechanisms and functional roles. *Prog. Neurobiol.* 119–120, 60–84. doi: 10.1016/j.pneurobio.2014.06.002

Ishibashi, K., Ishii, K., Oda, K., Kawasaki, K., Mizusawa, H., and Ishiwata, K. (2009). Regional analysis of age-related decline in dopamine transporters and dopamine D2-like receptors in human striatum. *Synapse* 63, 282–290. doi: 10.1002/syn.20603

Iwanami, J., Mogi, M., Tsukuda, K., Min, L. J., Sakata, A., Jing, F., et al. (2010). Low dose of telmisartan prevents ischemic brain damage with peroxisome proliferator-activated receptor-γ activation in diabetic mice. *J. Hypertens.* 28, 1730–1737. doi: 10.1097/hjh.0b013e32833a551a

Iwanami, J., Mogi, M., Tsukuda, K., Wang, X.-L., Nakaoka, H., Kan-no, H., et al. (2015). Direct angiotensin II type 2 receptor stimulation by compound 21 prevents vascular dementia. *J. Am. Soc. Hypertens.* 9, 250–256. doi: 10.1016/j.jash.2015.01.010

Jiang, C., Ting, A. T., and Seed, B. (1998). PPAR-γ agonists inhibit production of monocyte inflammatory cytokines. *Nature* 391, 82–86. doi: 10.1038/34184

Jin, C. Z., Jang, J. H., Wang, Y., Kim, J. G., Bae, Y. M., Shi, J., et al. (2012). Neuronal nitric oxide synthase is up-regulated by angiotensin II and attenuates NADPH oxidase activity and facilitates relaxation in murine left ventricular myocytes. *J. Mol. Cell. Cardiol.* 52, 1274–1281. doi: 10.1016/j.yjmcc.2012.03.013

Joglar, B., Rodriguez-Pallares, J., Rodriguez-Perez, A. I., Rey, P., Guerra, M. J., and Labandeira-Garcia, J. L. (2009). The inflammatory response in the MPTP model of Parkinson's disease is mediated by brain angiotensin: relevance to progression of the disease. *J. Neurochem.* 109, 656–669. doi: 10.1111/j.1471-4159.2009.05999.x

Jones, E. S., Vinh, A., McCarthy, C. A., Gaspari, T. A., and Widdop, R. E. (2008). AT2 receptors: functional relevance in cardiovascular disease. *Pharmacol. Ther.* 120, 292–316. doi: 10.1016/j.pharmthera.2008.08.009

Kehoe, P. G., and Wilcock, G. K. (2007). Is inhibition of the renin-angiotensin system a new treatment option for Alzheimer's disease? *Lancet Neurol.* 6, 373–378. doi: 10.1016/s1474-4422(07)70077-7

Kerr, D. S., Bevilaqua, L. R., Bonini, J. S., Rossato, J. I., Köhler, C. A., Medina, J. H., et al. (2005). Angiotensin II blocks memory consolidation through an AT2 receptor-dependent mechanism. *Psychopharmacology (Berl)* 179, 529–535. doi: 10.1007/s00213-004-2074-5

Kettenmann, H., Hanisch, U.-K., Noda, M., and Verkhratsky, A. (2011). Physiology of microglia. *Physiol. Rev.* 91, 461–553. doi: 10.1152/physrev.00011.2010

Kigerl, K. A., Gensel, J. C., Ankeny, D. P., Alexander, J. K., Donnelly, D. J., and Popovich, P. G. (2009). Identification of two distinct macrophage subsets with divergent effects causing either neurotoxicity or regeneration in the injured mouse spinal cord. *J Neurosci* 29, 13435–13444. doi: 10.1523/JNEUROSCI.3257-09.2009

Kim, J. Y., Kim, N., and Yenari, M. A. (2015). Mechanisms and potential therapeutic applications of microglial activation after brain injury. *CNS Neurosci. Ther.* 21, 309–319. doi: 10.1111/cns.12360

Koenigsknecht-Talboo, J., and Landreth, G. E. (2005). Microglial phagocytosis induced by fibrillar β-amyloid and IgGs are differentially regulated by proinflammatory cytokines. *J. Neurosci.* 25, 8240–8249. doi: 10.1523/JNEUROSCI.1808-05.2005

Kong, J., Zhang, K., Meng, X., Zhang, Y., and Zhang, C. (2015). Dose-dependent bidirectional effect of angiotensin IV on abdominal aortic aneurysm via variable angiotensin receptor stimulation. *Hypertension* 66, 617–626. doi: 10.1161/HYPERTENSIONAHA.115.05482

Kostenis, E., Milligan, G., Christopoulos, A., Sanchez-Ferrer, C. F., Heringer-Walther, S., Sexton, P. M., et al. (2005). G-protein-coupled receptor Mas is a physiological antagonist of the angiotensin II type 1 receptor. *Circulation* 111, 1806–1813. doi: 10.1161/01.cir.0000160867.23556.7d

Kubis, N., Faucheux, B. A., Ransmayr, G., Damier, P., Duyckaerts, C., Henin, D., et al. (2000). Preservation of midbrain catecholaminergic neurons in very old human subjects. *Brain* 123, 366–373. doi: 10.1093/brain/123.2.366

Kumar, A., Rassoli, A., and Raizada, M. K. (1988). Angiotensinogen gene expression in neuronal and glial cells in primary cultures of rat brain. *J. Neurosci. Res.* 19, 287–290. doi: 10.1002/jnr.490190302

Labandeira-García, J. L., Garrido-Gil, P., Rodriguez-Pallares, J., Valenzuela, R., Borrajo, A., and Rodríguez-Perez, A. I. (2014). Brain renin-angiotensin system and dopaminergic cell vulnerability. *Front. Neuroanat.* 8:67. doi: 10.3389/fnana.2014.00067

Labandeira-Garcia, J. L., Rodriguez-Pallares, J., Dominguez-Meijide, A., Valenzuela, R., Villar-Cheda, B., and Rodriguez-Perez, A. I. (2013). Dopamine-angiotensin interactions in the basal ganglia and their relevance for Parkinson's disease. *Mov. Disord.* 28, 1337–1342. doi: 10.1002/mds.25614

Labandeira-Garcia, J. L., Rodriguez-Perez, A. I., Valenzuela, R., Costa-Besada, M. A., and Guerra, M. J. (2016). Menopause and Parkinson's disease. Interaction between estrogens and brain renin-angiotensin system in dopaminergic degeneration. *Front. Neuroendocrinol.* 43, 44–59. doi: 10.1016/j.yfrne.2016.09.003

Labandeira-Garcia, J. L., Rodríguez-Perez, A. I., Villar-Cheda, B., Borrajo, A., Dominguez-Meijide, A., and Guerra, M. J. (2015). Rho kinase and dopaminergic degeneration: a promising therapeutic target for Parkinson's disease. *Neuroscientist* 21, 616–629. doi: 10.1177/1073858414554954

Lawson, L. J., Perry, V. H., Dri, P., and Gordon, S. (1990). Heterogeneity in the distribution and morphology of microglia in the normal adult mouse brain. *Neuroscience* 39, 151–170. doi: 10.1016/0306-4522(90)90229-w

Liu, M., Shi, P., and Sumners, C. (2016). Direct anti-inflammatory effects of angiotensin-(1–7) on microglia. *J. Neurochem.* 136, 163–171. doi: 10.1111/jnc.13386

Liu, J., Zhang, P.-S., Yu, Q., Liu, L., Yang, Y., Guo, F.-M., et al. (2012). Losartan inhibits conventional dendritic cell maturation and Th1 and Th17 polarization responses: novel mechanisms of preventive effects on lipopolysaccharide-induced acute lung injury. *Int. J. Mol. Med.* 29, 269–276. doi: 10.3892/ijmm.2011.818

Lopes, K. O., Sparks, D. L., and Streit, W. J. (2008). Microglial dystrophy in the aged and Alzheimer's disease brain is associated with ferritin immunoreactivity. *Glia* 56, 1048–1060. doi: 10.1002/glia.20678

Lopez-Real, A., Rey, P., Soto-Otero, R., Mendez-Alvarez, E., and Labandeira-Garcia, J. L. (2005). Angiotensin-converting enzyme inhibition reduces oxidative stress and protects dopaminergic neurons in a 6-hydroxydopamine rat model of Parkinsonism. *J. Neurosci. Res.* 81, 865–873. doi: 10.1002/jnr.20598

Lu, J., Wu, L., Jiang, T., Wang, Y., Zhao, H., Gao, Q., et al. (2015). Angiotensin AT2 receptor stimulation inhibits activation of NADPH oxidase and ameliorates oxidative stress in rotenone model of Parkinson's disease in CATH.a cells. *Neurotoxicol. Teratol.* 47, 16–24. doi: 10.1016/j.ntt.2014.11.004

Ma, L.-J., Corsa, B. A., Zhou, J., Yang, H., Li, H., Tang, Y.-W., et al. (2011). Angiotensin type 1 receptor modulates macrophage polarization and renal injury in obesity. *Am. J. Physiol. Renal Physiol.* 300, F1203–F1213. doi: 10.1152/ajprenal.00468.2010

MacMicking, J., Xie, Q. W., and Nathan, C. (1997). Nitric oxide and macrophage function. *Annu. Rev. Immunol.* 15, 323–350. doi: 10.1146/annurev.immunol.15.1.323

Mandrekar-Colucci, S., Karlo, J. C., and Landreth, G. E. (2012). Mechanisms underlying the rapid peroxisome proliferator-activated receptor-γ-mediated amyloid clearance and reversal of cognitive deficits in a murine model of Alzheimer's disease. *J. Neurosci.* 32, 10117–10128. doi: 10.1523/JNEUROSCI.5268-11.2012

Mantovani, A., Sica, A., Sozzani, S., Allavena, P., Vecchi, A., and Locati, M. (2004). The chemokine system in diverse forms of macrophage activation and polarization. *Trends Immunol.* 25, 677–686. doi: 10.1016/j.it.2004.09.015

Maul, B., Krause, W., Pankow, K., Becker, M., Gembardt, F., Alenina, N., et al. (2005). Central angiotensin II controls alcohol consumption via its AT1 receptor. *FASEB J.* 19, 1474–1481. doi: 10.1096/fj.05-3742com

McCormack, A. L., Di Monte, D. A., Delfani, K., Irwin, I., DeLanney, L. E., Langston, W. J., et al. (2004). Aging of the nigrostriatal system in the squirrel monkey. *J. Comp. Neurol.* 471, 387–395. doi: 10.1002/cne.20036

McGuire, S. O., Ling, Z. D., Lipton, J. W., Sortwell, C. E., Collier, T. J., and Carvey, P. M. (2001). Tumor necrosis factor α is toxic to embryonic mesencephalic dopamine neurons. *Exp. Neurol.* 169, 219–230. doi: 10.1006/exnr.2001.7688

Mehlhase, J., Gieche, J., Widmer, R., and Grune, T. (2006). Ferritin levels in microglia depend upon activation: modulation by reactive oxygen species. *Biochim. Biophys. Acta* 1763, 854–859. doi: 10.1016/j.bbamcr.2006.04.012

Mehta, P. K., and Griendling, K. K. (2007). Angiotensin II cell signaling: physiological and pathological effects in the cardiovascular system. *Am. J. Physiol. Cell Physiol.* 292, C82–C97. doi: 10.1152/ajpcell.00287.2006

Mendelsohn, F. A., Jenkins, T. A., and Berkovic, S. F. (1993). Effects of angiotensin II on dopamine and serotonin turnover in the striatum of conscious rats. *Brain Res.* 613, 221–229. doi: 10.1016/0006-8993(93)90902-y

Milsted, A., Barna, B. P., Ransohoff, R. M., Brosnihan, K. B., and Ferrario, C. M. (1990). Astrocyte cultures derived from human brain tissue express angiotensinogen mRNA. *Proc. Natl. Acad. Sci. U S A* 87, 5720–5723. doi: 10.1073/pnas.87.15.5720

Min, L. J., Mogi, M., Iwai, M., and Horiuchi, M. (2009). Signaling mechanisms of angiotensin II in regulating vascular senescence. *Ageing Res. Rev.* 8, 113–121. doi: 10.1016/j.arr.2008.12.002

Mittelbronn, M., Dietz, K., Schluesener, H. J., and Meyermann, R. (2001). Local distribution of microglia in the normal adult human central nervous system differs by up to one order of magnitude. *Acta Neuropathol.* 101, 249–255. doi: 10.1007/s004010000284

Miyoshi, M., Miyano, K., Moriyama, N., Taniguchi, M., and Watanabe, T. (2008). Angiotensin type 1 receptor antagonist inhibits lipopolysaccharide-induced stimulation of rat microglial cells by suppressing nuclear factor κB and activator protein-1 activation. *Eur. J. Neurosci.* 27, 343–351. doi: 10.1111/j.1460-9568.2007.06014.x

Mogi, M., Harada, M., Riederer, P., Narabayashi, H., Fujita, K., and Nagatsu, T. (1994). Tumor necrosis factor-α (TNF-α) increases both in the brain and in the cerebrospinal fluid from parkinsonian patients. *Neurosci. Lett.* 165, 208–210. doi: 10.1016/0304-3940(94)90746-3

Mogi, M., and Horiuchi, M. (2009). Effects of angiotensin II receptor blockers on dementia. *Hypertens. Res.* 32, 738–740. doi: 10.1038/hr.2009.110

Morale, M. C., Serra, P. A., L'Episcopo, F., Tirolo, C., Caniglia, S., Testa, N., et al. (2006). Estrogen, neuroinflammation and neuroprotection in Parkinson's disease: glia dictates resistance versus vulnerability to neurodegeneration. *Neuroscience* 138, 869–878. doi: 10.1016/j.neuroscience.2005.07.060

Mrak, R. E., and Landreth, G. E. (2004). PPARγ, neuroinflammation and disease. *J. Neuroinflammation* 1:5. doi: 10.1186/1742-2094-1-5

Muñoz, A., Rey, P., Guerra, M. J., Mendez-Alvarez, E., Soto-Otero, R., and Labandeira-Garcia, J. L. (2006). Reduction of dopaminergic degeneration and oxidative stress by inhibition of angiotensin converting enzyme in a MPTP model of parkinsonism. *Neuropharmacology* 51, 112–120. doi: 10.1016/j.neuropharm.2006.03.004

Münzel, T., and Keaney, J. F. Jr. (2001). Are ACE inhibitors a "magic bullet" against oxidative stress? *Circulation* 104, 1571–1574. doi: 10.1161/hc3801.095585

Nadjar, A., Berton, O., Guo, S., Leneuve, P., Dovero, S., Diguet, E., et al. (2009). IGF-1 signaling reduces neuro-inflammatory response and sensitivity of neurons to MPTP. *Neurobiol. Aging* 30, 2021–2030. doi: 10.1016/j.neurobiolaging.2008.02.009

Nguyen, G. (2011). Renin, (pro)renin and receptor: an update. *Clin. Sci. (Lond)* 120, 169–178. doi: 10.1042/CS20100432

Nguyen, G., and Contrepas, A. (2008). The (pro)renin receptors. *J. Mol. Med. (Berl)* 86, 643–646. doi: 10.1007/s00109-008-0319-1

Nguyen, G., Delarue, F., Burcklé, C., Bouzhir, L., Giller, T., and Sraer, J. D. (2002). Pivotal role of the renin/prorenin receptor in angiotensin II production and cellular responses to renin. *J. Clin. Invest.* 109, 1417–1427. doi: 10.1172/jci0214276

Nimmerjahn, A., Kirchhoff, F., and Helmchen, F. (2005). Resting microglial cells are highly dynamic surveillants of brain parenchyma *in vivo*. *Science* 308, 1314–1318. doi: 10.1126/science.1110647

Orihuela, R., McPherson, C. A., and Harry, G. J. (2016). Microglial M1/M2 polarization and metabolic states. *Br. J. Pharmacol.* 173, 649–665. doi: 10.1111/bph.13139

Oro, C., Qian, H., and Thomas, W. G. (2007). Type 1 angiotensin receptor pharmacology: signaling beyond G proteins. *Pharmacol. Ther.* 113, 210–226. doi: 10.1016/j.pharmthera.2006.10.001

Ouchi, Y., Yoshikawa, E., Sekine, Y., Futatsubashi, M., Kanno, T., Ogusu, T., et al. (2005). Microglial activation and dopamine terminal loss in early Parkinson's disease. *Ann. Neurol.* 57, 168–175. doi: 10.1002/ana.20338

Pang, T., Benicky, J., Wang, J., Orecna, M., Sanchez-Lemus, E., and Saavedra, J. M. (2012). Telmisartan ameliorates lipopolysaccharide-induced innate immune response through peroxisome proliferator-activated receptor-γ activation in human monocytes. *J. Hypertens.* 30, 87–96. doi: 10.1097/HJH.0b013e32834dde5f

Peng, J., Kimura, B., and Phillips, M. I. (2002). The predominant role of brain angiotensinogen and angiotensin in environmentally induced hypertension. *Regul. Pept.* 110, 25–32. doi: 10.1016/s0167-0115(02)00156-8

Phillips, M. I., and de Oliveira, E. M. (2008). Brain renin angiotensin in disease. *J. Mol. Med. (Berl)* 86, 715–722. doi: 10.1007/s00109-008-0331-5

Platten, M., Youssef, S., Hur, E. M., Ho, P. P., Han, M. H., Lanz, T. V., et al. (2009). Blocking angiotensin-converting enzyme induces potent regulatory T cells and modulates TH1- and TH17-mediated autoimmunity. *Proc. Natl. Acad. Sci. U S A* 106, 14948–14953. doi: 10.1073/pnas.0903958106

Plumb, R. D., El-Sherbeeny, N. A., Dixon, L. J., Hughes, S. M., Devine, A. B., Leahey, W. J., et al. (2005). NAD(P)H-dependent superoxide production in platelets: the role of angiotensin II and protein kinase C. *Clin. Biochem.* 38, 607–613. doi: 10.1016/j.clinbiochem.2005.04.012

Porrini, V., Lanzillotta, A., Branca, C., Benarese, M., Parrella, E., Lorenzini, L., et al. (2015). CHF5074 (CSP-1103) induces microglia alternative activation in plaque-free Tg2576 mice and primary glial cultures exposed to β-amyloid. *Neuroscience* 302, 112–120. doi: 10.1016/j.neuroscience.2014.10.029

Prinz, M., and Priller, J. (2014). Microglia and brain macrophages in the molecular age: from origin to neuropsychiatric disease. *Nat. Rev. Neurosci.* 15, 300–312. doi: 10.1038/nrn3722

Puche, J. E., García-Fernández, M., Muntané, J., Rioja, J., González-Barón, S., and Castilla Cortazar, I. (2008). Low doses of insulin-like growth factor-I induce mitochondrial protection in aging rats. *Endocrinology* 149, 2620–2627. doi: 10.3748/wjg.14.2731

Qin, L., Liu, Y., Wang, T., Wei, S. J., Block, M. L., Wilson, B., et al. (2004). NADPH oxidase mediates lipopolysaccharide-induced neurotoxicity and proinflammatory gene expression in activated microglia. *J. Biol. Chem.* 279, 1415–1421. doi: 10.1074/jbc.M307657200

Qin, L., Wu, X., Block, M. L., Liu, Y., Breese, G. R., Hong, J. S., et al. (2007). Systemic LPS causes chronic neuroinflammation and progressive neurodegeneration. *Glia* 55, 453–462. doi: 10.1002/glia.20467

Quesada, A., Romeo, H. E., and Micevych, P. (2007). Distribution and localization patterns of estrogen receptor-β and insulin-like growth factor-1 receptors in neurons and glial cells of the female rat substantia nigra: localization of ERβ and IGF-1R in substantia nigra. *J. Comp. Neurol.* 503, 198–208. doi: 10.1002/cne.21358

Rajaram, M. V., Brooks, M. N., Morris, J. D., Torrelles, J. B., Azad, A. K., and Schlesinger, L. S. (2010). Mycobacterium tuberculosis activates human macrophage peroxisome proliferator-activated receptor γ linking mannose receptor recognition to regulation of immune responses. *J. Immunol.* 185, 929–942. doi: 10.4049/jimmunol.1000866

Ransohoff, R. M., and Brown, M. A. (2012). Innate immunity in the central nervous system. *J. Clin. Invest.* 122, 1164–1171. doi: 10.1172/JCI58644

Ransohoff, R. M., and Perry, V. H. (2009). Microglial physiology: unique stimuli, specialized responses. *Annu. Rev. Immunol.* 27, 119–145. doi: 10.1146/annurev.immunol.021908.132528

Re, R. N. (2004). Tissue renin angiotensin systems. *Med. Clin. North Am.* 88, 19–38. doi: 10.1016/S0025-7125(03)00124-X

Reeves, E. P., Lu, H., Jacobs, H. L., Messina, C. G., Bolsover, S., Gabella, G., et al. (2002). Killing activity of neutrophils is mediated through activation of proteases by K^+ flux. *Nature* 416, 291–297. doi: 10.1038/416291a

Rey, P., Lopez-Real, A., Sanchez-Iglesias, S., Muñoz, A., Soto-Otero, R., and Labandeira-Garcia, J. L. (2007). Angiotensin type-1-receptor antagonists reduce 6-hydroxydopamine toxicity for dopaminergic neurons. *Neurobiol. Aging* 28, 555–567. doi: 10.1016/j.neurobiolaging.2006.02.018

Ricote, M., Li, A. C., Willson, T. M., Kelly, C. J., and Glass, C. K. (1998). The peroxisome proliferator-activated receptor-γ is a negative regulator of macrophage activation. *Nature* 391, 79–82. doi: 10.1038/34178

Rietdijk, C. D., Van Wezel, R. J. A., Garssen, J., and Kaneveld, A. D. (2016). Neuronal toll-like receptors and neuro-immunity in Parkinson's disease, Alzheimer's disease and stroke. *Neuroimmunol. Neuroinflammation* 3, 27–37. doi: 10.20517/2347-8659.2015.28

Rodriguez-Pallares, J., Parga, J. A., Joglar, B., Guerra, M. J., and Labandeira-Garcia, J. L. (2012). Mitochondrial ATP-sensitive potassium channels enhance angiotensin-induced oxidative damage and dopaminergic neuron degeneration. Relevance for aging-associated susceptibility to Parkinson's disease. *Age (Dordr)* 34, 863–880. doi: 10.1007/s11357-011-9284-7

Rodriguez-Pallares, J., Parga, J. A., Muñoz, A., Rey, P., Guerra, M. J., and Labandeira-Garcia, J. L. (2007). Mechanism of 6-hydroxydopamine neurotoxicity: the role of NADPH oxidase and microglial activation in 6-hydroxydopamine-induced degeneration of dopaminergic neurons. *J. Neurochem.* 103, 145–156. doi: 10.1111/j.1471-4159.2007.04699.x

Rodriguez-Pallares, J., Quiroz, C. R., Parga, J. A., Guerra, M. J., and Labandeira-Garcia, J. L. (2004). Angiotensin II increases differentiation of dopaminergic neurons from mesencephalic precursors via angiotensin type 2 receptors. *Eur. J. Neurosci.* 20, 1489–1498. doi: 10.1111/j.1460-9568.2004.03621.x

Rodriguez-Pallares, J., Rey, P., Parga, J. A., Muñoz, A., Guerra, M. J., and Labandeira-Garcia, J. L. (2008). Brain angiotensin enhances dopaminergic cell death via microglial activation and NADPH-derived ROS. *Neurobiol. Dis.* 31, 58–73. doi: 10.1016/j.nbd.2008.03.003

Rodriguez-Perez, A. I., Borrajo, A., Diaz-Ruiz, C., Garrido-Gil, P., and Labandeira-Garcia, J. L. (2016). Crosstalk between insulin-like growth factor-1 and angiotensin-II in dopaminergic neurons and glial cells: role in neuroinflammation and aging. *Oncotarget* 7, 30049–30067. doi: 10.18632/oncotarget.9174

Rodriguez-Perez, A. I., Borrajo, A., Rodriguez-Pallares, J., Guerra, M. J., and Labandeira-Garcia, J. L. (2015a). Interaction between NADPH-oxidase and Rho-kinase in angiotensin II-induced microglial activation. *Glia* 63, 466–482. doi: 10.1002/glia.22765

Rodriguez-Perez, A. I., Borrajo, A., Valenzuela, R., Lanciego, J. L., and Labandeira-Garcia, J. L. (2015b). Critical period for dopaminergic neuroprotection by hormonal replacement in menopausal rats. *Neurobiol. Aging* 36, 1194–1208. doi: 10.1016/j.neurobiolaging.2014.10.028

Rodriguez-Perez, A. I., Dominguez-Meijide, A., Lanciego, J. L., Guerra, M. J., and Labandeira-Garcia, J. L. (2013). Inhibition of Rho kinase mediates the neuroprotective effects of estrogen in the MPTP model of Parkinson's disease. *Neurobiol. Dis.* 58, 209–219. doi: 10.1016/j.nbd.2013.06.004

Rodriguez-Perez, A. I., Valenzuela, R., Villar-Cheda, B., Guerra, M. J., and Labandeira-Garcia, J. L. (2012). Dopaminergic neuroprotection of hormonal replacement therapy in young and aged menopausal rats: role of the brain angiotensin system. *Brain* 135, 124–138. doi: 10.1093/brain/awr320

Rodriguez-Perez, A. I., Valenzuela, R., Villar-Cheda, B., Guerra, M. J., Lanciego, J. L., and Labandeira-Garcia, J. L. (2010). Estrogen and angiotensin interaction in the substantia nigra. Relevance to postmenopausal Parkinson's disease. *Exp. Neurol.* 224, 517–526. doi: 10.1016/j.expneurol.2010.05.015

Rompe, F., Artuc, M., Hallberg, A., Alterman, M., Ströder, K., Thöne-Reineke, C., et al. (2010). Direct angiotensin II type 2 receptor stimulation acts anti-inflammatory through epoxyeicosatrienoic acid and inhibition of nuclear factor kappaB. *Hypertension* 55, 924–931. doi: 10.1161/HYPERTENSIONAHA.109.147843

Ruiz-Ortega, M., Lorenzo, O., Suzuki, Y., Rupérez, M., and Egido, J. (2001). Proinflammatory actions of angiotensins. *Curr. Opin. Nephrol. Hypertens.* 10, 321–329. doi: 10.1097/00041552-200105000-00005

Saab, Y. B., Gard, P. R., Yeoman, M. S., Mfarrej, B., El-Moalem, H., and Ingram, M. J. (2007). Renin-angiotensin-system gene polymorphisms and depression. *Prog. Neuropsychopharmacol. Biol. Psychiatry* 31, 1113–1118. doi: 10.1016/j.pnpbp.2007.04.002

Saavedra, J. M. (2012). Angiotensin II AT_1 receptor blockers as treatments for inflammatory brain disorders. *Clin. Sci.* 123, 567–590. doi: 10.1042/CS20120078

Sánchez-Iglesias, S., Rey, P., Méndez-Alvarez, E., Labandeira-García, J. L., and Soto-Otero, R. (2007). Time-course of brain oxidative damage caused by intrastriatal administration of 6-hydroxydopamine in a rat model of Parkinson's disease. *Neurochem. Res.* 32, 99–105. doi: 10.1007/s11064-006-9232-6

Santos, R. A., Simoes e Silva, A. C., Maric, C., Silva, D. M., Machado, R. P., de Buhr, I., et al. (2003). Angiotensin-(1–7) is an endogenous ligand for the G protein-coupled receptor Mas. *Proc. Natl. Acad. Sci. U S A* 100, 8258–8263. doi: 10.1073/pnas.1432869100

Savaskan, E. (2005). The role of the brain renin-angiotensin system in neurodegenerative disorders. *Curr. Alzheimer Res.* 2, 29–35. doi: 10.2174/1567205052772740

Schintu, N., Frau, L., Ibba, M., Caboni, P., Garau, A., Carboni, E., et al. (2009). PPAR-γ-mediated neuroprotection in a chronic mouse model of Parkinson's disease. *Eur. J. Neurosci.* 29, 954–963. doi: 10.1111/j.1460-9568.2009.06657.x

Seshiah, P. N., Weber, D. S., Rocic, P., Valppu, L., Taniyama, Y., and Griendling, K. K. (2002). Angiotensin II stimulation of NAD(P)H oxidase activity: upstream mediators. *Circ. Res.* 91, 406–413. doi: 10.1161/01.res.0000033523.08033.16

Shan, Z., Cuadra, A. E., Sumners, C., and Raizada, M. K. (2008). Characterization of a functional (pro)renin receptor in rat brain neurons. *Exp. Physiol.* 93, 701–708. doi: 10.1113/expphysiol.2008.041988

Sheh, Y. L., Hsu, C., Chan, S. H., and Chan, J. Y. (2007). NADPH oxidase- and mitochondrion-derived superoxide at rostral ventrolateral medulla in endotoxin-induced cardiovascular depression. *Free Radic. Biol. Med.* 42, 1610–1623. doi: 10.1016/j.freeradbiomed.2007.02.019

Shi, P., Grobe, J. L., Desland, F. A., Zhou, G., Shen, X. Z., Shan, Z., et al. (2014). Direct pro-inflammatory effects of prorenin on microglia. *PLoS One* 9:e92937. doi: 10.1371/journal.pone.0092937

Shrestha, S., Noh, J. M., Kim, S. Y., Ham, H. Y., Kim, Y. J., Yun, Y. J., et al. (2016). Angiotensin converting enzyme inhibitors and angiotensin II receptor antagonist attenuate tumor growth via polarization of neutrophils toward an antitumor phenotype. *Oncoimmunology* 5:e1067744. doi: 10.1080/2162402x.2015.1067744

Sica, A., and Bronte, V. (2007). Altered macrophage differentiation and immune dysfunction in tumor development. *J. Clin. Invest.* 117, 1155–1166. doi: 10.1172/JCI31422

Sica, A., and Mantovani, A. (2012). Macrophage plasticity and polarization: *in vivo* veritas. *J. Clin. Invest.* 122, 787–795. doi: 10.1172/JCI59643

Sohn, H. Y., Raff, U., Hoffmann, A., Gloe, T., Heermeier, K., Galle, J., et al. (2000). Differential role of angiotensin II receptor subtypes on endothelial superoxide formation. *Br. J. Pharmacol.* 131, 667–672. doi: 10.1038/sj.bjp.0703566

Sonsalla, P. K., Coleman, C., Wong, L. Y., Harris, S. L., Richardson, J. R., Gadad, B. S., et al. (2013). The angiotensin converting enzyme inhibitor captopril protects nigrostriatal dopamine neurons in animal models of parkinsonism. *Exp. Neurol.* 250, 376–383. doi: 10.1016/j.expneurol.2013.10.014

Stegbauer, J., Lee, D. H., Seubert, S., Ellrichmann, G., Manzel, A., Kvakan, H., et al. (2009). Role of the renin-angiotensin system in autoimmune inflammation of the central nervous system. *Proc. Natl. Acad. Sci. U S A* 106, 14942–14947. doi: 10.1073/pnas.0903602106

Stornetta, R. L., Hawelu-Johnson, C. L., Guyenet, P. G., and Lynch, K. R. (1988). Astrocytes synthesize angiotensinogen in brain. *Science* 242, 1444–1446. doi: 10.1126/science.3201232

Sugama, S., Yang, L., Cho, B. P., DeGiorgio, L. A., Lorenzl, S., Albers, D. S., et al. (2003). Age-related microglial activation in 1-methyl-4-phenyl-1,2,3,6-tetrahydropyridine (MPTP)-induced dopaminergic neurodegeneration in C57BL/6 mice. *Brain Res.* 964, 288–294. doi: 10.1016/s0006-8993(02)04085-4

Suh, Y., Atzmon, G., Cho, M. O., Hwang, D., Liu, B., Leahy, D. J., et al. (2008). Functionally significant insulin-like growth factor I receptor mutations in centenarians. *Proc. Natl. Acad. Sci. U S A* 105, 3438–3442. doi: 10.1073/pnas.0705467105

Suh, H. S., Zhao, M. L., Derico, L., Choi, N., and Lee, S. C. (2013). Insulin-like growth factor 1 and 2 (IGF1, IGF2) expression in human microglia: differential regulation by inflammatory mediators. *J. Neuroinflammation* 10:37. doi: 10.1186/1742-2094-10-37

Suzuki, S., Brown, C. M., Dela Cruz, C. D., Yang, E., Bridwell, D. A., and Wise, P. M. (2007). Timing of estrogen therapy after ovariectomy dictates the efficacy of its neuroprotective and antiinflammatory actions. *Proc. Natl. Acad. Sci. U S A* 104, 6013–6018. doi: 10.1073/pnas.0610394104

Suzuki, Y., Ruiz-Ortega, M., Lorenzo, O., Ruperez, M., Esteban, V., and Egido, J. (2003). Inflammation and angiotensin II. *Int. J. Biochem. Cell Biol.* 35, 881–900. doi: 10.1016/S1357-2725(02)00271-6

Tang, Y., and Le, W. (2016). Differential roles of M1 and M2 microglia in neurodegenerative diseases. *Mol. Neurobiol.* 53, 1181–1194. doi: 10.1007/s12035-014-9070-5

Tannahill, G. M., Iraci, N., Gaude, E., Frezza, C., and Pluchino, S. (2015). Metabolic reprograming of mononuclear phagocytes in progressive multiple sclerosis. *Front. Immunol.* 6:106. doi: 10.3389/fimmu.2015.00106

Tao, Y., Pinzi, V., Bourhis, J., and Deutsch, E. (2007). Mechanisms of disease: signaling of the insulin-like growth factor 1 receptor pathway—therapeutic perspectives in cancer. *Nat. Clin. Pract. Oncol.* 4, 591–602. doi: 10.1038/ncponc0934

Tao, L., Qiu, Y., Fu, X., Lin, R., Lei, C., Wang, J., et al. (2016). Angiotensin-converting enzyme 2 activator diminazene aceturate prevents lipopolysaccharide-induced inflammation by inhibiting MAPK and NF-κB pathways in human retinal pigment epithelium. *J. Neuroinflammation* 13:35. doi: 10.1186/s12974-016-0489-7

Thomas, W. G., Greenland, K. J., Shinkel, T. A., and Sernia, C. (1992). Angiotensinogen is secreted by pure rat neuronal cell cultures. *Brain Res.* 588, 191–200. doi: 10.1016/0006-8993(92)91575-y

Thompson, M. M., Oyama, T. T., Kelly, F. J., Kennefick, T. M., and Anderson, S. (2000). Activity and responsiveness of the renin-angiotensin system in the aging rat. *Am. J. Physiol. Regul. Integr. Comp. Physiol.* 279, R1787–R1794. doi: 10.1007/978-1-60761-186-8_16

Torika, N., Asraf, K., Roasso, E., Danon, A., and Fleisher-Berkovich, S. (2016). Angiotensin converting enzyme inhibitors ameliorate brain inflammation associated with microglial activation: possible implications for Alzheimer's disease. *J. Neuroimmune Pharmacol.* 11, 774–785. doi: 10.1007/s11481-016-9703-8

Touyz, R. M. (2004). Reactive oxygen species and angiotensin II signaling in vascular cells—implications in cardiovascular disease. *Braz. J. Med. Biol. Res.* 37, 1263–1273. doi: 10.1590/s0100-879x2004000800018

Tran, D., Bergholz, J., Zhang, H., He, H., Wang, Y., Zhang, Y., et al. (2014). Insulin-like growth factor-1 regulates the SIRT1–p53 pathway in cellular senescence. *Aging Cell* 13, 669–678. doi: 10.1111/acel.12219

Umemoto, S. (2008). Angiotensin II type 1 (AT1) receptor deficiency halts the progression of age-related atherosclerosis in hypercholesterolemia: molecular link between the AT1 receptor and hypercholesterolemia. *Hypertens. Res.* 31, 1495–1497. doi: 10.1291/hypres.31.1495

Unger, T., Chung, O., Csikos, T., Culman, J., Gallinat, S., Gohlke, P., et al. (1996). Angiotensin receptors. *J. Hypertens. Suppl.* 14, S95–S103.

Valenzuela, R., Barroso-Chinea, P., Villar-Cheda, B., Joglar, B., Muñoz, A., Lanciego, J. L., et al. (2010). Location of prorenin receptors in primate substantia nigra: effects on dopaminergic cell death. *J. Neuropathol. Exp. Neurol.* 69, 1130–1142. doi: 10.1097/NEN.0b013e3181fa0308

Valenzuela, R., Costa-Besada, M. A., Iglesias-Gonzalez, J., Perez-Costas, E., Villar-Cheda, B., Garrido-Gil, P., et al. (2016). Mitochondrial angiotensin receptors in dopaminergic neurons. Role in cell protection and aging-related vulnerability to neurodegeneration. *Cell Death Dis.* 7:e2427. doi: 10.1038/cddis.2016.327

Vegeto, E., Benedusi, V., and Maggi, A. (2008). Estrogen anti-inflammatory activity in brain: a therapeutic opportunity for menopause and neurodegenerative diseases. *Front. Neuroendocrinol.* 29, 507–519. doi: 10.1016/j.yfrne.2008.04.001

Villapol, S., and Saavedra, J. M. (2015). Neuroprotective effects of angiotensin receptor blockers. *Am. J. Hypertens.* 28, 289–299. doi: 10.1093/ajh/hpu197

Villar-Cheda, B., Dominguez-Meijide, A., Joglar, B., Rodriguez-Perez, A. I., Guerra, M. J., and Labandeira-Garcia, J. L. (2012a). Involvement of microglial RhoA/Rho-kinase pathway activation in the dopaminergic neuron death. Role of angiotensin via angiotensin type 1 receptors. *Neurobiol. Dis.* 47, 268–279. doi: 10.1016/j.nbd.2012.04.010

Villar-Cheda, B., Valenzuela, R., Rodriguez-Perez, A. I., Guerra, M. J., and Labandeira-Garcia, J. L. (2012b). Aging-related changes in the nigral angiotensin system enhances proinflammatory and pro-oxidative markers and 6-OHDA-induced dopaminergic degeneration. *Neurobiol. Aging* 33, 204.e1–204.e11. doi: 10.1016/j.neurobiolaging.2010.08.006

Villar-Cheda, B., Dominguez-Meijide, A., Valenzuela, R., Granado, N., Moratalla, R., and Labandeira-Garcia, J. L. (2014). Aging-related dysregulation of dopamine and angiotensin receptor interaction. *Neurobiol. Aging* 35, 1726–1738. doi: 10.1016/j.neurobiolaging.2014.01.017

Villar-Cheda, B., Rodríguez-Pallares, J., Valenzuela, R., Muñoz, A., Guerra, M. J., Baltatu, O. C., et al. (2010). Nigral and striatal regulation of angiotensin receptor expression by dopamine and angiotensin in rodents: implications for progression of Parkinson's disease. *Eur. J. Neurosci.* 32, 1695–1706. doi: 10.1111/j.1460-9568.2010.07448.x

Villar-Cheda, B., Sousa-Ribeiro, D., Rodriguez-Pallares, J., Rodriguez-Perez, A. I., Guerra, M. J., and Labandeira-Garcia, J. L. (2009). Aging and sedentarism decrease vascularization and VEGF levels in the rat substantia nigra. Implications for Parkinson's disease. *J. Cereb. Blood Flow Metab.* 29, 230–234. doi: 10.1038/jcbfm.2008.127

Villela, D., Leonhardt, J., Patel, N., Joseph, J., Kirsch, S., Hallberg, A., et al. (2015). Angiotensin type 2 receptor (AT2R) and receptor Mas: a complex liaison. *Clin. Sci. (Lond)* 128, 227–234. doi: 10.1042/CS20130515

Vinciguerra, M., Santini, M. P., Claycomb, W. C., Ladurner, A. G., and Rosenthal, N. (2009). Local IGF-1 isoform protects cardiomyocytes from hypertrophic and oxidative stresses via SirT1 activity. *Aging (Albany NY)* 2, 43–62. doi: 10.18632/aging.100107

Von Bohlen und Halbach, O., Walther, T., Bader, M., and Albrecht, D. (2000). Interaction between *Mas* and the angiotensin AT1 receptor in the amygdala. *J. Neurophysiol.* 83, 2012–2021.

Vowinckel, E., Reutens, D., Becher, B., Verge, G., Evans, A., Owens, T., et al. (1997). PK11195 binding to the peripheral benzodiazepine receptor as a marker of microglia activation in multiple sclerosis and experimental autoimmune encephalomyelitis. *J. Neurosci. Res.* 50, 345–353. doi: 10.1002/(SICI)1097-4547(19971015)50:2<345::AID-JNR22>3.3.CO;2-S

Wang, Y., Chan, G. L., Holden, J. E., Dobko, T., Mak, E., Schulzer, M., et al. (1998). Age-dependent decline of dopamine D1 receptors in human brain: a PET study. *Synapse* 30, 56–61. doi: 10.1002/(SICI)1098-2396(199809)30:1<56::AID-SYN7>3.0.CO;2-J

Wang, J., Pang, T., Hafko, R., Benicky, J., Sanchez-Lemus, E., and Saavedra, J. M. (2014). Telmisartan ameliorates glutamate-induced neurotoxicity: roles of AT(1) receptor blockade and PPARγ activation. *Neuropharmacology* 79, 249–261. doi: 10.1016/j.neuropharm.2013.11.022

West, A. P., Brodsky, I. E., Rahner, C., Woo, D. K., Erdjument-Bromage, H., Tempst, P., et al. (2011). TLR signalling augments macrophage bactericidal activity through mitochondrial ROS. *Nature* 472, 476–480. doi: 10.1038/nature09973

Wright, J. W., Kawas, L. H., and Harding, J. W. (2015). The development of small molecule angiotensin IV analogs to treat Alzheimer's and Parkinson's diseases. *Prog. Neurobiol.* 125, 26–46. doi: 10.1016/j.pneurobio.2014.11.004

Wu, L., Iwai, M., Li, Z., Shiuchi, T., Min, L. J., Cui, T. X., et al. (2004). Regulation of inhibitory protein-kappaB and monocyte chemoattractant protein-1 by angiotensin II type 2 receptor-activated Src homology protein tyrosine phosphatase-1 in fetal vascular smooth muscle cells. *Mol. Endocrinol.* 18, 666–678. doi: 10.1210/me.2003-0053

Wu, D. C., Teismann, P., Tieu, K., Vila, M., Jackson-Lewis, V., Ischiropoulos, H., et al. (2003). NADPH oxidase mediates oxidative stress in the 1-methyl-4-phenyl-1,2,3,6-tetrahydropyridine model of Parkinson's disease. *Proc. Natl. Acad. Sci. U S A* 100, 6145–6150. doi: 10.1073/pnas.0937239100

Xu, Y., Xu, Y., Wang, Y., Wang, Y., He, L., Jiang, Z., et al. (2015). Telmisartan prevention of LPS-induced microglia activation involves M2 microglia polarization via CaMKKβ-dependent AMPK activation. *Brain Behav. Immun.* 50, 298–313. doi: 10.1016/j.bbi.2015.07.015

Yan, J., Zhou, X., Guo, J. J., Mao, L., Wang, Y. J., Sun, J., et al. (2012). Nogo-66 inhibits adhesion and migration of microglia via GTPase Rho pathway *in vitro*. *J. Neurochem.* 120, 721–731. doi: 10.1111/j.1471-4159.2011.07619.x

Yang, J., Chen, C., Ren, H., Han, Y., He, D., Zhou, L., et al. (2012). Angiotensin II AT(2) receptor decreases AT$_1$ receptor expression and function via nitric oxide/cGMP/Sp1 in renal proximal tubule cells from Wistar-Kyoto rats. *J. Hypertens.* 30, 1176–1184. doi: 10.1097/HJH.0b013e3283532099

Zalba, G., San José, G., Moreno, M. U., Fortuño, M. A., Fortuño, A., Beaumont, F. J., et al. (2001). Oxidative stress in arterial hypertension: role of NAD(P)H oxidase. *Hypertension* 38, 1395–1399. doi: 10.1161/hy1201.099611

Zawada, W. M., Banninger, G. P., Thornton, J., Marriott, B., Cantu, D., Rachubinski, A. L., et al. (2011). Generation of reactive oxygen species in 1-methyl-4-phenylpyridinium (MPP+) treated dopaminergic neurons occurs as an NADPH oxidase-dependent two-wave cascade. *J. Neuroinflammation* 8:129. doi: 10.1186/1742-2094-8-129

Zecca, L., Gallorini, M., Schünemann, V., Trautwein, A. X., Gerlach, M., Riederer, P., et al. (2001). Iron, neuromelanin and ferritin content in the substantia nigra of normal subjects at different ages: consequences for iron storage and neurodegenerative processes. *J. Neurochem.* 76, 1766–1773. doi: 10.1046/j.1471-4159.2001.00186.x

Zhu, T., Miller, A. G., Deliyanti, D., Berka, D. R., Agrotis, A., Campbell, D. J., et al. (2015). Prorenin stimulates a pro-angiogenic and pro-inflammatory response in retinal endothelial cells and an M1 phenotype in retinal microglia. *Clin. Exp. Pharmacol. Physiol.* 42, 537–548. doi: 10.1111/1440-1681.12376

Permissions

All chapters in this book were first published by Frontiers; hereby published with permission under the Creative Commons Attribution License or equivalent. Every chapter published in this book has been scrutinized by our experts. Their significance has been extensively debated. The topics covered herein carry significant findings which will fuel the growth of the discipline. They may even be implemented as practical applications or may be referred to as a beginning point for another development.

The contributors of this book come from diverse backgrounds, making this book a truly international effort. This book will bring forth new frontiers with its revolutionizing research information and detailed analysis of the nascent developments around the world.

We would like to thank all the contributing authors for lending their expertise to make the book truly unique. They have played a crucial role in the development of this book. Without their invaluable contributions this book wouldn't have been possible. They have made vital efforts to compile up to date information on the varied aspects of this subject to make this book a valuable addition to the collection of many professionals and students.

This book was conceptualized with the vision of imparting up-to-date information and advanced data in this field. To ensure the same, a matchless editorial board was set up. Every individual on the board went through rigorous rounds of assessment to prove their worth. After which they invested a large part of their time researching and compiling the most relevant data for our readers.

The editorial board has been involved in producing this book since its inception. They have spent rigorous hours researching and exploring the diverse topics which have resulted in the successful publishing of this book. They have passed on their knowledge of decades through this book. To expedite this challenging task, the publisher supported the team at every step. A small team of assistant editors was also appointed to further simplify the editing procedure and attain best results for the readers.

Apart from the editorial board, the designing team has also invested a significant amount of their time in understanding the subject and creating the most relevant covers. They scrutinized every image to scout for the most suitable representation of the subject and create an appropriate cover for the book.

The publishing team has been an ardent support to the editorial, designing and production team. Their endless efforts to recruit the best for this project, has resulted in the accomplishment of this book. They are a veteran in the field of academics and their pool of knowledge is as vast as their experience in printing. Their expertise and guidance has proved useful at every step. Their uncompromising quality standards have made this book an exceptional effort. Their encouragement from time to time has been an inspiration for everyone.

The publisher and the editorial board hope that this book will prove to be a valuable piece of knowledge for researchers, students, practitioners and scholars across the globe.

List of Contributors

Li Zhong, Zhen-Lian Zhang, Xinxiu Li, Chunyan Liao, Pengfei Mou, Tingting Wang, Zongqi Wang, Zhe Wang and Min Wei
Fujian Provincial Key Laboratory of Neurodegenerative Disease and Aging Research, Institute of Neuroscience, Medical College, Xiamen University, Xiamen, China

Huaxi Xu
Fujian Provincial Key Laboratory of Neurodegenerative Disease and Aging Research, Institute of Neuroscience, Medical College, Xiamen University, Xiamen, China
Neuroscience and Aging Research Center, Sanford-Burnham-Prebys Medical Discovery Institute, La Jolla, CA, United States

Guojun Bu
Fujian Provincial Key Laboratory of Neurodegenerative Disease and Aging Research, Institute of Neuroscience, Medical College, Xiamen University, Xiamen, China
Department of Neuroscience, Mayo Clinic, Jacksonville, FL, United States

Xiao-Fen Chen
Fujian Provincial Key Laboratory of Neurodegenerative Disease and Aging Research, Institute of Neuroscience, Medical College, Xiamen University, Xiamen, China
Shenzhen Research Institute of Xiamen University, Shenzhen, China

Zongjian Liu, Yuanyuan Ran and Shuo Huang
China-America Institute of Neuroscience, Beijing Luhe Hospital, Capital Medical University, Beijing, China
Central Laboratory, Beijing Luhe Hospital, Capital Medical University, Beijing, China

Shaohong Wen, Wenxiu Zhang and Zhili Ji
Central Laboratory, Beijing Luhe Hospital, Capital Medical University, Beijing, China

Xiangrong Liu
Institute of Hypoxia Medicine, Xuanwu Hospital, Xuan Wu Hospital of the Capital Medical University, Beijing, China

Xiaokun Geng and Huishan Du
China-America Institute of Neuroscience, Beijing Luhe Hospital, Capital Medical University, Beijing, China

Xunming Ji and Rehana K. Leak
China-America Institute of Neuroscience, Beijing Luhe Hospital, Capital Medical University, Beijing, China
Institute of Hypoxia Medicine, Xuanwu Hospital, Xuan Wu Hospital of the Capital Medical University, Beijing, China

Xiaoming Hu
China-America Institute of Neuroscience, Beijing Luhe Hospital, Capital Medical University, Beijing, China
Pittsburgh Institute of Brain Disorders and Recovery, and Department of Neurology, University of Pittsburgh School of Medicine, Pittsburgh, PA, United States

Gyun Jee Song and Kyoungho Suk
BK21 Plus KNU Biomedical Convergence Program, Department of Pharmacology, Brain Science & Engineering Institute, School of Medicine, Kyungpook National University, Daegu, South Korea

Hassan Boukhaddaoui, Pauline Auzer and Nicolas Tricaud
Institut National de la Santé et de la Recherche Médicale, U1051, Montpellier, France

Guillaume Saint-Martin
University of Montpellier, Montpellier; Institut National de la Santé et de la Recherche Médicale, U1198, Montpellier; École Pratique des Hautes Études, Paris, France
Charles Coulomb Laboratory, UMR 5221 Centre National de la Recherche Scientifique, Montpellier, France

Rahima Sidiboulenouar, Eric Alibert, Christophe Goze-Bac and Christophe Coillot
Charles Coulomb Laboratory, UMR 5221 Centre National de la Recherche Scientifique, Montpellier, France

Nicolas Lonjon
University of Montpellier, Montpellier; Institut National de la Santé et de la Recherche Médicale, U1198, Montpellier; École Pratique des Hautes Études, Paris, France
Centre Hospitalier Universitaire de Montpellier (CHRU), Gui de Chauliac Hospital, Montpellier, France

Ngan Pan Bennett Au
Department of Biomedical Sciences, City University of Hong Kong, Kowloon Tong, Hong Kong

Chi Him Eddie Ma
Department of Biomedical Sciences, City University of Hong Kong, Kowloon Tong, Hong Kong
Centre for Biosystems, Neuroscience, and Nanotechnology, City University of Hong Kong, Kowloon Tong, Hong Kong
State Key Laboratory in Marine Pollution, City University of Hong Kong, Kowloon Tong, Hong Kong

Björn Spittau
Department of Molecular Embryology, Faculty of Medicine, Institute for Anatomy and Cell Biology, University of Freiburg, Freiburg, Germany
Institute of Anatomy, University of Rostock, Rostock, Germany

Emiliano Peña-Altamira, Sabrina Petralla, Francesca Massenzio, Marco Virgili, Maria L. Bolognesi and Barbara Monti
Department of Pharmacy and Biotechnology, University of Bologna, Bologna, Italy

Juliane Obst, Emilie Simon, Renzo Mancuso and Diego Gomez-Nicola
Biological Sciences, University of Southampton, Southampton General Hospital, Southampton, United Kingdom

Feng Zhang, Rujia Zhong, Song Li, Zhenfa Fu and Cheng Cheng
Liaoning Provincial Center for Clinical Research on Neurological Diseases, The First Affiliated Hospital, Dalian Medical University, Dalian, China
Liaoning Provincial Key Laboratory for Research on the Pathogenic Mechanisms of Neurological Diseases, The First Affiliated Hospital, Dalian Medical University, Dalian, China

Huaibin Cai
Laboratory of Neurogenetics, National Institute on Aging, National Institutes of Health, Bethesda, MD, United States

Weidong Le
Liaoning Provincial Center for Clinical Research on Neurological Diseases, The First Affiliated Hospital, Dalian Medical University, Dalian, China
Liaoning Provincial Key Laboratory for Research on the Pathogenic Mechanisms of Neurological Diseases, The First Affiliated Hospital, Dalian Medical University, Dalian, China
Collaborative Innovation Center for Brain Science, The First Affiliated Hospital, Dalian Medical University, Dalian, China

Cornelius K. Donat, Gregory Scott, Steve M. Gentleman and Magdalena Sastre
Division of Brain Sciences, Department of Medicine, Imperial College London, London, United Kingdom

Maria Concetta Geloso, Valentina Corvino, Elisa Marchese and Alessia Serrano
Institute of Anatomy and Cell Biology, Università Cattolica del Sacro Cuore, Rome, Italy

Fabrizio Michetti
Institute of Anatomy and Cell Biology, Università Cattolica del Sacro Cuore, Rome, Italy
IRCCS San Raffaele Scientific Institute, Università Vita-Salute San Raffaele, Milan, Italy

Nadia D'Ambrosi
Department of Biology, University of Rome Tor Vergata, Rome, Italy

Valentina Salvi
Department of Molecular and Translational Medicine, University of Brescia, Brescia, Italy

Francesca Sozio, Silvano Sozzani and Annalisa Del Prete
Department of Molecular and Translational Medicine, University of Brescia, Brescia, Italy
IRCCS-Humanitas Clinical and Research Center, Rozzano-Milano, Italy

Harald Lund, Melanie Pieber and Robert A. Harris
Department of Clinical Neuroscience, Karolinska Institutet, Centre for Molecular Medicine, Karolinska Hospital at Solna, Solna, Sweden

Sudhakar R. Subramaniam and Howard J. Federoff
Department of Neurology, University of California, Irvine, Irvine, CA, United States

Ana I. Ramirez, Rosa de Hoz and Juan J. Salazar
Instituto de Investigaciones Oftalmológicas Ramón Castroviejo. Universidad Complutense de Madrid, Madrid, Spain
Departamento de Oftalmología y ORL, Facultad de Óptica y Optometría, Universidad Complutense de Madrid (UCM), Madrid, Spain

Elena Salobrar-Garcia, Blanca Rojas, Alberto Triviño and José M. Ramírez
Instituto de Investigaciones Oftalmológicas Ramón Castroviejo. Universidad Complutense de Madrid, Madrid, Spain
Departamento de Oftalmología y ORL, Facultad de Medicina, Universidad Complutense de Madrid (UCM), Madrid, Spain

Daniel Ajoy and Inés López-Cuenca
Instituto de Investigaciones Oftalmológicas Ramón Castroviejo. Universidad Complutense de Madrid, Madrid, Spain

Pilar Rojas
Instituto de Investigaciones Oftalmológicas Ramón Castroviejo. Universidad Complutense de Madrid,

Madrid, Spain
Servicio de Oftalmología, Hospital Gregorio Marañón, Madrid, Spain

Anna-Elisa Roser and Paul Lingor
Department of Neurology, University Medicine Göttingen, Göttingen, Germany
DFG Cluster of Excellence Nanoscale Microscopy and Molecular Physiology of the Brain (CNMPB), University Medicine Göttingen, Göttingen, Germany

Lars Tönges
Department of Neurology, Ruhr-Universität Bochum, Bochum, Germany

Vanessa Porrini, Mariana Mota, Edoardo Parrella, Arianna Bellucci, Marina Benarese and Lara Faggi
Laboratory of Pharmacology, Department of Molecular and Translational Medicine, University of Brescia, Brescia, Italy

Paolo Tonin
IRCCS, San Camillo Hospital, Venice, Italy

Pier F. Spano and Marina Pizzi
Laboratory of Pharmacology, Department of Molecular and Translational Medicine, University of Brescia, Brescia, Italy
IRCCS, San Camillo Hospital, Venice, Italy

Jose L. Labandeira-Garcia, Ana I. Rodríguez-Perez, Pablo Garrido-Gil, Jannette Rodriguez-Pallares and Maria J. Guerra
Laboratory of Neuroanatomy and Experimental Neurology, Department of Morphological Sciences, Center for Research in Molecular Medicine and Chronic Diseases (CIMUS), University of Santiago de Compostela, Santiago de Compostela, Spain
Networking Research Center on Neurodegenerative Diseases (CIBERNED), Madrid, Spain

Jose L. Lanciego
Networking Research Center on Neurodegenerative Diseases (CIBERNED), Madrid, Spain
Neurosciences Division, Center for Applied Medical Research (CIMA), University of Navarra, Pamplona, Spain

Index

Printed in the USA
CPSIA information can be obtained
at www.ICGtesting.com
LVHW060411221124
797340LV00005B/12
* 9 7 9 8 8 8 7 4 0 3 0 3 8 *